I0066284

Skin Diseases: Clinical Dermatology

Skin Diseases: Clinical Dermatology

Editor: Derek Kennedy

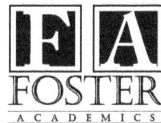

FA FOSTER
A C A D E M I C S

www.fosteracademics.com

www.fosteracademics.com

F A
FOSTER
A C A D E M I C S

Cataloging-in-Publication Data

Skin diseases : clinical dermatology / edited by Derek Kennedy.
    p. cm.
Includes bibliographical references and index.
ISBN 978-1-63242-620-8
1. Dermatology. 2. Skin--Diseases. I. Kennedy, Derek.
RL72 .S55 2019
616.5--dc23

© Foster Academics, 2019

Foster Academics,
118-35 Queens Blvd., Suite 400,
Forest Hills, NY 11375, USA

ISBN 978-1-63242-620-8 (Hardback)

This book contains information obtained from authentic and highly regarded sources. Copyright for all individual chapters remain with the respective authors as indicated. All chapters are published with permission under the Creative Commons Attribution License or equivalent. A wide variety of references are listed. Permission and sources are indicated; for detailed attributions, please refer to the permissions page and list of contributors. Reasonable efforts have been made to publish reliable data and information, but the authors, editors and publisher cannot assume any responsibility for the validity of all materials or the consequences of their use.

Trademark Notice: Registered trademark of products or corporate names are used only for explanation and identification without intent to infringe.

Contents

Preface...IX

Chapter 1 **Anaphylaxis to Iodinated Contrast Media: Clinical Characteristics Related with Development of Anaphylactic Shock**...1
Min-Hye Kim, Suh-Young Lee, Seung-Eun Lee, Min-Suk Yang, Jae-Woo Jung, Chang Min Park, Whal Lee, Sang-Heon Cho and Hye-Ryun Kang

Chapter 2 **Polymorphisms in the *CYP2E1* and *GSTM1* Genes as Possible Protection Factors for Leprosy Patients**...7
Pablo Pinto, Claudio Guedes Salgado, Ney Santos, Dayse O. Alencar, Sidney Santos, Mara H. Hutz and Ândrea Ribeiro-dos-Santos

Chapter 3 **Predictors of Fatigue Severity in Early Systemic Sclerosis: A Prospective Longitudinal Study of the GENISOS Cohort**...13
Shervin Assassi, Astrud L. Leyva, Maureen D. Mayes, Roozbeh Sharif, Deepthi K. Nair, Michael Fischbach, Ngan Nguyen, John D. Reveille, Emilio B. Gonzalez and Terry A. McNearney

Chapter 4 **IL-27 Regulates IL-18 Binding Protein in Skin Resident Cells**............................22
Miriam Wittmann, Rosella Doble, Malte Bachmann, Josef Pfeilschifter, Thomas Werfel and Heiko Mühl

Chapter 5 **γδ T Cells are Reduced and Rendered Unresponsive by Hyperglycemia and Chronic TNFα in Mouse Models of Obesity and Metabolic Disease**.....................31
Kristen R. Taylor, Robyn E. Mills, Anne E. Costanzo and Julie M. Jameson

Chapter 6 **Imaging Mass Spectrometry Visualizes Ceramides and the Pathogenesis of Dorfman-Chanarin Syndrome Due to Ceramide Metabolic Abnormality in the Skin**..47
Naoko Goto-Inoue, Takahiro Hayasaka, Nobuhiro Zaima, Kimiko Nakajima, Walter M. Holleran, Shigetoshi Sano, Yoshikazu Uchida and Mitsutoshi Setou

Chapter 7 **Dysregulation of Suppressor of Cytokine Signaling 3 in Keratinocytes Causes Skin Inflammation Mediated by Interleukin-20 Receptor-Related Cytokines**.................................57
Ayako Uto-Konomi, Kosuke Miyauchi, Naoko Ozaki, Yasutaka Motomura, Yoshie Suzuki, Akihiko Yoshimura, Shinobu Suzuki, Daniel Cua and Masato Kubo

Chapter 8 **Filaggrin Genotype Determines Functional and Molecular Alterations in Skin of Patients with Atopic Dermatitis and Ichthyosis Vulgaris**...............................69
Mårten C. G. Winge, Torborg Hoppe, Berit Berne, Anders Vahlquist, Magnus Nordenskjöld, Maria Bradley and Hans Törmä

Chapter 9 **Targeting the Neurokinin Receptor 1 with Aprepitant: A Novel Antipruritic Strategy**..77
Sonja Ständer, Dorothee Siepmann, Ilka Herrgott, Cord Sunderkötter and Thomas A. Luger

Chapter 10   **Differences between the Glycosylation Patterns of Haptoglobin Isolated from Skin Scales and Plasma of Psoriatic Patients**..82
Bernardetta Maresca, Luisa Cigliano, Maria Stefania Spagnuolo, Fabrizio Dal Piaz, Maria M. Corsaro, Nicola Balato, Massimiliano Nino, Anna Balato, Fabio Ayala and Paolo Abrescia

Chapter 11   **Skin-Targeted Inhibition of PPAR β/δ by Selective Antagonists to Treat PPAR β/δ – Mediated Psoriasis-Like Skin Disease *In Vivo***..93
Katrin Hack, Louise Reilly, Colin Palmer, Kevin D. Read, Suzanne Norval, Robert Kime, Kally Booth and John Foerster

Chapter 12   **Novel Sulfated Polysaccharides Disrupt Cathelicidins, Inhibit RAGE and Reduce Cutaneous Inflammation in a Mouse Model of Rosacea**..104
Jianxing Zhang, Xiaoyu Xu, Narayanam V. Rao, Brian Argyle, Lindsi McCoard, William J. Rusho, Thomas P. Kennedy, Glenn D. Prestwich and Gerald Krueger

Chapter 13   **L-selectin and Skin Damage in Systemic Sclerosis**..118
James V. Dunne, Stephan F. van Eeden and Kevin J. Keen

Chapter 14   ***In Vivo* Dioxin Favors Interleukin-22 Production by Human CD4+ T Cells in an Aryl Hydrocarbon Receptor (AhR)-Dependent Manner**..126
Nicolò Costantino Brembilla, Jean-Marie Ramirez, Rachel Chicheportiche, Olivier Sorg, Jean-Hilaire Saurat and Carlo Chizzolini

Chapter 15   **Distinct Effects of Different Phosphatidylglycerol Species on Mouse Keratinocyte Proliferation**..133
Ding Xie, Mutsa Seremwe, John G. Edwards, Robert Podolsky and Wendy B. Bollag

Chapter 16   **Increased Levels of Eotaxin and MCP-1 in Juvenile Dermatomyositis Median 16.8 Years after Disease Onset; Associations with Disease Activity, Duration and Organ Damage**..142
Helga Sanner, Thomas Schwartz, Berit Flatø, Maria Vistnes, Geir Christensen and Ivar Sjaastad

Chapter 17   ***In Vitro* Differential Diagnosis of Clavus and Verruca by a Predictive Model Generated from Electrical Impedance**..149
Chien-Ya Hung, Pei-Lun Sun, Shu-Jen Chiang and Fu-Shan Jaw

Chapter 18   **Persistent Release of IL-1s from Skin is Associated with Systemic Cardio-Vascular Disease, Emaciation and Systemic Amyloidosis: The Potential of Anti-IL-1 Therapy for Systemic Inflammatory Diseases**..156
Keiichi Yamanaka, Takehisa Nakanishi, Hiromitsu Saito, Junko Maruyama, Kenichi Isoda, Ayumu Yokochi, Kyoko Imanaka-Yoshida, Kenshiro Tsuda, Masato Kakeda, Ryuji Okamoto, Satoshi Fujita, Yoichiro Iwakura, Noboru Suzuki, Masaaki Ito, Kazuo Maruyama, Esteban C. Gabazza, Toshimichi Yoshida, Motomu Shimaoka and Hitoshi Mizutani

Chapter 19   **Chronic Stress Suppresses the Expression of Cutaneous Hypothalamic–Pituitary–Adrenocortical Axis Elements and Melanogenesis**......................167
Silin Pang, Huali Wu, Qian Wang, Minxuan Cai, Weimin Shi and Jing Shang

Chapter 20   **The Flavonoid Luteolin Inhibits Fcγ-Dependent Respiratory Burst in Granulocytes, but not Skin Blistering in a New Model of Pemphigoid in Adult Mice** 178
Eva Oswald, Alina Sesarman, Claus-Werner Franzke, Ute Wölfle,
Leena Bruckner-Tuderman, Thilo Jakob, Stefan F. Martin and Cassian Sitaru

Chapter 21   **Activation of PPARβ/δ Causes a Psoriasis-Like Skin Disease In Vivo** 189
Malgorzata Romanowska, Louise Reilly, Colin N. A. Palmer,
Mattias C. U. Gustafsson and John Foerster

Permissions

List of Contributors

Index

Preface

A skin condition is a medical condition, which affects the integumentary system that comprises of the hair, nails, skin and related glands and muscles. The diagnosis of skin conditions is built on a physical examination of the skin, skin appendages and mucous membranes. The clinical observation typically addresses the configuration, morphology and the distribution of the lesion. Lesions can be classified into primary and secondary lesions. Primary lesions can be tumors, macules, patches, plaques, cysts, etc. Secondary lesions include crust, lichenification, maceration, umbilication, excoriation, etc. Lesions can be clustered into annular, arciform, gyrate, linear, reticular organizations, etc. Dermatological therapies typically involve laser therapy, allergy testing, topical therapies, intralesional treatment, hair transplantation, besides many others. Some dermatological drugs include Dextranomer, Ingenol mebutate, Mederma, Dixanthogen, etc. This book unravels the recent studies in the field of dermatology. Also included in this book is a detailed explanation of the various diagnotic techniques and therapies used in dermatology. The extensive content of this book provides the readers with a thorough understanding of the subject.

After months of intensive research and writing, this book is the end result of all who devoted their time and efforts in the initiation and progress of this book. It will surely be a source of reference in enhancing the required knowledge of the new developments in the area. During the course of developing this book, certain measures such as accuracy, authenticity and research focused analytical studies were given preference in order to produce a comprehensive book in the area of study.

This book would not have been possible without the efforts of the authors and the publisher. I extend my sincere thanks to them. Secondly, I express my gratitude to my family and well-wishers. And most importantly, I thank my students for constantly expressing their willingness and curiosity in enhancing their knowledge in the field, which encourages me to take up further research projects for the advancement of the area.

Editor

Anaphylaxis to Iodinated Contrast Media: Clinical Characteristics Related with Development of Anaphylactic Shock

Min-Hye Kim[1,2,3,4], **Suh-Young Lee**[1,2], **Seung-Eun Lee**[1,2], **Min-Suk Yang**[1,2,5], **Jae-Woo Jung**[2,6], **Chang Min Park**[7], **Whal Lee**[7], **Sang-Heon Cho**[1,2,3], **Hye-Ryun Kang**[1,2,3]∗

1 Department of Internal Medicine, Division of Allergy and Clinical Immunology, Seoul National University Hospital, Seoul, Republic of Korea, 2 Institute of Allergy and Clinical Immunology, Seoul National University Medical Research Center, Seoul, Republic of Korea, 3 Seoul National University Hospital Regional Pharmacovigilance Center, Seoul, Republic of Korea, 4 Department of Internal Medicine, Ewha Womans University School of Medicine, Seoul, Republic of Korea, 5 Department of Internal Medicine, SMG-SNU Boramae Medical Center, Seoul, Republic of Korea, 6 Department of Internal Medicine, Chung-Ang University College of Medicine, Seoul, Republic of Korea, 7 Department of Radiology and Institute of Radiation Medicine, Seoul National University College of Medicine, Seoul, Republic of Korea

Abstract

Objective: Anaphylaxis is the most severe form of radiocontrast media (RCM) induced hypersensitivity and can be life-threatening if profound hypotension is combined. With increased use of iodine based RCM, related hypersensitivity is rapidly growing. However, the clinical characteristics and risk factors of RCM induced anaphylaxis accompanied by hypotension (anaphylactic shock) are not clearly defined. This study was performed to investigate the risk factors of RCM induced anaphylactic shock and the clinical value of RCM skin testing to identify causative agents in affected patients.

Methods: We analyzed the data of RCM induced anaphylaxis monitored by an inhospital pharmacovigilance center at a tertiary teaching hospital from January 2005 to December 2012 and compared the clinical features and skin test results according to the accompanying hypotension.

Results: Among total of 104 cases of RCM induced anaphylaxis, 34.6% of patients, developed anaphylaxis on their first exposure to RCM. Anaphylactic patients presenting with shock were older (57.4 vs. 50.1 years, $p = 0.026$) and had a history of more frequently exposure to RCM (5.1 ± 7.8 vs. 1.9 ± 3.3, $p = 0.004$) compared to those without hypotension. Among RCMs, hypotension was more frequent in anaphylaxis related to iopromide compared to other agents (85.0% vs. 61.4%, $p = 0.011$). Skin tests were performed in 51 patients after development of RCM induced anaphylaxis. Overall skin test positivity to RCM was 64.7% and 81.8% in patients with anaphylactic shock.

Conclusion: RCM induced anaphylactic shock is related to multiple exposures to RCM and most patients showed skin test positivity to RCM.

Editor: Jacques Zimmer, Centre de Recherche Public de la Santé (CRP-Santé), Luxembourg

Funding: This research was supported by a grant from Ministry of Food and Drug Safety to operation of the regional pharmacovigilance center in 2014. The funders had no role in study design, data collection and analysis, decision to publish, or preparation of the manuscript.

Competing Interests: The authors have declared that no competing interests exist.

∗ E-mail: helenmed@snu.ac.kr

Introduction

Anaphylaxis is a rapid-onset severe hypersensitivity reaction that can be fatal. Although death from anaphylaxis is not common and most episodes of anaphylaxis can be reversed by a single dose of epinephrine, severe anaphylaxis accompanied with cardiovascular collapse can be resistant to treatment and result in death.

As the use of computed tomography (CT) is rapidly growing, iodine based radiocontrast media (RCM) is administered about 75,000,000 times per year worldwide [1]. As low osmolality non-ionic contrast agents replaced high-osmolality ionic ones, the incidence of immediate RCM hypersensitivity diminished remarkably from 3.8–12.7% to 0.7–3.1% [2–4]. Similarly, the incidence of severe immediate RCM hypersensitivity also decreased from 0.1–0.4% to 0.01–0.04%. However, anaphylactic deaths still occur in 1–3 per 100,000–1,000,000 administrations regardless of ionicity [5,6]. Presently, the clinical characteristics and risk factors for the development of anaphylactic shock are not clearly defined.

The principle of post-anaphylaxis management is to avoid the causative agents. Although other imaging can be used as an alternative test in RCM hypersensitivity patients, CT imaging has its own advantage and unavoidable in some clinical situations. Although antihistamines and systemic steroids can be used as preventive measures, they cannot ensure complete prevention of RCM induced anaphylaxis [7,8]. Currently, there are no established guidelines on premedication for RCM induced anaphylaxis [9]. Therefore, information on a causal agent and safer substitutes will be very useful for patients who need contrast enhanced CT scan despite previous history of RCM induced anaphylaxis. Until recently, diagnostic value of RCM skin test has been underestimated and there are only a limited number of studies which evaluated the sensitivity of RCM skin testing to various RCM [10–12].

This study was performed to investigate the risk factors for the development of hypotension and the clinical value of RCM skin testing to identify causative agents in RCM induced anaphylaxis.

Methods

1. Study Subjects

This study protocol was approved by the institutional review board (IRB) of Seoul National University Hospital. Informed consents of patients were exempted from IRB because this study only used retrospective chart review data and all personal data was eliminated and coded as arbitrary number which were not personally-identifiable. Research data was accessed only by researchers using password.

We extracted all the cases of RCM induced hypersensitivity based on ATC code of causative agents (V08A: X-ray contrast media, iodinated, V08B: X-ray contrast media, non-iodinated)' and WHOART (ARRN: 0712 allergic reaction, 0713 anaphylactic shock, 0714 anaphylactoid reaction, 2237 anaphylactic reaction, 2268 documented hypersensitivity to administered drug) from our inhospital pharmacovigilance database collected from January 2005 to December 2012 at Seoul National University Hospital, in Seoul, Korea. Demographic and clinical data of affected patients such as age, sex, number of contrast exposures, laboratory test results, and underlying diseases based on ICD-10 were collected from electronic medical records. This study dealt

only with CT procedures, not with other procedures such as cardiac catheterization or coronary angiography.

All the medical records were thoroughly re-evaluated by two allergy specialists to assess clinical features of anaphylaxis and the presence of previous contrast hypersensitivity reactions. Anaphylaxis was diagnosed if cases satisfied the criteria of anaphylaxis suggested by the National Institute of Allergy and Infectious Disease and Food Allergy and the Anaphylaxis Network [13]. Hypotension was considered as a systolic blood pressure less than 90 mmHg or greater than 30% decrease from an individual's baseline. [13] Hypotension unrelated with underlying diseases or other drugs was considered a manifestation of anaphylaxis.

After completing review, patients with anaphylaxis were classified into two groups depending on combined hypotension. We analyzed the data to identify risk factors for the development of anaphylactic shock by comparing anaphylactic patients combined with and without hypotension.

2. Skin Tests with Iodinated Contrast Agents

Skin tests were carried out after experiencing RCM induced anaphylaxis for those patients who agreed to undergo skin testing. Skin prick and intradermal tests were performed on the volar part of the forearm with 6 different RCM used in our hospital - iopromide (Ultravist®, Bayer Healthcare, Brussels, Belgium), iopamidol (Pamiray®, Dongkook Pharm. Co., Ltd, Korea), iomeprol (Iomeron®, Bracco, Milan, Italy), iohexol (Omnipaque®, Armersham Health, Princeton, NJ), iodixanol (Visipaque®, Armersham Health, Princeton, NJ), and iobitridol (Xenetics®, Guerbet, Gorinchem, Netherlands). Undiluted solution and 1:10 diluted solution were used for the skin prick test and intradermal

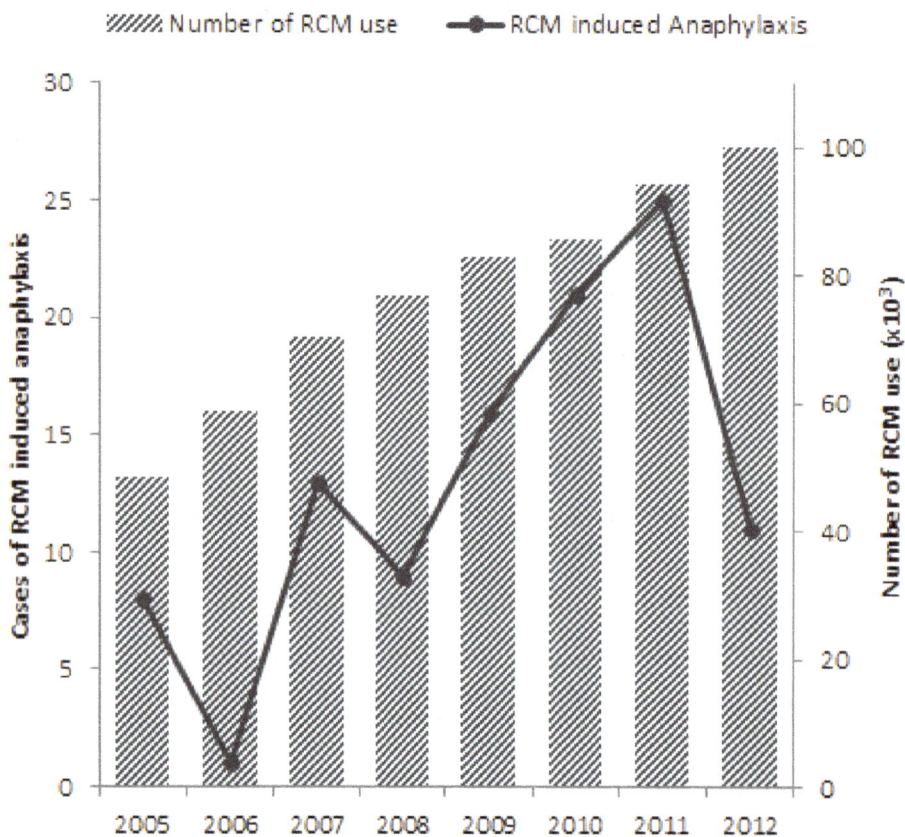

Figure 1. Anaphylactic reactions and total number of RCM use in every year of the study period.

Table 1. Clinical characteristics according to the development of hypotension.

	Total (N, %)	Anaphylactic shock (N, %)	Normotensive anaphylaxis (N, %)	P-value
Number	104	78	26	
Age (years)*	55.6±13.4	57.4±13.2	50.1±13.0	0.024
Male gender, %	43 (41.3)	35 (44.9)	8 (30.8)	0.254
Number of previous exposure to RCM*	4.3±7.1	5.1±7.8	1.9±3.3	0.004
None	36 (34.6)	24 (30.8)	12 (46.2)	0.369
1	17 (16.3)	13 (16.7)	4 (15.4)	
≥2	51 (49.0)	41 (52.6)	10 (38.5)	
Previous RCM reactions	21/68 (30.9)	18/54 (33.3)	3/14 (21.4)	0.362
WBC count (/µL)	5,844.7±1,883.8	5,886±1,921	5,617±1,720	0.668
Eosinophil count (/µL)	62.0±84.4	64.2±86.9	50.0±71.4	0.574
Hypersensitivity Symptoms				
Skin symptoms	69 (66.3)	49 (62.8)	20 (76.9)	0.235
Urticaria/erythema	53 (51.0)	36 (46.2)	17 (65.4)	0.114
Angioedema	34 (32.7)	21 (26.9)	13 (50.0)	0.052
Respiratory symptoms*	50 (48.1)	32 (41.0)	18 (69.2)	0.022
Dyspnea[†]	42 (40.4)	24 (30.8)	18 (69.2)	0.001
Cardiovascular symptoms[†]	88 (84.6)	78 (100.0)	10 (38.5)	<0.001
Gastrointestinal symptoms	20 (19.2)	16 (20.5)	4 (15.4)	0.775
Underlying allergic diseases	12 (11.5)	8 (10.3)	4 (15.4)	0.464
Radiocontrast media[‡]				
Iopromide*	60 (57.7)	51 (65.4)	9 (34.6)	0.011
Iopamidol	12 (11.6)	8 (10.3)	4 (15.4)	0.726
Iomeprol	11 (10.6)	8 (10.3)	3 (11.5)	1.000
Iohexol	7 (6.7)	3 (3.8)	4 (15.4)	0.064
Iobitridol	3 (2.9)	3 (3.8)	0 (0.0)	0.571
Iodixanol	4 (3.8)	3 (3.8)	1 (3.8)	1.000
Unidentified agents*	7 (6.7)	2 (2.6)	5 (19.2)	0.010
Positive skin test[†]	33/51 (64.7)	27/33 (81.8)	6/18 (33.3)	0.001
Skin prick test	1/51 (2.0)	1/33 (3.0)	0/18 (0.0)	1.000
Intradermal test[†]	33/51 (64.7)	27/33 (81.8)	6/18 (33.3)	0.001

Continuous variables are expressed as mean ± standard deviation.
*P<0.05, [†]P<0.01. [‡]Among the total 104 subjects, radiocontrast media involved in anaphylaxis could not be identified in seven patients who had experienced anaphylaxis prior to the introduction of electronic medical recording system.

test, respectively, as used in previous studies [10,12,14,15]. Histamine and normal saline were used as positive and negative control, respectively. The results were interpreted 15 minutes after the prick or the intradermal injection. Skin prick test was determined to be positive when wheal diameter was greater than 3 mm, and intradermal test was determined to be positive when wheal diameter increased 3 mm or more than the initial bleb [12]. The rate and factors contributing to the positivity of RCM skin test were analyzed.

3. Statistical Analysis

SPSS (version 19.0) was used to analyze the data. To compare the clinical features of two groups, Student t-test or Mann-Whitney test was used for continuous variables, and Chi-square test or Fisher's exact test was used for categorical variables. To identify the risk factors related with anaphylactic shock and a positive skin test, multiple logistic regression was used. We included adjustment factors that had a P-value less than 0.1 in

the univariate analysis, and other clinically important factors such as age and sex. A P-value less than 0.05 was considered statistically significant.

Results

1. Clinical Characteristics of the Study Subjects and Accompanied Anaphylaxis

A total number of contrast-enhanced CT scans during the study period was 632,513. A total of 104 cases of RCM related anaphylaxis were monitored during the study period. The incidence of contrast-induced anaphylaxis was 0.016%. As the total number of RCM use increased over the study period, the RCM related anaphylaxis also showed increasing tendency in number (Figure 1). The mean age was 55.6±13.1 years and 41.3% (43/104) of them were male (Table 1).

The median number of previous RCM exposures was 1.0 (interquartile range (IQR), 0.0–5.0) before the development of the

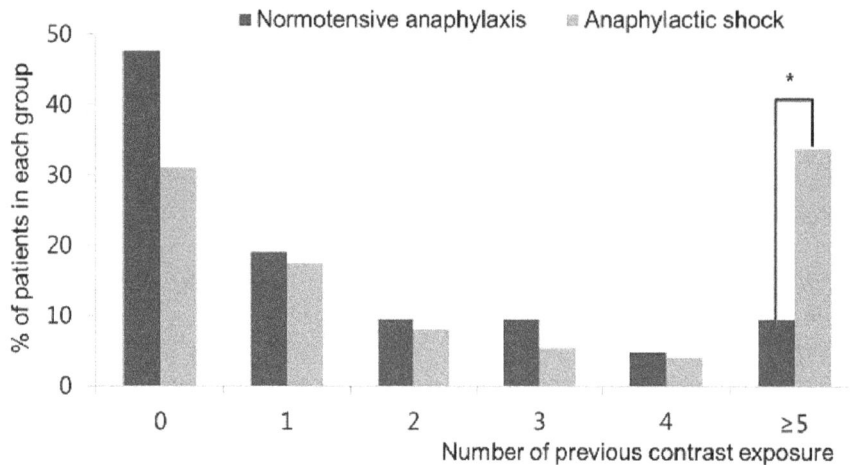

Figure 2. Comparison of the number of contrast exposures according to the presence of hypotension. *p<0.05.

first anaphylaxis. While anaphylaxis developed at the first exposure to RCM in 34.6% (36/104) of patients, 65.4% (68/104) of patients experienced anaphylaxis on repeated exposure to RCM and 21 of 68 (30.9%) had a milder form of hypersensitivity reactions in previous exposure to RCM.

Among hypersensitivity symptoms present in patients with anaphylaxis, cardiovascular symptoms were the most common (88/104, 84.6%), followed by skin symptoms (69/104, 66.3%) and respiratory symptoms (50/104, 48.1%) (Table 1). Most symptoms occurred within several minutes after the RCM injection. Seventy-eight patients experienced anaphylaxis with hypotension (anaphylactic shock) and 26 patients had anaphylaxis without hypotension.

2. Comparison of Clinical Characteristics According to the Development of Hypotension

Compared to anaphylactic patients without hypotension, patients who presented with anaphylactic shock were older (57.4 vs. 50.1 years, $p = 0.026$) and had significantly higher number of previous RCM exposures (5.1±7.8 vs. 1.9±3.3, $p = 0.004$). Of note, the number of patients who underwent previous CT more than two times was 52.6% and 38.5%, respectively in anaphylactic patients with and without hypotension. Especially, the proportion of previous exposure to RCM more than 5 times showed significant difference between anaphylactic patients with and without hypotension (35.4% vs. 9.1%, $p = 0.018$, Figure 2).

In terms of the causative contrast agent, hypotension was more frequent among anaphylaxis related to iopromide compared to other agents (85.0% vs. 61.4%, $p = 0.011$). Iopromide use was more frequently observed in patients with hypotension than in patients without it among patients with anaphylaxis (65.4% vs 34.6%, $p = 0.011$). With multiple logistic regression analysis after adjustment of age, sex, diabetes, and number of previous contrast exposure, iopromide use was still a risk factor for an anaphylactic shock (OR 3.088, 95% confidential interval (CI) = 1.078–8.843, $p = 0.036$).

3. Comparison of Clinical Characteristics According to Skin Test Positivity

Fifty-one patients with anaphylaxis followed the recommendation of allergists and underwent RCM skin test and the other 53 patients refused to perform skin test because they did not have a scheduled follow-up CT in the near future.

The mean interval between the time of anaphylaxis and skin test was 14.8 months (IQR 3.4–38.9). Skin test was performed in 41% of patients within one year since they experienced anaphylaxis. The remaining patients underwent skin test at the time when more than one year passed since anaphylaxis occurred (IQR 21.8–64.1).

Among those 51 patients with RCM skin test results, 33 (64.7%) had a positive response to at least one RCM while 18 patients (35.3%) did not show positivity to any RCM tested. In anaphylactic patients accompanied by hypotension, skin test showed 81.8% positivity. Among 33 patients with positive RCM skin test results, mean 1.1 contrast media (1.1±1.1) were positive per person.

Precise information on the culprit RCM was available in 29 patients. Twenty-two (75.9%) patients showed positivity to RCM including their culprit RCM; 14 patients showed single positivity to the culprit RCM; 8 patients showed positivity to other RCMs in addition to the culprit one. Another 7 patients responded to RCM agents other than the culprit one.

The positivity rate of skin test for each contrast agent is varied from 0.0% to 100.0% (Table 2). Iobitridol showed the highest sensitivity (100%) followed by iopromide (59.3%) and iodixanol (50.0%). However, all 5 patients who experienced iohexol induced anaphylaxis were negative in skin test with iohexol.

In patients with a positive RCM skin test, hypotension (79.4% vs. 35.3%, $p = 0.004$) and gastrointestinal symptoms (28.1% vs. 0.0%, $p = 0.047$) were more frequent compared to patients who had a negative RCM skin test. With multiple logistic regression analysis after adjustment by age, sex and diabetes, the presence of hypotension was a characteristic associated with a RCM skin test positivity (OR 10.0, 95% CI 2.105–47.098, $p = 0.004$). However, skin test positive rate was not different according to the history of previous RCM hypersensitivity reactions, accumulated number of exposures to the RCM, and underlying allergic disease.

Discussion

Incidence of anaphylaxis is increasing rapidly and known to be 4–50/100,000 person-years [16]. In adults, drugs are the most common cause of anaphylaxis [16,17] and radiocontrast media was the most commonly involved drug in a study of Korean tertiary care hospital [18]. Although the incidence of RCM hypersensitivity decreased as high-osmolality ionic contrasts were

Table 2. Sensitivity and false negative rate on skin test.

Causative RCM	Sensitivity		False negative rate	
	To any RCM N (%)	To culprit RCM N (%)	To any RCM N (%)	To culprit RCM N (%)
Iopromide	20/27 (74.1)	16/27 (59.3)	7/27 (25.9)	11/27 (40.7)
Iopamidol	2/5 (40.0)	1/5 (20.0)	3/5 (60.0)	4/5 (80.0)
Iomeprol	4/5 (80.0)	2/5 (40.0)	1/5 (20.0)	3/5 (60.0)
Iohexol	1/5 (20.0)	0/5 (0.0)	4/5 (80.0)	5/5 (100.0)
Iobitridol	2/2 (100.0)	2/2 (100.0)	0/2 (0.0)	0/2 (0.0)
Iodixanol	1/2 (50.0)	1/2 (50.0)	1/2 (50.0)	1/2 (50.0)
Total	30/46 (65.2)*	22/46 (47.8)	16/46 (32.6)	24/46 (52.1)

*Five patients in whom causal contrast media could not be identified were excluded from this analysis among 51 patients with skin test results.
Iopromide, iopamidol, iomeprol, iohexol, and iobitridol are low-osmolar contrast media. Iodixanol is an iso-osmolar contrast media.

replaced by low-osmolality non-ionic ones, anaphylactic death still occurred regardless of ionicity [5,6].

Traditionally, immediate hypersensitivity reactions to RCM were considered representative of non-IgE mediated 'anaphylactoid reaction' since it can occur on the first exposure and does not always recur on the repeated exposure [1,10,11,19]. However, a previous report showed that only 30% of immediate RCM hypersensitivity developed at the first exposure to RCM [20] and our study also revealed that only 35% of RCM induced anaphylaxis occurred at the first exposures to RCM. We found that milder hypersensitivity symptoms heralded anaphylaxis in 1/3 of the patients on preceding exposure to RCM. Multiple exposures and a previous hypersensitivity reaction prior to RCM induced anaphylaxis suggest that an immunologic mechanism may have some role in the development of some RCM induced anaphylaxis.

Anaphylaxis is a severe, life-threatening systemic hypersensitivity reaction involving at least two or more organs at the same time. However, diagnosis of anaphylaxis can be made if sudden hypotension develops after exposure to a known allergen. Based upon symptoms, anaphylaxis can be classified into mild, moderate, and severe grade. [21] When hypotension occurs as a manifestation of anaphylaxis either as a sole feature or with other symptoms, physicians should pay attention to the development of potential cardiovascular collapse which is the main cause of mortality in anaphylaxis [22]. There are several known risk factors for a severe RCM hypersensitivity such as previous history of RCM hypersensitivity, asthma, allergies requiring medical treatment, use of beta-adrenergic blockers, female gender, Indian and Mediterranean ethnicity, and malignant tumor [23]. However, there was no data on the risk factors for the development of hypotension in anaphylaxis. In this study, we reported risk factors for anaphylactic shock such as older age, previous multiple exposures to RCM, iopromide use. However, we do not have a clear picture of what the overall anaphylaxis rate is using iopromide or the other study contrast agents, since patients without anaphylaxis are not included in the study. Secondly, the number of administrations of other contrast agents was too small to provide statistically significant results. In other words, we cannot conclude from this study that iopromide is more likely to cause anaphylaxis than any of the other contrast agents, but among the anaphylactic patients, iopromide was associated with more severe forms of anaphylaxis (anaphylaxis with hypotension). In addition, anaphylaxis with hypotension showed stronger association with RCM skin test positivity than anaphylaxis without hypotension. Although skin test positivity might be the result of direct mast cell activation by

RCM, it is more likely that IgE mediated hypersensitivity may have a role in the development of RCM induced anaphylaxis when presented with hypotension.

Skin test is widely used to identify the causative agents in IgE mediated hypersensitivity [12,15,16]. Previously, sensitivity of the intradermal test was reported as high as 73% when performed with undiluted solutions [20]. However, this result may have been overestimated by irritation with undiluted RCM and a 1:10 solution has been preferred for intradermal test with RCM in general. The positive rate of the intradermal skin test was variable and reported as low as 4.2% among patients with RCM hypersensitivity [10]. On the other hand, data from the European Network of Drug Allergy multicentre study demonstrated a 50% positive rate of RCM skin test in immediate reactors [14]. Recently, Kim et al. reported that a significantly higher sensitivity positive rate of RCM skin test in severe immediate reactions (57.1%) compared with mild (12.9%) and moderate reactions (25.0%) and suggested their modest utility in evaluating severe adverse reactions retrospectively [24]. In this study, we observed much higher positive rate of RCM skin test in patient with RCM induced anaphylaxis (64.7%). Positive rate went up as high as 81.8% among patients with anaphylactic shock and it is the highest value ever reported in RCM hypersensitivity. Three quarter of patients who showed skin test positivity responded to the very same RCM used at the time of anaphylaxis and cross reactivity rate to other RCMs was low. These findings suggest that a substantial proportion of patients with RCM induced anaphylaxis, especially anaphylactic shock, may have specificity to causative agents and skin tests can provide information on the safe substitutes. However, considering negativity in one third of patients, skin test is not helpful to choose safe alternative RCMs in some populations and clinical reasoning is needed on interpreting the results.

Although we could not perform skin test in negative controls, skin test positivity in the negative control is known to be negligible. There are several studies which elucidated very low positivity of skin test in the negative controls. Brockow et al. reported that positivity of skin test was 0.0% (0/11)–4.2% (3/71) in the negative controls [14]. Kim et al. performed RCM skin testing on 1,048 Korean subjects before contrast-enhanced CT and found only 1 case of positive immediate skin test (0.09%) [24].

There are several limitations in this study. The main limitation is its retrospective design and underreporting of adverse reaction to spontaneous reporting systems. Another limitation is the lack of information on the number of individual RCM used in contrast-enhanced CT during the study period. Thus, large scale prospective studies including sufficient number of patients reacting to each RCM are needed in order to define the exact incidence and risk factors of RCM induced anaphylaxis.

Conclusion

RCM induced anaphylactic shock is related with multiple exposure to RCM and skin test positivity to RCM.

References

1. Brockow K, Ring J (2011) Anaphylaxis to radiographic contrast media. Curr Opin Allergy Clin Immunol 11: 326–331.
2. Kim MH, Park CH, Kim DI, Kim KM, Kim HK, et al. (2012) Surveillance of contrast-media-induced hypersensitivity reactions using signals from an electronic medical recording system. Ann Allergy Asthma Immunol 108: 167–171.
3. Katayama H (1990) Adverse reactions to contrast media. What are the risk factors? Invest Radiol 25 Suppl 1: S16–17.
4. Thomsen HS, Bush WH Jr (1998) Adverse effects of contrast media: incidence, prevention and management. Drug Saf 19: 313–324.
5. Cashman JD, McCredie J, Henry DA (1991) Intravenous contrast media: use and associated mortality. Med J Aust 155: 618–623.
6. Wysowski DK, Nourjah P (2006) Deaths attributed to X-ray contrast media on U.S. death certificates. AJR Am J Roentgenol 186: 613–615.
7. Williams AN, Kelso JM (2007) Radiocontrast-induced anaphylaxis despite pretreatment and use of iso-osmolar contrast. Ann Allergy Asthma Immunol 99: 467–468.
8. Davenport MS, Cohan RH, Caoili EM, Ellis JH (2009) Repeat contrast medium reactions in premedicated patients: frequency and severity. Radiology 253: 372–379.
9. Morcos SK, Thomsen HS, Webb JA (2001) Prevention of generalized reactions to contrast media: a consensus report and guidelines. Eur Radiol 11: 1720–1728.
10. Trcka J, Schmidt C, Seitz CS, Brocker EB, Gross GE, et al. (2008) Anaphylaxis to iodinated contrast material: nonallergic hypersensitivity or IgE-mediated allergy? AJR Am J Roentgenol 190: 666–670.
11. Brockow K, Ring J (2010) Classification and pathophysiology of radiocontrast media hypersensitivity. Chem Immunol Allergy 95: 157–169.
12. Caimmi S, Benyahia B, Suau D, Bousquet-Rouanet L, Caimmi D, et al. (2010) Clinical value of negative skin tests to iodinated contrast media. Clin Exp Allergy 40: 805–810.
13. Sampson HA, Munoz-Furlong A, Campbell RL, Adkinson NF Jr, Bock SA, et al. (2006) Second symposium on the definition and management of anaphylaxis: summary report–Second National Institute of Allergy and Infectious Disease/ Food Allergy and Anaphylaxis Network symposium. J Allergy Clin Immunol 117: 391–397.
14. Brockow K, Romano A, Aberer W, Bircher AJ, Barbaud A, et al. (2009) Skin testing in patients with hypersensitivity reactions to iodinated contrast media - a European multicenter study. Allergy 64: 234–241.
15. Goksel O, Aydin O, Atasoy C, Akyar S, Demirel YS, et al. (2011) Hypersensitivity reactions to contrast media: prevalence, risk factors and the role of skin tests in diagnosis–a cross-sectional survey. Int Arch Allergy Immunol 155: 297–305.
16. Lee JK, Vadas P (2011) Anaphylaxis: mechanisms and management. Clin Exp Allergy 41: 923–938.
17. Greenberger PA, Rotskoff BD, Lifschultz B (2007) Fatal anaphylaxis: postmortem findings and associated comorbid diseases. Ann Allergy Asthma Immunol 98: 252–257.
18. Yang MS, Lee SH, Kim TW, Kwon JW, Lee SM, et al. (2008) Epidemiologic and clinical features of anaphylaxis in Korea. Ann Allergy Asthma Immunol 100: 31–36.
19. Maddox TG (2002) Adverse reactions to contrast material: recognition, prevention, and treatment. Am Fam Physician 66: 1229–1234.
20. Dewachter P, Laroche D, Mouton-Faivre C, Bloch-Morot E, Cercueil JP, et al. (2011) Immediate reactions following iodinated contrast media injection: a study of 38 cases. Eur J Radiol 77: 495–501.
21. Muraro A, Roberts G, Clark A, Eigenmann PA, Halken S, et al. (2007) The management of anaphylaxis in childhood: position paper of the European academy of allergology and clinical immunology. Allergy 62: 857–871.
22. Khan BQ, Kemp SF (2011) Pathophysiology of anaphylaxis. Curr Opin Allergy Clin Immunol 11: 319–325.
23. Morcos SK (2005) Review article: Acute serious and fatal reactions to contrast media: our current understanding. Br J Radiol 78: 686–693.
24. Kim SH, Jo EJ, Kim MY, Lee SE, Kim MH, et al. (2013) Clinical value of radiocontrast media skin tests as a prescreening and diagnostic tool in hypersensitivity reactions. Ann Allergy Asthma Immunol 110: 258–262.

Author Contributions

Conceived and designed the experiments: H-RK S-HC. Performed the experiments: M-HK S-YL S-EL M-SY J-WJ. Analyzed the data: C-MP WL. Contributed reagents/materials/analysis tools: M-HK S-YL S-EL M-SY J-WJ C-MP WL S-HC H-RK. Wrote the paper: M-HK H-RK.

Polymorphisms in the *CYP2E1* and *GSTM1* Genes as Possible Protection Factors for Leprosy Patients

Pablo Pinto[1]**, Claudio Guedes Salgado**[2]**, Ney Santos**[1]**, Dayse O. Alencar**[1]**, Sidney Santos**[1]**, Mara H. Hutz**[3]**, Ândrea Ribeiro-dos-Santos**[1]*

1 Laboratório de Genética Humana e Médica, Instituto de Ciências Biológicas, Universidade Federal do Pará, Belém, Pará, Brasil, **2** Laboratório de Dermatoimunologia, Instituto de Ciências Biológicas, Universidade Federal do Pará, Belém, Pará, Brasil, **3** Instituto de Biociências, Departamento de Genética, Universidade Federal do Rio Grande do Sul, Rio Grande do Sol, Brasil

Abstract

Background: The *CYP2E1* and *GSTM1* genes encode metabolic enzymes that have key functions in drug modification and elimination.

Methodology/Principal Findings: We investigated the possible effects of *CYP2E1* and *GSTM1* polymorphisms in 71 leprosy patients and in 110 individuals from the general population. The *GSTM1*0* null allele and INDEL *CYP2E1*1D* mutant genotypes were analyzed by conventional PCR, while *CYP2E1* SNPs (1053C>T, 1293G>C and 7632T>A) were determined by RT-PCR. In leprosy patients, the *GSTM1*0* and *CYP2E1*5* alleles and the combined alleles *GSTM1*0/CYP2E1*6* and *GSTM1*0/CYP2E1*5* were significantly related to a baciloscopic index (BI) (BI<3), while the *CYP2E1*6* allele was related to a better clinical evolution in the leprosy spectrum.

Conclusions/Significance: Therefore, *GSTM1*0*, *CYP2E1*5* and *CYP2E1*6* may be possible protection factors for leprosy patients.

Editor: Tanya Parish, Queen Mary University of London, United Kingdom

Funding: This study was supported by FINEP (Financiadora de Estudos e Projetos), CNPq/Casadinho (Conselho Nacional de Desenvolvimento Científico e Tecnológico), CAPES (Coordenação de Aperfeiçoamento Pessoal de Nível Superior) and PROPES/UFPA (Universidade Federal do Pará), FADESP (Fundação de Amparo a Pesquisa). The funders had no role in study design, data collection and analysis, decision to publish, or preparation of the manuscript.

Competing Interests: The authors have declared that no competing interests exist.

* E-mail: akely@ufpa.br

Introduction

Leprosy is an insidious infectious disease caused by the obligate intracellular bacteria *Mycobacterium leprae* that affects the skin and peripheral nerves, causing a chronic granulomatous infection [1].

Multidrug therapy (MDT), the treatment recommended by the World Health Organization (WHO), has healed millions of patients since it was implemented in 1980s. MDT consists of the use of dapsone and rifampicin for 6 months in paucibacilary (PB) patients, or both along with a third drug, clofazimine, for 12 months in multibacilary (MB) cases [2].

Patients are classified as PB or MB using a simple system introduced by the WHO in 1982. Patients with 5 skin lesions or less are classified as PB, and those with more than 5 lesions are classified as MB [3,4]. Although this simple classification scheme is adequate for remote sites where the population has little or no access to health care, it is not detailed enough for more in-depth research surveys.

Another way to classify leprosy patients is based on a skin smear test, for which a positive result is classified as MB, and a negative result as PB. A trained laboratory technician can readily identify AFB (acid fast bacillus), making this test a very reliable method. However, cases initially classified as PB (AFB negative) can evolve to MB in the natural course of the disease [5]. This phenomenon is especially true for those patients classified as indeterminate (MHI) using the Madrid classification system.

The use of the Ridley-Jopling clinical, histological and immunological criteria further improves case definitions, with TT (tuberculoid-tuberculoid) patients exhibiting a strong cellular immune response (CIR) and a negative skin smear test, while LL (lepromatous-lepromatous) patients have a weak or absent CIR and a highly positive skin smear [6]. In the middle of the spectrum are a large number of borderline patients, varying from weak to strong CIR and from negative to positive skin smears.

Interestingly, neither the CIR status nor the skin smear test is predictive of leprosy reactions or of the progression of each case through the physical disabilities caused by the disease. To date, little is known about which factors are crucial to the development of these disabilities. All types of patients, TT, borderline or LL, can progress with highly incapacitating disabilities and chronic neuropathies with no single marker or criteria to predict patient outcome [2,3].

Dapsone (4,4′-diaminodiphenyl sulfone, DDS) is one of the primary drugs used in anti-leprosy therapeutics. It is a bacteriostatic agent that competes with para-aminobenzoic acid (PABA), diminishing or blocking the production of bacterial folic acid [5,7]. Clofazimine is a riminophenazine dye that has bactericidal and anti-inflammatory effects. It inhibits bacterial proliferation by binding to bacterial DNA and blocking its replication [8,9]. Rifampicin, or rifampin (RIF) has a well-proven bactericidal effect on *M. leprae*. It is a semisynthetic drug, originally derived from *Streptomyces mediterranei*, and it is widely used for treating leprosy and tuberculosis. RIF prevents protein production by inhibition of RNA polymerase in bacterial cells [10–16].

CYP-450 members of the heme protein superfamily are notable for their large spectrum of action and the distribution of their biological structures. These proteins participate in critical processes including the biosynthesis of steroidal hormones and the detoxification by conjugation with cellular components, such as glutathione [17].

CYP2E1 is found in various tissues including brain, lungs and kidneys, but it is most concentrated in the liver, where the majority of biotransformation occurs. Four main SNPs in the *CYP2E1* gene have been investigated in different populations, including tuberculosis (TB) patients [18–20], who often show 1053C>T and 1293G>C mutations, which together form the compound allele *CYP2E1*1A*, CG; *CYP2E1*5*, TC. Another SNP, 7632T>A, is located in the sixth intron of the *CYP2E1* gene and has two alleles, wild-type *CYP2E1*1A* (T) and mutant *CYP2E1*6* (A). Additionally, a 96-bp INDEL polymorphism with two alleles, wild-type *CYP2E1*1C* (DEL) and mutant *CYP2E1*1D* (INS), has also been described [18,19].

There are different glutathione S-transferase (GST) isoforms, including *GSTM1*, which is located on chromosome 1. More than 51 SNPs have been described within *GSTM1*, among which are two functional alleles, *GSTM1*A* and *GSTM1*B*, that have the same detoxification efficacy; one null (deletion) allele, *GSTM1*0*; and one duplication [21,22].

Two GSTM1 polymorphisms, *GSTM1*1*, which has normal activity, and *GSTM1*0*, which has no enzymatic activity because it is a complete gene deletion, have been well studied in different populations [23–25]. The presence of the null allele seems to be related to substrate conjugation and excretion; therefore, its presence can be an indicator for more rational drug dosages for various groups of patients [26].

We investigated a sample of MDT-treated leprosy patients ascertained at the Dr. Marcello Candia Reference Unit in the Sanitary Dermatology of the State of Pará (UREMC) with the aim of identifying associations among **CYP2E1** polymorphisms [including 1053 C>T, 1293G>C (*CYP2E1*1A*, *CYP2E1*5*); 7632T>A (*CYP2E1*1A*, *CYP2E1*6*); 96-bp INDEL *CYP2E1*1C* (DEL) and *CYP2E1*1D* (INS)] and **GSTM1** polymorphisms (*GSTM1*1* and *GSTM1*0*) and possible protection factors for leprosy patients.

Methods

Sample

We investigated 71 leprosy patients who attended the Dr. Marcello Candia Reference Unit in the Sanitary Dermatology of the State of Pará (UREMC) in Marituba, Pará, Brazil, from January 2008 to December 2009. In UREMC there are about 40,000 yearly consultations on different medicine specialties as, among others, leprology, dermatology, ophthalmology and orthopedics, besides nursery, physical therapy and other health professionals sessions. Since 2002, UREMC registered between 308 and 472 leprosy patients (mean: 408 cases/year). During years 2008 and 2009, 765 leprosy cases were registered, from those, 71 (9,28%) were randomly selected for this study.

All patients were evaluated neurologically by Semmes-Weinstein monofilament examination (SWME) for sensory testing, and by voluntary motor testing (VMT) for function assessment of

muscular force, as previously described [27]. They were classified according to the Ridley-Jopling system and were distributed in two groups depending on the progression of the disease: the positive (+) group consisted of PB patients skin smear negative Tuberculoid (TT) patients and MB skin smear negative Borderline-Tuberculoid (BT) patients, with or without leprosy reactions, with no sequel (defined by sensorial loss or motor deficit on hands or feet on Nerve Function Impairment (NFI) assessment), and the negative (−) group consisted of PB patients with or without leprosy reactions, but with sequel, together with all MB skin smear positive Borderline-Borderline (BB), Borderline-Lepromatous (BL) and Lepromatous-Lepromatous (LL) patients, regardless reactions or sequel. Additionally, in order to make other comparisons, patients were classified according to the baciloscopic index (BI), a group with a low (<3) BI (LBI), and a group with high (≥3) BI (HBI) [28]. A sample of 110 healthy individuals from the same geographic area were included in the study as controls. All patients were informed about the study before signing informed consent forms. The project was approved by the Pará Federal University ethics committee (N° 197/07).

DNA Extraction

DNA extraction was performed as previously described [29]. The DNA concentration was determined by spectrophotometry (Themo Scientific NanoDrop 1000, NanoDrop Technologies, Wilmington, US).

CYP2E1 Genotyping

Three *CYP2E1* polymorphisms, 1053C>T, 1293G>C and 7632T>A, were investigated using a TaqMan genotyping assay and analyzed by Real Time PCR 7500 (Life Technologies, CA, USA). The INDEL was investigated using conventional PCR methods, followed by visualization on an agarose gel. Specific PCR programs were established according to the annealing temperatures of the primers, and the amplifications were performed on a thermocycler Veriti 96 Well Thermal Cycler (Life Technologies, CA, USA). The alleles of the four *CYP2E1* polymorphisms investigated were defined using the official nomenclature, as described in http://www.cypalleles.ki.se/cyp2e1.htm.

GSTM1 Genotyping

For amplification, a set of primers for GSTM1F/GSTM1R was investigated using conventional PCR methods (thermocycler Veriti 96 Well Thermal Cycler - Life Technologies, CA, US), followed by visualization on an agarose gel.

Ancestry Informative Markers (AIM)

Individual interethnic admixture was estimated using a panel of 48 ancestry informative markers (AIMs), as previously described [30].

Statistical Analyses

Estimations of linkage disequilibrium (D and D') and haplotypes and allelic frequencies were estimated with the M. Locus v. 2.0 software [31]. All other statistical analyses were performed using SPSS v. 12.0 (SPSS, Chicago, IL, USA), and results were considered statistically significant at p<0.05.

Results

Demographic and clinical characteristics of the patients are shown in Table 1. Age, gender, sequel and clinical forms were all statistically significant when LBI and HBI were compared. Sequel

Table 1. Demographic and clinical characteristic of the sample according with Baciloscopic Index.

Variables	Baciloscopic Index[c] (N = 71)		p value (IC-95%)
	LBI n(%) = 32	HBI n(%) = 39	
Age[a]	35.2± 2.97	62.5± 3.42	<0.001
Gender[b] (M/F)	15(46.8%)/17(53.2%)	32(82%)/7(12%)	0.003
Sequel[b] (YES/NO)	12(37.5%)/20(62.5%)	30(76.9%)/9(23.1%)	0.001
Clinical Forms (PB/MB)[b]	10(31.2%)/22(68.8%)	0/39(100%)	0.002

[a]t-Test of Student;
[b]Fisher's Exact Test;
[c]Baciloscopic Index (LBI = Baciloscopic Index Low; HBI = Baciloscopic Index High).

occurred in 76.9% of the HBI patients whereas in the LBI group only 37.5% of the patients presented sequel.

There were 19 patients classified in the positive (+) group, of which nine were designated PB (two with reaction) and 10 were MB (four with reaction and all without sequel), while 52 patients comprised the negative (−) group, two of which were PB (all with reaction and sequel), and 50 were MB (35 with reaction and 40 with sequel) (Table 2). Concerning genotypic and allelic distribution of SNPs, a high (42.3%), statistically significant, frequency of the heterozygous genotype for the CYP2E1*6 allele was found among leprosy patients (Table 2). In the positive group, 63.2% (12 patients) exhibited this genotype, while in the negative group, a lower percentage (34.6%, 18 patients) was observed. The frequency of the wild-type CYP2E1*1A and mutant CYP2E1*6 alleles in this population was 0.789 and 0.211, respectively, which

was statistically significant when the positive and negative groups were compared (Table 2).

Leprosy patients were also divided into two groups according to the baciloscopic index (BI): a group with a low (<3) BI (LBI) and a group with high (≥3) BI (HBI). In addition to the analysis of the genotypic distribution of both CYP2E1 and GSTM1 markers in the LBI and HBI groups (Table 3), the combined effect of the two mutant alleles for the CYP2E1 and GSTM1 genes (CYP2E1*6/GSTM1*0 and CYP2E1*5/GSTM1*0) was also analyzed. The mutant CYP2E1*5 allele was present in 37.5% of the patients in the LBI group, while the wild-type CYP2E1*1A allele was observed in 92.3% of the patients in the HBI group. GSTM1 gene analysis demonstrated that the mutant GSTM1*0 allele was present in 56.2% of the LBI group patients and in 38.5% of the HBI group patients, while the wild-type GSTM1*1 allele was present in 61.5% of the HBI group patients (Table 3). The analysis of the combined

Table 2. Genotypic and allelic distribution of SNPs on CYP2E1 and GSTM1 genes among patients grouped according to clinical evolution.

Genotype	Patients with Leprosy (%) (n = 71)	Group (+) (%) (n = 19)	Group (−) (%) (n = 52)	P*[1]	OR(95% IC)*[2]
CYP2E1 (96 INDEL)					
*1C/*1C	64 (90.1%)	16 (84.2%)	48 (92.3%)		1 (reference)
*1C/*1D	7 (8.9%)	3 (15.8%)	4 (7.7%)	0.375	0.444(0.09–2.202)
CYP2E1*1C	0.951	0.921	0.962		
CYP2E1*1D	0.049	0.079	0.038		
CYP2E1 (7632)					
*1A/*1A	41 (57.7%)	7 (36.8%)	34 (65.4%)		1 (reference)
*1A/*6	30 (42.3%)	12 (63.2%)	18 (34.6%)	**0.03**	0.309(0.103–0.922)
CYP2E1*1A	0.789	0.684	0.827		
CYP2E1*6	0.211	0.316	0.173		
CYP2E1 (1053/1293)					
*1A/*1A	56 (78.9%)	13 (68.5%)	43 (82.6%)		1 (reference)
*1A/*5	15 (21.1%)	6 (31.5%)	9 (17.4%)	0.206	0.453(0.135–1.513)
CYP2E1*1A	0.894	0.842	0.914		
CYP2E1*5	0.106	0.158	0.086		
GSTM1					
GSTM1*1	38 (53.5%)	12 (63.2%)	26 (50%)		1 (reference)
GSTM1*0	33 (46.5%)	7 (36.8%)	26 (50%)	0.423	1.714 (0.583–5.043)

*[1]p-value;
*[2]OR-odds ratio, CI-confidence interval.

effect revealed that the *CYP2E1*6/GSTM1*0* genotypic combination was detected in 31.2% of the patients in the LBI group, while the *CYP2E1*5/GSTM1*0* genotypic combination was present in 28.1% of the patients in the LBI group; all were statistically significant when the different combinations were analyzed in the LBI or HBI groups.

Next, we performed a logistic regression analysis in which the two groups, LBI and HBI, were dependent variables and with covariables that could interfere with the results of PB and MB clinical forms. Although the results were not statistically significant for different variables, such as gender and sequel, they were significant when related to *CYP2E1*1A/*5* (p = 0.0266) and *GSTM1*0* (p = 0.0500) genotypes. These results suggest a strong association between both mutations and LBI (Table 4).

To evaluate the presence of population substructure, we compared the clinical progression of leprosy patients (positive and negative groups, as well as high and low baciloscopic index groups) with genomic ancestry, and the results showed no, significant. However, different frequencies were found for the investigated markers when leprosy patients were compared with a sample of healthy individuals from the same region (Table 5). The data showed that *CYP2E1*5* allele is more frequent among the healthy individuals than among patients (0.196 and 0.106, respectively; $X^2 = 6.85$; p = 0.032), while *CYP2E1*6* allele is more common among patients than in the control sample (0.211 e 0.090, respectively; $X^2 = 11.6$; p = 0.003).

Discussion

Loss of sensation is the hallmark of leprosy diagnosis. It is well known that both, MB and PB patients may evolve to nerve

Table 4. Logistic regression analysis of the association between genetic markers and LBI/HBI response in leprosy patients.

Variable	β	S.E.	Wald	df	P	O.R (95%CI)
Age	0.0363	0.0209	3.0109	1	**0.0012**	1.0562 (0.9953–1.0804)
Gender	0.8705	0.7327	1.4113	1	0.2348	2.3881 (0.5680–1.0407)
Sequel	0.8742	0.8405	1.0818	1	0.2983	2.3969 (0.4616–12.4468)
Clinical Form (PB/MB)	1.8598	1.1901	2.4421	1	0.1181	6.4226 (0.6233–66.1807)
CYP2E1 *1A/*5	−1.6341	0.8457	3.7339	1	**0.0266**	0.1198 (0.0184–0.7816)
CYP2E1 *1A/*6	1.0889	0.9079	1.4382	1	0.2304	2.9709 (0.5012–17.6087)
GSTM1*0	−1.3004	0.7025	3.4262	1	**0.05**	0.2724 (0.0687–1.0796)
African	−2.2083	1.8217	3.3266	1	0.4925	0.1099 (0.0002–60.2213)
European	0.9890	2.6275	0.1417	1	0.7066	2.6885 (0.0156–10.6548)
Amerindian	0.4674	2.5465	6.5769	1	0.8544	1.5958 (0.0108–11.0136)

β, Coefficient Stimation; **S.E.**, Standard Error; **df**, Degrees of Freedom; *p*, p-value; **OR**, Odds Ratio; **CI**, Confident Interval.

function impairment on the natural course of the disease [32]. It is usual - and comprehensible as an objective tool – to use BI to analyze the correlation between a specific gene or a genotypic combination and the evolution of leprosy. However, this cannot be the only parameter to evaluate in order to understand the disease behavior individually. HBI may indicate *M. leprae* ability to grow

Table 3. Combined and isolated genotypic distribution of *CYP2E1* gene (SNPs 1053T>C, 1293C>G and 7632T>A), and deletion (*GSTM1*1/GSTM1*0*) on gene *GSTM1* of patients classified accordingly to baciloscopic index BI (LBI and HBI).

Genotype	Leprosy patients (n = 71)	LBI (n = 32)	HBI (n = 39)	p*[1]	OR (95% IC)*[2]
CYP2E1 (7632)					
*1A/*1A	41 (57.74%)	16 (50%)	25 (64.1%)		1 (reference)
*1A/*6	30 (42.26%)	16 (50%)	14 (35.9%)	0.334	0.560 (0.216–1.452)
CYP2E1*1A	0.789	0.750	0.821		
CYP2E1*5	0.211	0.250	0.179		
CYP2E1 (1053/1293)					
*1A/*1A	56 (78.87%)	20 (62.5%)	36 (92.3%)		1 (reference)
*1A/*5	15 (21.13%)	12 (37.5%)	3 (7.7%)	**0.003**	0.139 (0.035–0.551)
CYP2E1*1A	0.894	0.813	0.962		
CYP2E1*5	0.106	0.187	0.038		
GSTM1					
GSTM1*1	38 (53.52%)	14 (43.8%)	24 (61.5%)		1 (reference)
GSTM1*0	33 (46.48%)	18 (56.2%)	15 (38.5%)	**0.0276**	0.486 (0.188–1.258)
*CYP2E1/GSTM1**[3]					
CYP2E1*1A/GSTM1*1	58 (81.7%)	22 (68.8%)	36 (92.3%)		1 (reference)
CYP2E1*6/GSTM1*0	13 (18.3%)	10 (31.2%)	3 (7.7%)	**0.012**	0.183(0.045–0.740)
CYP2E1*1A/GSTM1*1	62 (87.3%)	23 (71.9%)	39 (100%)		1 (reference)
CYP2E1*5/GSTM1*0	9 (12.7%)	9 (28.1%)	–	**<0.005**	0.371 (0.27–0.513)

*[1]p-value;
*[2]OR-odds ratio, CI-confidence interval;
*[3]Combined effect of mutant alleles of distinct genes.

Table 5. Allele and genotype distributions of CYP2E1 and GSTM1 genes within two samples from leprosy patients and healthy individuals.

Genotype	Patients with Leprosy (%) (n = 71)	Healthy Population (%) (n = 110)	χ^2	p
CYP2E1 (96 INDEL)				
*1C/*1C	64 (90.1%)	96 (87.3%)		
*1C/*1D	7 (8.9%)	12 (10.9%)		
*1D/*1D	–	2 (1.8%)		
CYP2E1*1C	0.951	0.927	1.376	0.743
CYP2E1*1D	0.049	0.073		
CYP2E1 (7632)				
*1A/*1A	41 (57.7%)	90 (81.8%)		
*1A/*6	30 (42.3%)	20 (17.2%)		
*6/*6	–	–		
CYP2E1*1A	0.789	0.909	11.673	**0.003**
CYP2E1*6	0.211	0.091		
CYP2E1 (1053/1293)				
*1A/*1A	56 (78.9%)	70 (63.6%)		
*1A/*5	15 (21.1%)	37 (33.6%)		
*5/*5	–	3 (2.8%)		
CYP2E1*1A	0.894	0.805	6.855	**0.032**
CYP2E1*5	0.106	0.195		
GSTM1				
GSTM1*1	38 (53.5%)	53 (48.2%)		
GSTM1*0	33 (46.5%)	57 (51.8%)	1.136	0.722

inside the host in order to keep transmission chain and strain survival, or may indicate the inability of the host in constrain bacterial growth.

Notwithstanding, the capacity of the human host immune system in dealing with leprosy infection with no sequel is rarely addressed. In the present study two groups of patients were examined, and a striking difference when BI or disease evolution were evaluated were observed in relation to the genes investigated herein. While $CYP2E1^{7632}*1A/*1A$ was associated to a worse disease progression, and the presence of the mutant $CYP2E1^{7632}*1A/*6$ was associated with a good evolution, however, none of them were related to LBI or HBI. These findings suggest that different genes may be related to disease progression or bacterial growth inhibition mechanisms. Furthermore, $CYP2E1^{1053/1293}*1A/*1A$ was associated with HBI, while there no significant association was observed for clinical evolution analyses., $CYP2E1^{1053/1293}*1A/*5$ was significantly associated with LBI and a better disease progression.

The availability of modern antibiotics can help us to better understand the disease, and it is reasonable to think that pharmacogenomics related genes may also be related to disease outcome in human hosts. One of these key drugs is rifampicin.

Rifampicin can be bacteriostatic at lower concentrations or bactericidal at higher concentrations. When used alone, mycobacterium can readily develop resistance to RIF, and therefore, treatment should not rely solely on this drug [15]. Its biotransformation occurs through a process of hepatic deacetylation, giving rise to the active metabolite desacetylrifampicin [26]. RIF has a high capacity for inducing CYP450 isoforms, which contributes to a 40% reduction in half-life during the first half month of treatment and the acceleration of RIF deacetylation.

Therefore, this drug is capable of intensifying its own biotransformation, diminishing its plasmatic half-life when administered in multiple doses [33]. Studies of the *CYP2E1* gene indicate that *CYP2E1*6* and *CYP2E1*5* alleles are associated with a higher level of transcription and microsomal enzyme activity; therefore, they are implicated in enzymatic biotransformation activity augmentation [34–36], consequently decreasing the half-life of RIF.

Our results show that among the patients grouped according to clinical progression, the heterozygous genotype *CYP2E1*1A/*6* was present in 63.2% of the individuals in the (+) group. The OR analysis of the *CYP2E1*6* allele demonstrated that this polymorphism provides protection to those individuals in the (+) group (Table 2).

We hypothesize that the *CYP2E1*6* allele could increased the rate of rifampicin metabolism. Augments the biotransformation by CYP450 enzymes and raising the levels of the active metabolite desacetylrifampicin, which has a higher bactericidal activity. Therefore, individuals with this mutation could more efficiently combat *M. leprae*.

A significant difference was found between healthy individuals and patients for the *CYP2E1*6* allele, which is more common among leprosy patients ($X^2 = 11.6$; p = 0.003). Since this association was unknown, more studies are necessary to confirm these results (Table 5).

Among leprosy patients, *CYP2E1*5* allele was more frequent in the LBI group. This allele was also more frequent in healthy subjects when compared to leprosy individuals. These results taken together suggest that *CYP2E1*5* is a protection factor that might be involved with bacterial growth inhibition (Table 5).

For the *GSTM1* gene, the null genotype *GSTM1*0* was present in 56.2% of the LBI group. The compound distribution of the two mutant alleles *CYP2E1*5/GSTM1*0* was present in 28.1% of LBI the patients, while *CYP2E1*6/GSTM1*0* was present in 31.2%. The estimated OR suggest that mutant alleles confer protection for LBI individuals.

Taken together, our results suggest that the *CYP2E1*5, CYP2E1*6* and *GSTM1*0* alleles may be considered as susceptibility markers for leprosy, and their distribution should be further investigated, as their presence seems to confer protection from *M. leprae.*

Acknowledgments

Special thanks the donors of samples (leprosy patients from northern Brazil), who enable this study to be carried out, CAPES (Coordenação de Aperfeiçoamento Pessoal de Nível Superior) and UFPA (Universidade Federal do Pará).

Author Contributions

Conceived and designed the experiments: CS SS MH ARS. Performed the experiments: PP CS DOA ARS. Analyzed the data: PP NS SS. Contributed reagents/materials/analysis tools: CS SS ARS. Wrote the paper: PP CS ARS.

References

1. Alcais A, Mira M, Casanova JI, Schurr E, Abel I (2005) Genetic dissection of immunity in leprosy. Current Opinion in Immunology 17: 44–48.
2. Moreira MBR, Pena GO, Pereira GFM, Madalena M (2002). Ministério da Saúde, Secretaria de Políticas de Saúde, Guia para o controle da hanseníase. ISBN 85-334-0346-1.
3. Stretch R (1999) Presentation and treatment of Hansen's disease. Nurs Times 95(29): 46–7.
4. Moreira AS, Ribeiro dos Santos RC, Bastos RR, Silva JV, Santos PM (2006) Conjunctival bacilloscopy in leprosy diagnosis and follow-up. Arq Bras Oftalmol 69(6): 865–9.
5. Goulart IMB, Arbex GL, Carneiro MH, Rodrigues MS, Gadia R (2002) Adverse effects of multidrug therapy in leprosy patients: a five-year survey at a Health. Rev Soc Bras Med Trop 35(5): 453–60.
6. Ridley DS, Jopling WH (1966) Classification of leprosy according to immunity: a five-group system. Inernational Journal of Leprosy Other Mycobact. Disease 34: 255–273.
7. Kaur MR, Lewis HM (2006) Hidradenitis suppurativa treated with dapsone: a case series of five patients. J Dermatol Treat 17: 211–213.
8. Morrison NE, Morley GM (1976) The mode of action of clofazimine: DNA binding studies. Int. J. Lepr 44: 133–135.
9. Yano T, Bratinova SK, Teh JS, Winkler J, Sullivan K, Isaacs A, et al. (2011) Reduction of Clofazimine by Mycobacterial Type 2 NADH:Quinone Oxido-reductase. Jour. Bio. Chem. 286: 10276–10287.
10. Jopling WH (1983) Side effects of antileprosy drugs in common use. Leprosy Review 54: 261–270.
11. Jopling WH (1985) References to "side-effects of antileprosy drugs in common use". Leprosy Review 56: 61–70.
12. Pfaltzgraff RE, Bryceson A (1985) Clinical Leprosy. In: Hastings RC. Leprosy. New York p.134–136.
13. Opromolla DVA (1997) Terapêutica da hanseníase. Medicina Ribeirão Preto 30: 345–350.
14. Souza CS (1997) Hanseníase: formas clínicas e diagnóstico diferencial. Medicina Ribeirão Preto 30: 325–334.
15. Rivers EC. Mancera RL (2008) New Anti-Tuberculosis Drugs with Novel Mechanisms of Action. Curr Med Chem; 15(19): 1956–67.
16. Rivera RC, López CR, Herranz AB, Cevallos MA (2010) Analysis of the Mechanism of Action of the Antisense RNA That Controls the Replication of the repABC Plasmid p42d. Journal of Bacteriology 192: 3268–3278.
17. -Hasler JA, Estabrook R, Murray M, Pikuleva I, Waterman M, Capdevila J, et al. (1999) Human cytochromes P450. Molecular Aspects of Medicine 20: 1–137.
18. Yamada S, Tang M, Richardson K, Halaschek-Wiener J, Chan M, et al. (2009) Genetic variations of NAT2 and CYP2E1 and isoniazid hepatotoxicity in a diverse population. Pharmacogenomics 10(9): 1433–45.
19. Kayaaltu Z, Söylemezoglu T (2010) Distribution of ADH1B, ALDH2, CYP2E1*6, and CYP2E1*7B genotypes in Turkish population. Alcohol 1: 9–12.
20. Uematsu F, Ikawa S, Kikuchi H, Sagami I, Kanamaru R, et al. (1994) Restriction fragment length polymorphism of the human CYP2E1 (cytochrome P450IIE1) gene and susceptibility to lung cancer: possible relevance to low smoking exposure. Pharmacogenetics 4(2): 58–63.
21. Widersten M, Pearson WR, Engstrom A, Mannervik B (1991) Heterologous expression of the allelic variant Mu-class glutathione transferases m and y. Biochemical Journal 276: 519–524.
22. Moyer AM, Salavaggione OE, Hebbring SJ (2007) Glutathione S-Transferase T1 and M1: Gene Sequence Variation and Functional Genomics. Clin Cancer Res 13: 7207–7216.
23. Li L, Yang L, Zhang Y, Xu Z, Qin T, et al. (2011) Detoxification and DNA repair genes polymorphisms and susceptibility of primary myelodysplastic syndromes in Chinese population. Leuk Res 35(6): 762–5.
24. Cho HR, Uhm YK, Kim HJ, Ban JY, Chung JH, et al. (2011) Glutathione S-transferase M1 (GSTM1) polymorphism is associated with atopic dermatitis susceptibility in a Korean population. Int J Immunogenet 38(2): 145–50.
25. Konwar R, Manchanda PK, Chaudhary P, Nayak VL, Singh V, et al. (2010) Glutathione S-transferase (GST) gene variants and risk of benign prostatic hyperplasia: a report in a North Indian population. Asian Pac J Cancer Prev 11(4): 1067–72.
26. Hardman JG, Limbird LE (2004) Goodman & Gilman as bases farmacológicas da terapêutica. Raven Press: Rio de Janeiro. 80 p.
27. Etienne D, Pieter F, Cairns S (2000) Report of theInternational Leprosy Association Technical Forum: Prevention of disabilities and rehabilitation. Lepr Rev73: S35–S43.
28. Vaishali BN, Usha BN, Swati M, Rao P (2011) Evaluation of significance of skin smears in leprosy for diagnosis follow-up, assessment of treatment outcome and relapse. Asiatic Jour. of Biotech. Resources 2(5): 547–552.
29. Sambrook J, Fritsch F, Maniatis T (1989) Molecular Cloning: A Laboratory Manual. Cold Spr Harb Laboratory, NY. 2nd edition.
30. Santos NPC, Ribeiro-Rodrigues EM, Ribeiro-dos-Santos AKC (2010) Assessing individual interethnic admixture and population substructure using a 48 insertion-deletion ancestry informative markers panel. Hum Mutat. 31(2): 184–90.
31. Long J (1999) Multiple Locus Haplotype Analysis, version 2.0. Software and documentation distributed by the author. Section on Population Genetics and Linkage, Laboratory of Neurogenetics, NIAAA, National Institutes of Health, Bethesda.
32. Crawford CL (2010) Historical aspects of leprosy. Clin Infect Dis 51: 476–7.
33. Douglas JG, Macleod MJ (1999) Pharmacokinetic factors in the modern drug treatment of tuberculosis. Clin Pharmacokinet 37: 127–46.
34. Tsutsumi M, Takada A, Wang JS (1994) Genetic polymorphisms of cytochrome P4502E1 related to the development of alcoholic liver disease. Gastroenterology 107: 1430–1435.
35. Yang BM, O'Reilly DA, Demaine AG, Kingsnorth AN (2001) Study of polymorphisms in the CYP2E1 gene in patients with alcoholic pancreatitis. Alcohol 23: 91–97.
36. Wang SM, Zhu AP, Li D, Wang Z, Zhang P, et al. (2009) Frequencies of genotypes and alleles of the functional SNPs in CYP2C19 and CYP2E1 in mainland Chinese Kazakh, Uygur and Han populations. J. Hum. Genet 54: 372–375.

Predictors of Fatigue Severity in Early Systemic Sclerosis: A Prospective Longitudinal Study of the GENISOS Cohort

Shervin Assassi[1][*][◑], Astrud L. Leyva[2][◑], Maureen D. Mayes[1], Roozbeh Sharif[1,2], Deepthi K. Nair[1], Michael Fischbach[3], Ngan Nguyen[1], John D. Reveille[1], Emilio B. Gonzalez[2], Terry A. McNearney[2][¤], for the GENISOS Study Group

1 Department of Medicine, Division of Rheumatology, University of Texas Health Science Center at Houston, Houston, Texas, United States of America, 2 Department of Medicine, University of Texas Medical Branch at Galveston, Galveston, Texas, United States of America, 3 Department of Medicine, Division of Rheumatology, University of Texas Health Science Center at San Antonio, San Antonio, Texas, United States of America

Abstract

Objectives: Longitudinal studies examining the baseline predictors of fatigue in SSc have not been reported. Our objectives were to examine the course of fatigue severity over time and to identify baseline clinical, demographic, and psychosocial predictors of sequentially obtained fatigue scores in early SSc. We also examined baseline predictors of change in fatigue severity over time.

Methods: We analyzed 1090 longitudinal Fatigue Severity Scale (FSS) scores belonging to 256 patients who were enrolled in the Genetics versus Environment in Scleroderma Outcomes Study (GENISOS). Predictive significance of baseline variables for sequentially obtained FSS scores was examined with generalized linear mixed models. Predictors of change in FSS over time were examined by adding an interaction term between the baseline variable and time-in-study to the model.

Results: The patients' mean age was 48.6 years, 47% were Caucasians, and 59% had diffuse cutaneous involvement. The mean disease duration at enrollment was 2.5 years. The FSS was obtained at enrollment and follow-up visits (mean follow-up time = 3.8 years). Average baseline FSS score was 4.7($\pm$0.96). The FSS was relatively stable and did not show a consistent trend for change over time (p = 0.221). In a multivariable model of objective clinical variables, higher Medsger Gastrointestinal (p = 0.006) and Joint (p = 0.024) Severity Indices, and anti-U1-RNP antibodies (p = 0.024) were independent predictors of higher FSS. In the final model, ineffective coping skills captured by higher Illness Behavior Questionnaire scores (p<0.001), higher self-reported pain (p = 0.006), and higher Medsger Gastrointestinal Severity Index (p = 0.009) at enrollment were independent predictors of higher longitudinal FSS scores. Baseline DLco % predicted was the only independent variable that significantly predicted a change in FSS scores over time (p = 0.013), with lower DLco levels predicting an increase in FSS over time.

Conclusions: This study identified potentially modifiable clinical and psychological factors that predict longitudinal fatigue severity in early SSc.

Editor: Carol Feghali-Bostwick, University of Pittsburgh, United States of America

Funding: This study was supported by the National Institutes of Health (NIH) Center for Research Translation P50AR054144 (Arnett and MDM); NIH-KL2RR024149-04 (SA); NIH -5T32-AR052283-03(JDR); University Clinic Research Center Grants: M01-RR00073 (UTMB) and M01-RR01346 (UT-HSC-SA); the NIH Clinical and Translational Sciences Award UL1-RR024148; and TL1 RR024147 from the National Center for Research Resources. The funders had no role in study design, data collection, and analysis, decision to publish, or preparation of the manuscript. The content is solely the responsibility of the authors and does not necessarily represent the official views of the National Center for Research Resources or the National Institutes of Health. Terry A McNearney is an employee of Eli Lilly and Company and contributed to the design and analysis of the study, the performing of experiments and writing of the manuscript.

Competing Interests: The authors wish to declare the following competing interest: Dr. Terry A. McNearney is an employee of Eli Lilly and Company. There are no patents, products, in development or marketed products to declare. Dr. McNearney was the former principal investigator of GENISOS study at University of Texas Medical Branch at Galveston. Eli Lilly and Company did not have any role in study design, data collection, analysis of the data, and writing the manuscript. Other authors have nothing to declare.

* E-mail: shervin.assassi@uth.tmc.edu

◑ These authors contributed equally to this work.

¤ Current address: Eli Lilly and Company, Indianapolis, Indiana, United States of America

Introduction

Systemic sclerosis (scleroderma, SSc) is an autoimmune disease in which fibrosis of the skin and internal organs occurs in association with small vessel vasculopathy and autoantibody production. Organ-specific and non-organ specific impairments lead to a spectrum of mild to severe limitations in physical, work and social activities, ultimately influencing health-related quality of life [1–3]. Fatigue is increasingly recognized as a common debilitating symptom reported by patients with SSc [4–7]. Fatigue was rated by SSc patients as the most bothersome symptom [8]. In a Canadian National survey, SSc patients considered fatigue as their most prevalent symptom that had at least moderate impact on activities of daily living [9]. The fatigue severity among SSc patients is similar to fatigue experienced by patients with rheumatoid arthritis (RA), ankylosing Spondylitis, and systemic lupus erythematosus (SLE) [10].

In a large cross sectional study, gastrointestinal (GI) symptoms, perceived dyspnea, number of comorbidities and current smoking were significant correlates of four fatigue related items collected as part of the vitality domain of the SF-36 [4] . To our knowledge, there are no published longitudinal studies of fatigue severity and its predictors in SSc.

The pathophysiology of fatigue in chronic diseases is not well understood, although several causative factors have been identified. These include anemia, malnutrition, nausea and other GI symptoms, cytokine imbalance, sleep disturbances, deconditioning, lifestyle and psychological factors [11].

In the current study, characteristics of fatigue were prospectively measured in SSc patients enrolled in the Genetics versus ENvironment In Scleroderma Outcomes Study (GENISOS) cohort, using the 29-item Fatigue Severity Scale (FSS) [12]. The FSS was designed for determining the impact of fatigue symptoms and severity in chronic diseases and has been extensively utilized in SLE and multiple sclerosis [12–14].

The objectives of current study were to examine the course of fatigue severity over time and to identify the baseline demographic, clinical, and psychosocial factors that predict sequentially obtained fatigue scores in early SSc. Furthermore, we examined the predictive significance of the baseline variables for the rate of change in FSS over time.

Methods

GENISOS is a multicenter prospective study of patients with early SSc. It is conducted at three sites: the University of Texas Medical Branch at Galveston (UTMB), the University of Texas Health Science Center at Houston (UTHSC-H), and the University of Texas Health Science Center at San Antonio (UTHSC-SA). Study recruitment started in January 1998 and is ongoing. The institutional review boards of all participating sites approved the study and written informed consent was obtained according to the declaration of Helsinki from all subjects. The description of the study, cost, risks and discomforts, benefits, and study withdrawal were included in the informed consent. Study investigators and coordinators interviewed all study subjects at each study site.

Patient Selection

Details of patient recruitment have been formerly reported [15–18]. Patients were enrolled if they met the following criteria: 1) age ≥18 years; 2) diagnosis according to the American College of Rheumatology (formerly the American Rheumatism Association) criteria or at least 3 of the 5 CREST syndrome features (**C**alcinosis, **R**aynaud's Phenomenon, **E**sophageal dysmotility, **S**clerodactyly, **T**eleangiectasia) ; 3) disease onset (defined as the time of onset of the first non-Raynaud's symptom) within five years of enrollment; and 4) defined ethnicity. All enrolled patients at the time of analysis were included in this study.

Data collection

As previously described [15–18], the demographic information, clinical manifestations, patient-reported clinical and psychosocial

data were obtained at the baseline visit and then on subsequent semi-annual visits.

Outcome variable. Fatigue was ascertained with Fatigue Severity Scale (FSS), a 29-item validated questionnaire [12] that reflects how fatigue influences motivation, exercise, physical functioning, daily activities, interference with work, family, or social life. Each item is scored on a scale of zero (completely disagree) to seven (completely agree). A higher score indicates more fatigue severity. The final score is the average of all scores, ranging from 0 to 7. Each patient answered the questionnaire at enrollment and subsequent follow-up visits.

Independent variable. To determine the predictors of fatigue severity in the course of disease, we investigated a comprehensive array of potential independent variables from the following domains: demographic information, clinical manifestations, patient-reported clinical and psychosocial data.

Demographic information. Age, gender, ethnicity, marital status, educational level, and health habits were recorded. Marital status data were dichotomized as being married or in a marriage-like relationship of cohabitation versus being single, divorced, separated, or never married. We categorized the educational level as holding an associate degree (2 years of college education) and above versus high school diploma and below. Moreover, patients were interviewed by the study coordinators, about their smoking and exercise habits, at each visit. Specifically, patients were asked whether they are currently exercising or smoking cigarettes.

Clinical manifestations. Disease type based on the extent of skin involvement [19], duration, and antibody profile were recorded. The disease duration was determined by the study investigators based on patient interview or review of medical records utilizing two different methods: from the first non-Raynaud's phenomenon symptom attributable to SSc and from the first symptom attributable to SSc (Raynaud's or non- Raynaud's phenomenon symptoms) to the time of visit. History, physical examination findings, modified Rodnan Skin Score (mRSS) [20], and Medsger Severity Index (SI) [21] were recorded. Laboratory studies, EKG, and pulmonary function tests (PFT) were obtained at enrollment and annually thereafter. SSc cardiac involvement was defined as having clinically significant arrhythmia (arrhythmia requiring treatment) or ejection fraction ≤40%. All pulmonary function tests were reviewed by a pulmonologist and studies that did not fulfill the American Thoracic Society/European Respiratory Society (ATS/ERS) were excluded [22]. Myositis was diagnosed if the patient had proximal muscle weakness with at least one of the following: elevated levels of muscle enzymes, myopathic changes on electromyography, and/or a characteristic muscle biopsy. Furthermore, we calculated the number of co-morbid conditions in each patient based on the patients' history of cardiovascular disease, hypertension, diabetes mellitus, stroke, lung disease, malignancy, kidney disease, SLE, RA, thyroid disease, osteoarthritis, fibromyalgia, peptic ulcer disease, obesity (body mass index ≥30), depression, and other neuropsychiatric disorders.

Patient-reported clinical outcomes. We recorded pain and dyspnea on visual analogue scales (length 10 cm). The anchors of the VAS were 0 (no pain or shortness of breath) to 100 (very severe pain or shortness of breath).The severity of symptoms was measured with a metric ruler in centimeters. A higher score indicated more severe pain or dyspnea.

Patient-reported dyspnea was investigated only in the univariable model. This variable was not included in the subsequent multivariable models because we assumed that there is a strong bidirectional relationship between the perceived dyspnea and fatigue which would inflate the association between those variables.

Patient-reported psychosocial data. We hypothesized based on previously published studies in SLE [23] and SSc [5] that coping skills and social support are possible determinants of fatigue severity. Illness behavior and social support were recorded by standard psychometric instruments. Coping with disease was evaluated with the Illness Behavior Questionnaire (IBQ) [24]. IBQ is a 62-item instrument with a summary score ranging from zero to 35. Higher scores indicate less appropriate illness behaviors. Social support was assessed by the Interpersonal Support Evaluation List (ISEL), a 40-item validated instrument with summary score of zero to ten [25]. Higher scores indicated better social support.

In confirmation of our previous findings [17], Fatigue Severity Scale and all psychometric instruments demonstrated adequate internal consistency reliability in the GENISOS cohort. FSS showed an adequate internal consistency as demonstrated by a Cronbach's Alpha value of 0.9. Social support measured by the ISEL questionnaire had a Cronbach's Alpha of 0.87. IBQ showed Cronbach's Alphas of 0.85.

Statistical analysis

The investigated outcome was the sequentially obtained FSS scores. We utilized generalized linear mixed models (GLMMS) for all our analyses to evaluate the effects of the measured baseline variables on sequentially obtained FSS scores. We treated patients as a sample from a larger population and modeled between patient variability in FSS as a random intercept. We also modeled between patient variability in the change of FSS over time by a random slope (i.e., we estimated a separate slope for each patient). We accounted for the correlations among random effect parameters by an independent covariance matrix. Exchangeable or unstructured covariance matrices did not improve model fit evaluated by the Bayesian Information Criterion (BIC). Generally, mixed-effect models allow inclusion of all data points in the analysis and can also be used when some data points are missing.

We first investigated the relationship of baseline demographic, clinical, and psychosocial variables to sequentially obtained FSS in the univariable model. Subsequently, we built a multivariable model of objective clinical data. In general, this multivariable model is less susceptible to problems arising from a bidirectional relationship between the independent variables and the FSS than models that include patient-reported independent variables. We first included all objective clinical variables showing a univariable association with p<0.1 in the multivariable model. Then, the number of variables was reduced utilizing a forward hierarchical variable selection strategy. This variable selection approach was chosen to decrease the effect of multi-colinearity in our analysis.

We next conducted a hierarchical modeling with successive conceptual blocks to evaluate whether demographic, clinical and psychosocial variables independently contribute to FSS. The independent variables with a p<0.1 in the univariable analysis were added into the analysis in the following successive conceptual blocks: demographic variables, objective clinical manifestations, self-reported clinical outcomes (pain), and psychosocial variables (Figure S1). The model fit was assessed after addition of each conceptual block by using Bayesian Information Criterion (BIC). Lower BIC values indicate better model fit. BIC values are interpreted as very strong evidence for better fit if the new value is >10 lower than the previous value. This approach tested the proposition that each conceptual block independently predicts the sequentially obtained FSS scores and is not merely a mediator of the previous variable blocks.

The final multivariable model was built following the above described forward hierarchical variable selection strategy after inclusion of relevant demographic, clinical and psychosocial variables.

We also investigated the predictors of rate of change in FSS over time. For this purpose, the interaction term of the independent variable with the time-in-study was investigated. A baseline variable considered a predictor of change in FSS over time if the interaction term between the variable and the time-in-study was significant. The sign and magnitude of the interaction term coefficient show the direction and magnitude of the change over time.

All the statistical analyses were performed with STATA 11 (StataCorp, College Station, TX). The hypothesis testing was 2-sided with a p≤0.05 significance level.

Results

Sample characteristics

Between January 1998 and October 2009, 266 patients were enrolled in the GENISOS cohort. The mean (SD) follow-up time was 3.8 (3.4) years, ranging up to 11.4 years. The FSS measurement was not available in 10 patients. In this study, 1090 FSS scores belonging to 256 patients were analyzed. A total of 213 patients had at least one follow up FSS measurement. Out of remaining 43 patients, 6 were recent enrollees, 15 died, and 22 were lost to follow up.

The mean age (SD) of patients was 48.6 (13.3) years at enrollment, 83% were female. The proportions of Caucasian, African American and Hispanic patients were 47%, 20% and 29%, respectively. About 41% had limited cutaneous involvement. The mean disease duration (SD) at enrollment was 2.5 (1.6) years. Table 1 presents the baseline demographic, clinical, psychosocial characteristics of GENISOS cohort. Further details have been published previously.

Progression of fatigue over time

At enrollment, the mean FSS (SD) score was 4.7 (0.9), ranging from 1.1 to 6.6. To determine if FSS scores change over time in SSc patients, sequentially obtained FSS scores from each individual in the GENISOS cohort were plotted over time in

Table 1. Population characteristics at baseline study visit.

Age, mean (SD), years	48.6(13.3)
Gender, female, n (%)	221 (83.1)
Ethnicity, n (%)	
Caucasian	125 (46.9)
Hispanic	77 (28.9)
African-American	54 (20.3)
Other	10 (3.9)
Disease duration, mean (SD), years	2.5 (1.6)
Cutaneous involvement, diffuse, n (%)	156 (58.6)
Autoantibody profile, n (%)	
Anti-centromere antibody	32 (12.0)
Anti-topoisomerase antibody	49 (18.4)
Anti-polymerase III antibody	62 (23.3)
Anti-ribonucleic protein antibody	30 (11.3)
Modified Rodnan Skin Score (MRSS), mean (SD)	15.8 (11.8)
Fatigue Severity Scale (FSS) score, mean (SD)	4.7 (0.9)
Interpersonal Support Evaluation List (ISEL) score, mean (SD)	8.1 (1.6)

Figure 1. This demonstrated that the FSS score fluctuated in some individuals over time but the FSS levels did not show a consistent trend of change during the follow up time in the overall cohort. This was verified by the fact that time-in-study was not associated with a decline or increase in the sequentially obtained FSS levels (p = 0.221). Figure 2 graphically illustrates that the FSS scores did not change in 2-year intervals of follow-up time. Furthermore, our data did not indicate that mortality has influenced the observed course of fatigue because the vital status (dead versus alive) was neither predictive of differential levels of serially measured FSS (p = 0.761), nor it was a predictor of change in FSS (p = 0.992).

Based on the first and last available FSS measurement, 108 patients (50.7%) showed improved fatigue severity while 103 (48.4%) experienced worsening of fatigue severity. Two patients (0.9%) had the same FSS level on the last follow up visit. A minimally clinically important difference (MCID) for FSS has not been defined for patients with SSc. Therefore, we cannot report what percentage of patients had a clinically important change in FSS over time.

Univariable predictors of sequentially obtained FSS

Among demographic variables, only current exercise was a significant predictor of sequentially obtained FSS scores (negative relationship) while gender, age, current smoking and ethnicity did not show a significant relationship to the outcome variable.

The presence of the following baseline clinical variables was a significant predictor of longitudinal FSS measurements: Diarrhea, dysphagia, anti-U1 RNP antibody, small joint contracture, higher serum creatinine level, and higher Medsger Gastrointestinal Index were associated with higher sequentially obtained FSS scores (increasing fatigue severity).

Both patient-reported clinical outcomes (VAS pain and dyspnea) were also associated with higher FSS. Among baseline psychosocial measures, maladaptive behavior (higher IBQ) was a significant predictor of higher longitudinal FSS scores. Detailed results of univariable analyses are shown in Table 2 and Table S1.

Independent clinical predictors of sequentially obtained FSS

We next identified independent objective clinical correlates of sequentially obtained FSS, utilizing a forward hierarchical variable selection. In this multivariable analysis, higher Medsger Gastrointestinal (p = 0.006) and Joint (p = 0.024) Severity Indices and presence of anti-U1 RNP antibodies (p = 0.024) were independent predictors of higher FSS (Table 3).

Successive conceptual blocks predicting sequentially obtained FSS

We next examined the predictive significance of baseline characteristics grouped in the following conceptual blocks: 1) demographic; 2) objective clinical manifestations; 3) patient-reported clinical outcomes; 4) psychosocial variables. In the following models, only the baseline variables were included that predicted the longitudinal FSS with p-values<0.1 in the univariable analysis. The results of this successive conceptual block modeling are shown in Figure S1 and Table S2.

In model 1, the relevant demographic variables were examined. This model had a BIC of 2381 (p = 0.007). In model 2, the relevant clinical variables were added to the previous model which resulted in an improved BIC of 2181 (delta = 200, p<0.001). This indicated that the addition of objective clinical variables led to a substantially better model fit. In model 3, we added the patient-reported clinical outcome, VAS for pain to the previous two blocks. This model also resulted in a better model fit as indicated by a BIC of 2132 (delta = 49, p<0.001). The VAS dyspnea was not included in this model because of concerns regarding a strong bidirectional relationship between perceived dyspnea and fatigue severity. In the last model, the relevant patient-reported psychosocial data were added to the previous conceptual blocks. Model 4 had the lowest BIC (2117) and showed a strong evidence for better model fit compared to Model 3 (delta = 15, p<0.001).

This blockwise hierarchical modeling strategy indicated that each successive block (demographic, objective clinical, patient-

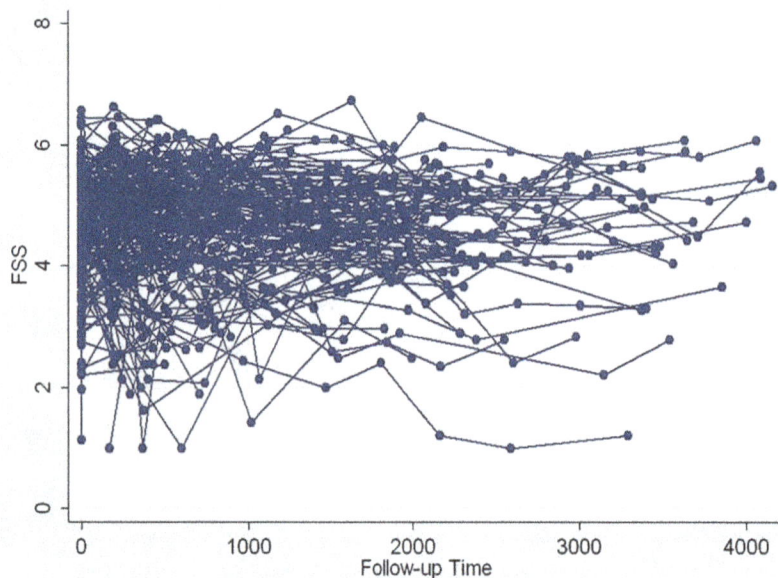

Figure 1. Course of Fatigue Severity Scale (FSS) scores in individual patients followed in the GENISOS cohort. X axis: follow-up time in days; Y axis: FSS scores.

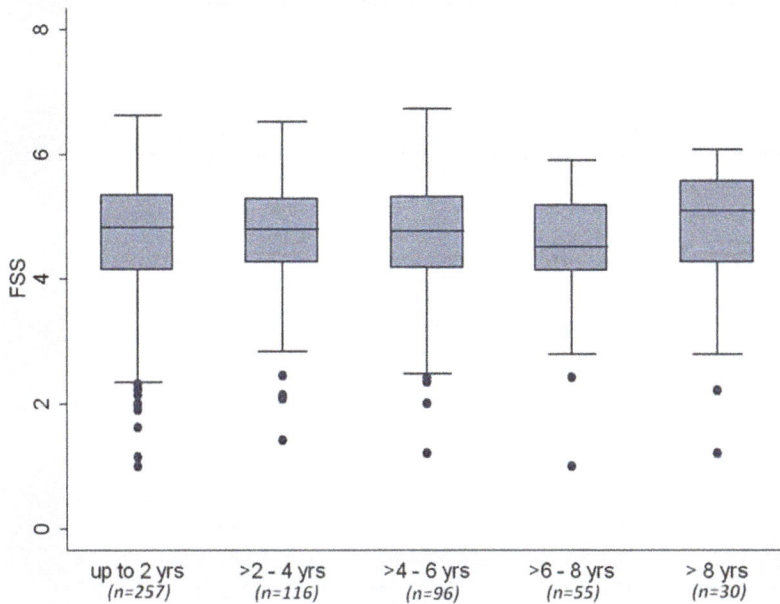

Figure 2. Course of Fatigue Severity Scale (FSS) scores over 2 year intervals of follow up time. Data are presented in box plots. Each box represents the 25th to 75th percentile. The length of the box is the interquartile range (IQR). The line inside the box represents the median. Whiskers reprsent 1.5 times the upper and lower IQRs. Circles indicate individual outliers. N is the number of patients who had at least one FSS measurement during the time interval.

reported clinical, and psychosocial variables) had independent predictive significance for sequentially obtained FSS and was not merely a mediator of previous blocks.

Independent predictors of sequentially obtained FSS (final model)

All relevant demographic, clinical, and psychosocial variables were included in the final model (Table 4). Following a forward variable selection strategy, VAS for pain (p = 0.006), maladaptive coping skills captured by higher IBQ score (p<0.001), and Medsger Gastrointestinal Severity Index (p = 0.009) were independent predictors of higher sequentially obtained FSS scores.

Predictor of rate of change in FSS over time

In the last step, we investigated the predictive significance of baseline variables for rate of change in FSS over time. As shown in Table 2 and Table S1, patient's baseline DLco% predicted level was the only significant predictor of change in FSS over time (p = 0.013). Patients with higher DLco% predicted levels had a decline in FSS whereas patients with lower DLco% predicted levels experienced an increase in FSS over time. Similar trends were observed for baseline FVC% predicted (p = 0.06).

Discussion

In this study, we examined the course of fatigue severity in a large, multi-ethnic cohort of early SSc patients. To our knowledge, the current study represents the first longitudinal examination of fatigue in SSc. FSS levels did not increase or decrease during the follow up time in the overall cohort, though patients with lower baseline DLco levels experienced an increase in their fatigue severity over time. Demographic, clinical, and psychosocial variables were all independent predictors of sequentially obtained FSS scores. Severity of GI and joint involvement and presence of

anti-U1 RNP antibodies were independent predictors of FSS in the multivariable model of clinical factors. Baseline perceived pain levels, coping skills (IBQ), and GI involvement were independent predictors of longitudinal FSS in the final extended multivariable model.

Higher baseline scores of the Medsger Gastrointestinal Severity Index were predictive of higher FSS scores. This supports a reported association of GI involvement and higher fatigue scores in a cross sectional study of SSc patients [4]. GI involvement is very common in SSc patients and its strong association with depression has been previously reported [26,27]. The association of GI dysmotility with fatigue severity may have several direct and indirect causes. Patients with diarrhea and decreased intestinal absorption might develop nutritional deficiencies with subsequent muscular and electrolyte abnormalities. Moreover, diarrhea and abdominal pain might interfere with sleep, resulting in higher fatigue scores. In patients with chronic fatigue syndrome, abdominal pain was stressful, but nocturnal diarrhea was found to further disrupt an already disrupted sleep pattern [28]. Fatigue is also a prominent feature of autoimmune diseases with primary GI manifestation such as Crohn's disease. In a randomized controlled study examining the effects of adalimumab therapy in patients with moderate to severe Crohn's disease, adalimumab maintenance therapy provided sustained improvement in fatigue severity compared to conventional immunosuppressive therapy [29].

In the current study, higher Medsger Joint Severity Index predicted higher FSS scores. The role of joint involvement as contributor to fatigue severity in SSc has not been previously reported. However, fatigue is also a prominent feature of other autoimmune diseases that primarily affect joints such as rheumatoid arthritis (RA) [30]. The effect of conventional disease modifying antirheumatic drugs (DMARD) on fatigue severity compared to placebo in RA has not been investigated but a

Table 2. Univariable analysis of demographic, clinical manifestation, patient-reported clinical outcomes, and psychosocial variables.

Independent Variable	Main effect b (95% CI)	p-value	Interaction between independent variable and time-in-study b (95% CI)	p-value
Follow-up time	−0.01 (−0.04, 0.01)	0.221		
Demographic				
Age	0.01 (−0.01, 0.01)	0.793	0.01 (−0.01,0.01)	0.31
Gender, female	0.08 (−0.20, 0.35)	0.579	−0.03(−0.09, 0.02)	0.255
Ethnicity, Caucasian	0.17 (−0.04, 0.37)	0.111	0.02(−0.02, 0.07)	0.287
Exercise habits	−0.31 (−0.52, −0.09)	0.004	0.02 (−0.02, 0.07)	0.367
Marital Status	−0.18 (−0.38−0.03)	0.093	0.01 (−0.04, 0.05)	0.919
Clinical manifestations				
Disease duration	0.01 (−0.05, 0.08)	0.658	0.01 (−0.01, 0.02)	0.752
Diffuse cutaneous involvement	−0.20 (−0.41, 0.01)	0.059	−0.01 (−0.05, 0.04)	0.971
Dysphagia	0.27 (0.07, 0.47)	0.009	−0.03 (−0.07, 0.02)	0.232
Diarrhea	0.28 (0.08, 0.48)	0.006	−0.03 (−0.07, 0.02)	0.221
BMI[*]	0.01 (−0.01, 0.02)	0.554	0.01 (−0.01, 0.01)	0.401
Small joint contracture	0.32 (0.05, 0.59)	0.021	−0.02 (−0.08, 0.04)	0.587
mRSS[**]	0.01 (−0.01, 0.02)	0.251	−0.01 (−0.01, 0.01)	0.947
No of comorbidities	0.06 (−0.01, 0.12)	0.089	0.01 (−0.01, 0.02)	0.954
Serum creatinine level	0.19 (0.02, 0.36)	0.033	−0.01 (−0.07, 0.06)	0.928
Hematocrit	0.01 (−0.02, 0.03)	0.889	0.01 (−0.01, 0.01)	0.106
Cardiac involvement	0.31 (−0.01, 0.62)	0.051	−0.02 (−0.1, 0.05)	0.538
Antibody profile				
Anti-centromere antibody	−0.16 (−0.47, 0.16)	0.329	0.01(−0.06, 0.08)	0.782
Anti-topoisomerase antibody	−0.12 (−0.39, 0.14)	0.359	0.03 (−0.03, 0.09)	0.298
Anti-polymerase III antibody	0.04 (−0.20, 0.27)	0.774	0.01 (−0.05, 0.05)	0.948
U1-RNP	0.42 (0.09, 0.74)	0.012	−0.04 (−0.12, 0.04)	0.376
FVC[†] % predicted value	−0.01 (−0.01, 0.01)	0.204	−0.01 (−0.01, 0.01)	0.06
DLco[‡] % predicted value	−0.01 (−0.01, 0.01)	0.135	−0.01 (−0.01, 0)	0.013
Medsger Severity Index				
General	0.02 (−0.11, 0.15)	0.721	0.01 (−0.03, 0.03)	0.969
Perivascular	0.01 (−0.09, 0.10)	0.956	−0.01 (−0.03, 0.12)	0.447
Skin	0.07 (−0.05, 0.19)	0.259	0.01 (−0.03, 0.03)	0.992
Joint	0.08 (−0.01, 0.16)	0.059	0.01 (−0.02, 0.02)	0.915
Muscle	0.19 (−0.06, 0.43)	0.133	0.01 (−0.04, 0.06)	0.713
GI Tract	0.23 (0.08, 0.39)	0.004	0.01 (−0.4, 0.05)	0.819
Lung	0.04 (−0.05, 0.14)	0.346	0.01 (−0.01, 0.03)	0.250
Heart	0.06 (−0.09, 0.19)	0.439	0.03 (−0.01, 0.07)	0.208
Kidney	0.20 (−0.03, 0.44)	0.090	0.06 (−0.03, 0.15)	0.21
Patient-reported clinical outcome				
VAS[β] for pain	0.06 (0.03, 0.09)	<0.001	−0.01 (−0.01, 0.01)	0.522
VASβ for dypnea	0.09 (0.05, 0.12)	<0.001	−0.01 (−0.01, 0.01)	0.994
Psychosocial measures				
IBQ[Ω]	0.06 (0.04, 0.08)	<0.001	−0.01 (−0.01, 0.01)	0.093
ISEL[Ψ]	−0.01 (−0.08, 0.06)	0.787	−0.01 (−0.02, 0.02)	0.959

*BMI: Body mass index;
**mRSS: modified Rodnan Skin Score;
[†]FVC: Forced vital capacity;
[‡]DLco: Diffuse capacity of the lung for carbon monoxide;
[β]VAS: Visual Analogue Scale;
[Ω]IBQ: Illness Behavior Questionnaire;
[Ψ]ISEL: Interpersonal Support Evaluation List.

Table 3. Multivariable analysis of objective clinical predictors of sequentially obtained FSS.

	Regression coefficient (95% CI)	p-value
Medsger Severity Index - GI tract	0.22 (0.06, 0.38)	0.006
Medsger Severity Index - Joint	0.09 (0.01, 0.17)	0.024
U1-RNP*	0.37 (0.05, 0.7)	0.024

*U1-RNP: Anti-U1 ribonucleoprotein antibodies.

significant improvement in fatigue severity in patients with moderate to severe RA was reported with adalimumab treatment compared to conventional DMARD therapy [31]. Furthermore, aerobic exercise, with most regimens consisting of 3 times weekly for 30–60 minutes exercises, was effective in treatment of fatigue in patients with RA (reviewed in [32]). Similar to RA, exercise habits were the only demographic variable predictive of fatigue severity in our study. This finding supports future interventional studies examining the efficacy of exercise regimens for treatment of fatigue in SSc.

Presence of U1-RNP antibodies were predictive of higher sequentially obtained FSS levels. Autoantibodies are important predictors of various disease manifestations in SSc [33,34]. The association of SSc-related antibodies with fatigue severity has not been examined in previous publications. The U1-RNP antibodies are associated with overlap cases of SSc with other connective tissue diseases such as SLE and polymyositis. It is possible that experiencing features of multiple connective tissue diseases can lead to more severe fatigue.

In the final model, two patient-reported outcomes (pain and IBQ) were predictive of higher FSS levels. The blockwise hierarchical analysis indicated that patient-reported variables contributed to fatigue beyond the effect of clinical and demographic factors. Although the relationship of the patient-reported variables to FSS might be bidirectional (e.g. pain and IBQ influence FSS and vice versa). The reported multivariable model with objective clinical variables is least susceptible to problems arising from the bidirectional relationship between the predictor and outcome variables. However, we did not confine our study to objective clinical predictors because this would have ignored important subjective determinants of FSS. Furthermore, we did not only investigate the relationship of the above mentioned independent variables with the concomitantly obtained FSS levels

Table 4. Multivariable analysis of independent demographics, clinical, and patient-reported clinical outcome, and psychosocial predictors of longitudinally obtained FSS scores.

	Regression coefficient (95% CI)	p-value
VAS* for pain	0.04 (0.01, 0.07)	0.006
IBQ**	0.05 (0.03, 0.07)	<0.001
Medsger Severity Index - GI tract	0.2 (0.05, 0.35)	0.009

*VAS: Visual Analogue Scale.
**IBQ: Illness behavior questionnaire.

but we also investigated whether they have predictive significance for FFS levels obtained on subsequent visits.

Inappropriate illness behavior (coping) captured by a higher IBQ score was an independent predictor of longitudinal FSS. The IBQ assesses a spectrum of illness behaviors or modes of perceiving, evaluating, or acting in relation to one's own state of health that may be in contradistinction to an accurate appraisal of the condition and prescribed treatment [24]. Similar to our results, the LUMINA study has demonstrated the association of higher IBQ scores with higher scores of perceived fatigue in SLE [23]. Furthermore, it has also been shown that higher IBQ scores reflecting worse coping behavior can affect the quality of life in SLE patients [14] . In patients with RA, group cognitive behavioral therapy for fatigue self-management (coping) was found be effective in treating fatigue severity in a recently published randomized controlled trial [35]. Our study provides further support for similar interventional studies in SSc, examining the efficacy of self management and coping strategies for treatment of fatigue.

Pain was another patient-reported variable that predicted higher FSS levels in our study. This finding is in agreement with longitudinal studies of fatigue in patient with SLE [23]. Pain in SSc can be caused by various disease manifestations such as joint pain, digital ulcer, heartburn, and tendon friction rub [36]. Better treatment of pain and more effective management of its underlying causes might alleviate fatigue severity in patient with SSc.

FSS scores did not increase or decrease during the follow up time in the overall cohort. Factors leading to worsening fatigue such as increasing age and disease damage might be counterbalanced by improving adaptive behaviors leading to stable longitudinal fatigue severity in SSc. A study of a longitudinal cohort of 122 patients with RA also reported that FSS scores did not change appreciably over time [37]. Furthermore, studies in patients with chronic fatigue syndrome indicated that patients with longer disease duration had better adaptive coping strategies than those with shorter disease duration, supporting the hypothesis that patients with chronic illnesses develop better coping skills for dealing with fatigue over time. Another possible explanation for stable longitudinal fatigue levels is that fatigue might be related to inherent perceived health or coping mechanisms. Although the success of exercise regimens [32], behavioral [35] and pharmacological [29,31] interventions for treatment of fatigue in other rheumatic diseases indicates that this disease manifestation is modifiable and not solely related to related inherent and non-modifiable patient characteristics.

DLco% predicted was the only baseline variable that was predictive of change in fatigue severity. A similar trend was observed for FVC although it did not reach statistical significance. This finding indicates that patients with more extensive lung involvement are more likely to experience an increase in their fatigue levels over time. Several medications are effective in treatment of pulmonary arterial hypertension (reviewed in [38]) and cyclophosphamide is beneficial for treatment of interstitial lung disease in SSc [39]. It is unclear whether treatment with these agents can lead to a reduction in fatigue severity in SSc. Furthermore, the role of pulmonary rehabilitation in treatment of lung impairment and fatigue also has not been investigated in SSc. In patients with chronic obstructive pulmonary disease, pulmonary rehabilitation for 3 months was effective for treatment of dyspnea and fatigue [40].

The current study had some limitations. The majority of study subjects were recruited from tertiary medical centers, which might skew the study population toward patients with more severe involvement. Furthermore, we did not have information on sleep disturbances in the GENISOS cohort, a factor that might be an independent predictor of fatigue in SSc. Furthermore, we did not use a designated questionnaire for capturing depressive symptoms in the GENISOS.

Fatigue is a prominent and debilitating problem for a large number of SSc patients. Our results indicate that potentially modifiable clinical and psychological factors predict longitudinal fatigue severity. Measures to decrease physical burden of disease such as respiratory, GI and joint involvement, as well as interventions focusing on improving coping skills and pain could potentially improve fatigue severity in SSc.

Supporting Information

Figure S1　Model structure of the blockwise hierarchical analysis.

Table S1　Univariable analysis of demographic, clinical, patient-reported clinical, and psychosocial variables. Abbreviations: BMI: Body mass index; MRSS: modified Radnon Skin Score; FVC: Forced vital capacity; DLco = Diffuse capacity

of the lung for carbon monoxide; VAS: visual analogue scale; IBQ: Illness Behavior Questionnaire; ISEL: Interpersonal Support Evaluation List.

Table S2　Blockwise modeling of demographic, clinical, patient-reported clinical, and psychosocial predictors of longitudinal FSS (*variables with p<0.1 included*). *BIC: Bayesian Information Criterion.

Acknowledgments

The authors thank Alison Z. Brown, Samuel Theodore, and Barbara A. Boyle for their assistance in data collection.

Author Contributions

Conceived and designed the experiments: SA ALL MDM RS JDR EBG TAM. Performed the experiments: SA ALL MDM RS DKN MF NN JDR EBG TAM. Analyzed the data: SA ALL MDM RS JDR EBG TAM. Contributed reagents/materials/analysis tools: SA ALL MDM RS DKN MF NN JDR EBG TAM. Wrote the paper: SA ALL MDM RS JDR EBG TAM.

References

1. Khanna D, Furst DE, Clements PJ, Park GS, Hays RD, et al. (2005) Responsiveness of the SF-36 and the Health Assessment Questionnaire Disability Index in a systemic sclerosis clinical trial. J Rheumatol 32: 832–840. 0315162X-32-832 [pii].

2. Del RA, Boldrini M, D'Agostino D, Placidi GP, Scarpato A, et al. (2004) Health-related quality of life in systemic sclerosis as measured by the Short Form 36: relationship with clinical and biologic markers. Arthritis Rheum 51: 475–481. doi:10.1002/art.20389.

3. Danieli E, Airo P, Bettoni L, Cinquini M, Antonioli CM, et al. (2005) Health-related quality of life measured by the Short Form 36 (SF-36) in systemic sclerosis: correlations with indexes of disease activity and severity, disability, and depressive symptoms. Clin Rheumatol 24: 48–54. doi: 10.1007/s10067-004-0970-z.

4. Thombs BD, Hudson M, Bassel M, Taillefer SS, Baron M, et al. (2009) Sociodemographic, disease, and symptom correlates of fatigue in systemic sclerosis: evidence from a sample of 659 Canadian Scleroderma Research Group Registry patients. Arthritis Rheum 61: 966–973. doi:10.1002/art.24614.

5. Sharif R, Mayes MD, Nicassio PM, Gonzalez EB, Draeger H, et al. (2011) Determinants of Work Disability in Patients with Systemic Sclerosis: A Longitudinal Study of the GENISOS Cohort. Semin Arthritis Rheum 41: 38–47. S0049-0172(11)00005-9 [pii]; doi:10.1016/j.semarthrit.2011.01.002.

6. Sandusky SB, McGuire L, Smith MT, Wigley FM, Haythornthwaite JA (2009) Fatigue: an overlooked determinant of physical function in scleroderma. Rheumatology (Oxford) 48: 165–169. ken455 [pii]; doi:10.1093/rheumatology/ken455.

7. Sandqvist G, Scheja A, Eklund M (2008) Working ability in relation to disease severity, everyday occupations and well-being in women with limited systemic sclerosis. Rheumatology (Oxford) 47: 1708–1711. ken359 [pii]; doi:10.1093/rheumatology/ken359.

8. van Lankveld WG, Vonk MC, Teunissen H, van den Hoogen FH (2007) Appearance self-esteem in systemic sclerosis–subjective experience of skin deformity and its relationship with physician-assessed skin involvement, disease status and psychological variables. Rheumatology (Oxford) 46: 872–876. kem008 [pii]; doi:10.1093/rheumatology/kem008.

9. Bassel M, Hudson M, Taillefer SS, Schieir O, Baron M, et al. (2011) Frequency and impact of symptoms experienced by patients with systemic sclerosis: results from a Canadian National Survey. Rheumatology (Oxford) 50: 762–767. keq310 [pii]; doi:10.1093/rheumatology/keq310.

10. Thombs BD, Bassel M, McGuire L, Smith MT, Hudson M, et al. (2008) A systematic comparison of fatigue levels in systemic sclerosis with general population, cancer and rheumatic disease samples. Rheumatology (Oxford) 47: 1559–1563. ken331 [pii]; doi:10.1093/rheumatology/ken331.

11. Wagner LI, Cella D (2004) Fatigue and cancer: causes, prevalence and treatment approaches. Br J Cancer 91: 822–828. doi:10.1038/sj.bjc.6602012;6602012 [pii].

12. Schwartz JE, Jandorf L, Krupp LB (1993) The measurement of fatigue: a new instrument. J Psychosom Res 37: 753–762. 0022-3999(93)90104-N [pii].

13. Krupp LB, LaRocca NG, Muir-Nash J, Steinberg AD (1989) The fatigue severity scale. Application to patients with multiple sclerosis and systemic lupus erythematosus. Arch Neurol 46: 1121–1123.

14. Sanchez ML, McGwin G, Jr., Duran S, Fernandez M, Reveille JD, et al. (2009) Factors predictive of overall health over the course of the disease in patients with

systemic lupus erythematosus from the LUMINA cohort (LXII): use of the SF-6D. Clin Exp Rheumatol 27: 67–71. 2559 [pii].

15. Assassi S, Del JD, Sutter K, McNearney TA, Reveille JD, et al. (2009) Clinical and genetic factors predictive of mortality in early systemic sclerosis. Arthritis Rheum 61: 1403–1411.

16. Assassi S, Sharif R, Lasky RE, McNearney TA, Estrada YMR, et al. (2010) Predictors of interstitial lung disease in early systemic sclerosis: a prospective longitudinal study of the GENISOS cohort. Arthritis Res Ther 12: R166.

17. McNearney TA, Hunnicutt SE, Fischbach M, Friedman AW, Aguilar M, et al. (2009) Perceived functioning has ethnic-specific associations in systemic sclerosis: another dimension of personalized medicine. J Rheumatol 36: 2724–2732. jrheum.090295 [pii]; doi:10.3899/jrheum.090295.

18. Reveille JD, Fischbach M, McNearney T, Friedman AW, Aguilar MB, et al. (2001) Systemic sclerosis in 3 US ethnic groups: a comparison of clinical, sociodemographic, serologic, and immunogenetic determinants. Semin Arthritis Rheum 30: 332–346.

19. Leroy EC, Black C, Fleischmajer R, Jablonska S, Krieg T, et al. (1988) Scleroderma (systemic sclerosis): classification, subsets and pathogenesis. J Rheumatol 15: 202–205.

20. Clements P, Lachenbruch P, Siebold J, White B, Weiner S, et al. (1995) Inter and intraobserver variability of total skin thickness score (modified Rodnan TSS) in systemic sclerosis. J Rheumatol 22: 1281–1285.

21. Medsger TA, Jr., Silman AJ, Steen VD, Black CM, Akesson A, et al. (1999) A disease severity scale for systemic sclerosis: development and testing. J Rheumatol 26: 2159–2167.

22. Wanger J, Clausen JL, Coates A, Pedersen OF, Brusasco V, et al. (2005) Standardisation of the measurement of lung volumes. Eur Respir J 26: 511–522.

23. Burgos PI, Alarcon GS, McGwin G, Jr., Crews KQ, Reveille JD, et al. (2009) Disease activity and damage are not associated with increased levels of fatigue in systemic lupus erythematosus patients from a multiethnic cohort: LXVII. Arthritis Rheum 61: 1179–1186. doi:10.1002/art.24649.

24. Pilowsky I, Spence N, Cobb J, Katsikitis M (1984) The Illness Behavior Questionnaire as an aid to clinical assessment. Gen Hosp Psychiatry 6: 123–130.

25. Cohen S, Mermelstein R, Kamarck T, Hoberman H (1985) Measuring the Functional Components of Social Support. In: Sarason I, Sarason B, eds. Social support: theory, research, and applications. Boston: Martinus Nijhoff. pp 73–94.

26. Bodukam V, Hays RD, Maranian P, Furst DE, Seibold JR, et al. (2011) Association of gastrointestinal involvement and depressive symptoms in patients with systemic sclerosis. Rheumatology (Oxford) 50: 330–334. keq296 [pii]; doi:10.1093/rheumatology/keq296.

27. Thombs BD, Taillefer SS, Hudson M, Baron M (2007) Depression in patients with systemic sclerosis: a systematic review of the evidence. Arthritis Rheum 57: 1089–1097. doi:10.1002/art.22910.

28. Burnet RB, Chatterton BE (2004) Gastric emptying is slow in chronic fatigue syndrome. BMC Gastroenterol 4: 32. 1471-230X-4-32 [pii]; doi:10.1186/1471-230X-4-32.

29. Loftus EV, Feagan BG, Colombel JF, Rubin DT, Wu EQ, et al. (2008) Effects of adalimumab maintenance therapy on health-related quality of life of patients with Crohn's disease: patient-reported outcomes of the CHARM trial. Am J Gastroenterol 103: 3132–3141. AJG2175 [pii]; doi:10.1111/j.1572-0241.2008.02175.x.

30. Gossec L, Dougados M, Rincheval N, Balanescu A, Boumpas DT, et al. (2009) Elaboration of the preliminary Rheumatoid Arthritis Impact of Disease (RAID) score: a EULAR initiative. Ann Rheum Dis 68: 1680–1685. ard.2008.100271 [pii];10.1136/ard.2008.100271 [doi].

31. Yount S, Sorensen MV, Cella D, Sengupta N, Grober J, et al. (2007) Adalimumab plus methotrexate or standard therapy is more effective than methotrexate or standard therapies alone in the treatment of fatigue in patients with active, inadequately treated rheumatoid arthritis. Clin Exp Rheumatol 25: 838–846. 2213 [pii].

32. Neill J, Belan I, Ried K (2006) Effectiveness of non-pharmacological interventions for fatigue in adults with multiple sclerosis, rheumatoid arthritis, or systemic lupus erythematosus: a systematic review. J Adv Nurs 56: 617–635. JAN4054 [pii]; doi:10.1111/j.1365-2648.2006.04054.x.

33. Steen VD, Powell DL, Medsger TA, Jr. (1988) Clinical correlations and prognosis based on serum autoantibodies in patients with systemic sclerosis. Arthritis Rheum 31: 196–203.

34. Steen VD (2005) Autoantibodies in systemic sclerosis. Semin Arthritis Rheum 35: 35–42.

35. Hewlett S, Ambler N, Almeida C, Cliss A, Hammond A, et al. (2011) Self-management of fatigue in rheumatoid arthritis: a randomised controlled trial of group cognitive-behavioural therapy. Ann Rheum Dis 70: 1060–1067. ard.2010.144691 [pii]; doi:10.1136/ard.2010.144691.

36. Steen VD, Medsger TA, Jr. (1997) The value of the Health Assessment Questionnaire and special patient-generated scales to demonstrate change in systemic sclerosis patients over time. Arthritis Rheum 40: 1984–1991.

37. Mancuso CA, Rincon M, Sayles W, Paget SA (2006) Psychosocial variables and fatigue: a longitudinal study comparing individuals with rheumatoid arthritis and healthy controls. J Rheumatol 33: 1496–1502. 06/13/0618 [pii].

38. Lambova S, Muller-Ladner U (2010) Pulmonary arterial hypertension in systemic sclerosis. Autoimmun Rev 9: 761–770. S1568-9972(10)00124-2 [pii]; doi:10.1016/j.autrev.2010.06.006.

39. Tashkin DP, Elashoff R, Clements PJ, Goldin J, Roth MD, et al. (2006) Cyclophosphamide versus placebo in scleroderma lung disease. N Engl J Med 354: 2655–2666.

40. Maltais F, Bourbeau J, Shapiro S, Lacasse Y, Perrault H, et al. (2008) Effects of home-based pulmonary rehabilitation in patients with chronic obstructive pulmonary disease: a randomized trial. Ann Intern Med 149: 869–878. 149/12/869 [pii].

IL-27 Regulates IL-18 Binding Protein in Skin Resident Cells

Miriam Wittmann[1,2]*, **Rosella Doble**[3], **Malte Bachmann**[4], **Josef Pfeilschifter**[4], **Thomas Werfel**[5], **Heiko Mühl**[4]

1 Leeds Institute of Molecular Medicine, LMBRU LTHT, Division of Rheumatic and Musculoskeletal Disease, University of Leeds, Leeds, United Kingdom, **2** Centre for Skin Sciences, School of Life Sciences, University of Bradford, Bradford, United Kingdom, **3** Institute of Molecular and Cellular Biology, Faculty of Biological Sciences, University of Leeds, Leeds, United Kingdom, **4** Pharmazentrum Frankfurt/ZAFES, University Hospital Goethe-University Frankfurt, Frankfurt am Main, Germany, **5** Division of Immunodermatology and Allergy Research, Department of Dermatology, Hannover Medical School, Hannover, Germany

Abstract

IL-18 is an important mediator involved in chronic inflammatory conditions such as cutaneous lupus erythematosus, psoriasis and chronic eczema. An imbalance between IL-18 and its endogenous antagonist IL-18 binding protein (BP) may account for increased IL-18 activity. IL-27 is a cytokine with dual function displaying pro- and anti-inflammatory properties. Here we provide evidence for a yet not described anti-inflammatory mode of action on skin resident cells. Human keratinocytes and surprisingly also fibroblasts (which do not produce any IL-18) show a robust, dose-dependent and highly inducible mRNA expression and secretion of IL-18BP upon IL-27 stimulation. Other IL-12 family members failed to induce IL-18BP. The production of IL-18BP peaked between 48–72 h after stimulation and was sustained for up to 96 h. Investigation of the signalling pathway showed that IL-27 activates STAT1 in human keratinocytes and that a proximal GAS site at the IL-18BP promoter is of importance for the functional activity of IL-27. The data are in support of a significant anti-inflammatory effect of IL-27 on skin resident cells. An important novel property of IL-27 in skin pathobiology may be to counter-regulate IL-18 activities by acting on keratinocytes and importantly also on dermal fibroblasts.

Editor: Pierre Bobé, Institut Jacques Monod, France

Funding: This study was supported by Royal Society Joint grant JP081045 and the Leeds Foundation for Dermatological Research. The funders had no role in study design, data collection and analysis, decision to publish, or preparation of the manuscript.

Competing Interests: The authors have declared that no competing interests exist.

* E-mail: M.Wittmann@leeds.ac.uk

Introduction

IL-27 is a member of the IL-12 family of cytokines and has been described to have opposing actions in inflammation. Both IL-27 receptor subunits WSX-1 and gp130 participate in signalling upon binding of IL-27 [1,2]. IL-27 consists of two subunits, EBV-induced gene 3 (EBI3) and p28 [3], and has been shown to possess unique features in the IL-12 family such as upregulation of the high affinity IL-12R expression important for Th1 lineage polarisation [2,3,4,5] or priming of antigen presenting cells (APC) for IL-23 production [6]. In human macrophages, monocytes and keratinocytes IL-27 has been shown to have a pro-inflammatory effect through the induction of CXCL10 [6,7]. This property of IL-27 has been proposed to be of significance for the inflammatory course of eczema [7] and psoriasis [8]. CXCL10 produced by skin resident cells attracts CXCR3 expressing, predominantly IFNγ producing cells.

However, in murine models IL-27 has been shown to have anti-inflammatory effects in later stages of infection [9,10,11,12]. IL-27−/− mice have been shown to be more susceptible to experimental autoimmune encephalomyelitis [11] and MRL/lpr mice overexpressing WSX-1 show reduced lupus like symptoms [12]. IL-27 has been described to inhibit Th17 differentiation in a signal transducer and activator of transcription 1 (STAT1)-dependent but IFNγ-independent manner in murine models [11].

Furthermore, IL-27 seems to stimulate murine (but not human [6,13]) cells for IL-10 production.

IL-18 is a member of the IL-1 family and is known to have potent pro-inflammatory effects by initiating an inflammatory cytokine cascade [14,15,16,17]. It supports differentiation and activation of either Th1 or Th2 cells depending on the surrounding cytokine environment and is recognised as an important regulator of both innate and acquired immunity [15,18]. Mice deficient in IL-18 show a largely reduced IFNγ production, NK cell activity [19] and reduced chronic inflammation and airway remodelling in asthma models [20].

A number of publication have described that high levels of IL-18 and/or IL-18R [21] are expressed in lesional skin of chronic inflammatory diseases such as psoriasis and cutaneous lupus erythematosus (CLE) [22,23,24,25]. We have previously shown that skin epithelial cells from CLE patients are more susceptible to IL-18 stimulation resulting in an increased TNFα production and TNFα dependent apoptosis. IL-18 is produced by skin resident dendritic cells as well as by the most abundant cell type of upper skin layers, the keratinocytes [26,27,28,29,30] but not by fibroblasts. An important proinflammatory property of IL-18 in the skin compartment may also be assumed due to the fact that skin-tropic viruses (e.g. Molluscum contagiosum, HPV) either produce a viral antagonist (vIL-18BP) or induce the production of endogenous IL-18BP [31,32,33,34,35]. It has been suggested that

IL-18 plays an important role in chronification of inflammatory diseases [17,20] and it contributes to the inflammation-fibrosis cascade in lung, kidney and cardiac pathologies [36,37,38,39]. Stimulation of normal keratinocytes with IL-18 results in the production of CXCR3 ligands such as CXCL10 [21,40] and increased surface expression of major histocompatibility complex (MHC) I and II [21,23].

IL-18 binding protein (BP) [41] is an endogenous antagonist with high neutralising capacity that inhibits the action of IL-18 by preventing interaction with its cell surface receptors [14]. At a molar excess of two, IL-18BP neutralises IL-18 to >95% [42]. IFNγ has been described as an inducer for IL-18BP production in various cell types [43]. IL-18 and IL-18BP are both up-regulated in inflammatory conditions which suggest that IL-18BP acts as a negative feedback response in pathologies with high IFNγ levels. It has however been illustrated that the neutralising capacity of IL-18BP may not be sufficient and/or that the balanced expression of IL-18/IL-18BP may be dysregulated in a number of viral, inflammatory or fibrosing disorders [17,33,36,37,44].

IFNγ is so far the only described robust inducer of IL-18BP expression thereby acting in particular on diverse non-leukocytic cell types, among others colon carcinoma cells, HaCaT keratinocyte [43,45], fibroblast-like synovial cells [46], and HepG2 cells [47]. By using DLD1 colon carcinoma cells, we have previously shown that STAT1 binding to a gamma-activated sequence (GAS) element in the IL-18BP promoter plays a pivotal role in the regulation of IL-18BP [48]. The significance of CCAATenhancer binding protein beta (CEBPbeta) that directs IL-18BP activation in hepatoma cells [47] and murine cardiomyocytes [49] remains to be fully elucidated in the context of skin resident cells.

Here we present data for a yet not described action of IL-27 on the induction and release of IL-18BP from human skin resident cells. These results may be helpful in understanding the potentially disturbed IL-18/IL-18BP balance in some inflammatory conditions as well as in the development of strategies for therapeutic induction of endogenous IL-18BP in inflammatory skin diseases such as CLE or psoriasis.

Results

Skin resident cells are known producers of a wide range of molecules involved in microbial defence and inflammatory responses. Here we were interested in molecules which could lead to an increased expression of the potent IL-18 neutralising molecule IL-18BP. So far, IFNγ is the only described cytokine to upregulate IL-18BP in tissue resident cells including fibroblasts and epithelial cells [43,45,46,47]. We analysed a number of ligands for pattern recognition receptors (Malp-2, Poly I:C, Murabutide) as well as cytokines belonging to the IL-12 family, oncostatin M, IL-1β, TNFα, curcurmin, prolactin, hydrocortisone, IL-15 and salbutamol. Some of these mediators have been chosen due to their capacity to activate c/EBP, binding sites for which have been identified in the IL-18BP promoter [47,49].

Apart from IFNγ the only other stimuli which markedly upregulated IL-18BP in human primary keratinocytes (HPK) were found to be IFNß and IL-27 (Figure 1A). IL-27 was the only IL-12 family member to regulate IL-18BP (Figure 1B). Since upregulation of IL-18BP by type I IFN has been observed previously [50] we chose to focus herein on IL-18BP regulation by IL-27. At a concentration of 50 ng/ml IFNγ showed approximately 100 fold stronger response than IL-27. 1 ng/ml IFNγ had an equal potency to induce IL-18BP as 50 ng/ml of IL-27 in HPK. Increasing doses of IL-27 yielded in high production of IL-18BP (Figure 1C). Secretion of protein showed no further increase at concentration

higher than 100 ng/ml (data not shown). Among all cell types analysed, HPK were the only ones to produce basal levels of IL-18BP. The human keratinocyte cell line HaCat (Figure 1D) displays a very similar IL-18BP response pattern upon IL-27 (and IFNγ) stimulation as primary cells. The measured levels of IL-18BP secreted from HaCat were much higher than those seen in stimulated HPK. In HaCat cells, a dose-dependent increase of IL-18BP production could be observed for up to 200 ng/ml (mean for 200 ng/ml = 4268 pg/m, SD 1498) of IL-27 but higher concentration (e.g. 300 ng/ml) showed no further increase in the production.

Human primary dermal fibroblasts (Figure 2A) were found to produce unexpectedly high amounts of the IL-18BP. Fibroblasts seem very sensitive to IL-27 with around 70% of the donors responding to IL-27 concentration of 1 ng/ml (between 50 and up to 800 pg/ml IL-18BP). For fibroblasts the potency of 50 ng/ml IL-27 was in the same range as seen with equal concentration of IFNγ (Figure 2B) which was markedly different from keratinocytes. Concentration higher than 100 ng/ml (e.g. 200 and 300 ng/ml) did not further increase IL-18BP production.

In fibroblasts, time kinetic experiments with IL-27 stimulated cells point to a peak in the production between 24 and 48 h of incubation and sustained production for up to 96 h (Figure 3A). The same time kinetic profile was observable for HPK (not shown) and HaCaT keratinocytes (Figure 3B). Both IL-27 and IFNγ stimulation resulted in very similar time kinetic profiles with IFNγ resulting in higher protein content in the supernatant of stimulated keratinocytes but not fibroblasts. Time periods longer than 96 h are difficult to follow up in in-vitro experiments. From experiments performed for 120 h we deduce that the production of IL-18BP reaches a plateau around 96 h.

All cell types showed a robust upregulation of mRNA expression after IL-27 stimulation. The maximum induction after stimulation with either IL-27 or IFNγ occurred with some delay. Keratinocytes and fibroblasts showed higher induction levels after overnight stimulation as compared to 5 h stimulation (Figures 4 A,B and 5B). The inducibility of fibroblasts (fold induction up to 100 fold) was much higher in fibroblasts than in keratinocytes (10 fold in both HPK and HaCat). mRNA stability assays performed with fibroblasts using actinomycin D showed that IL-18BP mRNA was as "unstable" as IL-8 mRNA determined in the same samples (Figure 4C).

In order to further decipher the signalling pathways leading to increased IL-18BP production we analysed HaCat cells which showed a robust induction of IL-18BP similar to HPK. These cells respond to IL-27 with an activation of STAT1 (Figure 5A). STAT1 activationby IL-27 or IFNγ was associated with significant IL-18BP mRNA induction (Figure 5B). Luciferase reporter assays were performed in order to analyse IL-18BP promoter activation under the influence of IL-27. Figure 5C demonstrates induction of the IL-18BP wild type promoter (pGL3-BPwt) in HaCat cells in response to IL-27. Promoter activation was significantly reduced in the context of a mutated proximal GAS site (pGL3-BPmt/prox). By contrast, a dysfunctional distal GAS site (pGL3-BPmt/dist) left the induction unaffected whereas the double mutation (pGL3-BPmt/prox/dist) resulted in similar suppression of the reporter gene activity as the single proximal mutation. These results show that the proximal GAS site at the IL-18BP promoter is crucial for gene activation in response to IL-27.

Discussion

In most chronic inflammatory skin disease tissue resident cells over-express IL-1 family members, T cell attracting chemokines,

a

b

c

d

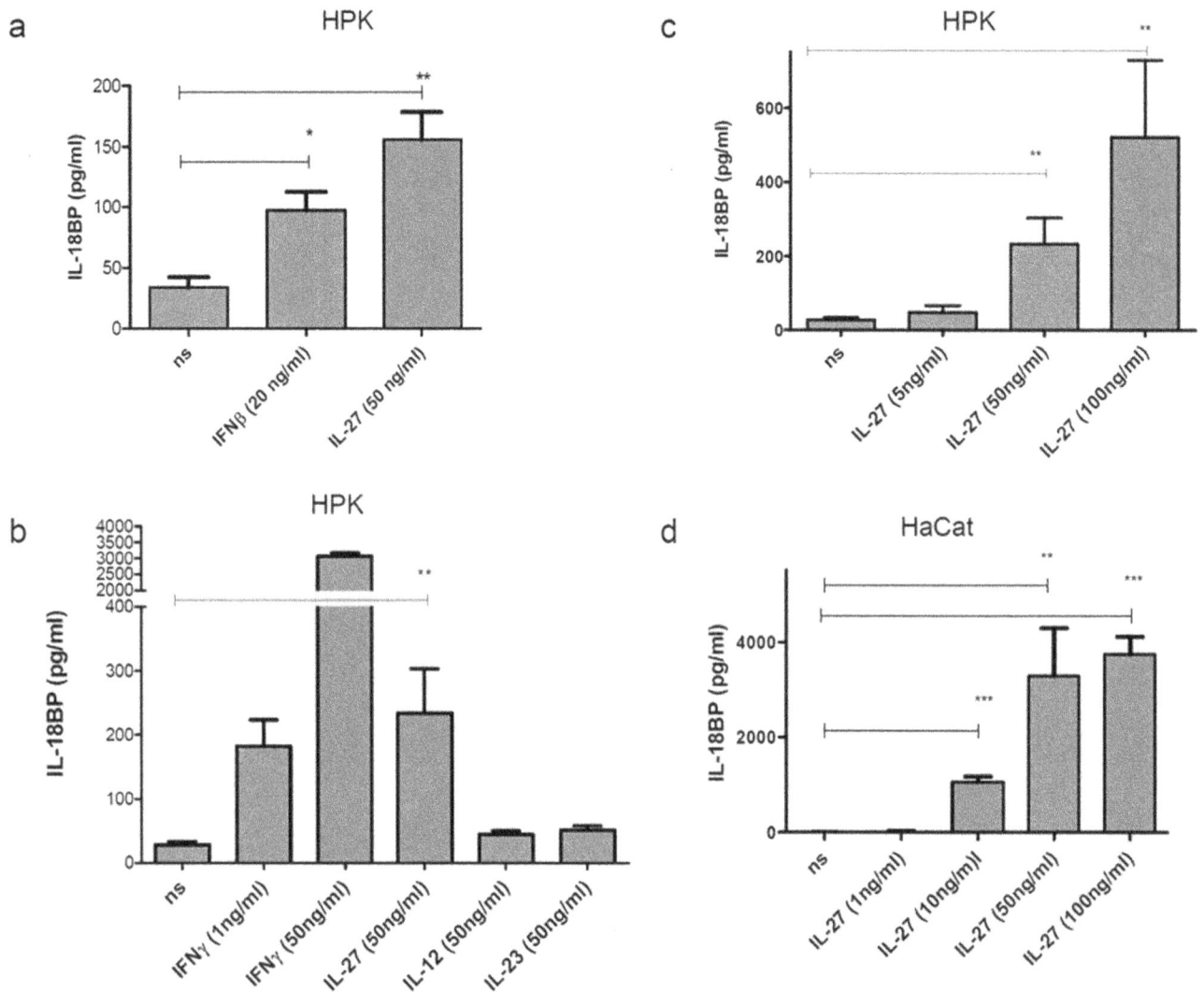

Figure 1. IL-27 dose-depenently induces IL-18BP secretion in human keratinocytes. Human primary keratinocytes (a, b, c) or HaCat (d) were stimulated for 48 h. Cell free supernatant was harvested and IL-18BP content was determined by Elisa. Independent experiments were performed. (a) n = 4 different experiments and donors; (b) n = 7 different experiments and donors; (c) n = 3 different experiments and donors; (d) n = 3. Mean and SEM are depicted. ns = non stimulated, HPK = human primary keratinocytes.

proteases (e.g. MMPs) and/or TNFα. One factor for diseases such as cutaneous lupus erythematosus, psoriasis and eczema to become chronic is the disturbed balance in producing pro- and anti-inflammatory molecules by infiltrating leukocytes and tissue cells. An inflammatory response to a given stimulus is normally counter-regulated, once the causing agent is removed. However, in a number of diseases at epithelial surfaces, the pro-inflammatory response is ongoing. IL-18BP may to be of high importance in balancing skin inflammatory responses as supported by the fact that a number skin-tropic viruses induce or express this IL-18 neutralising molecule.

IL-18 seems to play an important pathogenic role with regard to maintaining inflammatory responses. It induces TNFα and favours the release of IFNγ by infiltrating lymphocytes. IL-18 is highly expressed in chronic phases of skin diseases such as eczema, lupus erythematosus and psoriasis but also in e.g. lupus nephritis, chronic joint diseases and graft-versus-host disease [17,24,25,26,51,52,53,54,55,56,57]. It has been suggested that in allergic contact eczema IL-18 may act upstream of IL-1ß and

TNFα in the induction of Langerhans cell migration [58] and its potential role in allergic contact dermatitis is highlighted by the fact that measurement of IL-18 has been suggested as a tool for the identification of substances with high sensitising potential [51]. We lack precise information on the (dys)balanced expression of IL-18 and its natural antagonist IL-18BP in pathological conditions and the need to determine "free" IL-18 activity has been pointed out by Favilli et al. [59]. An elevation of IL-18 and IL-18BP has been described in chronic liver disease by Ludwiczek et al. [60], and the levels reflect the severity of disease. This study suggests that in the patients suffering from advanced cirrhotic disease stages the levels of IL-18BP may not be sufficient to counteract the pro-inflammatory actions of IL-18. Patients with heart failure have also been reported to show increased IL-18 but decreased IL-18BP levels [61].

Basal levels of IL-18BP can be found in the "circulation". Keratinocytes seem to contribute to a basal level in the skin organ. These cells along with resident and infiltrating APCs do express IL-18. It is important to note, that the here presented data point to

a

b

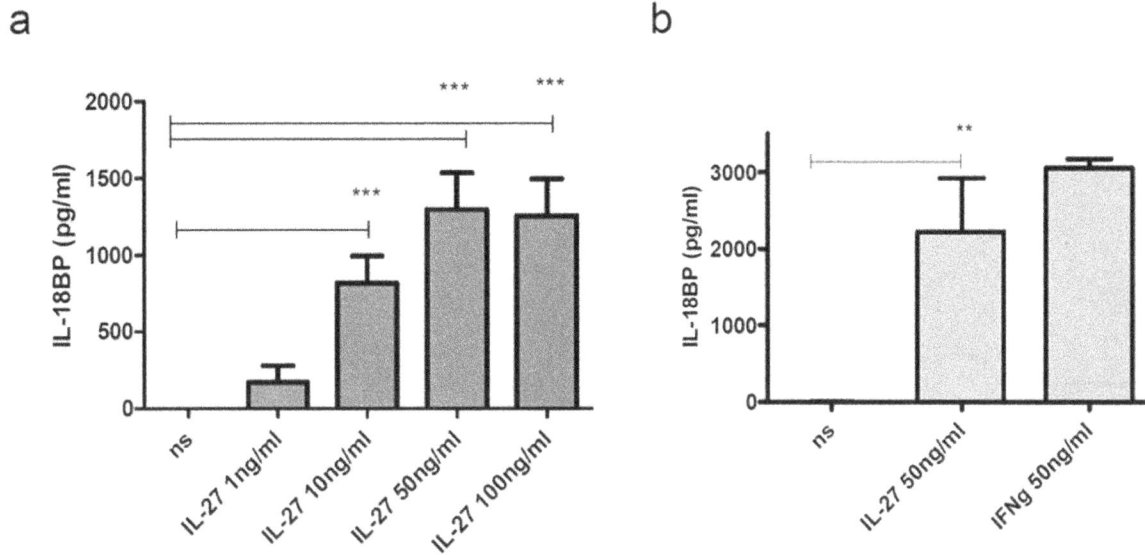

Figure 2. Human fibroblasts are very responsive to IL-27 stimulation. Stimulation of primary human skin fibroblasts was performed for 48 h and cell-free supernatants were analysed for IL-18BP by Elisa. Results are given as mean and SEM. (a) n = 7 (b) n = 4, ns = non stimulated.

dermal fibroblasts as a significant source of inducible IL-18BP production. These cells do not express IL-18. This further highlights the complex interaction between different tissue cell types in maintaining a fine-tuned mediator network balance and highlight fibroblasts as important "regulators".

Our data support the view that the proximal GAS site in the IL-18BP promoter [47,48] is crucial for IL-18BP induction. Besides IFNγ, IL-27 is a novel player determining cytokine-induced IL-18BP expression. It has been shown to promote a pro-inflammatory response by priming keratinocytes, macrophages or inflammatory dendritic epidermal cells (IDEC) for TNFα, CXCL10 and IL-23 production respectively, and therefore may contribute to the elicitation of inflammatory skin diseases [6,7,8,13]. On the other hand, it has been shown that IL-27 also

suppresses the development of Th1, Th2 and Th17 subsets in later phases of infection. Yoshimura et al. [10] found that IL-27 suppresses the production of e.g. IL-2, IL-4, IFNγ and IL-17 by fully activated CD4+ T cells. These and other findings suggest that in early phases of immune responses, IL-27 may act as an amplifier to achieve a robust response to pathogen associated stimuli, whereas in later phases of immune response, the role of IL-27 seems to be regulatory.

To comprehend the complex actions of IL-27, the understanding of its signalling pathways is crucial. The IL-27 receptor composed of the WSX-1 and the common gp130 chain is widely expressed. Downstream of the IL27R, STAT1 and STAT3 are activated and may coordinate the pleiotropic effects of IL-27. However, it has been shown that STAT3 does not affect IL-18BP

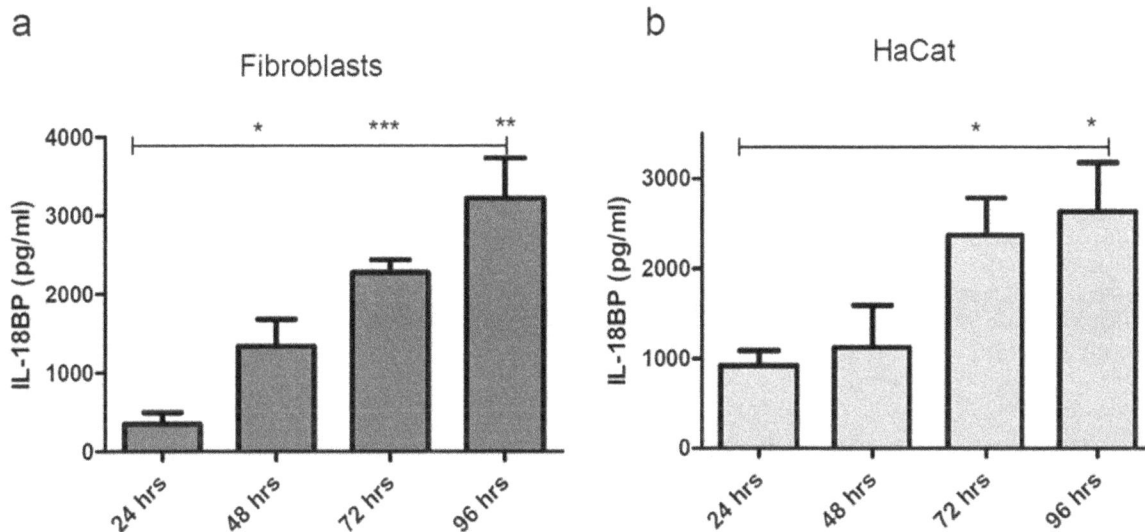

a

Fibroblasts

b

HaCat

Figure 3. Time course of IL-18BP release by IL-27 stimulated skin cells. Fibroblasts (a) and HaCat cells (b) were cultured for up to 96 h after initial stimulation with IL-27 (50 ng/ml). Supernatants were collected at the indicated time points. Levels of IL-18BP for non stimulated cells were below the detection limit of the ELISA. n = 4 (a, b).

a **Fibroblasts**

b **HPK**

c **Fibroblasts**

- IL-18BP
- IL-8

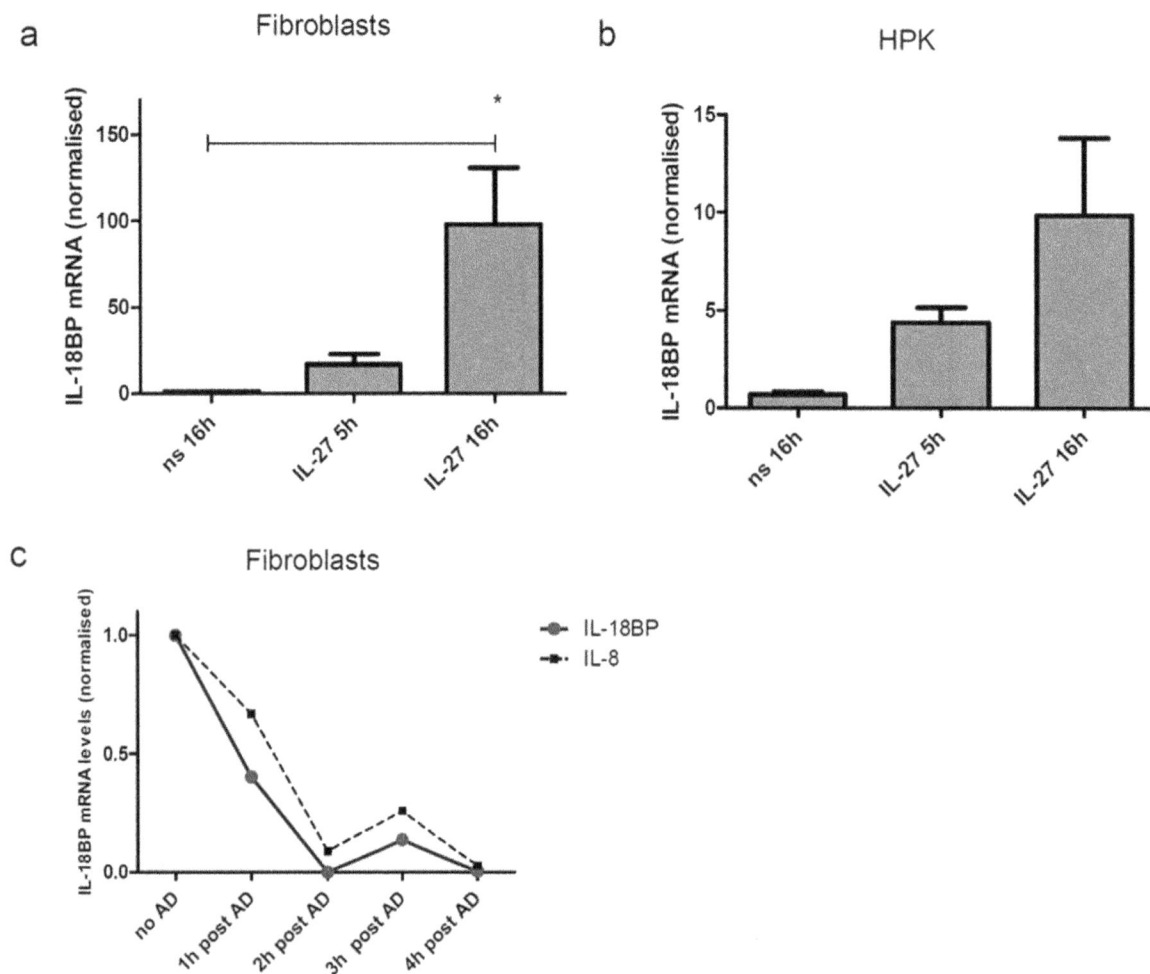

Figure 4. IL-18BP mRNA induction by IL-27. Fibroblasts (a,c) and HaCat cells (b) were stimulated with IL-27 (50 ng/ml) for 5 h or overnight (16 h). qRT-PCR was performed and results were normalised to the expression of the housekeeping gene U6. The result obtained for non stimulated cells (5 h; not depicted) was used as "calibrator" (defined as 1). Stability of the IL-18BP and IL-8 mRNA stability was analysed in IL-27 (50 ng/ml) stimulated cells using actinomycin D (AD). Results were normalised to the expression of the housekeeping gene U6snRNA and the value obtained for cells not treated with AD (= no AD) was used as "calibrator" and defined as 1. (a) n = 3, (b) n = 2, (c) one out of 2 independent experiments is depicted. ns = non stimulated.

expression in colon carcinoma cells [62]. In those cells IL-18BP induction depends in large part on STAT1 binding to the proximal GAS element [48].

In a recent study Murray et al. [49] show that in cardiac cardiomyocytes ß2-adrenergic receptor triggering activates a signalling cascade which ultimately leads to a CREB and c/EBPß dependent increased IL-18BP promoter activity. These findings support data by Hurgin et al. [47] who described c/EBPß as important transcription factor binding to the afore-mentioned proximal GAS site in the IL-18BP promoter of HepG2 cells. We have stimulated keratinocytes with salbutamol (a beta2 adrenergic agonist) and failed to see any increase in IL-18BP production (data not shown). Taken together these findings indicate that cell type specific differences may exist between primary human tissue cells, murine cells and transfected HepG2 cells with regard to IL-18BP promoter activation. It would be interesting to further investigate potential differences in different cell types and to further elucidate the significance of c/EBPß dependent IL-18BP regulation in human tissues and diseases such as hypertrophic cardiomyopathies.

Our data confirm and expand the current knowledge on IL-18BP regulation in the skin. IL-18BP is highly regulated at transcriptional level. We also demonstrate herein the crucial role of the proximal GAS element for IL-18BP promoter activation in response to IL-27. As upon stimulation IL-18BP is produced with some delay (max. production around 48 h after stimulation) but in a prolonged manner (up to 120 h) we were surprised to see that the stability of the mRNA in fibroblasts was not greater than that of IL-8 (known to be "not" stable). However, the protein seem to be rather stable once produced and Hurgin et al. [47] have already pointed to the fact that it accumulates in the supernatants of cultured cells. It has been described that IFNα induces IL-18BP in chronic hepatitis C patients [50]. IL-18BP upregulation by IL-27 could therefore be regulated by endogenous IFNs. In our experimental setup we failed to detect increased IL-27 induced mRNA levels of IFNλ by keratinocytes or fibroblasts and could not detect elevated levels of IFNα in the supernatant of stimulated cells. IFNγ, which is an extremly potent inducer of IL-18BP, is not expressed by human keratinocytes or fibroblasts. We can, however, not fully exclude that type I IFN, namely IFNß, or type III IFN may contribute to the IL-27 effect on IL-18BP

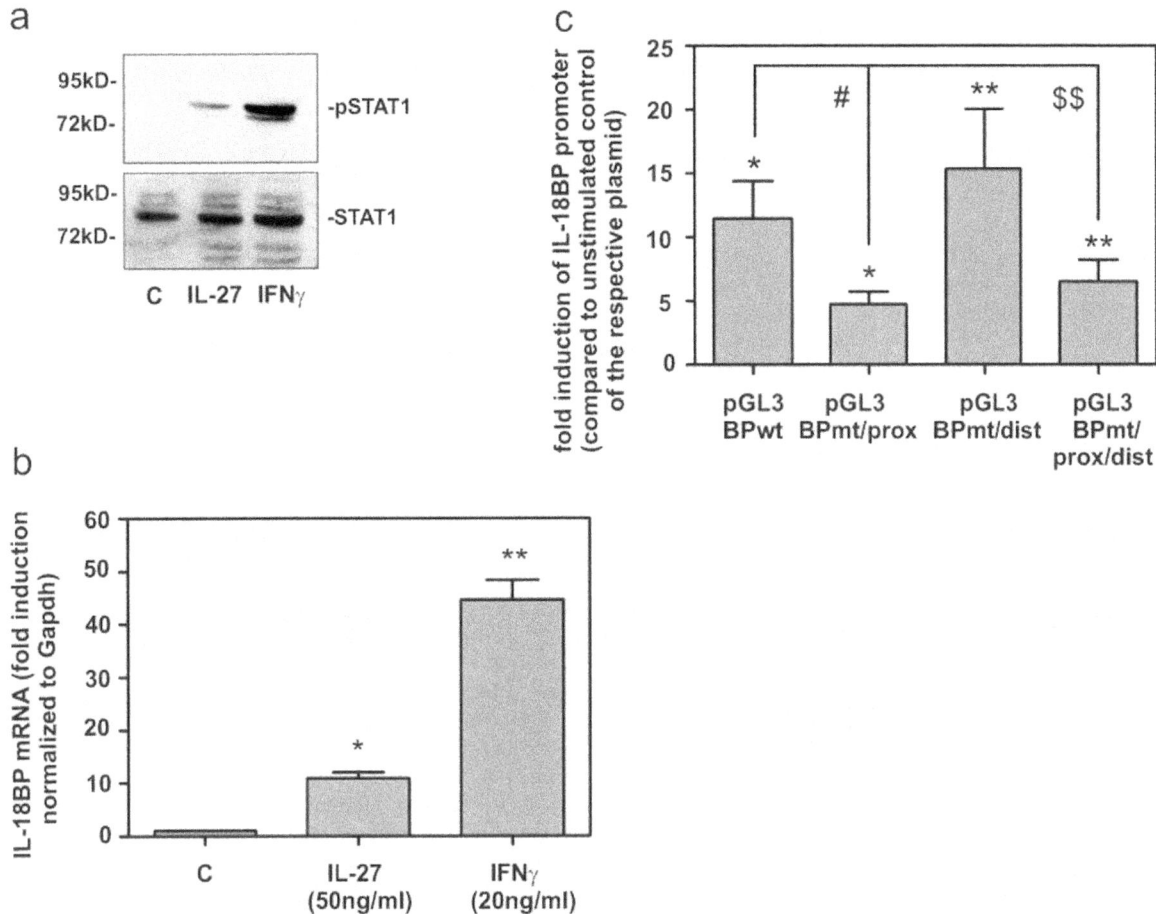

Figure 5. IL-27 induced IL-18BP activation pathway in HaCat cells. (a) HaCat cells were stimulated for 30 min with IL-27 (100 ng/ml), IFNγ (20 ng/ml) or used as non stimulated control, lysed and the obtained nuclear extract analysed by western blot using antibodies specific for total STAT1 and pSTAT1-Y701. One representative of three independently performed experiments is shown. (b) HaCat cells were stimulated for 24 h with with IL-27 (50 ng/ml), IFNγ (20 ng/ml) or used as unstimulated control and mRNA expression of IL-18BP was determined by qRT-PCR. IL-18BP mRNA was normalized to that of GAPDH and is shown as mean fold induction compared to unstimulated control ± S.D. (n = 6). (c) HaCat cells were transfected with the indicated IL-18BP promoter constructs. After 24 h, cells were kept as non-stimulated control or stimulated with IL-27 (100 ng/ml). After another 24 h, cells were harvested and luciferase assays were performed. Data are expressed as mean fold-luciferase induction ± SD (compared to the non-stimulated control transfected with the same plasmid) obtained from 4 independent experiments. *p<0.05 and **p<0.01 compared to non stimulated control of the respective plasmid; #p<0.05 compared pGL3-BPwt under the influence of IL-27, $$p<0.01 compared to pGL3-BPmt/dist under the influence of IL-27.

upregulation. We seek to investigate how IL-27 interacts with the IFN system in inflammatory skin diseases such as psoriasis and lupus erythematosus in future studies.

It seems of great interest to therapeutically manipulate the IL-18/IL-18BP system. A phase I study [63], has shown that in healthy volunteers, rheumatoid arthritis and psoriasis patients subcutaneous injections of IL-18BP are well tolerated and within 1–2 weeks show steady levels of the protein in serum. This suggests that there is therapeutic viability for this protein. However, efficacy of the drug in chronic inflammation needs to be further established. In viral infections it seems favourable to reduce IL-18BP expression and thereby to enhance antiviral IL-18 activity. On the contrary, in chronic inflammatory diseases associated with tissue remodelling local counterregulation of IL-18 bioactivity may be highly beneficial. However, increasing IL-18BP by pharmacological means might not be advised under all pathophysiological conditions. In fact, recent data indicate that high levels of IL-18BP, by scavenging immunosuppressive IL-37 [64,65], may even have a pathogenic pro-inflammatory side. Thus, it appears that

tissue IL-18BP needs to be tightly balanced in order to achieve the desired anti-inflammatory effect. IL-27 is an interesting molecule with "regulatory" potential. However, we need to better understand the fine tuned regulation of different effector molecules and the crosstalk between different tissue cells before proposing this molecule as valuable for therapeutic intervention in humans.

Materials and Methods

Cytokines and Reagents

All cytokines were used as purified recombinant human preparations. IL-27, IL-12, IL-23 and IFNγ/ß were purchased from eBioscience (Hatfield, UK) or RnD Systems (Abingdon, UK).

Cell Isolation and Culture

Cultures of human primary keratinocytes (HPK) and fibroblasts were prepared from foreskin as described previously [23]. All patients gave written conformed consent to participate in the study. The procedure to use foreskin from anonymised patients was approved by the Ethical Committee of Hannover Medical School, Hannover, Germany. HPK were cultured in Keratinocyte Growth Medium Kit II (PromoCell, Heidelberg, Germany). HaCat cells as well as fibroblasts were grown in DMEM with 4.5 g/L of glucose and L-Glutamine (Lonza, Slough, UK) supplemented with fetal calf serum (10%) (PromoCell), 0.05 mg/ml streptomycin and 50 U/ml penicillin. Culture medium was changed every second to third day. When the fibroblasts reached 90% confluency (HPK: 60–70% and HaCaT: 70–80% confluency) they were passaged and 20 000 cells were plated into each well of a 24 well plate for stimulation. They were left at least for 24 hours at 37°C after plating before medium was changed and stimulation was carried out. Stimulation of keratinocytes was performed in the absence of hydrocortisone and EGF. For experiment depicted in Figure 5 HaCaT keratinocytes were maintained in DMEM (Invitrogen, Karlsruhe, Germany) supplemented with 100 units/ml penicillin, 100 µg/ml streptomycin, and 10% heat-inactivated FCS (GIBCO-BRL, Eggenstein, Germany). For experiments, HaCat keratinocytes were seeded on 6-well polystyrene plates (Greiner, Frickenhausen, Germany) in the aforementioned culture medium.

Quantitative Real Time PCR

qRT-PCR for fibroblasts was performed on a RotorGen (Qiagen, Hilden, Germany) using a $\Delta\Delta$CT-analysis based on the generation of standard curves for both the housekeeping gene (U6snRNA) and the target gene (IL-18BP, QuantiTect Primer Assay, Qiagen). For RNA isolation Quick-RNA MiniPrep (Zymo Research, Cambridge Bioscience, Cambridge, UK) was used. First strand cDNA synthesis kit (Fermentas/Thermo Fisher Scientific, Loughborough, UK) was used for reverse transcription. Quanti-Fast SYBR green PCR (Qiagen) was used to carry out the RT-PCR.

For IL-18BP mRNA expression in HaCat keratinocytes, total RNA was isolated and transcribed using TRI-Reagent (Sigma-Aldrich), random hexameric primers, and Moloney virus reverse transcriptase (Applied Biosystems, Weiterstadt, Germany) according to the manufacturers' instructions. During realtime PCR, changes in fluorescence were caused by the Taq-polymerase degrading the probe that contains a fluorescent dye (FAM used for IL-18BP, VIC for GAPDH) and a quencher (TAMRA). Primers and probe for IL-18BPa were designed using Primer Express (Applied Biosystems) according to AF110798: forward, 5'-ACCTCCCAGGCCGACTG-3'; reverse, 5'-CCTTGCA-CAGCTGCGTACC-3'; probe 5'-CACCAGCCGG-GAACGTGGGA-3'. Amplification of genomic DNA was avoided by selecting an amplicon that crosses an exon/intron boundary. For GAPDH pre-developed assay reagents were used (4310884E; Applied Biosystems). Assay-mix was used from Thermo Fisher Scientific. qRT-PCR was performed on AbiPrism 7500 Fast Sequence Detector (Applied Biosystems): One initial step at 95°C for 5 min was followed by 40 cycles at 95°C for 2 s and 60°C for 25 s. Detection, calculation of threshold cycles (Ct values), and data analysis were performed by Sequence Detector software. mRNA was quantified by use of cloned cDNA standards for IL-18BP and GAPDH. Data for IL-18BP were normalized to those of GAPDH.

Determination of RNA Stability

Fibroblasts were stimulated for 4 h. Actinomycin D (Sigma) was added 30 minutes before stimulation. mRNA expression was monitored for up to 4 h by qRT-PCR. Samples were normalised to U6snRNA which remained stable over the time course measured. QuantiTect Primer Assay for IL-8 was purchased from Qiagen.

Elisa

Cell-free supernatant was collected, stored at −20 (short term) or −80°C and analysed for the content of IL-18BP using a DuoSet human IL-18BP ELISA kit (RnD Systems, Abingdon, UK) following the manufacturer's instructions.

Luciferase Reporter Assay

An IL-18BP promoter fragment was cloned into pGL3-Basic (Promega, Mannheim, Germany) and entitled pGL3-BPwt as previously described [48]. Site directed mutagenesis was performed by using the QuikChange site-directed mutagenesis kit (Stratagene, Amsterdam, Netherlands) in order to generate promoter fragments that show a dysfunctional proximal γ-activated sequence (GAS) (pGL3-BPmt/prox, located at −25 bp to −33 bp), a dysfunctional putative distal GAS site (pGL3-BPmt/dist, located at −625 bp to −633), and a double-mutation of both GAS sites (pGL3-BPmt/dist/prox) as previously described. For each transfection experiment 4 µg of the indicated plasmids were transfected using Nucleofector Technology according to the manufacturer's instructions (Amaxa, Cologne, Germany). For control of transfection efficiency 0.2 µg pRL-TK (Promega) coding for *Renilla* luciferase were cotransfected. After rest of 24 h, cells were either kept as unstimulated control or stimulated with IL-27 (100 ng/ml). After a 24 h stimulation period, cells were harvested and fold-induction of luciferase activity by IL-27 with control conditions was determined by using the dual reporter gene system (Promega) and an automated chemiluminescence detector (Berthold, Bad Wildbad, Germany) (unstimulated cells transfected with the same respective promoter fragment) set to 1.

Western Blot

To detect total STAT1 and activated phosphorylated pSTAT1, nuclear extracts of HaCat cells were isolated as previously described [66]. For detection of total nuclear STAT1, blots were stripped and reprobed. Antibodies: Total STAT1, rabbit polyclonal antibody (Santa Cruz Biotechnology, Heidelberg, Germany); pSTAT1-Y701, rabbit polyclonal antibody (Cell Signaling, Frankfurt, Germany).

Statistical Analysis

Raw data were analysed by non-paired student's t-test (GraphPad Prism 5.03, GraphPad Software, San Diego, CA).

Author Contributions

Conceived and designed the experiments: MW HM. Performed the experiments: MB RD. Analyzed the data: MW HM RD MB. Contributed reagents/materials/analysis tools: JP TW HM MW. Wrote the paper: MW HM RD TW.

References

1. Pflanz S, Hibbert L, Mattson J, Rosales R, Vaisberg E, et al. (2004) WSX-1 and glycoprotein 130 constitute a signal-transducing receptor for IL-27. J Immunol 172: 2225–2231.
2. Takeda A, Hamano S, Yamanaka A, Hanada T, Ishibashi T, et al. (2003) Cutting edge: role of IL-27/WSX-1 signaling for induction of T-bet through activation of STAT1 during initial Th1 commitment. J Immunol 170: 4886–4890.
3. Pflanz S, Timans JC, Cheung J, Rosales R, Kanzler H, et al. (2002) IL-27, a heterodimeric cytokine composed of EBI3 and p28 protein, induces proliferation of naive CD4(+) T cells. Immunity 16: 779–790.

4. Lucas S, Ghilardi N, Li J, de Sauvage FJ (2003) IL-27 regulates IL-12 responsiveness of naive CD4+ T cells through Stat1-dependent and - independent mechanisms. Proc Natl Acad Sci U S A 100: 15047–15052.

5. Hibbert L, Pflanz S, De Waal Malefyt R, Kastelein RA (2003) IL-27 and IFN-alpha signal via Stat1 and Stat3 and induce T-Bet and IL-12Rbeta2 in naive T cells. J Interferon Cytokine Res 23: 513–522.

6. Zeitvogel J, Werfel T, Wittmann M (submitted) IL-27 acts as a Priming Signal for IL-23 but not IL-12 production on human antigen presenting cells. submitted.

7. Wittmann M, Zeitvogel J, Wang D, Werfel T (2009) IL-27 is expressed in chronic human eczematous skin lesions and stimulates human keratinocytes. J Allergy Clin Immunol 124: 81–89.

8. Shibata S, Tada Y, Kanda N, Nashiro K, Kamata M, et al. (2010) Possible roles of IL-27 in the pathogenesis of psoriasis. J Invest Dermatol 130: 1034–1039.

9. Stumhofer JS, Laurence A, Wilson EH, Huang E, Tato CM, et al. (2006) Interleukin 27 negatively regulates the development of interleukin 17-producing T helper cells during chronic inflammation of the central nervous system. Nat Immunol 7: 937–945.

10. Yoshimura T, Takeda A, Hamano S, Miyazaki Y, Kinjyo I, et al. (2006) Two-sided roles of IL-27: induction of Th1 differentiation on naive CD4+ T cells versus suppression of proinflammatory cytokine production including IL-23-induced IL-17 on activated CD4+ T cells partially through STAT3-dependent mechanism. J Immunol 177: 5377–5385.

11. Batten M, Li J, Yi S, Kljavin NM, Danilenko DM, et al. (2006) Interleukin 27 limits autoimmune encephalomyelitis by suppressing the development of interleukin 17-producing T cells. Nat Immunol 7: 929–936.

12. Sugiyama N, Nakashima H, Yoshimura T, Sadanaga A, Shimizu S, et al. (2008) Amelioration of human lupus-like phenotypes in MRL/lpr mice by over-expression of interleukin 27 receptor alpha (WSX-1). Ann Rheum Dis 67: 1461–1467.

13. Kalliolias GD, Ivashkiv LB (2008) IL-27 activates human monocytes via STAT1 and suppresses IL-10 production but the inflammatory functions of IL-27 are abrogated by TLRs and p38. J Immunol 180: 6325–6333.

14. Arend WP, Palmer G, Gabay C (2008) IL-1, IL-18, and IL-33 families of cytokines. Immunol Rev 223: 20–38.

15. McInnes IB, Liew FY, Gracie JA (2005) Interleukin-18: a therapeutic target in rheumatoid arthritis? Arthritis Res Ther 7: 38–41.

16. Muhl H, Pfeilschifter J (2004) Interleukin-18 bioactivity: a novel target for immunopharmacological anti-inflammatory intervention. Eur J Pharmacol 500: 63–71.

17. Wittmann M, Macdonald A, Renne J (2009) IL-18 and skin inflammation. Autoimmun Rev 9: 45–48.

18. Akira S (2000) The role of IL-18 in innate immunity. Curr Opin Immunol 12: 59–63.

19. Takeda K, Tsutsui H, Yoshimoto T, Adachi O, Yoshida N, et al. (1998) Defective NK cell activity and Th1 response in IL-18-deficient mice. Immunity 8: 383–390.

20. Yamagata S, Tomita K, Sato R, Niwa A, Higashino H, et al. (2008) Interleukin-18-deficient mice exhibit diminished chronic inflammation and airway remodelling in ovalbumin-induced asthma model. Clin Exp Immunol 154: 295–304.

21. Wittmann M, Purwar R, Hartmann C, Gutzmer R, Werfel T (2005) Human keratinocytes respond to interleukin-18: implication for the course of chronic inflammatory skin diseases. J Invest Dermatol 124: 1225–1233.

22. Gangemi S, Merendino RA, Guarneri F, Minciullo PL, DiLorenzo G, et al. (2003) Serum levels of interleukin-18 and s-ICAM-1 in patients affected by psoriasis: preliminary considerations. J Eur Acad Dermatol Venereol 15: 42–46.

23. Wang D, Drenker M, Eiz-Vesper B, Werfel T, Wittmann M (2008) Evidence for a pathogenetic role of interleukin-18 in cutaneous lupus erythematosus. Arthritis Rheum 58: 3205–3215.

24. Companjen A, van der Wel L, van der Fits L, Laman J, Prens E (2004) Elevated interleukin-18 protein expression in early active and progressive plaque-type psoriatic lesions. Eur Cytokine Netw 15: 210–216.

25. Johansen C, Moeller K, Kragballe K, Iversen L (2007) The activity of caspase-1 is increased in lesional psoriatic epidermis. J Invest Dermatol 127: 2857–2864.

26. Ohta Y, Hamada Y, Katsuoka K (2001) Expression of IL-18 in psoriasis. Arch Dermatol Res 293: 334–342.

27. Naik SM, Cannon G, Burbach GJ, Singh SR, Swerlick RA, et al. (1999) Human keratinocytes constitutively express interleukin-18 and secrete biologically active interleukin-18 after treatment with pro-inflammatory mediators and dinitro-chlorobenzene. J Invest Dermatol 113: 766–772.

28. Companjen AR, Prens E, Mee JB, Groves RW (2000) Expression of IL-18 in human keratinocytes. J Invest Dermatol 114: 598–599.

29. Gutzmer R, Langer K, Mommert S, Wittmann M, Kapp A, et al. (2003) Human dendritic cells express the IL-18R and are chemoattracted to IL-18. J Immunol 171: 6363–6371.

30. Kampfer H, Muhl H, Manderscheid M, Kalina U, Kauschat D, et al. (2000) Regulation of interleukin-18 (IL-18) expression in keratinocytes (HaCaT): implications for early wound healing. Eur Cytokine Netw 11: 626–633.

31. Esteban DJ, Buller RM (2004) Identification of residues in an orthopoxvirus interleukin-18-binding protein involved in ligand binding and species specificity. Virology 323: 197–207.

32. Reading PC, Smith GL (2003) Vaccinia virus interleukin-18-binding protein promotes virulence by reducing gamma interferon production and natural killer and T-cell activity. J Virol 77: 9960–9968.

33. Xiang Y, Moss B (1999) IL-18 binding and inhibition of interferon gamma induction by human poxvirus-encoded proteins. Proc Natl Acad Sci U S A 96: 11537–11542.

34. Xiang Y, Moss B (2003) Molluscum contagiosum virus interleukin-18 (IL-18) binding protein is secreted as a full-length form that binds cell surface glycosaminoglycans through the C-terminal tail and a furin-cleaved form with only the IL-18 binding domain. J Virol 77: 2623–2630.

35. Lee SJ, Cho YS, Cho MC, Shim JH, Lee KA, et al. (2001) Both E6 and E7 oncoproteins of human papillomavirus 16 inhibit IL-18-induced IFN-gamma production in human peripheral blood mononuclear and NK cells. J Immunol 167: 497–504.

36. Bani-Hani AH, Leslie JA, Asanuma H, Dinarello CA, Campbell MT, et al. (2009) IL-18 neutralization ameliorates obstruction-induced epithelial-mesenchymal transition and renal fibrosis. Kidney Int 76: 500–511.

37. Hayashi N, Yoshimoto T, Izuhara K, Matsui K, Tanaka T, et al. (2007) T helper 1 cells stimulated with ovalbumin and IL-18 induce airway hyperresponsiveness and lung fibrosis by IFN-gamma and IL-13 production. Proc Natl Acad Sci U S A 104: 14765–14770.

38. Xing SS, Bi XP, Tan HW, Zhang Y, Xing QC, et al. (2010) Overexpression of interleukin-18 aggravates cardiac fibrosis and diastolic dysfunction in fructose-fed rats. Mol Med 16: 465–470.

39. Yu Q, Vazquez R, Khojeini EV, Patel C, Venkataramani R, et al. (2009) IL-18 induction of osteopontin mediates cardiac fibrosis and diastolic dysfunction in mice. Am J Physiol Heart Circ Physiol 297: H76–85.

40. Kanda N, Shimizu T, Tada Y, Watanabe S (2007) IL-18 enhances IFN-gamma-induced production of CXCL9, CXCL10, and CXCL11 in human keratinocytes. Eur J Immunol 37: 338–350.

41. Novick D, Kim SH, Fantuzzi G, Reznikov LL, Dinarello CA, et al. (1999) Interleukin-18 binding protein: a novel modulator of the Th1 cytokine response. Immunity 10: 127–136.

42. Kim SH, Eisenstein M, Reznikov L, Fantuzzi G, Novick D, et al. (2000) Structural requirements of six naturally occurring isoforms of the IL-18 binding protein to inhibit IL-18. Proc Natl Acad Sci U S A 97: 1190–1195.

43. Muhl H, Kampfer H, Bosmann M, Frank S, Radeke H, et al. (2000) Interferon-gamma mediates gene expression of IL-18 binding protein in nonleukocytic cells. Biochem Biophys Res Commun 267: 960–963.

44. Iannello A, Boulassel MR, Samarani S, Tremblay C, Toma E, et al. (2010) HIV-1 causes an imbalance in the production of interleukin-18 and its natural antagonist in HIV-infected individuals: implications for enhanced viral replication. J Infect Dis 201: 608–617.

45. Paulukat J, Bosmann M, Nold M, Garkisch S, Kampfer H, et al. (2001) Expression and release of IL-18 binding protein in response to IFN-gamma. J Immunol 167: 7038–7043.

46. Moller B, Paulukat J, Nold M, Behrens M, Kukoc-Zivojnov N, et al. (2003) Interferon-gamma induces expression of interleukin-18 binding protein in fibroblast-like synoviocytes. Rheumatology (Oxford) 42: 442–445.

47. Hurgin V, Novick D, Rubinstein M (2002) The promoter of IL-18 binding protein: activation by an IFN-gamma -induced complex of IFN regulatory factor 1 and CCAAT/enhancer binding protein beta. Proc Natl Acad Sci U S A 99: 16957–16962.

48. Bachmann M, Paulukat J, Pfeilschifter J, Muhl H (2009) Molecular mechanisms of IL-18BP regulation in DLD-1 cells: pivotal direct action of the STAT1/GAS axis on the promoter level. J Cell Mol Med 13: 1987–1994.

49. Murray DR, Mummidi S, Valente AJ, Yoshida T, Somanna NK, et al. (2011) beta2 adrenergic activation induces the expression of IL-18 binding protein, a potent inhibitor of isoproterenol induced cardiomyocyte hypertrophy in vitro and myocardial hypertrophy in vivo. J Mol Cell Cardiol 52: 206–218.

50. Kaser A, Novick D, Rubinstein M, Siegmund B, Enrich B, et al. (2002) Interferon-alpha induces interleukin-18 binding protein in chronic hepatitis C patients. Clin Exp Immunol 129: 332–338.

51. Corsini E, Mitjans M, Galbiati V, Lucchi L, Galli CL, et al. (2009) Use of IL-18 production in a human keratinocyte cell line to discriminate contact sensitizers from irritants and low molecular weight respiratory allergens. Toxicol In Vitro 23: 789–796.

52. Dinarello CA (2007) Interleukin-18 and the pathogenesis of inflammatory diseases. Semin Nephrol 27: 98–114.

53. Park HJ, Kim JE, Lee JY, Cho BK, Lee WJ, et al. (2004) Increased expression of IL-18 in cutaneous graft-versus-host disease. Immunol Lett 95: 57–61.

54. Calvani N, Tucci M, Richards HB, Tartaglia P, Silvestris F (2005) Th1 cytokines in the pathogenesis of lupus nephritis: the role of IL-18. Autoimmun Rev 4: 542–548.

55. Lotito AP, Silva CA, Mello SB (2007) Interleukin-18 in chronic joint diseases. Autoimmun Rev 6: 253–256.

56. Hu D, Liu X, Chen S, Bao C (2010) Expressions of IL-18 and its binding protein in peripheral blood leukocytes and kidney tissues of lupus nephritis patients. Clin Rheumatol 29: 717–721.

57. Novick D, Elbirt D, Miller G, Dinarello CA, Rubinstein M, et al. (2010) High circulating levels of free interleukin-18 in patients with active SLE in the presence of elevated levels of interleukin-18 binding protein. J Autoimmun 34: 121–126.

58. Antonopoulos C, Cumberbatch M, Mee JB, Dearman RJ, Wei XQ, et al. (2008) IL-18 is a key proximal mediator of contact hypersensitivity and allergen-induced Langerhans cell migration in murine epidermis. J Leukoc Biol 83: 361–367.

59. Favilli F, Anzilotti C, Martinelli L, Quattroni P, De Martino S, et al. (2009) IL-18 activity in systemic lupus erythematosus. Ann N Y Acad Sci 1173: 301–309.

60. Ludwiczek O, Kaser A, Novick D, Dinarello CA, Rubinstein M, et al. (2002) Plasma levels of interleukin-18 and interleukin-18 binding protein are elevated in patients with chronic liver disease. J Clin Immunol 22: 331–337.

61. Mallat Z, Heymes C, Corbaz A, Logeart D, Alouani S, et al. (2004) Evidence for altered interleukin 18 (IL)-18 pathway in human heart failure. FASEB J 18: 1752–1754.

62. Ziesche E, Bachmann M, Kleinert H, Pfeilschifter J, Muhl H (2007) The interleukin-22/STAT3 pathway potentiates expression of inducible nitric-oxide synthase in human colon carcinoma cells. J Biol Chem 282: 16006–16015.

63. Tak PP, Bacchi M, Bertolino M (2006) Pharmacokinetics of IL-18 binding protein in healthy volunteers and subjects with rheumatoid arthritis or plaque psoriasis. Eur J Drug Metab Pharmacokinet 31: 109–116.

64. Boraschi D, Lucchesi D, Hainzl S, Leitner M, Maier E, et al. (2011) IL-37: a new anti-inflammatory cytokine of the IL-1 family. Eur Cytokine Netw 22: 127–147.

65. Nold MF, Nold-Petry CA, Zepp JA, Palmer BE, Bufler P, et al. (2010) IL-37 is a fundamental inhibitor of innate immunity. Nat Immunol 11: 1014–1022.

66. Sadik CD, Bachmann M, Pfeilschifter J, Muhl H (2009) Activation of interferon regulatory factor-3 via toll-like receptor 3 and immunomodulatory functions detected in A549 lung epithelial cells exposed to misplaced U1-snRNA. Nucleic Acids Res 37: 5041–5056.

γδ T Cells Are Reduced and Rendered Unresponsive by Hyperglycemia and Chronic TNFα in Mouse Models of Obesity and Metabolic Disease

Kristen R. Taylor, Robyn E. Mills, Anne E. Costanzo, Julie M. Jameson*

Department of Immunology and Microbial Science, The Scripps Research Institute, La Jolla, California, United States of America

Abstract

Epithelial cells provide an initial line of defense against damage and pathogens in barrier tissues such as the skin; however this balance is disrupted in obesity and metabolic disease. Skin γδ T cells recognize epithelial damage, and release cytokines and growth factors that facilitate wound repair. We report here that hyperglycemia results in impaired skin γδ T cell proliferation due to altered STAT5 signaling, ultimately resulting in half the number of γδ T cells populating the epidermis. Skin γδ T cells that overcome this hyperglycemic state are unresponsive to epithelial cell damage due to chronic inflammatory mediators, including TNFα. Cytokine and growth factor production at the site of tissue damage was partially restored by administering neutralizing TNFα antibodies *in vivo*. Thus, metabolic disease negatively impacts homeostasis and functionality of skin γδ T cells, rendering host defense mechanisms vulnerable to injury and infection.

Editor: Nick Gay, University of Cambridge, United Kingdom

Funding: This work is supported by National Institutes of Health (NIH) grant DK073098 and DK080048 (J.M.J), a Scripps Translational Science Institute Award from NIH UL1 RR055774 (J.M.J.), The Leukemia and Lymphoma Society (J.M.J.) and a Department of Immunology Institutional Training Grant 5T32 AI007244-24 (K.R.T.). The funders had no role in study design, data collection and analysis, decision to publish, or preparation of the manuscript.

Competing Interests: The authors have declared that no competing interests exist.

* E-mail: jamesonj@scripps.edu

Introduction

Resident intraepithelial γδ T cells are responsible for maintaining epithelial integrity, regulating homeostasis and providing a first line of defense against pathogens and injury in mice and humans [1,2,3]. γδ T cells arise in the thymus during ontogeny and migrate, in waves, to epithelial tissues such as the skin, lung, intestine and reproductive tract where they populate these tissues for the life of the animal [4,5]. In addition to their role in the innate immune response, γδ T cells regulate the subsequent recruitment of inflammatory cells to sites of injury and infection [6,7,8]. Murine skin resident T cells express a canonical Vγ3Vδ1 T cell receptor (TCR) and respond to a proposed, yet unknown, self antigen expressed by stressed or damaged keratinocytes [9,10]. Skin γδ T cells display a dendritic morphology, retract their dendrites following activation and are critical for epidermal homeostasis and wound repair through their production of cytokines and regulation of inflammatory cells [1,6,11,12,13,14,15]. Mice deficient in γδ T cells exhibit disrupted skin homeostasis, impaired barrier function and delayed wound healing [1,15,16,17]. In humans, the epidermis consists of a mixed resident αβ and γδ T cell population [18]. Similar to observations in mice, skin-resident Vδ1+ γδ T cells in humans produce cytokines and growth factors after activation and participate in wound repair [19].

In obesity and metabolic syndrome, the epidermal barrier is disrupted and skin complications can ultimately result in chronic and debilitating non-healing wounds and persistent infections [20]. Chronic wounds in obese and diabetic patients show diminished or altered levels of growth factors, impaired leukocyte infiltration and function and the absence of cell growth and migration over the wound [20]. Even with medical treatment, these chronic non-healing wounds may ultimately result in amputation of extremities [21]. Recent work has focused on the initiation of chronic inflammation in adipose tissue in obesity. An increase in effector CD8+ T cells and a decrease in CD4+ and T regulatory cells in adipose tissue have been shown to correlate with exacerbated adipocyte inflammation and metabolic disease progression [22,23,24]. However, the consequence of obesity and metabolic disease on the function of skin resident lymphocyte populations and how this contributes to skin complications associated with obesity and metabolic disease are unknown.

In this study we investigated how skin γδ T cell function becomes altered in obesity and metabolic disease. We show that the progression of metabolic disease impacts both the homeostasis and wound healing response of skin γδ T cells. Correlating with early hyperglycemia, the proliferation of skin γδ T cells is impaired, which ultimately results in a reduction in tissue-resident epidermal T cell numbers. The remaining skin γδ T cells overcome this hyperglycemic state, but exhibit altered metabolic and nutrient sensing pathways. The chronic inflammatory environment, specifically elevated TNFα, renders the remaining skin γδ T cells dysfunctional to tissue damage. In this inflammatory environment, skin γδ T cells are unresponsive to keratinocyte stimulation and unable to produce cytokines and epithelial regulating factors such as TGFβ1. We can improve skin γδ T cells function *in vivo* by blocking TNFα, providing evidence that chronic TNFα in metabolic syndrome contributes to skin γδ T cell dysfunction in wound healing.

Results

Skin γδ T cells are unable to maintain epidermal numbers in obesity

Skin γδ T cells arise in the thymus during fetal development, migrate to the skin and actively expand to reach a maximum of ~5% of the total cells in the epidermis. After this early migration, the epidermal skin γδ T cell compartment is maintained through self-renewal. To determine the impact of obesity and metabolic disease on skin γδ T cell survival and maintenance, we quantified γδ T cell numbers in epidermal sheets and analyzed their morphology starting at 6-weeks of age and continuing out to 14-weeks of age. Epidermal sheets from 6-week old $db/+$ (lean control) and db/db mice demonstrated that skin γδ T cells seeded the epidermis, were present in expected numbers and exhibited their characteristic dendritic morphology (**Figure 1A**). However, at this 6-week time point, a slight decrease in γδ T cell numbers was observed. By 8- and 10-weeks of age a pronounced decrease in skin γδ T cell numbers was apparent in obese db/db mice (**Figure 1A and 1B**). Following this rapid decline, epidermal γδ T cells stabilized at 10-weeks of age and remained reduced out to 14-weeks of age (**Figure 1A and 1B**).

In addition to the lymphocyte population, a resident dendritic cell population, the Langerhans cells (LC), also resides in the skin.

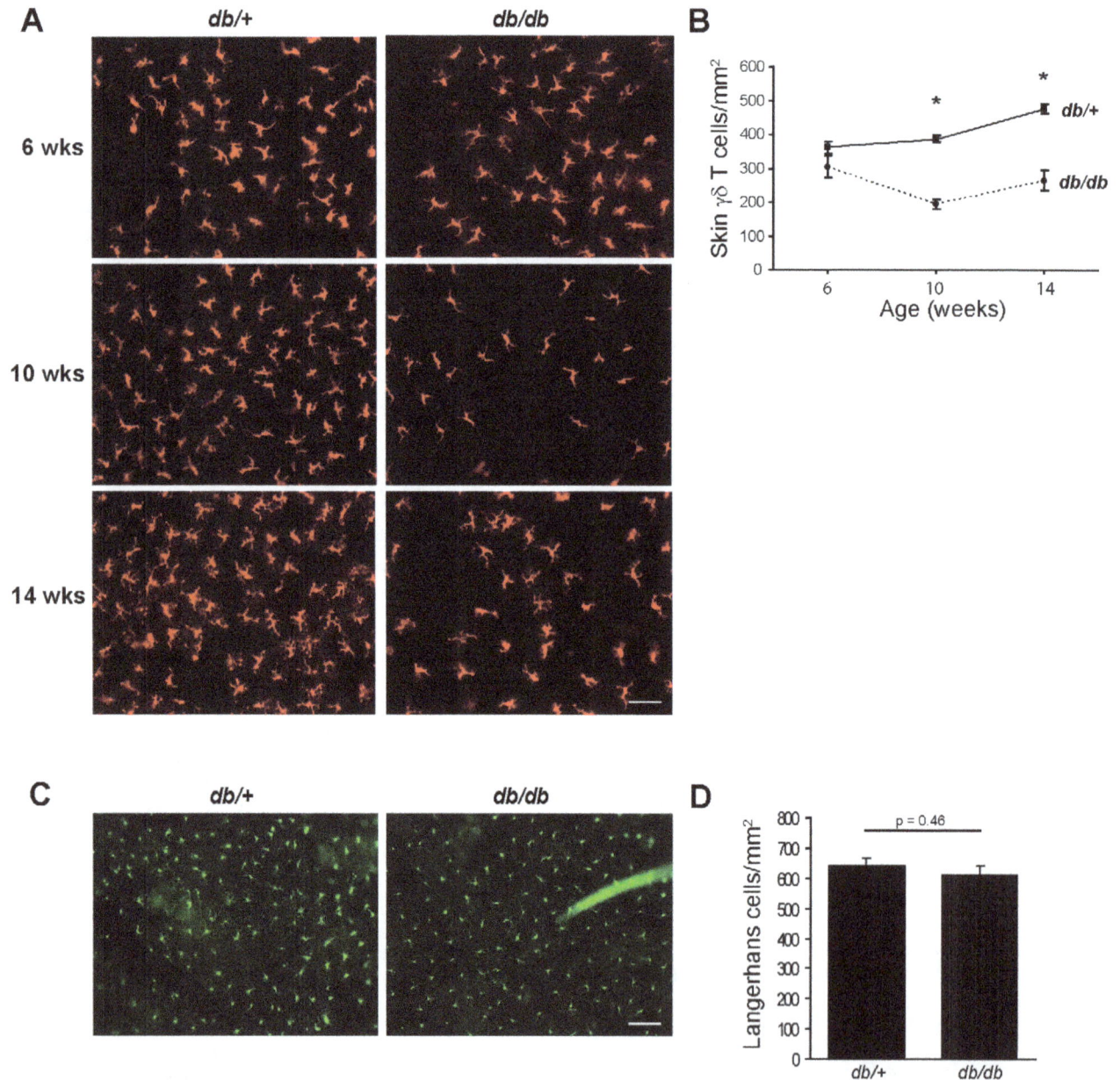

Figure 1. Reduced numbers of skin γδ T cells during obesity and metabolic disease is associated with hyperglycemia. (**A**) γδ TCR immunofluorescence staining of epidermal sheets from BKS $db/+$ and db/db mice at 6-, 10- and 14-weeks of age. (**B**) Graphical representation of the number of epidermal γδ T cells in $db/+$ (solid line) and db/db (dashed line) mice at each age. *p<0.005. (**C**) Epidermal sheets from 10-week old BKS $db/+$ and db/db mice immunostained for the LC marker, langerin. (**D**) Graphical representation of the number of Langerhans cells at 10-weeks of age. All microscopy images were acquired at ×200. The bar represents 0.05 μm. Data (mean ± SEM) are representative of three independent experiments for each age group and a minimum of 15 fields per mouse.

To determine the impact of obesity and metabolic disease on another skin-resident immune population, we examined LC numbers using anti-langerin and anti-CD45.2 antibodies to stain epidermal sheets [25]. Obese *db/db* mice had similar numbers of LC in the epidermis as compared to lean *db/+* control mice at all ages tested (**Figure 1C and 1D**). Our data suggest that the early progression of obesity and metabolic syndrome are marked by a selective inability of skin γδ T cells to maintain homeostatic numbers within the epidermis.

To address the possible contribution of leptin receptor deficiency on skin γδ T cells from *db/db* animals, we investigated the expression of leptin (Lep) and two leptin receptor isoforms (Lepr) in skin γδ T cells. No expression of either leptin or two leptin receptor isoforms, Ob-Ra and Ob-Rb, was detected in mRNA from skin γδ T cells isolated directly *ex vivo* or in the γδ 7–17 cell line *in vivo* (**Figure S1**).

Hyperglycemia alters STAT5 signaling and impedes γδ T cell proliferation

Between 6- and 10-weeks of age, BKS *db/db* mice are hyperglycemic and exhibit greater weight gain than their *db/+* control littermates (**Table S1**). To determine the impact of environmental factors that are present during this phase of disease, such as glucose and fatty acids, we tested whether the 7–17 skin γδ T cell line can maintain itself and survive when these factors are present and elevated. We found that 7–17 γδ T cells treated with 33.3 mM glucose resulted in a rapid decline of T cells within 24 to 48 hours of treatment (**Figure 2A**). However, treatment of 7–17 γδ T cells with fatty acids did not inhibit γδ T cell growth (**Figure S2**).

To investigate the impact of glucose on skin γδ T cell proliferation, 7–17 cells were maintained in IL-2, treated with elevated glucose and proliferation determined. As shown in **Figure 2B**, there was a dose dependent inhibition of γδ T cell proliferation 36 hours post-glucose treatment. In addition to the 7–17 γδ T cell line, freshly isolated skin γδ T cells were sorted from epidermal cell preparations from wild-type mice, placed into IL-2 containing media in the presence of baseline (11.2 mM) or elevated (33.3 mM) glucose. Similar to observations with the 7–17 γδ T cell line, freshly isolated skin γδ T cells also displayed reduced proliferation in the presence of elevated glucose (**Figure 2C**). This data suggests that skin γδ T cells are highly sensitive to elevations in glucose, affecting their ability to proliferate and maintain homeostatic numbers.

Since γδ T cells proliferate after stimulation with IL-2 in a glucose-sensitive manner, we next asked whether glucose treatment alters downstream IL-2 signaling. IL-2 receptor binding results in Jak1 and Jak3 activation, phosphorylation of STAT5 and translocation of the STAT5 complex to the nucleus where it regulates gene transcription [26]. Following stimulation of untreated skin γδ T cells with IL-2, phosphorylation of STAT5A and STAT5B peaked at 30 minutes, followed by a rapid decrease in phosphorylation (**Figure 2D**). However, in glucose-treated γδ T cells, STAT5A was rapidly phosphorylated to peak levels within 10 to 30 minutes after IL-2 stimulation but displayed altered kinetics and prolonged phosphorylation compared to untreated cells. In addition, glucose-treated γδ T cells had negligible phosphorylation of STAT5B after IL-2 stimulation (**Figure 2D**). This data suggests that diminished proliferation of skin γδ T cells may be due to altered IL-2 and STAT5 signaling in response to hyperglycemic conditions. Moreover, STAT5A/B signaling is critical to γδ T cell function as γδ T cells are absent in mice deficient in STAT5A/B [27].

To determine if diminished skin γδ T cell proliferation in BKS *db/db* mice accounts for the reduction in epidermal T cell numbers, we first had to investigate the rate of γδ T cell proliferation *in vivo*. Although long-lived, memory-like Vγ2+ T cells in the periphery have been shown to have very slow turnover [28], the rate of Vγ3+ T cell proliferation and homeostatic maintenance in the epidermis has yet to be defined. Unlike the rapid turnover of epithelial keratinocytes [29,30,31], LC turnover is much slower, between 5 and 10% of cells proliferating per week [32,33]. To determine the rate of γδ T cell proliferation in the epidermis, control BKS *db/+* mice were treated for one week with BrdU in the drinking water and skin γδ T cells were analyzed for BrdU incorporation at 6- and 10-weeks of age. Skin γδ T cell proliferation in 6- and 10-week old lean *db/+* mice averaged approximately 11% of the total cells proliferating per week (**Figure 2E, left panels**).

BrdU incorporation was then quantified in 6- and 10-week old BKS *db/db* mice to ascertain whether decreased proliferation accounts for diminished skin γδ T cell numbers in the *db/db* mouse. In contrast to the 10–12% BrdU incorporation of skin γδ T cells in 6-week old lean *db/+* mice, only half as many γδ T cells incorporated BrdU in *db/db* mice (**Figure 2E, right panel, and 2F**). This reduced percentage of γδ T cells isolated from 6-week old *db/db* mice indicates decreased skin γδ T cell turnover in the BKS *db/db* mouse. Turnover of epithelial keratinocytes confirmed that BrdU was reaching the skin and being incorporated at a similar rate in 6-week old BKS *db/+* and *db/db* (**Figure 2G**). In contrast to 6-week old mice, skin γδ T cells from obese 10-week old *db/db* mice had a similar percentage of skin γδ T cells incorporating BrdU as compared to control *db/+* mice (**Figure 2E, right panel, and 2F**). This correlates with the data presented in **Figure 1B**, which shows that γδ T cell numbers stabilize in 10-week old *db/db* mice.

To confirm that skin γδ T cells were not undergoing increased apoptosis in BKS *db/db* mice, freshly isolated γδ T cells from the epidermis were stained with annexin-V and subject to propidium iodide incorporation (PI). No significant changes in skin γδ T cell annexin+PI+ populations were detected between lean *db/+* and obese *db/db* animals at multiple ages (**Figure S3A**). Furthermore, to verify that skin γδ T cells in the obese environment were not migrating out of the epidermis, whole skin cross-sections were stained with γδ TCR-specific antibodies and analyzed by immunofluorescent microscopy. We established that γδ T cells in the BKS *db/db* mouse remained localized to the epidermis and hair follicles (**Figure S3B**) and were not found migrating into the dermis. Additionally, skin-specific Vγ3+ T cells were not detected in lymph nodes providing further evidence that they have not migrated out of the epidermis (**Figure S3C**).

Taken together, this data demonstrates that hyperglycemia impacts skin γδ T cell proliferation, specifically at 6-weeks of age, ultimately reducing the population of skin γδ T cells in the epidermis by half. However, by 10-weeks of age, the remaining skin γδ T cells in the *db/db* animals have overcome the impaired proliferation induced by hyperglycemia.

Skin γδ T cells are unresponsive to tissue damage in obesity

Since a population of skin γδ T cells survived the hyperglycemic environment, we next asked whether the remaining skin γδ T cells in the 10-week old *db/db* mice were able to respond to epithelial damage *in vivo*. One major function of skin γδ T cells is to recognize epithelial tissue damage and release cytokines and growth factors that facilitate wound repair. To investigate whether the remaining skin γδ T cells in the obese mouse are able to

A

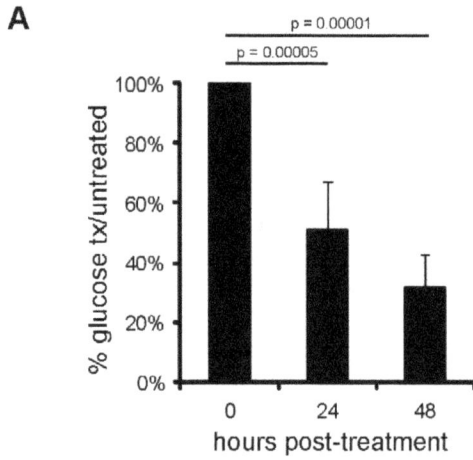

B

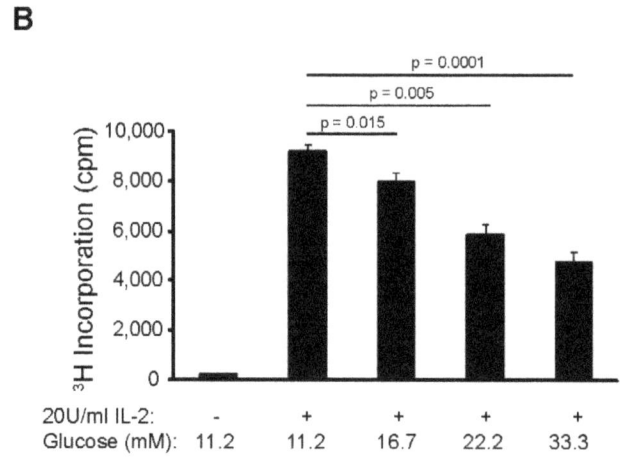

C

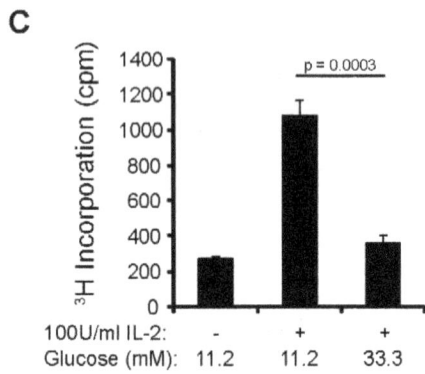

D

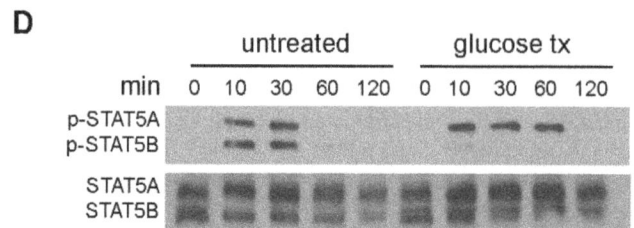

E

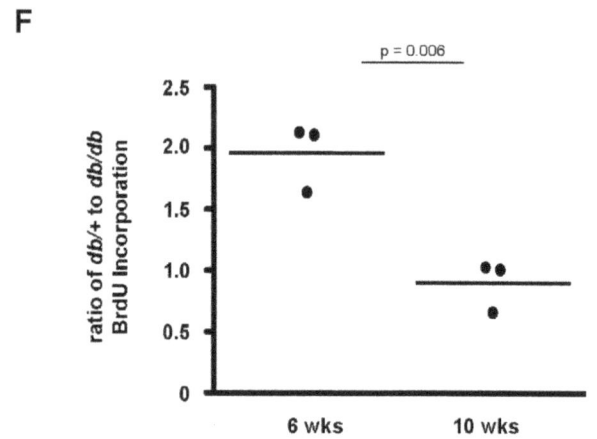

F

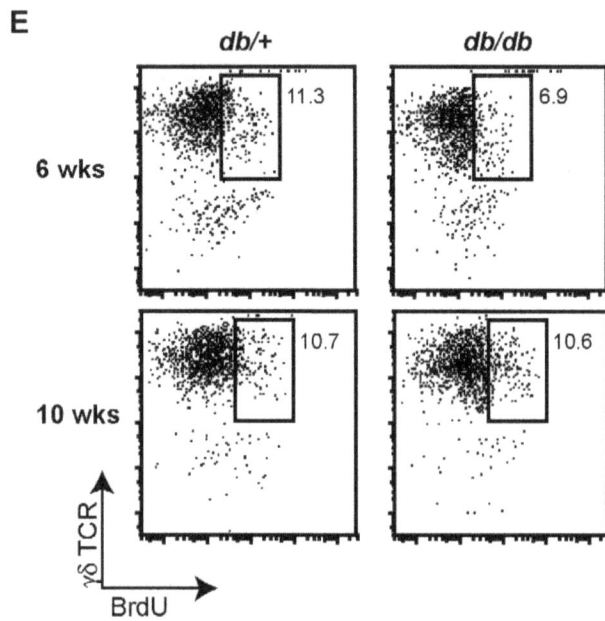

G

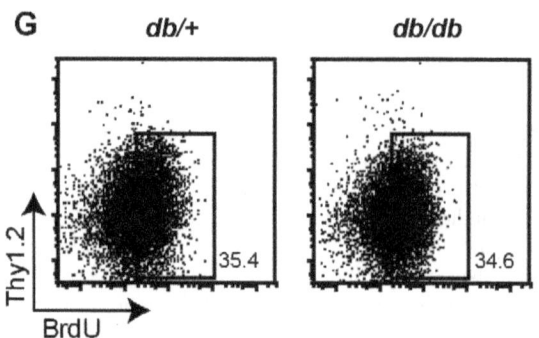

Figure 2. Regulation of skin γδ T cell proliferation by glucose is associated with decreased STAT5B phosphorylation. (A) *In vitro* growth of γδ 7–17 T cell line treated with 33.3 mM glucose at 0, 24 and 48 hours. Data (mean ± SD) presented as the % of glucose treated cells to untreated control cells. (B, C) Proliferation of (B) γδ 7–17 T cells and (C) freshly isolated γδ T cells sorted from wild-type B6 mice in IL-2 containing growth media supplemented with elevated glucose concentrations. Each experiment was performed in triplicate, data presented as mean ± SD. (D) The kinetics of expression of phosphorylated STAT5A and STAT5B following 40U/ml IL-2 stimulation in untreated and glucose treated γδ 7–17 T cells. Total STAT5 expression demonstrates even loading and expression. (E) Multiparameter flow cytometry of BrdU incorporation by skin γδ T cells isolated from 6- and 10-week old BKS *db/+* and *db/db* mice treated with BrdU for 7 days. The same number of events is presented for each dot plot, numbers indicate the percent of γδ T cells that have incorporated BrdU. Epidermal cells were gated on live Thy1.2$^+$ events for γδ T cells. (F) Graphical representation of the ratio of BrdU incorporation by γδ T cells in BKS *db/+* to *db/db* mice at 6-weeks and 10-weeks of age, n = 3 per strain and age. Shown are black dots to represent the ratio of each experiment, the black line represents the average of three experiments. (G) Multiparameter flow cytometry of BrdU incorporation by keratinocytes isolated from 6-week old BKS *db/+* and *db/db* mice treated with BrdU for 7 days. The same number of events is presented for each dot plot, numbers on the right indicate the percent of keratinocytes that have incorporated BrdU. Epidermal cells were gated on live γδ TCR$^-$ events for keratinocytes. Data are representative of five (**A, B**) or three (**C–G**) separate experiments.

rapidly respond following injury, we monitored the ability of skin γδ T cells to retract their dendrites at the wound edge. Following injury and activation through their TCR, γδ T cells round-up at the wound edge and lose their dendritic morphology [1]. Cells distal to the wound site remain dendritic [1], confirming that this is a localized response to tissue damage. Full-thickness punch biopsy wounds were performed on obese 10- to 14-week old BKS *db/db* mice and skin γδ T cell morphology was examined at various time points by immunofluorescent microscopy. Our data indicates that skin γδ T cells in the obese *db/db* mice were delayed in their ability to round following wounding as compared to lean *db/+* control mice (**Figure 3A**). These results were confirmed by quantifying the number of γδ T cells having retracted all their dendrites (**Figure 3B**).

Another characteristic feature of skin γδ T cell activation is the upregulation of several Th1-type proinflammatory cytokines, including TNFα [34]. To determine if skin γδ T cells in obese mice have lost their ability to produce cytokines, we examined TNFα production by γδ T cells located along the wound edge. Full-thickness punch biopsy wounds were performed, γδ T cells were isolated from the wound edge, treated with brefeldin A and immediately stained using intracellular cytokine staining. This technique allows for the examination of skin γδ T cell function immediately *ex vivo* without any additional stimulus beyond the wound. In wild-type mice, cytokine production (using TNFα as a readout) was upregulated in skin γδ T cells directly adjacent to the wound site in control BKS *db/+* mice (**Figure 3C**). However, γδ T cells isolated from the wounds of obese 10- to 14-week old BKS *db/db* mice did not produce TNFα (**Figure 3C**).

We confirmed our *in vivo* wound healing results in another mouse model of obesity, the diet-induced obesity (DIO) model. C57BL/6J mice were started on a 60% kcal fat diet (B6 HFD) at 6 weeks of age compared to the normal chow diet (B6 NCD) (**Table S1**). As shown in **Figure 3D**, γδ T cells isolated from B6 NCD mice upregulated TNFα production at the wound edge compared to non-wounded controls. However, similar to BKS *db/db* animals, skin γδ T cells isolated from 26- to 32-week old B6 HFD mice had little upregulation of TNFα at the wound edge (**Figure 3D**).

In addition to early release of proinflammatory molecules, growth factor production is another key function of skin γδ T cells in response to epithelial damage. We therefore reasoned that this functional response of skin γδ T cells was likely to be disrupted in skin γδ T cells in the obese environment. To address this directly, we investigated intracellular TGFβ1 production in skin γδ T cells isolated from wounded lean control and obese animals. Skin γδ T cells from control 10- to 14-week old BKS *db/+* animals increased TGFβ1 production at the wound edge 24 hours post-wounding (**Figure 3E**). However, skin γδ T cells from obese 10- to 14-week old *db/db* mice had little to no upregulation in TGFβ1 expression (**Figure 3E**). This defective TGFβ1 production was confirmed in

our second model of obesity, the DIO model. Skin γδ T cells isolated from the wound edge of B6 NCD mice upregulated TGFβ1 production, however, skin γδ T cells isolated from the wound edge of 26- to 32-week old B6 HFD mice had impaired TGFβ1 upregulation (**Figure 3F**). Therefore, in addition to defective cytokine production, skin γδ T cells in obesity and metabolic disease were unable to upregulate TGFβ1 production at the wound edge, an important growth factor in several aspects of wound repair.

Delayed rounding and the inability of skin γδ T cells to produce cytokines at the wound edge only occurred in obese 10- to 14-week old *db/db* animals. Skin γδ T cells in 6-week old *db/+* and *db/db* mice retracted their dendrites similarly within 4 hours post wounding and were able to upregulate TNFα adjacent to the wound edge (**data not shown**). Together, this data suggests two separate stages of disease: 1) an early defect in skin γδ T cell proliferation due to hyperglycemia that eventually results in half the number of skin γδ T cells residing in the epidermis and 2) a later defect characterized by the inability of skin γδ T cells to perform tissue repair functions *in vivo*.

Impaired skin γδ T cell nutrient sensing and activation in obesity

The inability of skin γδ T cells to be activated and produce cytokines and growth factors following epithelial damage occurred only in 10- to 14-week old BKS *db/db* and not 6-week old mice. This unresponsive state was not caused by hyperglycemia and suggests that other environmental factors, such as chronic inflammatory factors, or cell-intrinsic factors may be responsible for the lack of tissue damage responses. To better understand the impact of metabolic disease on skin γδ T cells, we performed microarray analysis on skin γδ T cells sorted from total epidermal cell preparations from 10-week old BKS lean *db/+* and obese *db/db* mice.

Based on the gene array, we found that skin γδ T cells differentially express NR4A1 and NR4A3, two orphan nuclear receptors which have been shown to sensitize muscle to insulin and have been reported to be underexpressed in obesity and type 2 diabetes [35]. We observed reduced expression of both NR4A1 and NR4A3 in γδ T cells isolated from obese *db/db* mice (**Figure 4A**), suggesting that skin γδ T cells residing in *db/db* animals have decreased insulin sensitivity. Additionally, Pdk1, a central molecule that regulates Akt function, and two members of the mTORC2 complex, Rictor and Sin 1 (Mapkap1), all display decreased gene expression in skin γδ T cells isolated from obese *db/db* mice (**Figure 4B**). Together these genes, which are necessary for the growth and function of γδ T cells [36], were altered in obese mice and reveal a breakdown in the normal signaling pathways required for skin γδ T cells homeostasis and function.

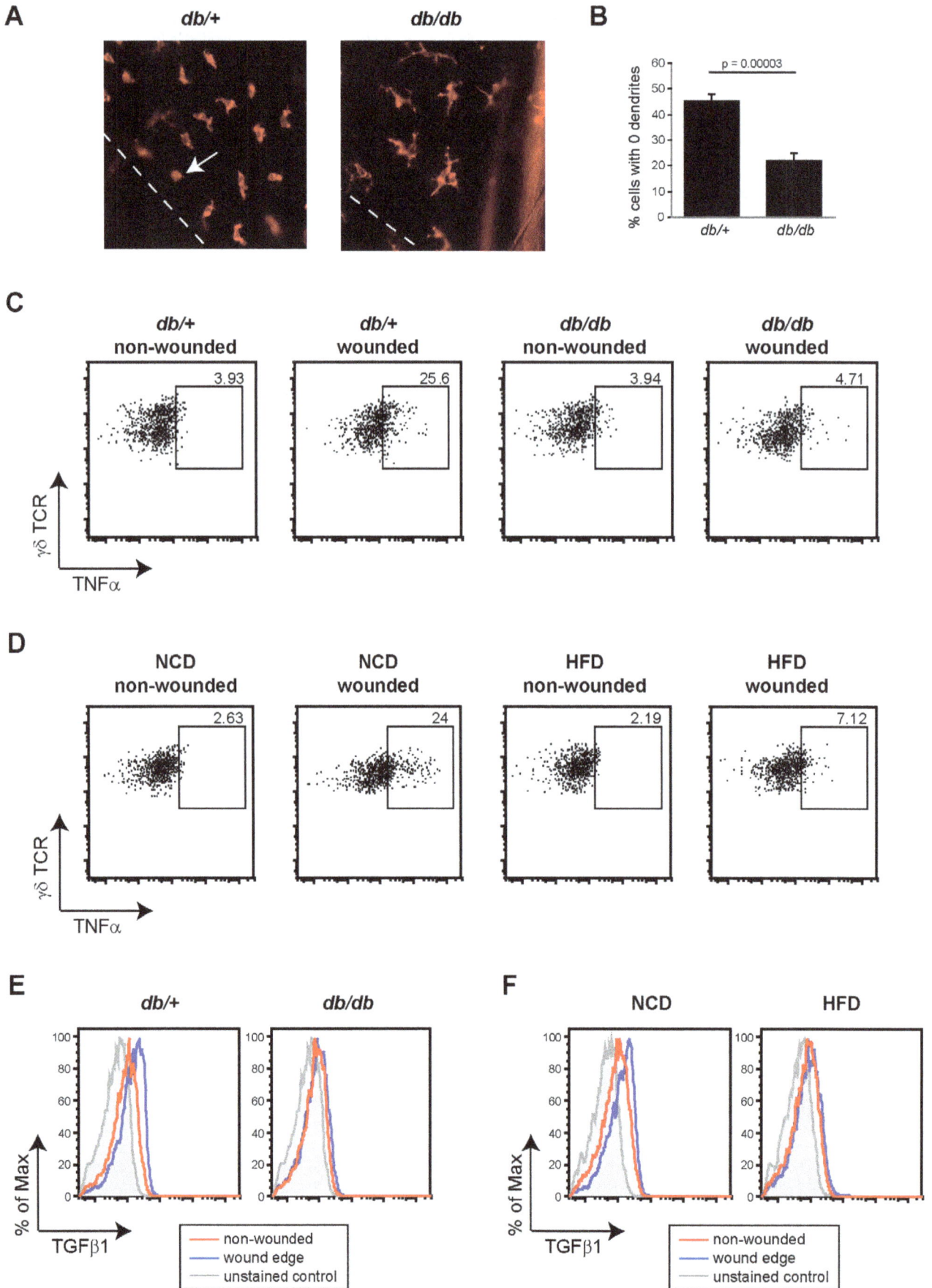

A

db/+   *db/db*

B

p = 0.00003

% cells with 0 dendrites

db/+   *db/db*

C

| *db/+* non-wounded | *db/+* wounded | *db/db* non-wounded | *db/db* wounded |

3.93   25.6   3.94   4.71

γδ TCR

TNFα

D

| NCD non-wounded | NCD wounded | HFD non-wounded | HFD wounded |

2.63   24   2.19   7.12

γδ TCR

TNFα

E

db/+   *db/db*

% of Max

TGFβ1

— non-wounded
— wound edge
— unstained control

F

NCD   HFD

% of Max

TGFβ1

— non-wounded
— wound edge
— unstained control

Figure 3. Obese mice display impaired skin γδ T cell wound healing functions after injury. (**A**) Immunofluorescent staining for γδ TCR in 12-week old lean BKS *db/+* and obese *db/db* mice four hours post-wounding. The white dashed line represents the wound edge and arrowheads depict γδ T cells that have rounded near the wound edge. A minimum of 10 images was acquired at the wound edge for each experiment and the number of dendrites was determined per cell, a minimum of 300 total cells were counted. (**B**) Shown is the percentage of γδ T cells with 0 dendrites per cell (mean ± SEM). All images were acquired at ×200 magnification. (**C, D**) Skin γδ T cell production of TNFα in non-wounded and wounded skin tissue of (**C**) 12-week old BKS *db/+* and *db/db* mice and (**D**) 27-week old B6 NCD and HFD mice. The numbers represent the percentage of cells expressing TNFα. Skin γδ T cell production of TGFβ1 in non-wounded and wounded skin tissue of (**E**) 12-week old BKS *db/+* and *db/db* mice and (**F**) 27-week old B6 NCD and HFD mice. The numbers represent the percentage of cells expressing TGFβ1. Epidermal cells were gated on live Thy1.2$^+$ and γδ TCR$^+$ to distinguish γδ T cells. Shown is one representative experiment, a minimum of three experiments were performed with similar results (**A–F**).

A breakdown in skin γδ T cell signaling pathways may result in changes to their characteristic innate T cell phenotype and function. Skin γδ T cells express a Vγ3Vδ1 TCR and constitutively elevated levels of the activation markers CD69 and CD25 (IL-2 receptor α), suggesting that they are primed to rapidly respond to TCR-mediated activation and growth factors, such as IL-2 [1,36,37]. No changes were observed in the expression of activation markers on skin γδ T cells isolated from 6-week old BKS *db/+* and *db/db* mice (**Figure S4A**). However, in obese *db/db* mice at 10-weeks of age, skin γδ T cells reproducibly displayed diminished levels of CD69, CD25 and CD103 (**Figure 4C**). Furthermore, γδ TCR expression was reproducibly decreased in 10-week old obese *db/db* mice (**Figure 4D**), but no decrease in γδ TCR expression was observed in 6-week old *db/db* mice (**Figure S4B**). Decreased expression of activation markers and γδ TCR may be due to overstimulation by stressed keratinocytes in obesity and metabolic disease.

γδ TCR does not contribute to epidermal T cell dysfunction in obesity

To investigate the contribution of the γδ TCR to the hyporesponsive state of skin γδ T cells in obesity, we crossed B6 δ$^{-/-}$ and B6 *db/+* animals to generate mice lacking γδ TCR that develop obesity and metabolic disease (**Figure 5A**). The epidermis of γδ T cell knockout mice (δ$^{-/-}$) lacks Vγ3$^+$ T cells but does have an αβ T cell population that takes up residence, however, these αβ T cells do not respond to keratinocyte damage [37]. No differences in breeding, litter size or growth of the animals were observed in the B6 δ$^{-/-}$ *db/db* mice as compared to B6 *db/db* animals. Both male and female B6 δ$^{-/-}$ *db/db* mice gained weight and became obese similar to B6 *db/db* mice (**Figure 5B**).

To determine the impact of the γδ TCR on maintenance of homeostatic numbers of epidermal T cells in δ$^{-/-}$ *db/db* animals, epidermal αβ T cells were visualized using immunofluorescent microscopy. In both δ$^{-/-}$ *db/+* control and δ$^{-/-}$ *db/db* mice, the only T cell population in the epidermis was CD3$^+$ αβ T cells; no γδ T cells or other CD3$^+$ populations were present, similar to the epidermal T cell makeup of B6 δ$^{-/-}$ mice (**data not shown**). However, in 14-week old obese δ$^{-/-}$ *db/db* mice there were ~30% fewer epidermal αβ T cells compared with lean δ$^{-/-}$ *db/+* control animals (**Figure 5C**). This suggests that the keratinocyte antigen-specific γδ TCR is not necessary for the decline in epidermal T cell numbers observed in obesity.

Although the epidermal αβ T cells identified in B6 δ$^{-/-}$ mice are not responsive to keratinocyte damage, they do express the activation markers CD69, CD25 and CD103 similar to γδ T cells in the skin [37]. Since expression of these molecules was diminished on γδ T cells in the obese environment, we determined whether activation markers on epidermal αβ T cells in the B6 δ$^{-/-}$ *db/db* mouse were similarly affected. Decreased expression of both CD69 (**Figure 5D**) and CD25 (**data not shown**) was observed on epidermal αβ T cells in 14-week old obese B6 δ$^{-/-}$ *db/db* mouse similar to that observed on epidermal γδ T cells in obese B6 *db/db* mice. Together, this data suggests that the

hyporesponsiveness observed in γδ T cells of obese mice is not TCR mediated or a direct consequence of overactivation by stressed keratinocytes. Therefore, dysfunction of skin γδ T cells in obesity and metabolic disease may be a direct consequence of the inflammatory milieu of the obese environment.

Rescue of skin γδ T cell function ex vivo

If the environment in obesity and metabolic disease contributes to skin γδ T cell dysfunction, we hypothesized that removal from this environment would improve skin γδ T cell function. To investigate whether the response of skin γδ T cells in obese mice can be restored by removal from their environment, we isolated epidermal sheets from 10- to 14-week old obese BKS *db/db* mice and lean *db/+* controls and stimulated the skin-resident T cells *in vitro* with anti-CD3ε antibody. After 6 hours in culture, we visualized epidermal sheets by immunofluorescent microscopy and quantified the number of dendrites per cell to determine cellular rounding after stimulation. The majority of γδ T cells in unstimulated epidermal sheets exhibited 3 or more dendrites per cell (**Figure 6A**). However, after anti-CD3ε stimulation, γδ T cells began to round up similarly in epidermal sheets isolated from obese *db/db* and control *db/+* mice, as indicated by the reduced number of skin γδ T cells with 3 or more dendrites per cell (**Figure 6A and 6B**). This indicates that removing epidermal cells from the obese *db/db* mouse, where they were unable to round upon wounding, restores the ability of γδ T cells to respond to stimulation.

Since stimulating epidermal sheets from obese *db/db* mice *ex vivo* restored the ability of skin γδ T cells to round, we next identified whether other γδ T cell functions could be rescued as well. To determine if cytokine production could be restored by removing γδ T cells from the obese environment, we isolated epidermal cells from 10- to 14-week old BKS lean *db/+* and obese *db/db* mice and cultured them in plates either coated with PBS (unstimulated) or anti-CD3ε antibody. Strikingly, upon removal from the obese environment, anti-CD3ε stimulated skin γδ T cells from obese *db/db* mice were able to produce cytokines, such as TNFα, and upregulate the activation marker CD25 to a similar degree as skin γδ T cells isolated from control *db/+* animals (**Figure 6C**). Together, these data demonstrate that the dysfunction of skin γδ T cells in the obese *db/db* mouse is not permanent. It suggests that by removing extrinsic factors present in obesity and metabolic disease through the isolation of these cells from the epidermis, the hyporesponsive state of skin γδ T cells can be reversed.

Blocking TNFα in obese mice restores skin γδ T cell function in epithelial repair

Increased plasma TNFα levels correlate with obesity and insulin resistance in both humans and animals [38]. Our microarray data revealed that several members of the TNFα signaling pathway were increased in skin γδ T cells isolated from obese *db/db* mice, including Traf2, Tradd and Ripk1 (**Figure 7A**), which lead to activation of NF-κB and Jun N-terminal kinase (JNK) [39]. As

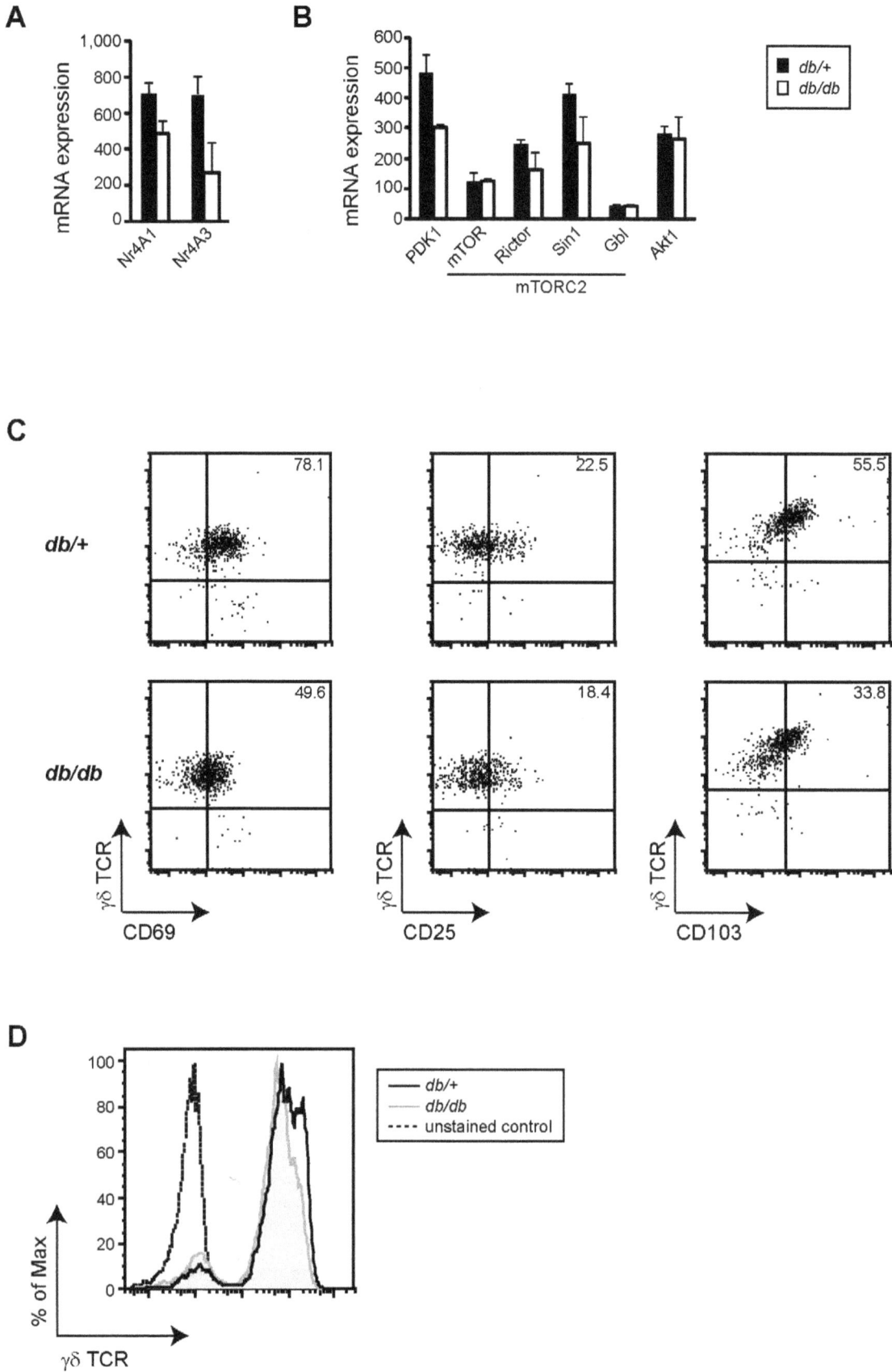

Figure 4. Impaired activation and nutrient sensing by skin γδ T cells in obese mice. (**A, B**) Microarray analysis of skin γδ T cells isolated from 10-week old BKS db/+ and db/db mice. Shown is gene expression of molecules associated with (**A**) insulin sensitivity and (**B**) PI3K/Akt/mTOR signaling. Data is presented as the mean of two independent experiments ± SEM. (**C**) Multiparameter flow cytometry of CD69, CD25 and CD103 on the cell surface of γδ T cells isolated from BKS db/+ and db/db in mice at 10-weeks of age. Numbers in the top right corners indicate percent of γδ T cells. (**D**) γδ TCR expression on γδ T cells isolated from BKS db/+ (solid line) and db/db (shaded gray) at 10-weeks of age. Dotted lines represent unstained controls. Epidermal cells were gated on live Thy1.2+ to distinguish γδ T cells. A minimum of three experiments were performed per age, shown is one representative experiment for each, the same number of events is presented for each dot plot.

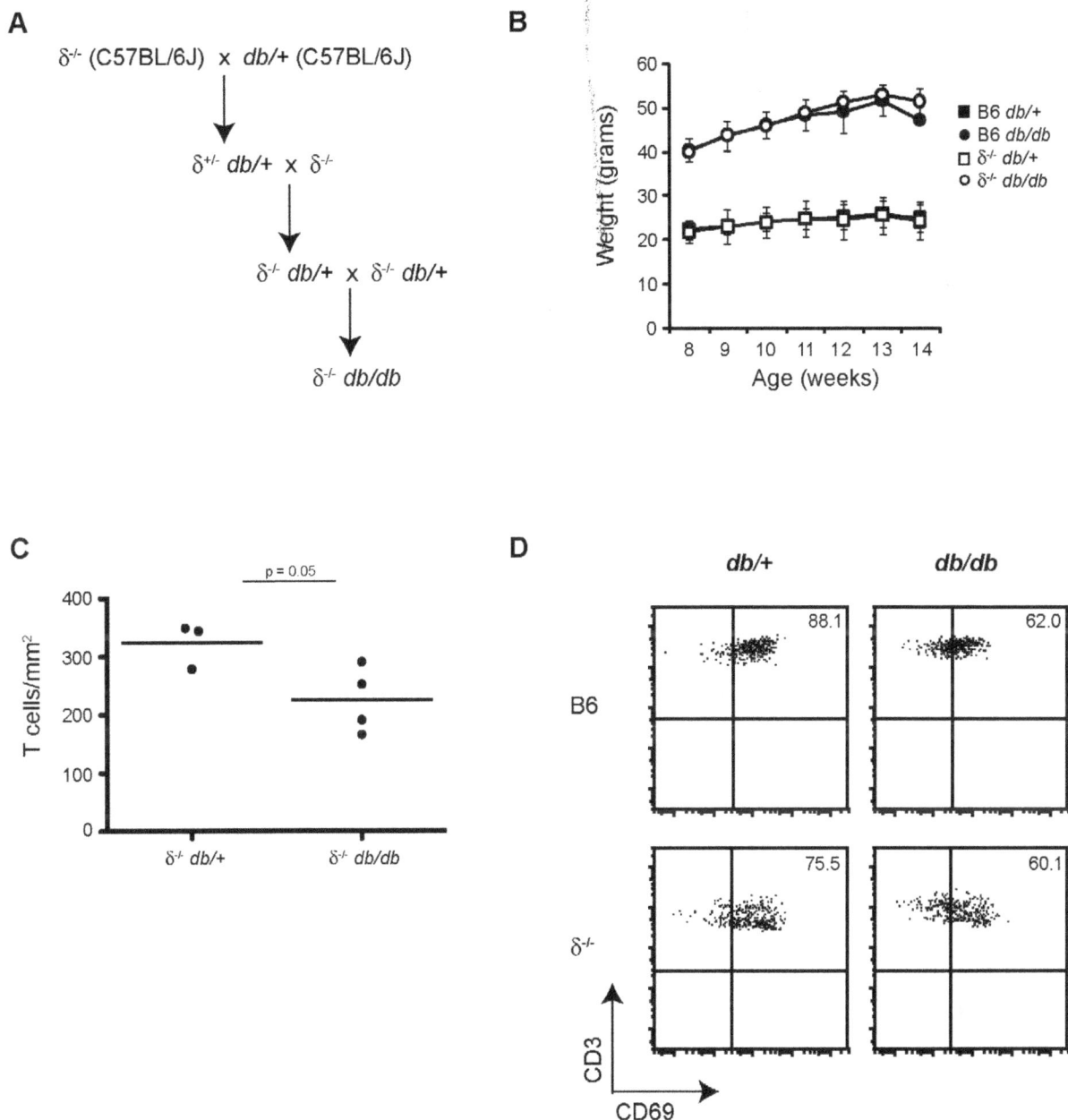

A

δ-/- (C57BL/6J) × db/+ (C57BL/6J)

↓

δ+/- db/+ × δ-/-

↓

δ-/- db/+ × δ-/- db/+

↓

δ-/- db/db

B

■ B6 db/+
● B6 db/db
□ δ-/- db/+
○ δ-/- db/db

C

p = 0.05

D

db/+   db/db

B6   88.1   62.0

δ-/-   75.5   60.1

CD3

CD69

Figure 5. γδ TCR does not contribute to defective skin γδ T cells in obese mice. (**A**) $\delta^{-/-}$ db/db mice were generated by breeding C57BL/6J $\delta^{-/-}$ mice with C57BL/6J db/+ mice. (**B**) Weight of $\delta^{-/-}$ db/db and B6 db/db obese mice compared to their $\delta^{-/-}$ db/+ and B6 db/+ lean littermates. Data is presented as the mean weight ± SD. Between two and eleven mice were weighed per age per strain. (**C**) Graphical representation of the number of epidermal T cells at 14-weeks of age. Skin γδ T cells were counted in epidermal ear sheets from three $\delta^{-/-}$ db/+ mice and four $\delta^{-/-}$ db/db mice. The mean was determined for each experiment (black dots) and the black line represents the average of all the experiments. A minimum of 15 fields were counted for each mouse per experiment, with a minimum of 500 cells per experiment, a minimum of three independent experiments were performed. (**D**) Multiparameter flow cytometry of CD69 expression on the cell surface of γδ T cells isolated from B6 db/+ and db/db and $\delta^{-/-}$ db/+ and db/db mice at 14-weeks of age. Numbers on the top right corner indicate percent of αβ T cells. Epidermal cells were gated on live CD3+ and Thy1.2+ to distinguish epidermal T cells. A minimum of three experiments were performed, shown is one representative experiment, the same number of events is presented for each dot plot.

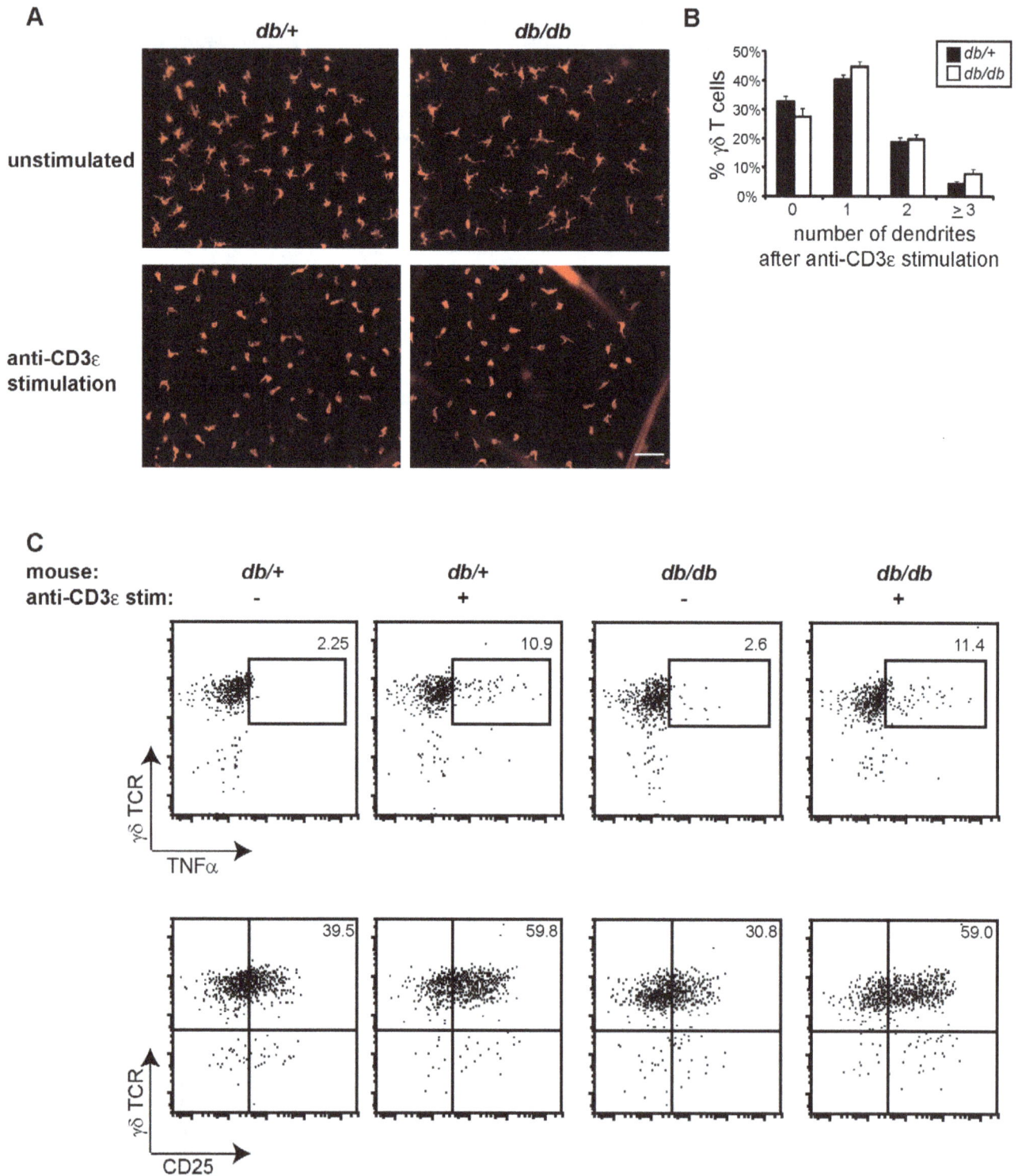

Figure 6. The obese environment inhibits skin γδ T cell function. (**A**) Skin γδ T cell morphology changes in epidermal sheets isolated from 10- to 14-week old BKS *db/+* and *db/db* following *in vitro* stimulation with 10 μg/ml anti-CD3ε antibody compared to unstimulated control. All microscopy images were acquired at ×200 and the bar represents 0.05 μm. (**B**) Shown is a graphical representation of the percentage of skin γδ T cells with 0, 1, 2 or ≥3 dendrites, which represent the degree of γδ T cell rounding (mean ± SEM), in epidermal ear sheets from 10- to 14-week old BKS *db/+* and obese *db/db* animals stimulated with 10 μg/ml anti-CD3ε antibody. Three independent experiments were performed, a minimum of 10 fields were counted for each, and this data represents the average of all 35 fields and approximately 1000 total cells. (**C**) Multiparameter flow cytometry of TNFα production and CD25 expression by γδ T cells isolated from 10- to 14-week old BKS *db/+* and *db/db* mice following overnight stimulation with 1 μg/ml anti-CD3ε. Numbers in the upper right corner indicate percent γδ T cells. Epidermal cells gated on live Thy1.2⁺ events. Data are representative of at least three independent experiments.

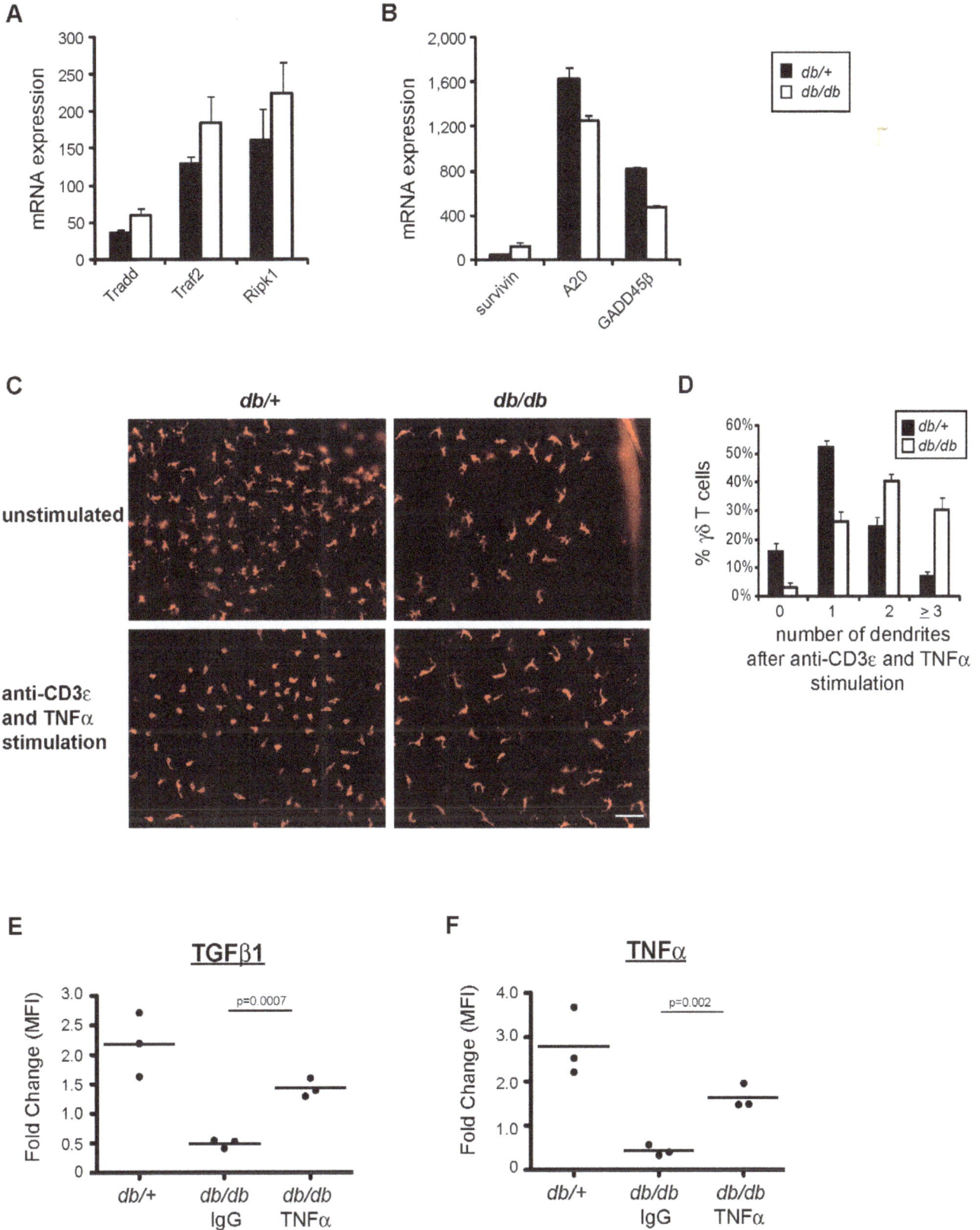

Figure 7. Neutralization of TNFα rescues skin γδ T cell function at the wound site. (A, B) Microarray analysis of skin γδ T cells isolated from 10-week old BKS db/+ and obese db/db mice. Shown is gene expression of molecules associated with TNFα signaling. Data is presented as the mean of two independent experiments ± SEM. (C) Epidermal sheets isolated from 10- to 14-week old BKS db/+ and obese db/db animals either unstimulated or stimulated with 10 μg/ml anti-CD3ε antibody and 100 ng/ml TNFα. All microscopy images were acquired at ×200 and the bar represents 0.05 μm. (D) Quantification of the percentage of skin γδ T cells with 0, 1, 2 or ≥3 dendrites, which represent the degree of γδ T cell rounding (mean ± SEM), in epidermal ear sheets from 10- to 14-week old BKS db/+ and obese db/db animals stimulated with 10 μg/ml anti-CD3ε

antibody and 100 ng/ml TNFα. Three independent experiments were performed, a minimum of 10 fields were counted for each, and this data represents the average of all 35 fields and approximately 1000 total cells. (**E, F**) Fold change in MFI of (**E**) TGFβ1 and (**F**) TNFα expression in skin γδ T cells isolated from the wound edge compared to non-wound edge cells. Skin γδ T cells from 10- to 14-week old BKS *db/+* mice were used as a positive control, 10- to 14-week old *db/db* mice were either treated with 1 mg/kg IgG control antibody or anti-TNFα antibody for a minimum of four days. Shown in fold change in MFI for 3 separate experiments, significance was determined by *t-test*.

shown in **Figure 7B**, downstream molecules contributing to survival, such as Birc5 (survivin), are increased in skin γδ T cells isolated from obese *db/db* animals. However, molecules that negatively regulate Ripk1 and Jnk signaling, such as Tnfaip3 (A20) and GADD45β respectively [40], are decreased in γδ T cells isolated from obese *db/db* mice.

Since elevated gene expression of TNFα signaling molecules was observed in skin γδ T cells isolated from obese *db/db* mice, we set out to determine the consequence of elevated and chronic TNFα levels on skin γδ T cell function. Exogenous TNFα was added to cultured epidermal sheets isolated from control and obese animals. If TNFα alone contributes to the suppressive inflammatory milieu, skin γδ T cells would remain impaired upon *ex vivo* stimulation in the presence of this cytokine. Epidermal sheets from 10- to 14-week old lean *db/+* mice, which have not been exposed to chronic TNFα in their environment, rounded when stimulated with anti-CD3ε antibody in the presence of acute TNFα (**Figure 7C and 7D**). However, γδ T cells in epidermal sheets isolated from obese *db/db* animals, which have been exposed to elevated and chronic TNFα in their environment, displayed delayed rounding when stimulated with anti-CD3ε antibody only if TNFα was present (**Figure 7C and 7D**). As shown in **Figure 6A**, epidermal sheets from obese *db/db* mice were able to round following stimulation with anti-CD3ε antibody alone. This suggests that TNFα alone alters the ability of skin γδ T cells to round following stimulation, providing a mechanism for skin γδ T cell dysfunction.

Due to the contribution of chronic TNFα to γδ T cell dysfunction, we investigated whether skin γδ T cell responses to tissue damage could be restored *in vivo* by treatment with neutralizing anti-TNFα antibody. 10- to 14-week old obese *db/db* animals were treated daily for a minimum of four days with 1 mg/kg anti-TNFα or IgG control antibody. On day 4, full-thickness punch biopsy wounds were performed on each animal and epidermal cells were isolated around the wound edge 24 hours post-wounding. Skin γδ T cells isolated from obese *db/db* animals treated with anti-TNFα antibody showed improved TGFβ1 production as compared to *db/db* animals treated with IgG control antibody (**Figure 7E**). Similar rescue of TNFα production was observed in skin γδ T cells isolated from *db/db* animals treated with anti-TNFα (**Figure 7F**). A significant improvement in skin γδ T cell function at the wound site suggests that chronic inflammatory conditions, specifically in the form of TNFα, contributes to skin γδ T cell hyporesponsiveness to *in vivo* wounding in obesity and metabolic disease.

Discussion

Skin γδ T cells contribute to homeostatic maintenance of the epidermis and respond early to epithelial damage. Skin complications associated with obesity, metabolic disease and type 2 diabetes include barrier dysfunction, chronic non-healing wounds and increased infection. Due to their role in epidermal homeostasis and early response to keratinocyte damage, we investigated whether skin γδ T cell are functional in mouse models of obesity and metabolic disease. Strikingly, we observed a biphasic progression of epidermal T cell dysfunction and the parameters responsible for each phase of T cell dysfunction were distinct. Hyperglycemia impacted early skin γδ T cell proliferation and homeostasis, ultimately resulting in reduced epidermal T cell numbers. Chronic inflammation, occurring later in metabolic disease, rendered skin γδ T cells hyporesponsive to *in vivo* stimulation. In spite of this, skin γδ T cell dysfunction was reversible as improved cytokine production to *in vivo* stimulation was restored by systemic anti-TNFα antibody treatment. To our knowledge, this is the first description correlating different stages of lymphocyte dysfunction to disease progression in obesity.

Nutrients, such as glucose, are critical for lymphocyte survival, proliferation, differentiation and function [41,42]. Many growth factors, such as insulin, IGF-1 and members of the common γc cytokine family (IL-2, IL-4, IL-7, IL-15) increase glucose uptake and metabolism via signaling through the PI3K/Akt pathway [42]. For example, IL-7 signaling in lymphocytes results in STAT5 and PI3K/Akt activation-induced glucose uptake [43]. However, we report here that during the first phase of dysfunction, skin γδ T cells are highly susceptible to alterations in glucose concentrations. Similarly, both αβ T cells and B cells have been shown to exhibit reduced proliferation when exposed to elevated glucose concentrations *in vitro* [43]. This suggests that although glucose and other nutrients may be critical for lymphocyte homeostasis and function, a chronic overabundance of nutrients is detrimental to the maintenance of γδ T cells in the epidermis.

Elevated glucose resulted in altered STAT5 phosphorylation after IL-2 stimulation *in vitro* and ultimately impaired γδ T cell proliferation. STAT5A/B signaling is critical to γδ T cells as mice deficient in STAT5A/B lack γδ T cells [27]. The inability of glucose-treated γδ T cells to phosphorylate STAT5B in response to IL-2 points directly to an effect on proliferation as mice expressing a constitutively active STAT5B have an expanded γδ T cell population [44]. Additionally, the severity of loss of skin γδ T cells in BKS *db/db* mice correlates with a period of rapid expansion of γδ T cells in the epidermis at 6-weeks of age. The hyperglycemic conditions during this seeding are severe in BKS *db/db* mice which may explain the sharp decrease in γδ T cells. Overall, these data demonstrate that skin γδ T cells are highly sensitive to metabolic changes, such as hyperglycemia, in the cellular environment and respond to this stress by shutting down nutrient sensing pathways, such as cytokine and growth factor signal reception, resulting in decreased homeostatic proliferation and a reduced epidermal T cell compartment.

In the next phase of metabolic disease, skin γδ T cells become unresponsive to tissue damage, resulting in reduced production of skin γδ T cell cytokines and growth factors. Skin γδ T cells are important mediators of inflammation and tissue repair as mice deficient in γδ T cells (δ−/− mice) exhibit delayed wound healing [1]. Additionally, skin-resident T cells in chronic wounds isolated from human patients do not upregulate growth factor production, which may contribute to the inability of chronic non-healing wounds to resolve [19]. In addition to the production of cytokines by skin γδ T cells early in tissue damage, skin γδ T cells also produce growth factors which are critical to skin homeostasis [16]. We observed a decrease in homeostatic TGFβ1 production by skin γδ T cells and an inability to upregulate TGFβ1 following injury in obesity and metabolic disease. In the skin, the effects of TGFβ1 are broad and contribute to various aspects of wound healing including inflammation, angiogenesis, tissue remodeling and reepithelialization [45]. Altered TGFβ1 production by skin γδ T cells in obesity and metabolic disease may impact multiple phases of epidermal homeostasis and early and late stages of tissue repair.

To understand how the environment impacts the ability of skin γδ T cells to respond to *in vivo* damage, we performed microarray analysis to investigate alterations in gene expression and found an increase in expression of molecules involved in TNFα signaling. In primary cells, TNFα induces NF-κB but not cell death pathways, and chronic TNFα would predictably result in chronic NF-κB activation, gene expression and survival [39]. This persistent activation leads to the induction of reactive oxygen species [39], which can attenuate T cell responses [46,47], and uncouple TCR signal transduction, resulting in lower cell surface expression of the TCR/CD3 complex [48]. This supports our observation that cell surface γδ TCR expression is decreased and downstream molecules regulating survival and negative feedback of NF-κB signaling were altered in skin γδ T cells isolated from obese mice.

In addition, chronic TNFα and persistent NF-κB activation negatively impact other cell signaling pathways, including PI3K/Akt/mTOR signaling [36,49,50]. TNFα and NF-κB suppress TSC1 inhibition of mTORC1, resulting in hyperactive mTORC1 activity, which contributes to insulin resistance [50]. Recently, mTORC1 has been shown to negatively inhibit mTORC2 signaling, a necessary complex for Akt activation, and may negatively inhibit growth factor signaling in pathways that don't require IRS-1 [51]. Furthermore, knockdown or deletion of mTORC2 complex molecules, including Rictor, Sin1 and Gbl, result in defective mTORC2 complex assembly and Akt activation [52,53,54]. Both mTORC1 and mTORC2 have been shown to be critical for skin γδ T cell homeostasis and *in vivo* wound healing response [36]. Chronic TNFα stimulation of skin γδ T cells results in direct effects, including alterations in TCR expression, and effects on other signaling pathways, including mTOR and Akt. These alterations in signaling ultimately render epidermal T cells hyporesponsive to barrier tissue disruption and keratinocyte damage.

Together, our data demonstrate that obesity and metabolic disease negatively impact the homeostasis and wound healing functions of γδ T cells located in the epidermal barrier. The impact of chronic TNFα on γδ T cells was reversible, suggesting that therapeutic strategies targeting the inflammatory environment and γδ T cell dysfunction may provide additional treatments for complications associated with obesity, metabolic disease and type 2 diabetes. In addition to the skin, intraepithelial γδ T cells reside in multiple barrier tissue locations, including the lung and intestinal tract, and the impact of metabolic disease on the function of other resident γδ T cell populations is unknown. The consequence of reduced numbers and unresponsiveness of γδ T cells in multiple barrier tissues would result in compromised ability to protect against damage or environmental insults and increased susceptibility to infection. This study demonstrates a previously unrecognized biphasic progression of skin γδ T cell dysfunction in obesity and metabolic disease, in which hyperglycemia impacts skin γδ T cell proliferation and homeostasis and chronic inflammatory mediators alter skin γδ T cell response to barrier damage.

Materials and Methods

Ethics Statement

All animals were handled in strict accordance with good animal practice as defined by the relevant national and/or local animal welfare bodies. All animal work was approved by The Scripps Research Institute Institutional Animal Care and Use Committee (protocol 08-0057).

Mice

Wild-type C57BLKS/J, BKS-*Lepr^db* heterozygous (C57BLKS/J *db/+*), and B6- *Lepr^db* heterozygous (C57BL/6J *db/+*) mice were purchased from The Jackson Laboratory (Bar Harbor) and were housed and bred at The Scripps Research Institute (TSRI). Wild-type C57BL/6J mice were bred at TSRI Rodent Breeding Colony. For high fat diet experiments, wild-type male C57BL/6J mice were placed on a 60 kcal% fat diet (Research Diets) at 6 weeks of age, control mice were maintained on a 5 kcal% (Harlan Laboratory) or a 10 kcal% (Research Diets) diet. To generate $\delta^{-/-}$ *db/db* mice, C57BL/6J $\delta^{-/-}$ were crossed with C57BL/6J *db/+* mice to generate $\delta^{-/-}$ *db/+* mice. All mice were periodically weighed and blood glucose monitored by an Ascensia Elite XL blood glucose monitor (Bayer). BKS *db/+* and *db/db* mice were assayed at 6 weeks and at 10- and 14-weeks of age. For HFD experiments, mice were assayed after 20 to 26 weeks on HFD. Mice were given access to food and water ad libitum and were housed in sanitized conditions.

Flow cytometry

FITC-, PE-, or allophycocyanin-conjugated monoclonal antibodies specific for γδ TCR (GL3), Vγ3+ (536), CD25 (PC61), TNFα (MP6-XT22), CD45.2, IL-4Rα and Thy1.2 (53.2.1) were purchased from BD Biosciences, CD69 (H1.2F3), CD103, CD3ε, and Langerin antibodies were purchased from eBioscience, and TGFβ1 was purchased from R&D Systems. The BD Bioscience Cytofix/Cytoperm kit was used for intracellular staining and Annexin-V/PI kit for flow cytometry. Cells were acquired with DiVa 5.0 software on a Digital LSRII (BD Biosciences) and analyzed with FlowJo software (Tree Star, Inc.). For FACS plots, gating was determined for each individual experiment using negative or isotype controls.

In vitro γδ 7–17 cell line

The skin γδ T-cell line 7–17 was maintained in complete RPMI (Mediatech, Inc.) supplemented with 10% heat-inactivated FBS and 20U/ml IL-2. For proliferation studies, 7–17 cells were plated at 1×10^5 cells per well in a 96 well flat bottom plate in IL-2 containing growth media with either glucose (MediaTech) or fatty acids (palmitic acid, oleic acid and linoleic acid (Sigma)). Cells were pulsed with 1 μCi/well [³H]thymidine (MP Biomedicals), harvested and incorporation of radioactive material was determined using a β-counter (Beckman). Fatty acids were prepared for cell culture assays as described elsewhere [55]. For analysis of phosphorylated STAT5A and STAT5B, 7–17 cells were pretreated with starvation media for 4 hours, then placed into IL-2 containing growth media supplemented with 33.3 mM glucose for 24 hours. Cells were starved for additional 4 hours +/− glucose, followed by treatment with 40U/ml IL-2. Cells were lysed in TritonX Lysis Buffer, analyzed by Western blot using antibodies against phosphorylated STAT5A/STAT5B (Tyr⁶⁹⁴) and total STAT5 (Cell Signaling), probed with secondary goat anti-rabbit IgG-HRP (Southern Biotech) and developed with Super Signal West Pico Chemiluminescence Kit (Thermo Scientific).

Epidermal cell preparation

Epidermal cells were isolated from mouse skin as described previously [1,37] and rested at 37°C for 3–16 hours followed by antibody staining and flow cytometric analysis. For *in vitro* stimulation experiments, epidermal cells were isolated from mouse epidermis and placed into culture in complete DMEM media (Mediatech, Inc.) supplemented with 10% heat-inactivated FBS (Omega Scientific) and stimulated overnight with pre-coated anti-CD3ε antibody at 1 µg/ml. Approximately 16 to 18 hours after culturing, cells were treated with 5 µg/ml brefeldin A (Sigma) for 4 hours at 37°C, isolated and stained intracellularly with antibodies for flow cytometry. All cells were cultured at 37°C and 5% CO_2.

Freshly isolated γδ T cells

Epidermal cell preparations were prepared from wild-type C57BL/6J mice as described above, and γδ T cells were sorted on a FACSAria (TSRI Flow Cytometry Lab) based on anti-Thy1.2 antibody staining to a minimum of 95% purity. Skin γδ T cells were collected into FCS, spun down and placed directly into 96 well round bottom plates in normal growth media (cRPMI with 10% FBS and 100U/ml IL-2) with baseline (11.1 mM) or elevated (33.3 mM) glucose. Cell proliferation was based on [³H] thymidine incorporation as described above.

BrdU treatment *in vivo*

Mice were given a one time i.p. injection of 3.3 mg/ml BrdU (Sigma) in PBS, followed by 7 days of BrdU in their drinking water at 0.8 mg/ml. Mice were euthanized on day 8 and epidermal cells were isolated as described above. BrdU incorporation was detected by using the FITC BrdU Flow Kit (BD Biosciences).

Epidermal ear sheet and whole skin immunofluorescence

Epidermal sheets were isolated and stained as described previously [1,37]. For *in vitro* stimulation assays, ears were removed from control *db/+* animals, separated in half and floated on DMEM media (supplemented with 10% FBS) and treated with 10 µg/ml anti-CD3ε antibody or 100 ng/ml recombinant TNFα (R&D Systems) as indicated. After indicated incubation at 37°C, ear sheet halves were removed, the epidermal sheet was separated from the dermis using ammonium thiocyanate and staining was performed. To visualize cross-sections of mouse skin, whole skin tissue was embedded in O.C.T. compound (Tissue-Tek), and 10 µm skin sections were cut on a Leica Cryostat. Sections were fixed with 4% paraformaldehyde for 10 minutes, and immunostained with γδ TCR and CD3ε antibodies. DAPI was used to counterstain the sections. Digital images were acquired (Zeiss AxioCam HRc) and analyzed using Photoshop CS2 software (Adobe). At least three separate experiments were performed for each time point and a minimum of 500 cells were quantified per experiment.

Animal dorsal and ear wounding protocols

Full-thickness biopsy punch wounds were performed on the dorsal surface and ears of mice as previously described [1,14]. At the indicated time after wounding, mice were euthanized and wounds were harvested. Epidermal sheets were isolated for analysis of γδ T cell rounding at the wound site by immunofluorescent microscopy. Epidermal cells were isolated using trypsin as described above, allowed to rest three hours in the presence of 5 µg/ml brefeldin A at 37°C, and followed by intracellular antibody staining for TNFα and/or TGFβ1 expression and analysis by flow cytometry. For anti-TNFα treatment, obese *db/db* animals were randomly assigned to a treatment group, then weighed and blood glucose determined before the start of experiment. Mice received 1 mg/kg either anti-TNFα or IgG control antibody (Biolegend) each day i.p. for a minimum of 4 days

total. On the final day of treatment, mice were euthanized and full-thickness punch biopsy wounds were administered as described above. Non-wounded skin and skin at the wound edge was removed 24 hours post-wounding and epidermal cells were isolated and stained for intracellular cytokine production as described above.

Microarray analysis

Epidermal cell preparations from mice were isolated and skin γδ T cells were sorted on a FACSAria as described above. Skin γδ T cells were collected directly into TRIzol LS reagent (Invitrogen), RNA was immediately isolated using the Qiagen RNeasy Micro RNA Kit and submitted to the TSRI DNA Array Core. 100 ng product was processed with GeneChip Whole Transcript Sense Target Labeling Assay (Affymetrix) and cDNA was hybridized overnight to the Mouse Gene 1.0ST Array (two independent data sets for each sample). Chips were scanned using the Affymetrix GeneChip Scanner 3000 7G with default settings and a target intensity of 250 for scaling. Data normalization was performed using RMA Express 1.0 with quantile normalization, median polish and background adjustment. This data has been deposited in NCBI's Gene Expression Omnibus and is accessible through GEO Series accession number GSE22196.

PCR determination of Lep and Lepr isoforms (Ob-Ra and Ob-Rb)

RNA was isolated from primary sorted skin γδ T cells or 7–17 cell lines with TRIzol reagent and transcribed into cDNA with reverse transcriptase (Invitrogen). 1 µl cDNA was amplified using PCR with primers directed against Ob-Ra and Ob-Rb for 35 cycles [56], leptin for 30 cycles [57] and β-actin controls [1]. A plasmid containing leptin cDNA was kindly provided by Dr. Luc Teyton (The Scripps Research Institute, La Jolla).

Lymph node staining

Lymph nodes were isolated from mice and pooled. Cells were mechanically disrupted from the tissue by gently agitating between two frosted slides in DMEM. Cells were stained for flow cytometric analysis using antibodies listed above.

Statistic analysis

Data are presented as mean ± SEM or mean ± SD and significance was determined using the *t-test* function of Microsoft Excel (two-tailed).

Supporting Information

Table S1
Found at: doi:10.1371/journal.pone.0011422.s001

Figure S1 Expression of Leptin and Leptin Receptor in skin γδ T cells. RT-PCR for expression of Lep mRNA in skin γδ T cells isolated from BKS db/+ and db/db mice, or from skin γδ 7-17 T cells ±1 µg/ml anti-CD3ε stimulation for 2 hours or 24 hours. Shown is Lep cDNA positive control and H2O negative control. Expression of Lepr isoforms, Ob-Ra and Ob-Rb, mRNA was not detected in mouse γδ T cells. RT-PCR for expression of Lepr in skin γδ T cells isolated from BKS db/+ and db/db mice, or in 7–17 skin γδ T cells ±1 µg/ml anti-CD3ε stimulation for 2 hours or 24 hours. Shown is whole liver positive control and H2O negative control. β-actin expression was used to control for all PCR reactions.
Found at: doi:10.1371/journal.pone.0011422.s002

Figure S2 Fatty acids do not inhibit skin γδ T cell growth. Proliferation of skin γδ 7–17 T cells in IL-2 containing growth media supplemented with palmitic, lineolic and oleic acid between 0 and 200 μM. Each experiment was performed in duplicate, data presented as mean ± SD.
Found at: doi:10.1371/journal.pone.0011422.s003

Figure S3 Skin γδ T cells in the db/db mouse are not undergoing apoptosis or migration. (A) Multiparameter flow cytometry of annexin-V/PI staining of skin γδ T cells, gated on Thy1.2+ expression, at 6-, 8- and 14-weeks of age. Numbers indicate the percent of γδ T cells. A minimum of two experiments were performed per time point, shown is one representative experiment. (B) Skin sections from 10- to 14-week old BKS db/+ and db/db mice were immunostained with γδ TCR (red) and dapi (blue). Three separate experiments were performed with similar results. Magnification is ×200, bar represents 0.05 μm. (C) γδ T cell populations in skin-draining lymph nodes isolated from 10- to 14-week old BKS db/+ and db/db animals. In the upper plots, live cells were gated on Thy1.2+ and Vγ3+, exclusive markers for skin-specific γδ T cells. In the lower plots, cells were gated on γδ TCR+ and CD3+ T cells to visualize the peripheral γδ T cell population. Numbers indicate percent γδ T cells. Data are representative of two independent experiments.
Found at: doi:10.1371/journal.pone.0011422.s004

Figure S4 Skin γδ T cell activation marker and γδ TCR expression is not altered by hyperglycemia. (A) Multiparameter

flow cytometry of CD69, CD25 and CD103 on the cell surface of γδ T cells isolated from BKS db/+ and db/db in mice at 6-weeks of age. Numbers in the top right corners indicate percent of γδ T cells. (B) γδ TCR expression on γδ T cells isolated from BKS db/+ (solid line) and db/db (shaded gray) at 6-weeks of age. Dotted lines represent unstained controls. Epidermal cells were gated on live Thy1.2+ to distinguish γδ T cells. A minimum of three experiments were performed per age, shown is one representative experiment for each, the same number of events is presented for each dot plot.
Found at: doi:10.1371/journal.pone.0011422.s005

Acknowledgments

We thank Drs. Deborah Witherden, Kerri Mowen, David Nemazee, H. Kiyomi Komori, Ryan Kelly, Stephanie Degner, Jared Purton and M. Rachel Richards for technical advice and manuscript review. We thank Sherry Torng, Alexandre Webster, Jennifer Hao and Max Rich for technical assistance and Steve Head of the TSRI DNA Array Core for microarray assistance. We thank Dr. Wendy Havran for her support and advice.

Author Contributions

Conceived and designed the experiments: KRT JMJ. Performed the experiments: KRT REM AEC. Analyzed the data: KRT REM AEC JMJ. Wrote the paper: KRT JMJ.

References

1. Jameson J, Ugarte K, Chen N, Yachi P, Fuchs E, et al. (2002) A role for skin γδ T cells in wound repair. Science 296: 747–749.
2. Cheroutre H (2005) IELs: enforcing law and order in the court of the intestinal epithelium. Immunol Rev 206: 114–131.
3. Komori HK, Meehan TF, Havran WL (2006) Epithelial and mucosal γδ T cells. Curr Opin Immunol 18: 534–538.
4. Xiong N, Raulet DH (2007) Development and selection of γδ T cells. Immunol Rev 215: 15–31.
5. Born WK, Jin N, Aydintug MK, Wands JM, French JD, et al. (2007) γδ T lymphocytes-selectable cells within the innate system? J Clin Immunol 27: 133–144.
6. Boismenu R, Feng L, Xia YY, Chang JC, Havran WL (1996) Chemokine expression by intraepithelial γδ T cells. Implications for the recruitment of inflammatory cells to damaged epithelia. J Immunol 157: 985–992.
7. Born WK, Lahn M, Takeda K, Kanehiro A, O'Brien RL, et al. (2000) Role of γδ T cells in protecting normal airway function. Respir Res 1: 151–158.
8. Nanno M, Shiohara T, Yamamoto H, Kawakami K, Ishikawa H (2007) γδ T cells: firefighters or fire boosters in the front lines of inflammatory responses. Immunol Rev 215: 103–113.
9. Garman RD, Doherty PJ, Raulet DH (1986) Diversity, rearrangement, and expression of murine T cell gamma genes. Cell 45: 733–742.
10. Havran WL, Chien YH, Allison JP (1991) Recognition of self antigens by skin-derived T cells with invariant γδ antigen receptors. Science 252: 1430–1432.
11. Hayday AC (2000) γδ cells: a right time and a right place for a conserved third way of protection. Annu Rev Immunol 18: 975–1026.
12. Girardi M (2006) Immunosurveillance and immunoregulation by γδ T cells. J Invest Dermatol 126: 25–31.
13. Jameson J, Havran WL (2007) Skin γδ T-cell functions in homeostasis and wound healing. Immunol Rev 215: 114–122.
14. Jameson JM, Cauvi G, Sharp LL, Witherden DA, Havran WL (2005) γδ T cell-induced hyaluronan production by epithelial cells regulates inflammation. J Exp Med 201: 1269–1279.
15. Daniel T, Thobe BM, Chaudry IH, Choudhry MA, Hubbard WJ, et al. (2007) Regulation of the postburn wound inflammatory response by γδ T-cells. Shock 28: 278–283.
16. Sharp LL, Jameson JM, Cauvi G, Havran WL (2005) Dendritic epidermal T cells regulate skin homeostasis through local production of insulin-like growth factor 1. Nat Immunol 6: 73–79.
17. Girardi M, Lewis JM, Filler RB, Hayday AC, Tigelaar RE (2006) Environmentally responsive and reversible regulation of epidermal barrier function by γδ T cells. J Invest Dermatol 126: 808–814.
18. Dupuy P, Heslan M, Fraitag S, Hercend T, Dubertret L, et al. (1990) T-cell receptor-γδ bearing lymphocytes in normal and inflammatory human skin. J Invest Dermatol 94: 764–768.

19. Toulon A, Breton L, Taylor KR, Tenenhaus M, Bhavsar D, et al. (2009) A role for human skin-resident T cells in wound healing. J Exp Med 206: 743–750.
20. Blakytny R, Jude E (2006) The molecular biology of chronic wounds and delayed healing in diabetes. Diabet Med 23: 594–608.
21. Cavanagh PR, Lipsky BA, Bradbury AW, Botek G (2005) Treatment for diabetic foot ulcers. Lancet 366: 1725–1735.
22. Nishimura S, Manabe I, Nagasaki M, Eto K, Yamashita H, et al. (2009) CD8+ effector T cells contribute to macrophage recruitment and adipose tissue inflammation in obesity. Nat Med 15: 914–920.
23. Winer S, Chan Y, Paltser G, Truong D, Tsui H, et al. (2009) Normalization of obesity-associated insulin resistance through immunotherapy. Nat Med 15: 921–929.
24. Feuerer M, Herrero L, Cipolletta D, Naaz A, Wong J, et al. (2009) Lean, but not obese, fat is enriched for a unique population of regulatory T cells that affect metabolic parameters. Nat Med 15: 930–939.
25. Henri S, Poulin LF, Tamoutounour S, Ardouin L, Guilliams M, et al. (2010) CD207+ CD103+ dermal dendritic cells cross-present keratinocyte-derived antigens irrespective of the presence of Langerhans cells. J Exp Med 207: 189–206, S181-186.
26. Hennighausen L, Robinson GW (2008) Interpretation of cytokine signaling through the transcription factors STAT5A and STAT5B. Genes Dev 22: 711–721.
27. Yao Z, Cui Y, Watford WT, Bream JH, Yamaoka K, et al. (2006) Stat5a/b are essential for normal lymphoid development and differentiation. Proc Natl Acad Sci U S A 103: 1000–1005.
28. Tough DF, Sprent J (1998) Lifespan of γδ T cells. J Exp Med 187: 357–365.
29. Reichelt J, Magin TM (2002) Hyperproliferation, induction of c-Myc and 14-3-3sigma, but no cell fragility in keratin-10-null mice. J Cell Sci 115: 2639–2650.
30. Raymond K, Kreft M, Janssen H, Calafat J, Sonnenberg A (2005) Keratinocytes display normal proliferation, survival and differentiation in conditional beta4-integrin knockout mice. J Cell Sci 118: 1045–1060.
31. Misawa M, Watanabe S, Ihara S, Muramatsu T, Matsuzaki T (2008) Accelerated proliferation and abnormal differentiation of epidermal keratinocytes in endo-beta-galactosidase C transgenic mice. Glycobiology 18: 20–27.
32. Merad M, Manz MG, Karsunky H, Wagers A, Peters W, et al. (2002) Langerhans cells renew in the skin throughout life under steady-state conditions. Nat Immunol 3: 1135–1141.
33. Poulin LF, Henri S, de Bovis B, Devilard E, Kissenpfennig A, et al. (2007) The dermis contains langerin+ dendritic cells that develop and function independently of epidermal Langerhans cells. J Exp Med 204: 3119–3131.
34. Boismenu R, Hobbs MV, Boullier S, Havran WL (1996) Molecular and cellular biology of dendritic epidermal T cells. Semin Immunol 8: 323–331.
35. Fu Y, Luo L, Luo N, Zhu X, Garvey WT (2007) NR4A orphan nuclear receptors modulate insulin action and the glucose transport system: potential role in insulin resistance. J Biol Chem 282: 31525–31533.

36. Mills RE, Taylor KR, Podshivalova K, McKay DB, Jameson JM (2008) Defects in skin γδ T cell function contribute to delayed wound repair in rapamycin-treated mice. J Immunol 181: 3974–3983.

37. Jameson JM, Cauvi G, Witherden DA, Havran WL (2004) A keratinocyte-responsive γδ TCR is necessary for dendritic epidermal T cell activation by damaged keratinocytes and maintenance in the epidermis. J Immunol 172: 3573–3579.

38. Wellen KE, Hotamisligil GS (2005) Inflammation, stress, and diabetes. J Clin Invest 115: 1111–1119.

39. Clark J, Vagenas P, Panesar M, Cope AP (2005) What does tumour necrosis factor excess do to the immune system long term? Ann Rheum Dis 64 Suppl 4: iv70–76.

40. Bubici C, Papa S, Pham CG, Zazzeroni F, Franzoso G (2004) NF-kappaB and JNK: an intricate affair. Cell Cycle 3: 1524–1529.

41. Frauwirth KA, Thompson CB (2004) Regulation of T lymphocyte metabolism. J Immunol 172: 4661–4665.

42. Maciver NJ, Jacobs SR, Wieman HL, Wofford JA, Coloff JL, et al. (2008) Glucose metabolism in lymphocytes is a regulated process with significant effects on immune cell function and survival. J Leukoc Biol 84: 949–957.

43. Wofford JA, Wieman HL, Jacobs SR, Zhao Y, Rathmell JC (2008) IL-7 promotes Glut1 trafficking and glucose uptake via STAT5-mediated activation of Akt to support T-cell survival. Blood 111: 2101–2111.

44. Burchill MA, Goetz CA, Prlic M, O'Neil JJ, Harmon IR, et al. (2003) Distinct effects of STAT5 activation on CD4+ and CD8+ T cell homeostasis: development of CD4+CD25+ regulatory T cells versus CD8+ memory T cells. J Immunol 171: 5853–5864.

45. Barrientos S, Stojadinovic O, Golinko MS, Brem H, Tomic-Canic M (2008) Growth factors and cytokines in wound healing. Wound Repair Regen 16: 585–601.

46. Cope AP, Londei M, Chu NR, Cohen SB, Elliott MJ, et al. (1994) Chronic exposure to tumor necrosis factor (TNF) in vitro impairs the activation of T cells through the T cell receptor/CD3 complex; reversal in vivo by anti-TNF antibodies in patients with rheumatoid arthritis. J Clin Invest 94: 749–760.

47. Cope AP, Liblau RS, Yang XD, Congia M, Laudanna C, et al. (1997) Chronic tumor necrosis factor alters T cell responses by attenuating T cell receptor signaling. J Exp Med 185: 1573–1584.

48. Isomaki P, Panesar M, Annenkov A, Clark JM, Foxwell BM, et al. (2001) Prolonged exposure of T cells to TNF down-regulates TCR zeta and expression of the TCR/CD3 complex at the cell surface. J Immunol 166: 5495–5507.

49. Ozes ON, Akca H, Mayo LD, Gustin JA, Maehama T, et al. (2001) A phosphatidylinositol 3-kinase/Akt/mTOR pathway mediates and PTEN antagonizes tumor necrosis factor inhibition of insulin signaling through insulin receptor substrate-1. Proc Natl Acad Sci U S A 98: 4640–4645.

50. Lee DF, Kuo HP, Chen CT, Wei Y, Chou CK, et al. (2008) IKKbeta suppression of TSC1 function links the mTOR pathway with insulin resistance. Int J Mol Med 22: 633–638.

51. Julien LA, Carriere A, Moreau J, Roux PP (2010) mTORC1-activated S6K1 phosphorylates Rictor on threonine 1135 and regulates mTORC2 signaling. Mol Cell Biol 30: 908–921.

52. Guertin DA, Stevens DM, Thoreen CC, Burds AA, Kalaany NY, et al. (2006) Ablation in mice of the mTORC components raptor, rictor, or mLST8 reveals that mTORC2 is required for signaling to Akt-FOXO and PKCalpha, but not S6K1. Dev Cell 11: 859–871.

53. Jacinto E, Facchinetti V, Liu D, Soto N, Wei S, et al. (2006) SIN1/MIP1 maintains rictor-mTOR complex integrity and regulates Akt phosphorylation and substrate specificity. Cell 127: 125–137.

54. Yang Q, Inoki K, Ikenoue T, Guan KL (2006) Identification of Sin1 as an essential TORC2 component required for complex formation and kinase activity. Genes Dev 20: 2820–2832.

55. Listenberger LL, Ory DS, Schaffer JE (2001) Palmitate-induced apoptosis can occur through a ceramide-independent pathway. J Biol Chem 276: 14890–14895.

56. Lee GH, Proenca R, Montez JM, Carroll KM, Darvishzadeh JG, et al. (1996) Abnormal splicing of the leptin receptor in diabetic mice. Nature 379: 632–635.

57. Yoshida T, Monkawa T, Hayashi M, Saruta T (1997) Regulation of expression of leptin mRNA and secretion of leptin by thyroid hormone in 3T3-L1 adipocytes. Biochem Biophys Res Commun 232: 822–826.

Imaging Mass Spectrometry Visualizes Ceramides and the Pathogenesis of Dorfman-Chanarin Syndrome Due to Ceramide Metabolic Abnormality in the Skin

Naoko Goto-Inoue[1], Takahiro Hayasaka[1], Nobuhiro Zaima[2], Kimiko Nakajima[3], Walter M. Holleran[4], Shigetoshi Sano[3], Yoshikazu Uchida[4*◗], Mitsutoshi Setou[1*◗]

1 Department of Cell Biology and Anatomy, Hamamatsu University School of Medicine, 1-20-1 Handayama, Higashi-ku, Hamamatsu, Shizuoka, Japan, 2 Department of Applied Biological Chemistry, Kinki University, Nara, Nara, Japan, 3 Department of Dermatology, Kochi Medical School, Kochi University, Kohasu, Okocho, Nankoku, Nankoku, Japan, 4 Department of Dermatology, School of Medicine, University of California San Francisco, Department of Veterans Affairs Medical Center, and Northern California Institute for Research and Education, San Francisco, California, United States of America

Abstract

Imaging mass spectrometry (IMS) is a useful cutting edge technology used to investigate the distribution of biomolecules such as drugs and metabolites, as well as to identify molecular species in tissues and cells without labeling. To protect against excess water loss that is essential for survival in a terrestrial environment, mammalian skin possesses a competent permeability barrier in the stratum corneum (SC), the outermost layer of the epidermis. The key lipids constituting this barrier in the SC are the ceramides (Cers) comprising of a heterogeneous molecular species. Alterations in Cer composition have been reported in several skin diseases that display abnormalities in the epidermal permeability barrier function. Not only the amounts of different Cers, but also their localizations are critical for the barrier function. We have employed our new imaging system, capable of high-lateral-resolution IMS with an atmospheric-pressure ionization source, to directly visualize the distribution of Cers. Moreover, we show an ichthyotic disease pathogenesis due to abnormal Cer metabolism in Dorfman–Chanarin syndrome, a neutral lipid storage disorder with ichthyosis in human skin, demonstrating that IMS is a novel diagnostic approach for assessing lipid abnormalities in clinical setting, as well as for investigating physiological roles of lipids in cells/tissues.

Editor: Leah J. Siskind, MUSC SC College of Pharmacy, United States of America

Funding: This work was supported by a Grant-in-Aid under the SENTAN program of the Japan Science and Technology Agency to TH, Grant-in-Aid for Scientific Research (C) for NG-I, Grant-in-aid for the scientific research project "Machinery of bioactive lipids in homeostatis and diseases" for MS, and National Institutes of Health Grant (AR051077 and AR062025) for YU. The funders had no role in study design, data collection and analysis, decision to publish, or preparation of the manuscript.

Competing Interests: The authors have declared that no competing interests exist.

* E-mail: uchiday@derm.ucsf.edu (YU); setou@hama-med.ac.jp (MS)

◗ These authors contributed equally to this work.

Introduction

Imaging mass spectrometry (IMS) has several advantages for exploring the two-dimensional distribution of lipids [1–3]: First, IMS does not require any labels or specific probes to investigate the localization; second, IMS is a non-targeted imaging method, allowing us to detect the localization of unexpected metabolites [4–7]. Finally, IMS allows the simultaneous imaging of many types of molecular species at once. Therefore, IMS has been a powerful technique for characterizing and/or determining the distribution of molecular species on tissue sections [8,9]. IMS has been applied to lipid imaging analysis because lipids have relatively small molecular sizes compared to proteins/peptides and lack specific probes for other imaging techniques. A technical difficulty of IMS exists in the ionization efficiency of some lipids, including ceramides (Cers). In addition, the resolution and sensitivities of IMS are based on laser and ionization methods. The recent experimental model of IMS demonstrates the highest resolution (<1 μm) [10], while conventional matrix-assisted laser desorption/ionization (MALDI) imaging mass spectrometers are equipped with lasers of diameter 10–100 μm [11–14]. We have developed the instrument composed of an atmospheric-pressure (AP) ion-source chamber for MALDI and a quadrupole ion trap time-of-flight (QIT-TOF) mass spectrometer [15]. Using a 10-μm-diameter laser, the instrument can visualize the distribution of biomolecules, including volatile molecules. Since this machine employs an AP ion-source chamber that utilizes soft ionization and a QIT that concentrates the specific ions to be analyzed, we hypothesize that ion suppression of Cers from other lipids is avoided in this case.

Mammalian skin possesses a competent barrier to prevent excess water loss, localized in the outer layer of the skin, the epidermis, predominantly consisting of keratinocytes. Keratinocytes proliferate at the stratum basale (SB), and migrate towards the skin surface to the stratum spinosum (SS), the stratum granulosum (SG), and then the stratum corneum (SC), in parallel with their differentiation (Fig. 1). The SC is largely responsible for the barrier function of the skin. This outermost epidermal layer is composed of terminally differentiated (denucleated) keratinocytes,

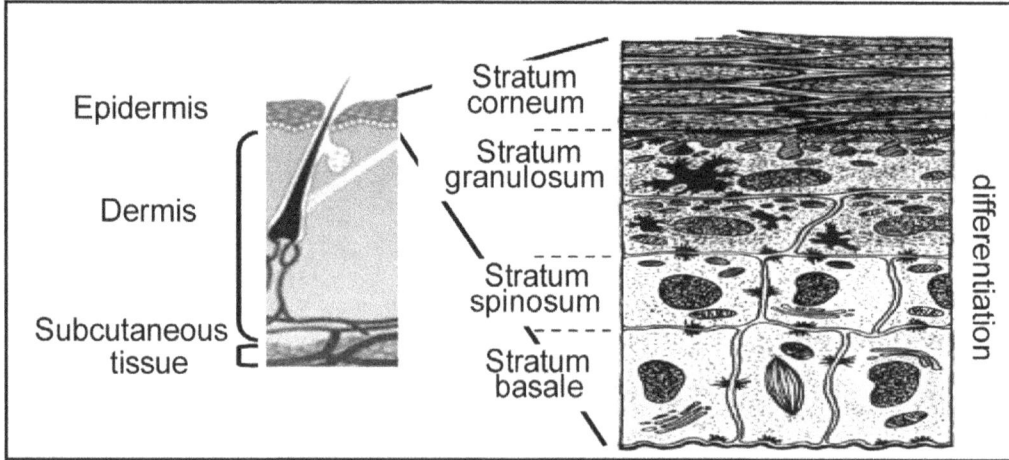

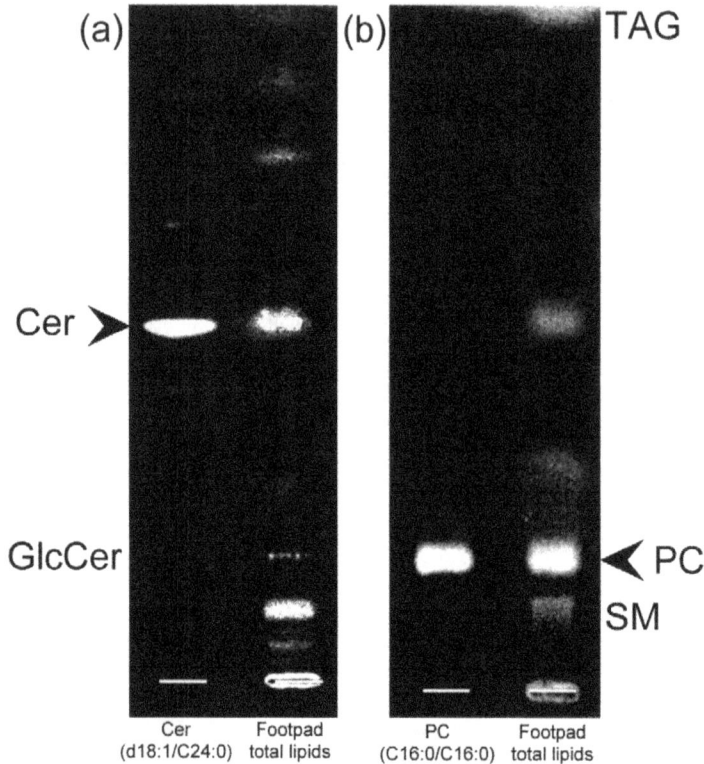

Figure 1. Skin structure and lipid composition of skin. Upper panel shows a model of the structure of the skin. Lower panel shows the results of thin-layer chromatographic analyses of lipid in mouse skin. We assessed lipid composition enriched in mouse footpad skin by TLC analysis. Cer and PC are shown as major lipid species. In addition we also detected GlcCer (a), SM, and TAG (b).The arrowhead shows the localization of standard, Cer (d18:1/C24:0) and PC (C16:0/C16:0).

and corneocytes, surrounded by a mixture of lipids (mainly Cers, cholesterol, and fatty acid), which together form continuous multilamellar membranes serving as a permeability barrier.

Cers are particularly unique in the epidermis in displaying molecular heterogeneity. At least ten molecular groups of species exist due to the variation of the sphingosine base and amide-linked fatty acids (Fig. S1). Ceramide-1-phosphate (Cer1P), which is a metabolite of Cer generated by ceramide kinase, is an anionic bioregulatory lipid that translocates and directly activates cytosolic phospholipase A2, making it a leading mediator of inflammatory

responses [16]. Yet, the roles of Cer1P in epidermal function are unknown.

Glucosylceramide (GlcCer) is a simple glycosphingolipid composed of one mole each of glucose and Cer. GlcCer is enriched in certain tissues, including mammalian skin, and is the major precursor for more complex glycosphingolipid. During differentiation, the most newly synthesized heterogeneous Cer species in the SG are glucosylated to GlcCer [17] or are phosphocholinated to sphingomyelin (SM), and then most are packed into lamellar bodies [18]. The lamellar body membrane fuses with the plasma membrane on the apical surface of the granular cells, at which point its contents are extruded into the interface between the SG and the SC. In parallel to the transition from SG to SC, the glucose moiety of GlcCer is hydrolyzed by ß- glucocerebrosidase, resulting in the production of Cer in the SC [19–21]. A deficiency of ß- glucocerebrosidase or inhibition of its activity in the epidermis decreases the amount of Cer in the SC and results in failure to form a competent epidermal permeability barrier [19,20]. Sphingomyelinase-mediated hydrolysis of SM also contributes to the barrier's homeostasis [22,23]. These prior studies indicate that both GlcCer and SM are immediate precursors for the Cers in the SC. Furthermore, previous studies have demonstrated that not only the total amount of Cers in the SC, but also the distribution of each Cer molecular species is important for the formation of lamellar structures in the SC [24]. Indeed, alteration of Cer composition has been reported in several skin diseases; i.e., atopic dermatitis, psoriasis, and certain ichthyoses that also display epidermal barrier abnormalities [25–28]. Little is known, however, about the mechanism(s) responsible for these alterations; i.e., abnormalities of localization and/or synthesis. Thus, characterization of the specific distribution of each Cer species is important in order to elucidate the relationship between Cers in the SC and the barrier defects of those skin diseases.

Attenuation of permeability barrier function, which not only affects skin (atopic dermatitis, psoriasis, and some ichthyoses), but also affects systemic issues (asthma, food allergy, infection) is a pathogenesis in a number of diseases. In addition, barrier abnormalities cause disease phenotype in several inherited cutaneous diseases, including Dorfman-Chanarin syndrome, a focus of this manuscript. Hence, an accurate, precise, and sensitive method for the quantification of Cer is required for not only investigation of the physiological function of distinct Cer, but also for clinical reasons, i.e., diagnosing Cer deficiencies in subjects provides both pathogenesis and potential therapeutic approaches. In addition, patients, their families, and communities need accurate diagnoses for many reasons, including proper therapy, minimization of disease development, and decreased risks of transfering diseases to the next generation. Currently, Cers are analyzed by enzymatic diacylglycerol kinase assay [29], thin-layer chromatography (TLC) detection [30], high-performance liquid chromatography (HPLC) [31,32], HPLC-mass spectrometry or tandem mass spectrometry [33,34], and gas chromatography mass spectrometry analysis [35]. These approaches of analyzing Cer levels in skin require large amounts of skin samples. In addition, these methods are not able to localize Cer species in the tissues/cells. Whereas immunoelectron microscopic analysis can localize total Cer species in cells and tissues, it cannot localize each molecular species of Cer. A recent study demonstrated skin lipid analysis of sphingolipids, including SM and Cer1P, but not Cer and GlcCer, using MALDI-IMS (spatial resolution is>30 μm) [36]. We here demonstrate that IMS characterizes the distribution of Cer species, as well as Cer1P, GlcCer, SM, and phosphatidylcholine (PC) using 3–5 mm diameter biopsy samples. In addition, our present study reveals new insights into epidermal lipids directly from mammalian tissues and the epidermal metabolic abnormality of a key Cer species, AcylCer, occurring in Dorfman-Chanarin syndrome, a neutral lipid storage disorder with ichthyosis in human skin.

Results

Lipid Composition on Mouse Footpad Skin

Because imaging mass spectra are directly acquired from a section of tissues which contain various amounts of substances, abundant molecules that have higher ionization efficiency are preferentially detected. Therefore, we first assessed lipid composition enriched in murine footpad skin by TLC analysis. The chromatograms showed that Cer (Fig. 1a) and PC (Fig. 1b) are major components. In addition, we also detected GlcCer (Fig 1a), SM, and triacylglycerol (TAG) (Fig 1b). While epidermal Cers comprise a number of heterogeneous species (Fig. S1) [37], one species, Cer (amide-linked non-hydroxy fatty acid and sphingosine) was detected as the major component in mouse footpads, having a similar mobility to the Cer standard (d18:1/C24:0).

The Detection of Ceramide Molecules on Tissue Sections

We first investigated the ionization patterns of the Cer standard (d18:1/C24:0). Figure 2a shows the mass spectrum of Cer (d18:1/C24:0) on stainless target plates with our AP ion-source instrument. We detected m/z 632.5 as a dominant peak; it was assigned to the $[M-H_2O+H]^+$ion. We applied the same scheme with the commercial intermediate vacuum-type MALDI instrument. Although signal intensity of Cer-related ions by vacuum-type MALDI instrument was higher than the AP ion-source instrument, there is no significant difference of a signal-to-noise (S/N) ratio between the two instruments. In contrast to AP ion-source instrument that showed single $[M-H_2O+H]^+$ion, multiple adduct ions, such as $[M-H2O+H]^+$, $[M-H2O+2Na-H]^+$, and $[M+2Na-H]^+$of Cer-related ions were detected in the vacuum-type MALDI instrument (Fig. 2b). Similar results were shown in another intermediate vacuum-type MALDI instrument (data not shown). Multiple substances on a tissue section interfere with and diminish each other's ionization. Therefore, we deposited the Cer standard (d18:1/C24:0) onto a mouse brain tissue section and acquired the mass spectrum of gray square area in the optical image (Fig. 2f). A mass signal, $[M-H_2O+H]^+$, was detected from deposited Cer (arrowhead) in addition to endogenous tissue-derived signals (closed circle) (Fig. 2c). On the contrary, a vacuum-type instrument showed various kinds of adduct ions of Cer, and resulted in a complicated spectrum (Fig. 2d). Subsequent tandem mass spectrometric analysis revealed the generation of stable product ions with m/z 282.3 and 264.3 corresponding to the loss of an amide-bound acyl group and one or two molecules of water, respectively [33] (Fig. 2e), indicating that the signal at m/z 632.5 detected on the brain tissue is a Cer molecule. Moreover, we also visualized ion images of major tissue-derived signals (m/z 638.9, 772.5, and 798.5), as well as Cer at m/z 632.5 (Fig. 2g) and assigned m/z 798.5 as PC (diacyl-16:0/18:1) (Fig. S3) as we reported previously [6]. Other molecules, at m/z 638.9 and 772.5, were not assigned (Fig. 2i, j, k). To verify mass accuracy, we also constructed an ion image at m/z 632.7 (Fig. 2h).

Imaging Mass Spectrometric Analysis of Ceramide Species in Mouse Footpad Skin

We demonstrated here the distribution of various kinds of Cer molecular species on the footpad skin by IMS. The optical image of skin sections, the HE staining images of serial sections and enlarged images are shown in Figures 3a, b, c. IMS analyses, using our AP ion-source instrument, detected some peaks enriched in the fine region of the epidermis. Taken together with tandem mass spectrometric analyses and prior studies that characterize mammalian epidermal Cer species [38,39], we constructed some ion images detected by IMS, as summarized in Table 1. Three Cer1P (m/z 618.40, 646.46, and 730.57) and three Cer peaks (m/z 630.50, 744.68, and 758.70) were deduced as Cer1P (d18:1/C16:0, d18:1/C18:0, d18:1/C24:0), and Cer (d18:1/C24:1, d18:1/C32:0, and d18:1/C32:1h), respectively (Figures 3d, e, f, g, h, i). By comparing the fragment patterns of standard Cer

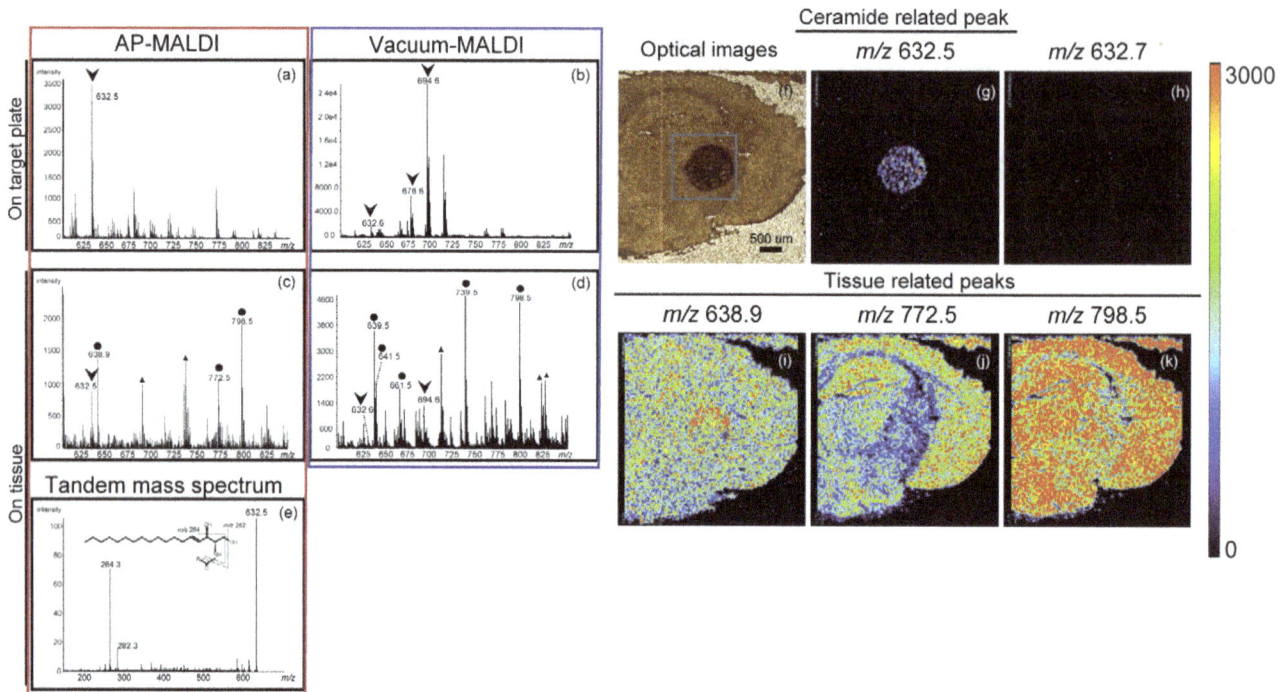

Figure 2. Detection of Ceramides by mass spectrometry. The ionization patterns of Cer standard (d18:1/C24:0) deposited on stainless-steel target plates with AP ion-source instrument (a) and vacuum-type instrument (b). The Cer standard (d18:1/C24:0) was deposited onto a mouse brain tissue section and the mass spectrum was acquired (c and d). A subsequent tandem mass spectrometric analysis of precursor ions at m/z 632.5 was shown (e). The optical image (f) and ion image revealed that m/z 632.5 was predominantly derived from exogenous Cer (g). The ion image at m/z 632.7 is also shown (h). Moreover, we visualized ion images of major tissue-derived signals (m/z 638.9, 772.5, and 798.5) (i–k). Color bar shows signal intensity.

(d18:1/C24:1) and Cer1P (d18:1/C18:0), we successfully confirmed these structures (Fig. S3).

Imaging Mass Spectrometric Analysis of Ceramide Precursors in Murine Footpad Skin

Both GlcCer and SM, which are immediate precursors that generate Cer in the SC, are converted to Cer during transition from SG/SS to SC in epidermis. The abnormality of these conversion has been shown in a pathological condition, such as hyperplasia, as well as inherited disease, *i.e.*, deficiencies of ß-glucoserebrosidase, activator protein of ß-glucoserebrosidase (sapocin C), or sphingomyelinase [40]. Therefore, assessments of GlcCer and SM are a diagnostic approach to these conditions. IMS analysis revealed the presence of at least three SM species (m/z 713.49, 741.51, and 769.52) (Fig. 3j, k, l) and four predictable GlcCer possible ions (m/z 866.65, 880.62 894.65, and 906.63) (Fig. 3p, q, r, s). For tandem mass spectrometric analyses of SM, we detected the neutral loss (NL) of 53 and 183 Da that corresponds to the trimethylamine [(CH3)3N] and the head group [(CH3)3N(CH2)2PO4H] of SM [41] and the fragment ion of d18:1 (m/z 305.0) (Fig. S3) [42], identifying these three as SM species (d18:1/C14:0, d18:1/C16:0, and d18:1/C18:0) (Table 1). Since similar to Cer, GlcCer is a difficult molecular species to ionize compared with other lipid species, to further increase the sensitivity of GlcCer, we minimized the mass range (m/z 800–1200) to allow the efficient accumulation of these ions into the quadrupole ion trap, and succeeded to get clear localization of GlcCers and reproducibility (Fig. 3, tu, v, w and Fig. S4). Tandem mass spectrometric analysis showed the neutral loss (NL) of glucose from a precursor ion and assigned m/z 732.6 as a (d18:1/C26:0h),

while tandem mass spectrometric analyses of other GlcCer species were not completed due to low signal intensities/sensitivity issues. Therefore, we deduced these ions as GlcCer possible species, *i.e.*, GlcCer (d18:1/C24:0h, d18:1/C26:1, d18:1/C26:0h, and d18:1/C28:0) (Table 1).

All SM species were distributed throughout epidermis and dermis. On the other hand, GlcCer, including GlcCer possible ions, were localized at epidermis specifically. In addition, interestingly the composition of FA is completely different between SM and GlcCer (Table 1).

Phosphatidylcholine Detection by Imaging Mass Spectrometry

As shown in Figure 1b, PCs are also major epidermal lipid species in the mouse footpad. IMS analysis shows that three molecular species of PCs, a major component of cellular membrane species, are localized across the skin, including the dermis and significantly decreased (or at trace levels) in the SC (Fig. 3m, n, o). These molecules are annotated based on previous reports [6] [43] and tandem mass spectrometric analyses. Tandem mass spectrometric analysis showed the NL of head group and fatty acids, respectively, and assigned molecular species (Fig. S3 and Table 1). Notably, the molecular ion at m/z 796.5 assigned as PC (diacyl 16:0–18:2) was detected epidermis main PC species, while m/z 798.5 assigned as PC (diacyl 16:0–18:1) was detected in both epidermis and dermis. Since PC is a major membrane constituent, membrane property likely differs in keratinocytes and fibroblasts, and it mainly constituted in epidermis and dermis, respectively.

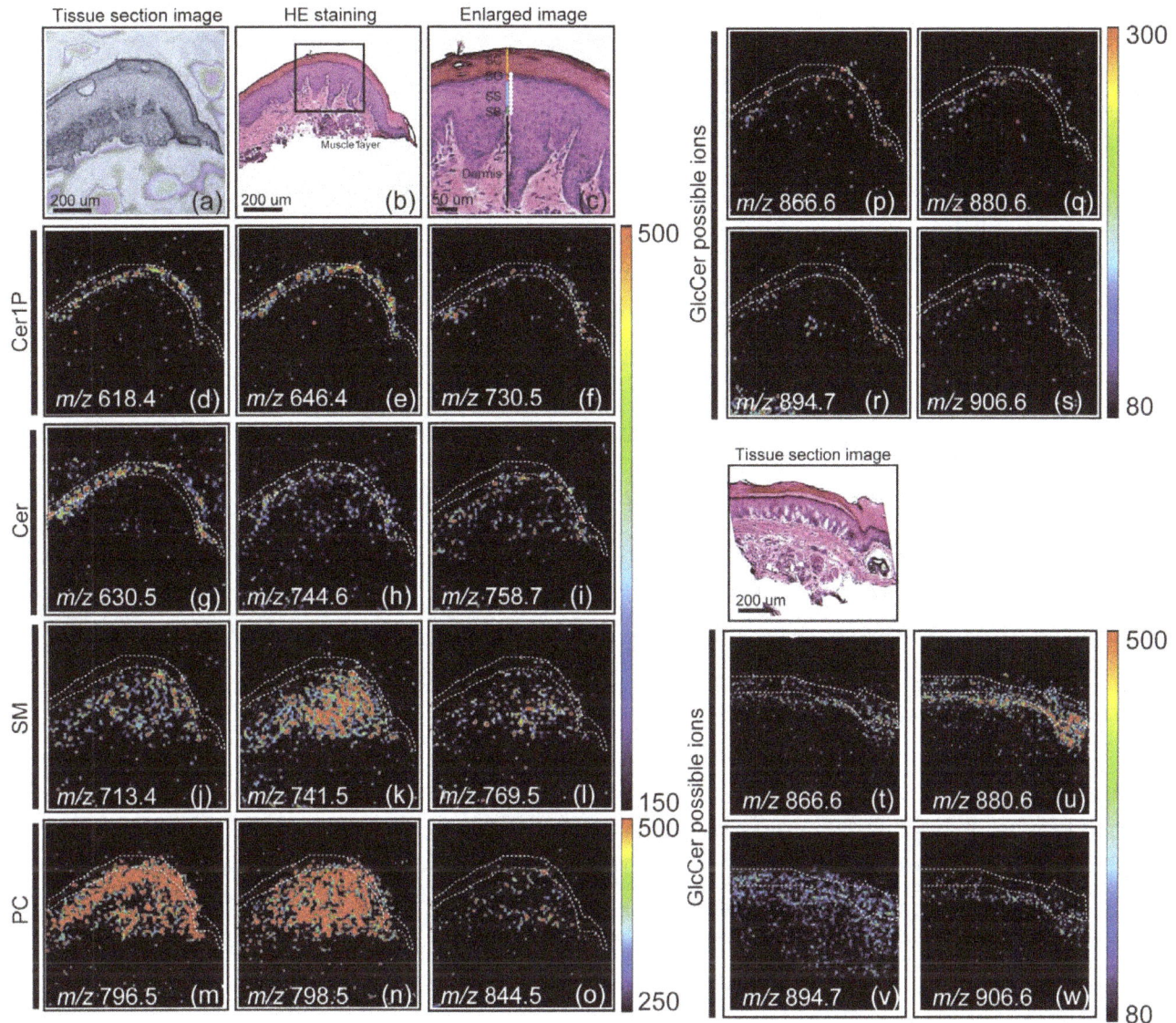

Figure 3. IMS analyses revealed the localization of Cer and Cer-related ions in a mouse footpad skin section. Optical image of mouse footpad section (a), the HE staining image of the serial section (b), the enlarged image (c) are shown. We could detect four layers in the epidermis: SC, SG, SS, and SB. Ion images of Cer1P (d–f), Cer (g–i), SM (j–l), PC (m–o) and GlcCer possible ions (p–s) are shown (SC indicated as a white line; SS and SG indicated as brown lines). We tried to increase sensitivities of GlcCer by limiting detection mass ranges, 800–1200 (t–w). The imaging pixel is 10 μm (a white dot indicates 10 μm, [c]). Color bar shows signal intensity.

Clinical Application of Imaging Mass Spectrometric Analyses

We recently found that AcylCer deficiencies occur in Dorfman–Chanarin syndrome (DCS), an autosomal recessive, neutral lipid storage disorder with ichthyosis, due to loss-of-function mutations in CGI-58 (α/β-hydrolase domain containing protein 5, ABHD5) in human skin [44]. Therefore, we performed IMS analyses of these skins for clinical application to assess whether TAG accumulation, including linoleate-containing species and AcylCer deficiencies, occur in the SC of DCS. To further increase the sensitivity of IMS, we minimized the mass range (m/z 800–1200 for TAG, and m/z 900–1200 for AcylCer) to allow the efficient accumulation of these ions into the quadrupole ion trap and to prevent ion suppression by other lipids. IMS analysis demonstrated that the ion signals of possible AcylCer were significantly attenuated, and conversely that TAGs accumulated in the SC of

the patient compared with the control (Fig. 4). Consistent with our prior lipid analysis of lipid extracts from control normal SC [44], the AcylCer-related ion (m/z 1048.7, d18:1/C34:1) was found to be present in the control normal SC. The AcylCer signal had only trace-level intensity in the patient (Fig. 4a). Moreover, tandem mass spectrometric analysis proved that the accumulation of TAG containing linoleate (m/z 895.7, C16:0/C18:2/C18:1) is one of the major molecular species in the SG, where AcylCer is synthesized, and is also retained in the SC (Fig. 4b). These results clarified that AcylCer deficiencies in the SC of DCS are caused by decreases of that synthesis, rather than misslocalization in the epidermis. Moreover, TAG accumulation does not significantly occur in extra SC regions in skin.

Table 1. List of the molecules observed in the mouse footpad.

Observed m/z	Theoletical m/z	tolerance	ion	possible molecular structure
618.4	618.48	0.08	$[M+H]^+$	Ceramide-1-phosphate (d18:1/C16:0)
630.5	630.62	0.12	$[M-H_2O+H]^+$	Ceramide (d18:1/C24:1)
646.46	646.51	0.05	$[M+H]^+$	Ceramide-1-phosphate (d18:1/C18:0)
713.49	713.49	0	$[M+K]^+$	Sphingomyelin (d18:1/C14:0)
730.57	730.63	0.06	$[M+H]^+$	Ceramide-1-phosphate (d18:1/C24:0)
741.51	741.53	0.02	$[M+K]^+$	Sphingomyelin (d18:1/C16:0)
744.68	744.72	0.04	$[M-H_2O+H]^+$	Ceramide (d18:1/C32:0)
758.7	758.72	0.02	$[M-H_2O+H]^+$	Ceramide (d18:1/C32:1h)
769.52	769.56	0.04	$[M+K]^+$	Sphingomyelin (d18:1/C18:0)
796.53	796.52	−0.01	$[M+K]^+$	Phosphatidylcholine (C16:0/C18:2)
798.55	798.54	−0.01	$[M+K]^+$	Phosphatidylcholine (C16:0/C18:1)
844.54	844.52	−0.02	$[M+K]^+$	Phosphatidylcholine (C16:0/C22:6)
866.65	866.67	0.02	$[M+K]^+$	Glucosylceramide (d18:1/C24:0h)
869.67	869.69	0.02	$[M+K]^+$	Triacylglycerol (C16:0/C16:0/C18:2)
880.62	880.69	0.07	$[M+K]^+$	Glucosylceramide (d18:1/C26:1)
895.64	893.71	0.07	$[M+K]^+$	Triacylglycerol (C16:0/C18:2/C18:1)
894.65	894.67	0.02	$[M+K]^+$	Glucosylceramide (d18:1/C26:0h), (t18:1/C26:1)
897.72	897.73	0.01	$[M+K]^+$	Triacylglycerol (C16:0/C18:1/C18:1)
906.63	906.7	0.07	$[M+K]^+$	Glucosylceramide (d18:1/C28:0)

Underlined molecules are only predicted molecules based on the localization and molecular mass.

Discussion

TLC analysis of extracted lipids suggests that Cers (amide-linked non-hydroxy fatty acid and sphingosine) were a primary target in the mouse footpad epidermis by IMS analysis because the relative amounts of Cer species were higher than the other lipids (Fig. 1). Since a previous report described that the AP ion source exhibits soft ionization [45], we compared ionization patterns of Cer between our AP ion-source instrument and vacuum-type instrument. We found that although the S/N ratio of the two instruments is nearly equal, the ionization tendency of the AP ion-source instrument is different from that of a vacuum-type instrument. As shown in Figure 2, the AP ion-source instrument demonstrated a simple ionization pattern of Cer; but the vacuum type showed multiple adduct ions, which made it complicated. Therefore, our developed instrument equipped with an AP ion-source chamber, which shows the most intense peak with the Cer $[M-H_2O+H]^+$ion, is suitable for ionization of Cer.

Next, we deposited the Cer standard onto a mouse brain tissue section to validate the ionization pattern on tissue sections. Three tissue-derived signals (m/z 638.9, 772.5, and 798.5) were thoroughly distributed in the brain sections. The background signals derived from matrix-related peaks (i.e., signals outside of the tissue) had a one or zero at the first decimal point, and the target lipid derived signals that we assigned showed 4 to 6 at the first decimal point. The mass tolerance of our machine was lower than 0.1 Da in the range of m/z 500–1200. Therefore, it is unlikely that lipid-derived signals overlapped with matrix signals. In contrast, the ion image at m/z 632.5 showed high intensity on the deposited area, revealing that the m/z 632.5 was exogenous Cer. Moreover, the ion image at m/z 632.7 showed a completely different image than m/z 632.5, meaning we could distinguish these ions individually (Fig. 2h). The mass range around 600–800 is complicated with various molecules especially with a vacuum-

type instrument, but not with an AP ion-source instrument (Fig. 2c, d). Because Cer display molecular heterogeneity in certain tissues, in particular epidermis, a simplified spectrum to distinguish their mass is an important requirement. These results suggest that IMS with AP ion-source instrument is appropriate to analyze Cer species on tissues.

Previous immunoelectron microscopic analysis using an anti-Cer antibody showed that anti-Cer staining on the human epidermis was abundantly concentrated at the cell membranes and/or intercellular space in the SC and in the perinuclear region of the cells in the lower SS [38]. A recent report of skin IMS demonstrated the presence of Cer1P (Cer has not been reported) [36]. However, the spatial resolution was not sufficient (30–150 μm), and plural molecular species have not yet been detected. We demonstrated here the distribution of various kinds of Cer molecular species, as well as Cer1P on the footpad skin by IMS (Fig. 3). All Cers were enriched at SC and SG (white-line area). These findings are consistent with the previous study by immunoelectron microscopic analysis [38], as well as lipid quantification from each epidermal layer [46], showing that the Cer content is high at differentiated layers of the epidermis, SC, SG and SS. We summarized the deduced molecular structures based on the previous report [36] compared with the theoretical mass (Table 1). Moreover, we also demonstrated a different localization of Cer-related species due to their amide-linked fatty acid composition (Fig. S2). The result suggested that each Cer-related species shows a different distribution, according to its fatty acid composition.

In the epidermis, some pools of GlcCer and SM localized in the SG are immediate precursors of Cer in the epidermis. As shown in Figure 3, GlcCer was fairly well detected in the brown-line area (SG and SS) but not in the dermis, while SM levels were the same throughout the epidermis and dermis. These results are consistent

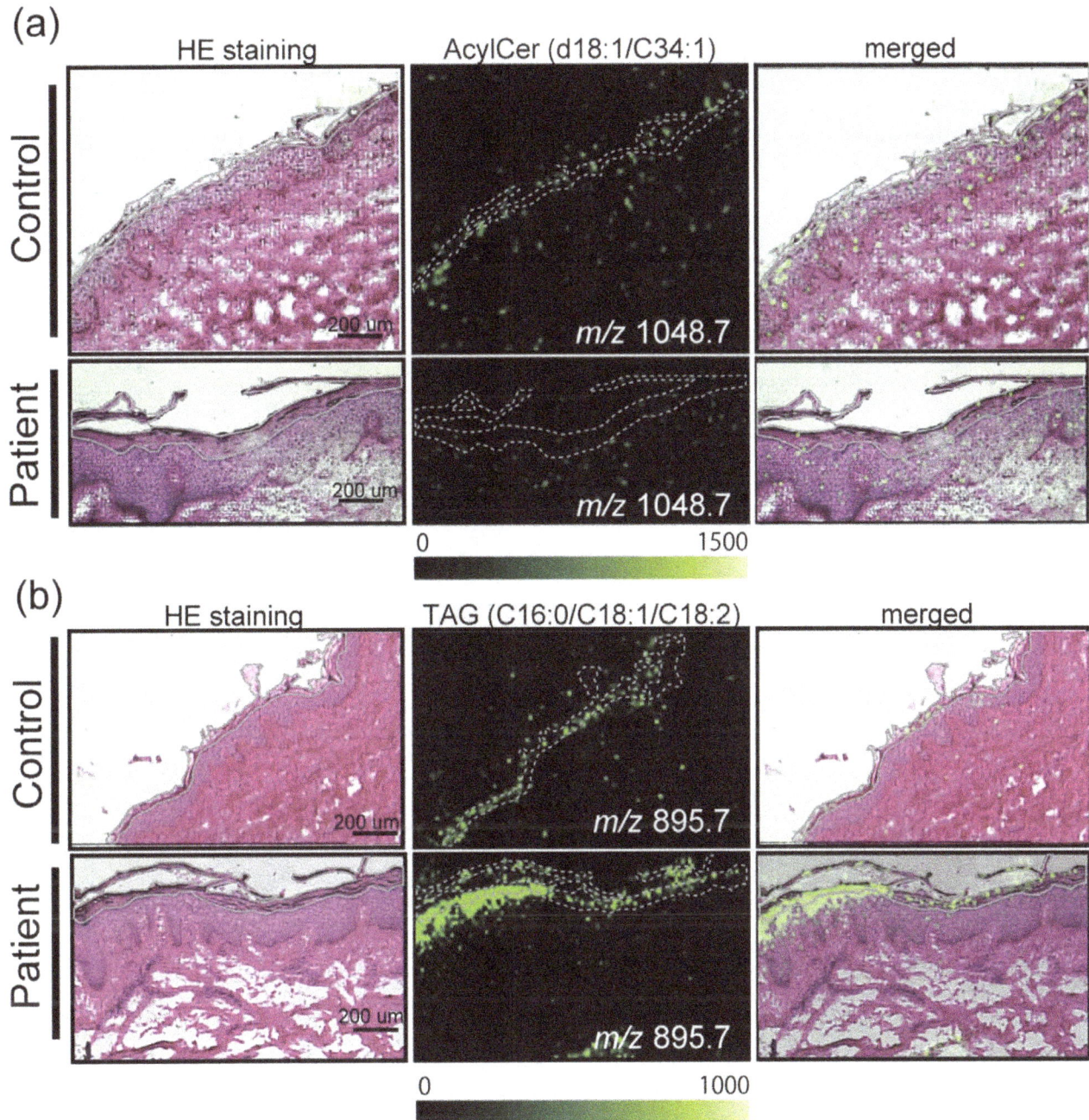

Figure 4. IMS analyses of clinical samples. IMS analysis demonstrates deficiencies of AcylCer (a) (S/N ratio: 9) and, conversely, the accumulation of TAG (b) in the SC (indicated as a gray line) of a DCS patient compared with a normal human subject. The scale bar shows 200 μm. The imaging pixel is 10 μm. Color bar shows signal intensity.

with prior biochemical analysis showing that GlcCer, but not SM, levels significantly increase during epidermal differentiation [47]. Importantly, our IMS analysis showed that the distribution of amide-linked fatty acid of GlcCer and SM species are C24–28 and C16–18, respectively, while the major epidermal Cer is C22–32 in SC, as elucidated by IMS (Table 1), suggesting that GlcCer rather than SM appears to the major pool for Cer species production in the SC (Fig. S1). These results are comparable with a previous study, which detected Cer but not GlcCer in the SC layers.

Out studies reveal that PCs are one of the major lipids in skins and are localized using IMS. Not only Cers, but also PC molecular species shows different signal patterns due to the FA composition. Consistent with prior studies analyzing lipid extracts of epidermal fractions, PC is trace (or not preset) in the SC, further validating the IMS alternative method.

We recently found that AcylCer deficiencies occur in DCS, due to loss-of-function mutations in CGI-58 in human skin [44]. In addition, *Cgi-58 null* mice display the same features, *i.e.*, lack of AcylCer in parallel with epidermal permeability barrier defects [48]. CGI-58 is a cofactor of adipose TAG lipase and other still unidentified TAG lipases. Indeed, oil red O-stained lipid droplets are present within keratinocytes in the SC, SG, and SB [48].

Because AcylCers are required for normal permeability barrier formation, AcylCer deficiencies most likely contribute to the barrier abnormalities in DCS [44], in addition to lamellar/nonlamellar phase separation due to accumulated TAG within the extracellular domains of the SC [49]. It has been suggested that linoleate from TAG is preferentially utilized for the acylation of ω-hydroxyCer to generate AcylCer. In this study, we showed that AcylCer deficiencies do occur at both the SG and SC, eliminating a possibility of misslocalization of AcylCer. As shown in Figure 4, the ion signals relating to AcylCer are significantly attenuated; on the other hand, TAGs were accumulated in the SC of DCS patients compared with the control. These results not only proved our previous findings, *i.e.*, the accumulation of TAG and deficiencies of AcylCer, but also demonstrated the distribution of AcylCer and TAG, their molecular species, and their abnormalities that likely contribute to permeability barrier defects in patient skin.

This is the first report to describe Cer imaging by MALDI-IMS and also to characterize the distribution of Cer species within the epidermal layers of clinical samples using our developed machine, which has an AP ion-source. We were able to obtain detailed distributions of Cers including Cer1P, AcylCer, GlcCer, as well as SM, PC, and TAG in murine and human skin. In contrast to conventional lipid analysis using lipid extracts, which requires large amounts of samples, IMS allows Cer analysis using 3–5 mm diameter biopsy samples. Therefore, IMS can minimize a limitation to assessing lipid profiles in cells/tissues, in particular human samples. IMS is a useful method for diagnosing lipid metabolic abnormalities in several cutaneous diseases and for investigating their pathogeneses that can lead to developing new therapeutic approaches. In summary, our study has illuminated a novel approach for investigating roles of Cer and other lipids in skin and/or diagnosis of diseases, as well as for further application of IMS technology in biomedical fields. Moreover, the IMS apparatus of an AP-MALDI and a QIT-TOF mass spectrometer, which output simple spectrum, is useful for imaging heterogeneous Cer species in cells and tissues.

Materials and Methods

Ethics Statement

For human samples, informed consent was obtained from all volunteers before participation. Subjects consented in written form to cooperate after they were informed. This study was specifically approved by the Institute Ethical Review Board of the Hamamatsu University School of Medicine, and performed according to the Declaration of Helsinki Principles. For animal samples, all experiments in this study were specifically approved by the Ethics Committee at the Hamamatsu University School of Medicine. And all efforts were made to minimize suffering.

Reagents and Materials

All solvents used for MS analyses were of HPLC grade and were purchased from Kanto Chemical Co., Inc. (Tokyo, Japan). Bradykinin and angiotensin-II were obtained from Sigma-Aldrich Japan (Tokyo, Japan) and used as calibration standards. 2, 5-Dihydroxy benzoic acid (DHB) was used as the matrix (Bruker Daltonics, Leipzig, Germany). Sodium carboxymethyl cellulose (CMC) was from Wako Pure Industries LTD (Osaka, Japan). C57BL/6Cr mice were from Japan SLC (Shizuoka, Japan). *Cer and PC standards were purchased from Toronto Research Chemicals Inc. (North York, Canada) and* Avanti Polar Lipids (Alabaster, AL, USA), respectively.

Clinical Samples

DCS patients' skin was obtained as described previously [44]. Briefly, collected tissues were embedded in 2% pre-cooled *CMC and were then* sectioned to a 10-μm thickness at −20°C using a Leica CM1950 cryostat (Leica *Microsystems*, Wetzlar, *Germany)*. The control skin was gifted from a volunteer without any skin diseases. We made three sections per person to get reproducibility of measurements.

Tissue Preparation

We used the footpad skin of 8-week-old C57BL/6Cr mice from Japan SLC (Shizuoka, Japan). The tissues were embedded in 2% pre-cooled *CMC and were then* sectioned to a 10-μm thickness at −20°C using a Leica CM1950 cryostat (Leica *Microsystems*, Wetzlar, *Germany)*. *The brain tissues were snap-frozen in liquid nitrogen directly and sectioned to a 10-*μm thickness. Frozen sections were thaw-mounted on indium-tin-oxide (ITO)-coated glass slides (Bruker Daltonics). We used a DHB solution (50 mg/mL in 70% methanol) as the matrix. The matrix solution was uniformly sprayed over the tissue surface using a 0.2-mm nozzle-caliber air brush (Procon Boy FWA Platinum; Mr. Hobby, Tokyo, Japan). Continuous frozen sections were also thaw-mounted on MAS-coated glass slides (Matsunami Glass Industries, Ltd., Osaka, Japan) for conventional hematoxylin-eosin (HE) staining. One μg of Cer standard was deposited on a brain section.

Thin-layer Chromatography

We used the footpad skin of 8-week-old C57BL/6Cr mice from Japan SLC (Shizuoka, Japan). Epidermal lipids were extracted from murine tissue using a 20-fold volume of solvent, incubated twice with chloroform/methanol (2:1, v/v) overnight at room temperature. Lipids were separated on a silica gel 60 HPTLC plates (Merck, Darmstadt, Germany) using methylacetate/propanol/chloroform/methanol/0.25% aqueous CaCl$_2$, (25/25/25/10/9, v/v/v/v) for separation of phospholipids. A four-sequence solvent system was used to isolate Cer species: 1) chloroform/methanol/water (40/10/1, v/v/v) 1.8 cm, 2) chloroform/methanol/water (40/10/1, v/v/v) 4.5 cm, 3) chloroform/methanol/acetic acid (47/2/0.5, v/v/v) 8.5 cm, and 4) n-hexane/diethylether/acetic acid (30/10/0.5, v/v/v) 8.5 cm. Lipids were visualized using 0.1% primuline reagent under UV light at 365 nm.

Mass Spectrometry

MALDI-TOF mass spectrometric analyses of vacuum-MALDI were performed using a MALDI-hybrid quadrupole TOF-type mass spectrometer (QSTAR Elite, AB Sciex, Foster City, CA) equipped with an orthogonal MALDI source and an Nd:YAG laser at a repetition rate of 200 Hz. Samples were analyzed in positive ion mode over the range of *m/z* 400–1000. The mass spectra were calibrated externally using a standard peptide calibration mixture containing 10 pmol/μl each of bradykinin peptide fragment (amino acid residue 1–7) ([M+H]$^+$, *m/z* 757.4) and human angiotensin-II peptide fragment ([M+H]$^+$, *m/z* 1046.5). A methanol/0.1% TFA solution (1/1, v/v) containing 10 mg/ml DHB was used as the matrix. For comparison with AP ion-source mass spectrometer, serial sections (n = 3) were prepared and were matrix sprayed at the same time. The spectra were extracted from same positions.

Imaging Mass Spectrometry

IMS analyses were performed by an AP ion-source mass spectrometer with a laser frequency of 1000 Hz (laser diameter of

10 μm). All analyses were performed in the positive-ion mode within the mass ranges of m/z 600–1200 for Cer, Cer1P, PC, and SM, m/z 800–1200 for TAG and GlcCer, and m/z 900–1200 for AcylCer. A 10-μm raster width was set to generate images of the skin, and a 50-μm raster width was set to generate the images of the brain. The ion images were constructed using BioMap software (Novartis, Basel, Switzerland). Embedded compounds are required to prepare skin section. We used 2% pre-cooled *CMC* for embedding compounds. Levels of signal on outside of the section, which is derived from CMC, were employed as the threshold, i.e., 150 to 500 for Cer1P, Cer, SM, and PC, and 50–200 for GlcCer. All spectra were normalized by total ion current.

Supporting Information

Figure S1   Generation of ceramide in stratum corneum. Abbreviations for Cer structures are according to (Motta et al., Biochim Biophys Acta 1182:147-151, 1993 and Robson et al., J Lipid Res 35:2060-2068,1994). N, A and EO indicate amide-linked fatty acid (FA) species: N, non-OH FA; A, 2-OH FA; EO,omega-O-esterified FA. S, sphingosine; P, phytosphingosine (or 4-hydoxysphinganine); H, 6-hydroxysphingosine indicate sphingosine base structures. Cer 2 (NS) are ubiquitously expressed in mammalian tissues, while late stages of differentiation produce heterogeneous Cer species. In particular, Cer 1 (EOS), Cer 4 (EOH) and Cer 9 (EOP) are unique to the epidermis.

Figure S2   Mass Microscope characterizes the different distribution of Cer Species in murine skin. The merged image of three Cer1P ion images shows their different distributions. We selected three Cer1P molecular species at m/z 618.4, 646.4, and 730.5 suggesting Cer1P (d18:1/C16:0), Cer1P (d18:1/C18:0), and Cer1P (d18:1/C24:0), respectively. The ion images at m/z 618.4 and m/z 646.4 were detected in the middle of SC regions, while the ion image at m/z 730.5 was detected in relatively lower SC. Scale bar showed 200 μm.

Figure S3   Tandem mass spectrometric analyses on tissue sections. Tandem mass spectrometric analyses of Cer, Cer1P, SM, PC, TAG and GlcCer were performed on tissue sections. (a) Tandem mass spectrum of m/z 646.4. (b) Tandem mass spectrum of m/z 630.5. The spectra (c) and (d) were standard mass spectrum of Cer1P and Cer, respectively. The fragment patterns of these spectra were compared and confirmed the structure. The tandem mass spectrometric analyses of representative SM (e), PC (f), TAG (g) and GlcCer (h) were also performed and confirmed their structures.

Figure S4   GlcCer distribution of other murine footpad sections. The signal intensity of GlcCer is very low and hard to get tandem mass spectrometric data. Therefore, we minimize the m/z range to concentrate these molecules in quadrupole ion trap. We made multiple sections and get reproducibility of these moelcular localization. As described, the signals are predominantly detected in SS and SG regions (white-line area). Lower pannels show the statistical analyses results of ion signal intensity between biological regions and out of sections. As shown in bar graph, the significant difference tendencis are existed (SM and PC: $p<0.05$, GlcCer: $p<0.1$).

Acknowledgments

We gratefully acknowledge the superb editorial assistance of Ms. Joan Wakefield, and appreciate the useful assistance of Ms. Yukiko Sugiyama.

Author Contributions

Conceived and designed the experiments: NG-I MS YU. Performed the experiments: NG-I. Analyzed the data: NG-I TH. Contributed reagents/materials/analysis tools: NZ KN WM-H SS. Wrote the paper: NG-I MS YU.

References

1. Shimma S, Sugiura Y, Hayasaka T, Zaima N, Matsumoto M, et al. (2008) Mass imaging and identification of biomolecules with MALDI-QIT-TOF-based system. Anal Chem. 80: 878–885.
2. Hayasaka T, Goto-Inoue N, Sugiura Y, Zaima N, Nakanishi H, et al. (2008) Matrix-assisted laser desorption/ionization quadrupole ion trap time-of-flight (MALDI-QIT-TOF)-based imaging mass spectrometry reveals a layered distribution of phospholipid molecular species in the mouse retina. Rapid Commun Mass Spectrom. 22: 3415–3426.
3. Cornett DS, Reyzer ML, Chaurand P, Caprioli RM (2007) MALDI imaging mass spectrometry: molecular snapshots of biochemical systems. Nat Methods. 4: 828–833.
4. Yao I, Takagi H, Ageta H, Kahyo T, Sato S, et al. (2007) SCRAPPER-dependent ubiquitination of active zone protein RIM1 regulates synaptic vesicle release. Cell. 130: 943–957.
5. Morita Y, Ikegami K, Goto-Inoue N, Hayasaka T, Zaima N, et al. (2010) Imaging mass spectrometry of gastric carcinoma in formalin-fixed paraffin-embedded tissue microarray. Cancer Sci. 101: 267–273.
6. Hayasaka T, Goto-Inoue N, Zaima N, Kimura Y, Setou M (2009) Organ-specific distributions of lysophosphatidylcholine and triacylglycerol in mouse embryo. Lipids. 44: 837–848.
7. Goto-Inoue N, Setou M, Zaima N (2010) Visualization of spatial distribution of gamma-aminobutyric acid in eggplant (Solanum melongena) by matrix-assisted laser desorption/ionization imaging mass spectrometry. Anal Sci. 26: 821–825.
8. Zaima N, Hayasaka T, Goto-Inoue N, Setou M (2009) Imaging of metabolites by MALDI mass spectrometry. J Oleo Sci. 58: 415–419.
9. Sugiura Y, Konishi Y, Zaima N, Kajihara S, Nakanishi H, et al. (2009) Visualization of the cell-selective distribution of PUFA-containing phosphatidylcholines in mouse brain by imaging mass spectrometry. J Lipid Res. 50: 1776–1788.
10. Spengler B, Hubert M (2002) Scanning microprobe matrix-assisted laser desorption ionization (SMALDI) mass spectrometry: instrumentation for sub-micrometer resolved LDI and MALDI surface analysis. J Am Soc Mass Spectrom. 13: 735–748.
11. Yang J, Caprioli RM (2011) Matrix sublimation/recrystallization for imaging proteins by mass spectrometry at high spatial resolution. Anal Chem. 83: 5728–5734.
12. Spraggins JM, Caprioli RM (2011) High-speed maldi-tof imaging mass spectrometry: rapid ion image acquisition and considerations for next generation instrumentation. J Am Soc Mass Spectrom. 22: 1022–1031.
13. Hankin JA, Farias SE, Barkley RM, Heidenreich K, Frey LC, et al. (2011) MALDI Mass Spectrometric Imaging of Lipids in Rat Brain Injury Models. J Am Soc Mass Spectrom. 22: 1014–1021.
14. Deutskens F, Yang J, Caprioli RM (2011) High spatial resolution imaging mass spectrometry and classical histology on a single tissue section. J Mass Spectrom. 46: 568–571.
15. Harada T, Yuba-Kubo A, Sugiura Y, Zaima N, Hayasaka T, et al. (2009) Visualization of volatile substances in different organelles with an atmospheric-pressure mass microscope. Anal Chem. 81: 9153–9157.
16. Pettus BJ, Bielawska A, Subramanian P, Wijesinghe DS, Maceyka M, et al. (2004) Ceramide 1-phosphate is a direct activator of cytosolic phospholipase A2. J Biol Chem. 279: 11320–11326.
17. Ponec M, Weerheim A, Kempenaar J, Mommaas AM, Nugteren DH (1988) Lipid composition of cultured human keratinocytes in relation to their differentiation. J Lipid Res. 29: 949–961.
18. Wertz PW, Downing DT (1982) Glycolipids in mammalian epidermis: structure and function in the water barrier. Science. 217: 1261–1262.
19. Holleran WM, Takagi Y, Menon GK, Legler G, Feingold KR, et al. (1993) Processing of Epidermal Glucosylceramides Is Required for Optimal Mammalian Cutaneous Permeability Barrier Function. J Clin Invest. 91: 1656–1664.
20. Holleran WM, Ginns EI, Menon GK, Grundmann JU, Fartasch M, et al. (1994) Consequences of Beta-Glucocerebrosidase Deficiency in Epidermis - Ultrastructure and Permeability Barrier Alterations in Gaucher Disease. J Clin Invest. 93: 1756–1764.

21. Elias PM, Menon GK (1991) Structural and lipid biochemical correlates of the epidermal permeability barrier. Adv Lipid Res. 24: 1–26.
22. Schmuth M, Man MQ, Weber F, Gao W, Feingold KR, et al. (2000) Permeability barrier disorder in Niemann-Pick disease: sphingomyelin-ceramide processing required for normal barrier homeostasis. J Invest Dermatol. 115: 459–466.
23. Jensen JM, Schutze S, Forl M, Kronke M, Proksch E (1999) Roles for tumor necrosis factor receptor p55 and sphingomyelinase in repairing the cutaneous permeability barrier. J Clin Invest. 104: 1761–1770.
24. Bouwstra JA, Gooris GS, Dubbelaar FE, Weerheim AM, Ijzerman AP, et al. (1998) Role of ceramide 1 in the molecular organization of the stratum corneum lipids. J Lipid Res. 39: 186–196.
25. Paige DG, Morse-Fisher N, Harper JI (1994) Quantification of stratum corneum ceramides and lipid envelope ceramides in the hereditary ichthyoses. Br J Dermatol. 131: 23–27.
26. Motta S, Monti M, Sesana S, Caputo R, Carelli S, et al. (1993) Ceramide composition of the psoriatic scale. Biochim Biophys Acta. 1182: 147–151.
27. Imokawa G, Abe A, Jin K, Higaki Y, Kawashima M, et al. (1991) Decreased level of ceramides in stratum corneum of atopic dermatitis: an etiologic factor in atopic dry skin? J Invest Dermatol. 96: 523–526.
28. Bleck O, Abeck D, Ring J, Hoppe U, Vietzke JP, et al. (1999) Two ceramide subfractions detectable in Cer(AS) position by HPTLC in skin surface lipids of non-lesional skin of atopic eczema. Journal of Investigative Dermatology. 113: 894–900.
29. Preiss JE, Loomis CR, Bell RM, Niedel JE (1987) Quantitative measurement of sn-1,2-diacylglycerols. Methods Enzymol. 141: 294–300.
30. Gorska M, Dobrzyn A, Zendzian-Piotrowska M, Namiot Z (2002) Concentration and composition of free ceramides in human plasma. Horm Metab Res. 34: 466–468.
31. Yano M, Kishida E, Muneyuki Y, Masuzawa Y (1998) Quantitative analysis of ceramide molecular species by high performance liquid chromatography. J Lipid Res. 39: 2091–2098.
32. Dobrzyn A, Gorski J (2002) Ceramides and sphingomyelins in skeletal muscles of the rat: content and composition. Effect of prolonged exercise. Am J Physiol Endocrinol Metab. 282: E277–285.
33. Kasumov T, Huang H, Chung YM, Zhang R, McCullough AJ, et al. (2010) Quantification of ceramide species in biological samples by liquid chromatography electrospray ionization tandem mass spectrometry. Anal Biochem.
34. Farwanah H, Pierstorff B, Schmelzer CE, Raith K, Neubert RH, et al. (2007) Separation and mass spectrometric characterization of covalently bound skin ceramides using LC/APCI-MS and Nano-ESI-MS/MS. J Chromatogr B Analyt Technol Biomed Life Sci. 852: 562–570.
35. Tserng KY, Griffin R (2003) Quantitation and molecular species determination of diacylglycerols, phosphatidylcholines, ceramides, and sphingomyelins with gas chromatography. Anal Biochem. 323: 84–93.
36. Hart PJ, Francese S, Claude E, Woodroofe MN, Clench MR (2011) MALDI-MS imaging of lipids in ex vivo human skin. Anal Bioanal Chem. 401: 115–125.
37. Uchida Y, Visireddy V, Gooris G, Alderson NI, Brown J, et al. (2008) ELOVL4 is required to generate epidermal-unique omega-O-(acyl)ceramides that form two structures critical for the epidermal permeability barrier. Journal of Investigative Dermatology. 128: S92–S92.
38. Vielhaber G, Pfeiffer S, Brade L, Lindner B, Goldmann T, et al. (2001) Localization of ceramide and glucosylceramide in human epidermis by immunogold electron microscopy. J Invest Dermatol. 117: 1126–1136.
39. Munoz-Garcia A, Ro J, Brown JC, Williams JB (2006) Identification of complex mixtures of sphingolipids in the stratum corneum by reversed-phase high-performance liquid chromatography and atmospheric pressure photospray ionization mass spectrometry. J Chromatogr A. 1133: 58–68.
40. Holleran WM, Takagi Y, Uchida Y (2006) Epidermal sphingolipids: metabolism, function, and roles in skin disorders. Febs Lett. 580: 5456–5466.
41. Kobayashi Y, Hayasaka T, Setou M, Itoh H, Kanayama N (2010) Comparison of phospholipid molecular species between terminal and stem villi of human term placenta by imaging mass spectrometry. Placenta. 31: 245–248.
42. Nakamura K, Suzuki Y, Goto-Inoue N, Yoshida-Noro C, Suzuki A (2006) Structural characterization of neutral glycosphingolipids by thin-layer chromatography coupled to matrix-assisted laser desorption/ionization quadrupole ion trap time-of-flight MS/MS. Anal Chem. 78: 5736–5743.
43. Zaima N, Goto-Inoue N, Hayasaka T, Setou M (2010) Application of imaging mass spectrometry for the analysis of Oryza sativa rice. Rapid Commun Mass Spectrom. 24: 2723–2729.
44. Uchida Y, Cho Y, Moradian S, Kim J, Nakajima K, et al. (2010) Neutral lipid storage leads to acylceramide deficiency, likely contributing to the pathogenesis of Dorfman-Chanarin syndrome. J Invest Dermatol. 130: 2497–2499.
45. Laiko VV, Baldwin MA, Burlingame AL (2000) Atmospheric pressure matrix-assisted laser desorption/ionization. Anal Chem. 72: 652–657.
46. Vietzke JP, Brandt O, Abeck D, Rapp C, Strassner M, et al. (2001) Comparative investigation of human stratum corneum ceramides. Lipids. 36: 299–304.
47. Hamanaka S, Nakazawa S, Yamanaka M, Uchida Y, Otsuka F (2005) Glucosylceramide accumulates preferentially in lamellar bodies in differentiated keratinocytes. Br J Dermatol. 152: 426–434.
48. Radner FP, Streith IE, Schoiswohl G, Schweiger M, Kumari M, et al. (2010) Growth retardation, impaired triacylglycerol catabolism, hepatic steatosis, and lethal skin barrier defect in mice lacking comparative gene identification-58 (CGI-58). J Biol Chem. 285: 7300–7311.
49. Demerjian M, Crumrine DA, Milstone LM, Williams ML, Elias PM (2006) Barrier dysfunction and pathogenesis of neutral lipid storage disease with ichthyosis (Chanarin-Dorfman syndrome). J Invest Dermatol. 126: 2032–2038.

Dysregulation of Suppressor of Cytokine Signaling 3 in Keratinocytes Causes Skin Inflammation Mediated by Interleukin-20 Receptor-Related Cytokines

Ayako Uto-Konomi[1,2], Kosuke Miyauchi[1], Naoko Ozaki[2], Yasutaka Motomura[1], Yoshie Suzuki[1], Akihiko Yoshimura[3], Shinobu Suzuki[2], Daniel Cua[4], Masato Kubo[1,5]*

1 Laboratory for Signal Network, Research Center for Allergy and Immunology, RIKEN Yokohama Institute, Yokohama, Kanagawa, Japan, 2 Department of Molecular and Cellular Biology, Kobe Pharma Research Institute, Nippon Boehringer Ingelheim Co., Ltd., Kobe, Hyogo, Japan, 3 Department of Microbiology and Immunology, Keio University School of Medicine, Tokyo, Japan, 4 Schering-Plough Biopharma, Palo Alto, California, United States, 5 Division of Molecular Pathology, Research Institute for Biological Science, Tokyo University of Science, Noda, Chiba, Japan

Abstract

Homeostatic regulation of epidermal keratinocytes is controlled by the local cytokine milieu. However, a role for suppressor of cytokine signaling (SOCS), a negative feedback regulator of cytokine networks, in skin homeostasis remains unclear. Keratinocyte specific deletion of *Socs3* (*Socs3* cKO) caused severe skin inflammation with hyper-production of IgE, epidermal hyperplasia, and S100A8/9 expression, although *Socs1* deletion caused no inflammation. The inflamed skin showed constitutive STAT3 activation and up-regulation of IL-6 and IL-20 receptor (IL-20R) related cytokines, IL-19, IL-20 and IL-24. Disease development was rescued by deletion of the *Il6* gene, but not by the deletion of *Il23*, *Il4r*, or *Rag1* genes. The expression of IL-6 in *Socs3* cKO keratinocytes increased expression of IL-20R-related cytokines that further facilitated STAT3 hyperactivation, epidermal hyperplasia and neutrophilia. These results demonstrate that skin homeostasis is strictly regulated by the IL-6-STAT3-SOCS3 axis. Moreover, the SOCS3-mediated negative feedback loop in keratinocytes has a critical mechanistic role in the prevention of skin inflammation caused by hyperactivation of STAT3.

Editor: Christianne Bandeira de Melo, Instituto de Biofisica Carlos Chagas Filho, Universidade Federal do Rio de Janeiro, Brazil

Funding: This work was supported by a grant from Grant in Aid for Scientific Research (B) and Grant in Aid for Scientific Research on Priority Areas of the Ministry of Education, Culture, Sports, Science, and Technology (Japan) and the Program for Promotion of Fundamental Studies in Health Sciences of the National Institute of Biomedical Innovation (NIBIO). The funders had no role in study design, data collection and analysis, decision to publish, or preparation of the manuscript.

Competing Interests: Ayako Uto-Konomi, Naoko Ozaki and Shinobu Suzuki are employed by Nippon Boehringer Ingelheim Co., Ltd., and Daniel Cua is employed by Schering-Plough Biopharma. There are no patents, products in development or marketed products to declare.

* E-mail: raysolfc@rcai.riken.jp

Introduction

The suppressor of cytokine signaling (SOCS) family of proteins plays a role in the negative regulation of cytokine-JAK-STAT signaling by inhibiting JAK tyrosine kinase activity. There are eight proteins in this family, each of which has a central SH2 domain and a C-terminal 40-amino-acid conserved domain called the SOCS box. SOCS1 inhibits STAT1 activation in the IFN-γ signaling cascade, while SOCS3 is a major negative regulator of IL-6-STAT3 signaling [1,2]. Additionally, SOCS3 negatively regulates skin wound healing through inhibition of the gp130-STAT3 pathway [3], suggesting a pivotal role for SOCS proteins in skin inflammatory responses. However, the regulatory role of SOCSs in the maintenance of skin homeostasis remains unclear.

The skin consists of two major layers, the epidermis and the dermis. The epidermis consists of keratinocytes, which proliferate in the basal layer and differentiate into cells that migrate towards the outer layer to form the stratified epithelium that provides the skin barrier. The epidermis is in a continuous equilibrium of growth and differentiation and has the remarkable capacity for complete self-renewal, relying on its rich reservoir of stem cells. The dermis contains mainly fibroblasts and a large population of immune cells, along with structures important for skin function including blood vessels, nerves, hair follicles, and glands. The dermis also provides the epidermis with mechanical support and nutrients [4],[5]. Epidermal homeostasis is dependent on proper repair after injury and on maintenance of a tight junction with the underlying basement membrane, both of which are precisely regulated by various cytokines. Keratinocytes are now proposed to play important roles in the regulation of skin homeostasis by producing a variety of cytokines [5]. TNF-α, IL-1 and IL-6 have been shown to have regulatory roles in skin wound healing, and also in skin permeability [6,7,8]. For example, IL-6 deficiency caused delayed skin repair, and topical application of IL-6 to barrier-disrupted skin enhanced repair of the skin barrier [8].

STAT3 is one of the key components for IL-6 receptor signaling, and it is thought to be an important transcription factor in skin homeostasis [8,9]. Activated (phosphorylated) STAT3 expression is enhanced at sites of injured epidermis compared with the normal epidermis, and STAT3 related signaling also affects the survival of keratinocyte stem cells, which are important for keratinocyte renewal and wound healing. Besides IL-6, other cytokines/growth factors also stimulate the phosphorylation of STAT3 and the subsequent STAT3 mediated nuclear signaling.

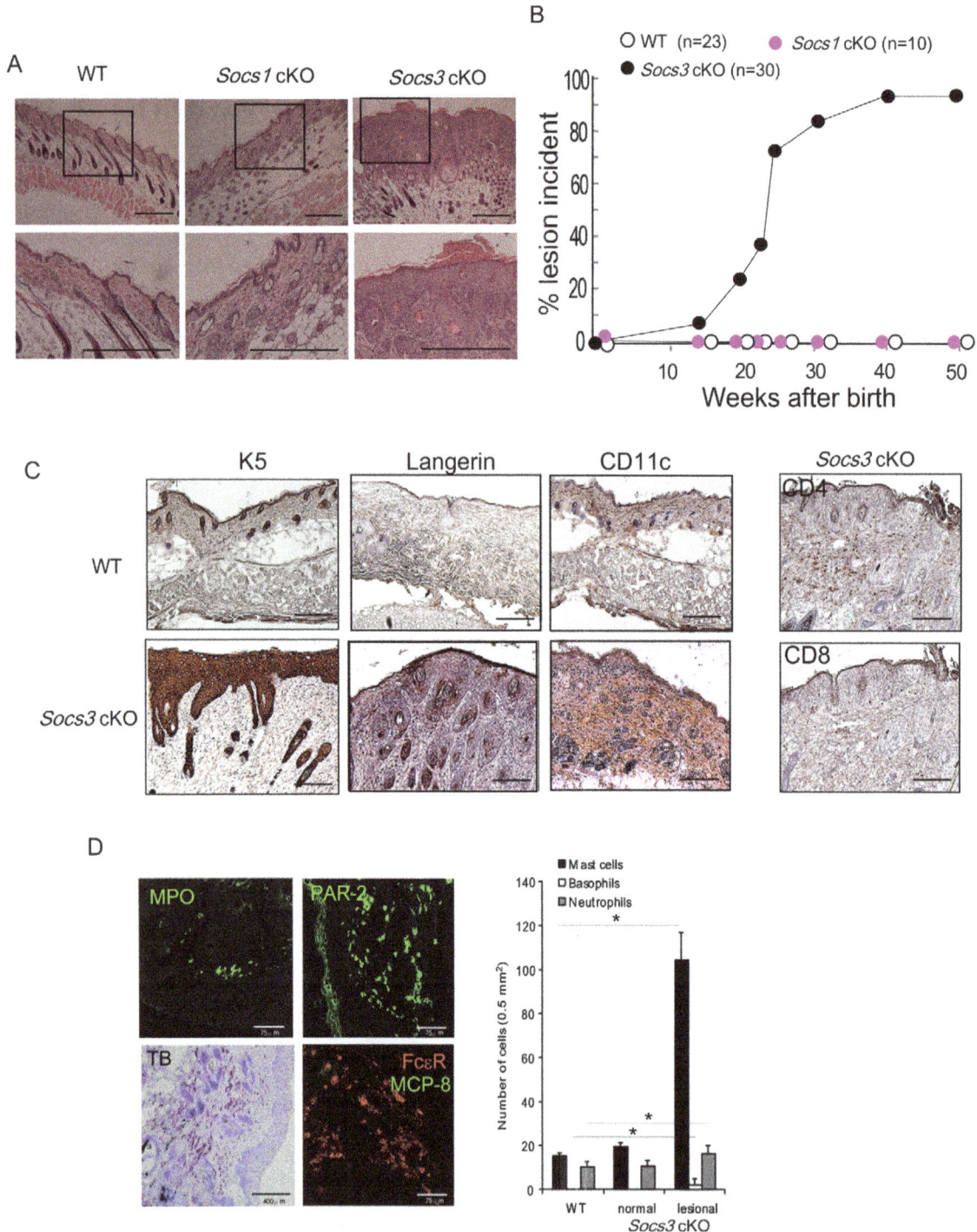

Figure 1. Socs3 cKO spontaneously developed epidermal hyperplasia and skin inflammation. A) Upper and bottom panels show histopathological analysis of K5-Cre (WT) (left), *Socs1* cKO (center) and *Socs3* cKO (right) mice skin with hematoxylin and eosin staining. Magnification of upper and lower panels are x40 and x100, respectively. Scale bar in each section indicates 750 υm. B) Percentage of mice showing skin lesion incidences in wild type (WT) (open circle), *Socs1* cKO (closed purple circle) and *Socs3* cKO (closed-black circle) mice. Disease incidence was monitored weekly up to 50 weeks after birth. Percentage of mice showing incidence of disease is shown on the Y axis at each time point. The number of mice used in each group is indicated in the figure. C) Localization of keratinocytes (K5), Langerhans cells (Langerin), and CD11c⁺ dendritic cells (CD11c) in epidermis and dermis of the diseased *Socs3* cKO skin was assessed by immunohistlogical staining (x40) (left panel). Wild type (WT) mice skin was stained as a control. CD4 and CD8 positive T cells were also identified in epidermis and dermis of the diseased *Socs3* cKO skin (right panel). Scale bar in each section indicates 750 υm. D) Neutrophil number was confirmed by counting MPO positive cells in epidermis and dermis of the diseased *Socs3* cKO skin by immunohistlogical staining (x400) (upper left panel). PAR-2, TB staining, FcεR and MCP-8 positive cells in epidermis and dermis of the diseased *Socs3* cKO skin are shown (upper right, lower left, and lower right panel, respectively). Scale bar in each section indicates 75 υm. Number of neutrophils, mast cells and basophils in epidermis and dermis are shown in the right bar graphs. *P<0.01. Data are the mean from three independent experiments. Error bars are SD.

Thus a sophisticated cytokine network is required for the homeostatic events in the proliferation and differentiation of keratinocytes. Disruption of this homeostasis has pathological consequences. For example, the overexpression of active-*Stat3* resulted in impaired wound healing and increased keloid pathogenesis [9] and augmented the development of spontaneous psoriatic skin disease [10]. Therefore, dysregulation of STAT3 activation results in the breakdown of keratinocyte homeostasis, sometimes leading the development of skin carcinogenesis [11].

Phosphorylation of STAT3 is regulated by IL-6, IL-10, EGF and many other cytokines, including the interleukin-20 receptor (IL-20R) related cytokines, IL-19, IL-20, and as well as IL-24 [12]. The IL-20RI is composed of two chains, IL-20RA and IL-20RB, and its ligands are IL-19, IL-20 and IL-24, which are highly expressed in keratinocytes [13]. These cytokines are important in the manifestation of psoriatic lesions [14] and, recently, an association of polymorphisms of IL-20 with psoriasis has been described [15]. IL-19, IL-20 and IL-24 are reported to induce epidermal hyperplasia and STAT3 activation in the reconstituted human epidermis [16], and are highly expressed in psoriatic inflammatory sites [17].

In the present study, we investigated the role of SOCS3 in keratinocyte function using keratinocyte-specific SOCS3 gene deficient mice, and found that these mice spontaneously developed a severe form of skin inflammation. Here we identified a critical role for SOCS3 as a negative regulator of STAT3 hyperactivation in keratinocytes that restored skin homeostasis. Moreover, in the absence of SOCS3, excessive IL-6 signaling resulted in skin lesions that were also strongly correlated with increased IL-19/IL-24 cytokines and the expression levels of anti-microbial peptides, β-defensin and S100A8/A9.

Results

Loss of SOCS3 in keratinocytes resulted in skin inflammation

To examine the role of SOCS proteins in the epidermis, we generated keratin 5-specific *Socs1* and *Socs3* conditional knockout mice (*Socs1* cKO and *Socs3* cKO respectively; See Materials and Methods). At age 40 weeks or older, mice lacking SOCS3 in keratinocytes spontaneously developed a severe form of skin inflammation, with a disease incidence of >90% (**Fig. 1A&B**). Histopathological analysis revealed epidermal hyperplasia and massive leukocyte infiltration in the skin of the *Socs3* cKO mice, whereas the deletion of *Socs1* did not cause such inflammation. These findings suggested that SOCS3 expression in keratinocytes is required for the maintenance of normal skin. Additionally, we analyzed the cell types in the skin lesions (**Fig. 1C&D**). Keratin 5 (K5) staining showed a thickened epithelium in *Socs3* cKO mice as a result of an extensive expansion of keratinocytes. Compared to the control K5-Cre mice (with a wild type *Socs3* locus), *Socs3* cKO mice displayed an increased infiltration of Langerin⁺ Langerhans cells and CD11c⁺ dendritic cells (DCs). We also identified an increased number of CD4⁺ but not CD8⁺ T cells in the dermis of *Socs3* cKO mice (**Fig. 1C, right panel**). In addition, we performed an immunohistochemical staining of neutrophils, connective tissue type mast cells and basophils in the epidermis and dermis of *Socs3* cKO mice, using toluidine blue or antibodies for myeloperoxidase (MPO), PAR-2, FcεR and MCP-8 (**Fig. 1D**). Compared to the wild type littermates, elevated numbers of mast cells were identified in both the epidermis and dermis of *Socs3* cKO mice, and there was also an increased infiltration of neutrophils and basophils. These findings indicated that the loss

of SOCS3 rendered the mice prone to spontaneous skin inflammation.

The skin inflammation in Socs3 cKO mice is T and B cell independent

We examined whether this skin inflammation was due to an atopic type Th2 response and, interestingly, we found that total serum levels of the prototypical Th2-type immunoglobulin, IgE, were markedly increased in the diseased *Socs3* cKO mice, but not in pre-disease *Socs3* cKO mice. Moreover, we observed that there was a positive correlation between the IgE levels and the severity of inflammation in the diseased *Socs3* cKO mice (**Fig. 2A**). Therefore, in order to understand if any atopic response associates with this skin pathology, the *Socs3* cKO mice were crossed with *Il4 receptor (Il4r)* KO mice and monitored for the spontaneous development of skin inflammation over time. We found that *Il4r* KO mice still developed skin lesions similar to those observed in *Il4r*⁺/⁻ mice, even with complete attenuation of the increased serum IgE levels (**Fig. 2B**). This further demonstrates that the skin inflammation observed in *Socs3* cKO mice completely segregated from the IgE-mediated as well as the IL-4/IL-13-mediated responses.

As shown in Fig. 1D, we found massive infiltration of CD4⁺ cells but not CD8⁺ T cells in the dermis of the diseased skin. We therefore asked whether T cells were involved in the actual development of skin lesions, or were only needed for maintenance of the disease situation in an ongoing inflammation. To answer the question, we crossed *Socs3* cKO mice onto a *Rag1* KO background, in which T and B cells were completely absent. Interestingly, spontaneous skin lesions still occurred in these mice (**Fig. 2C**). Our results indicate that the development of skin lesion in *Socs3* cKO mice was independent of CD4 T cells, and that CD4 T cells in the lesions might accumulate locally as a result of the inflammation.

Cytokine profile in the lesional skin of Socs3 cKO mice

To understand the mechanism underlying the development of skin inflammation in *Socs3* cKO mice, we examined the cytokine profiles. Cytokines, cytokine receptors, and anti-microbial peptide gene panels, that are known to play a role in skin homeostasis or diseases, were analyzed by quantitative real-time PCR in normal skin from controls and *Socs1* cKO mice, as well as in the inflamed skin of *Socs3* cKO mice. We found clear induction of IL-1β, IL-4, IL-6, IL-19, IL-20 and IL-24 expression in *Socs3* cKO derived skin (**Fig. 3A&B**). It has been reported that the cytokines IL-19, IL-20 and IL-24 are highly expressed in the inflammatory sites of psoriasis, and may thus mediate the progression of psoriasis [13,17]. Only STAT3, but no other STAT family member (STAT1, STAT5, or STAT6), is highly phosphorylated in the skin of *Socs3* cKO mice (**Fig. 3C, Fig. S1**). Immunohistochemical analysis revealed that IL-6, IL-19 and IL-24 protein levels are also elevated in *Socs3* cKO mouse skin (**Fig. 3D**). However, the inflamed skin had no expression of IL-23, IL-17A, IL-17F, IL-22, and RORγt (**Fig. 3A&B Fig. S2**), which are known to be expressed by Th17 cells, a critical helper T cell population in various inflammatory conditions including psoriasis [18]. On the other hand, the inflamed skin expressed significantly high levels of the anti-microbial peptides; S100A8, S100A9, and β-defensin (**Fig. 3A&B**)

IL-6 plays a regulatory role in skin wound healing through its effect on skin barrier homeostasis [8]. This indicates that IL-6 might be a key cytokine to enhance the hyperactivation of STAT3 in the skin of *Socs3* cKO mice. IL-23 is also well known to be an important STAT3 cytokine related to skin disorders such as

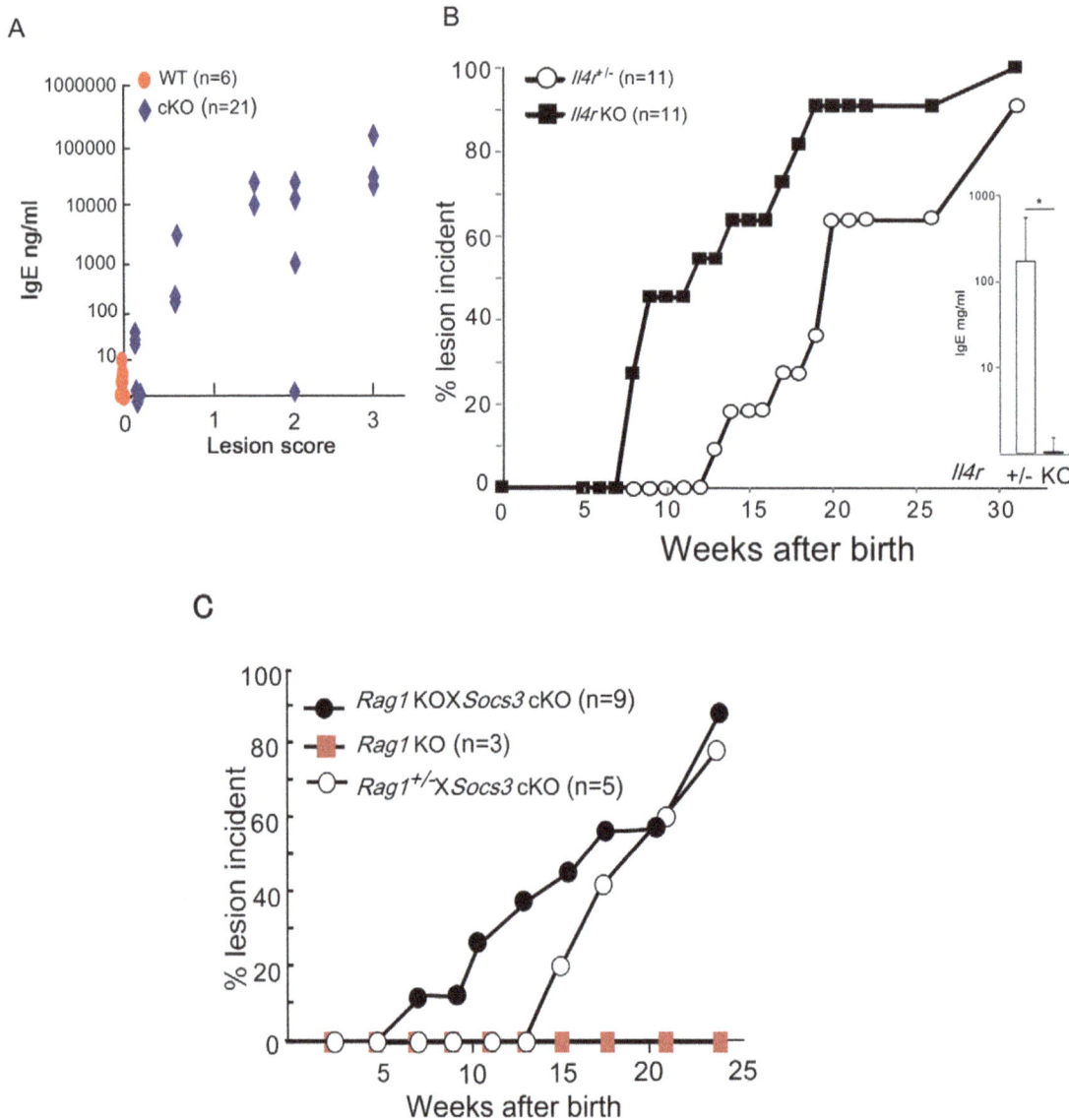

Figure 2. T cell responses are not required for initiation of the skin disease in Socs3cKOmice. A) Serum level of IgE was measured in wild type (WT) and *Socs3* cKO mice and is shown on the Y axis. X axis indicates skin disease severity (Lesion score). Red symbols indicate WT mice (n = 6) and blue symbols indicate *Socs3* cKO with or without skin lesions (n = 21). B) Lesion incidence was examined in *Socs3* cKO with *Il4r*[+/−] (shown as *Il4r*[+/−] in the figure, open circle, n = 11) and *Il4r* null *Socs3* cKO (shown as *Il4* KO in the figure, closed circle, n = 11). Serum IgE in individual *Socs3* cKO with *Il4r*[+/−] (+/−) and *Socs3* cKO with *Il4r* KO mice (KO) was measured at 30 weeks of age and the mean +/− SD is shown (right). C) Role of T-B cells in the development of the skin lesions in *Socs3* cKO mice. Lesion incidence was examined in *Rag1* KO (red-square, n = 3), *Socs3* cKO with *Rag1* KO (Rag1 KOX*Socs3* cKO, closed circles, n = 9), and *Socs3* cKO with *Rag1*[+/−] (*Rag1*[+/−]X*Socs3* cKO, open circles, n = 5) mice. Each mouse strain was monitored until 24 weeks after birth (X axis). The percentage of mice with lesions is shown on the Y axis at each time point after birth.

psoriasis [19,20,21]. Therefore, we tested *Socs3* cKO mice crossed with either *Il6* KO or *Il23* KO mice to identify which cytokine is more important for disease development. We found that crossing *Socs3* cKO mice with *Il6* KO mice markedly restored the skin condition (**Fig. 4A**). By contrast, skin from *Socs3* cKO mice crossed with *Il23* KO mice did not show any improvement in disease development (**Fig. 4B**). These results demonstrate that IL-6 is a key cytokine for the regulation of homeostasis in keratinocytes, and that STAT3 activation and aberrant expression of IL-19 and IL-24 may promote development of skin inflammation.

IL-6 induces IL-20-RI related cytokines in Socs3 KO keratinocytes

As shown in Fig. 3C, the STAT3 pathway is highly active in *Socs3* deficient skin. To confirm the prolonged activation of STAT3 in the SOCS3 deficient condition, keratinocytes were isolated from wild type and pre-diseased *Socs3* cKO mice and cultured with IL-6 before analyzing their STAT3 phosphorylation status. Ten minute stimulation of KO keratinocytes induced similar levels of STAT3 phosphorylation to that of wild type keratinocytes. However, after 60 min, there was a significant reduction in STAT3 phosphorylation in control keratinocytes, whereas the phosphorylation levels in KO keratinocytes was markedly sustained (**Fig. 5A**).

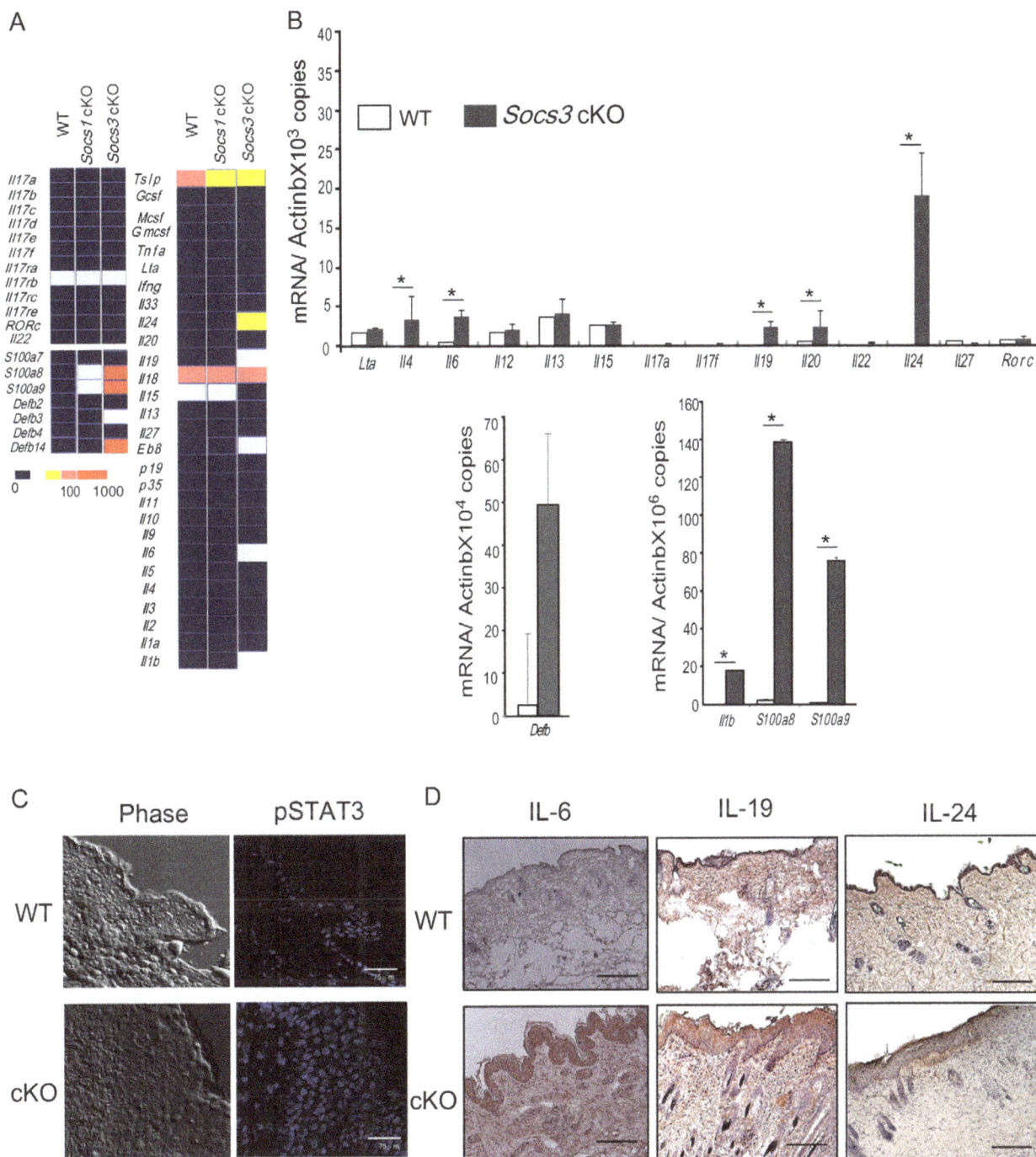

Figure 3. Cytokine expression in the diseased skin. A) Expression profiles. RNA was prepared from skin of K5-Cre (WT), *Socs1* cKO, and the diseased *Socs3* cKO mice, and analyzed using a TAQMAN™ real-time quantitative PCR system. Copy numbers are depicted by the color indicators shown on the lower left. B) Quantitative RT-PCR analysis of the cytokine and *Rorc* panel (upper), *Defb* (lower left) and *S100a8* and *S100a9* (lower right) expression. Skin from K5-Cre (WT, open column) and *Socs3* cKO (closed column) mice was analyzed by SYBR green real-time qPCR. Data are normalized to β-actin mRNA copy number and the mean and SEM (n = 5) are indicated. Statistical significance was determined using the Student's t-test. * $p < 0.05$. C) Skin sections from K5-Cre control (WT) and the diseased *Socs3* cKO mice (cKO) were stained with Alexa 488 labeled anti-pSTAT3. Left panels represent phase contrast of skin section, and right panels represent pSTAT3 (green) in the skin section (x400). Scale bar in each section indicates 75 υm. D) Protein expression of IL-6, IL-19, and IL-24 in the frozen skin sections from K5-Cre (WT) and the diseased *Socs3* cKO mice were analyzed by immunohistochemical staining (x40). Scale bar in each section indicates 750 υm.

We further examined the effect of IL-6 on *Socs3* deficient keratinocytes in the induction of expression of IL-20R related cytokine genes, *Il19*, *Il20* and *Il24*. Socs3 deficient keratinocytes showed much higher IL-20RI related cytokine mRNA levels than the control keratinocytes (**Fig. 5B**). Our results revealed a prolonged STAT3 activation in response to IL-6 in the *Socs3* deficient keratinocytes, eventually leading to the expression of IL-19, IL-20 and IL-24 by keratinocytes. Furthermore, we found

A

B

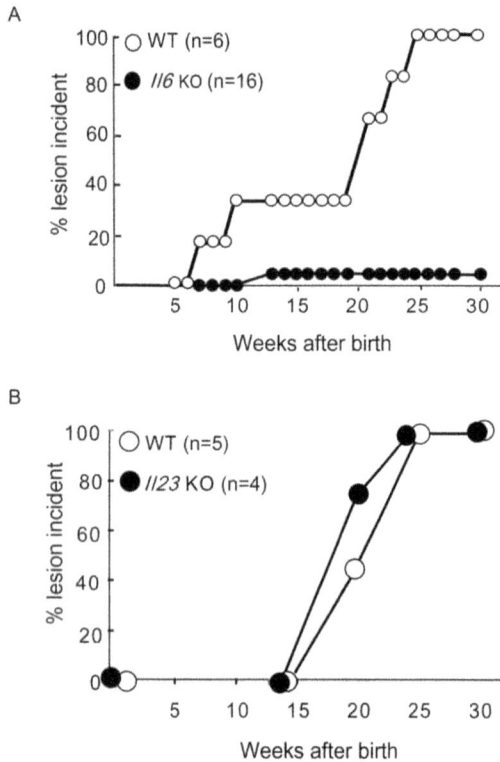

Figure 4. Lesion incidences in Socs3 cKO mice and in combined Il6$^{-/-}$- or Il23$^{-/-}$-Socs3 cKO mice. A) Lesion incidences were examined in K5-Cre mice (WT, open circle, n = 6) and Il6$^{-/-}$ Socs3 cKO (Il6 KO, closed circle, n = 16) mice. Each mouse strain was monitored up to 30 weeks after birth. The percentage of the mice showing disease incidence is shown on the Y axis in all examined mice at each time point. B) Lesion incidences were examined in K5-Cre mice (WT, open circle, n = 5) and Il23$^{-/-}$ Socs3 cKO (Il23 KO, closed circle, n = 4) mice. Each mouse strain was monitored for up to 30 weeks after birth. The percentage of the mice showing disease incidence is shown on the Y axis in all examined mice at each time point.

enhanced expression of IL-20R2, the receptor for IL-19, IL-20, and IL-24, on the keratinocytes of the diseased Socs3 cKO mice (**Fig. 5C**).

IL-20R related cytokines induce epidermal hyperplasia in Socs3 cKO skin

Up-regulation of IL-20R related cytokines, IL-19, IL-20 and IL-24, has often been reported in several skin diseases [22]. We therefore examined the effect of IL-20R related cytokines on skin pathology using the air pouch system. Recombinant IL-19 was injected into the air space generated in the skin of control and Socs3 cKO mice. Interestingly, treatment with IL-19 in the pouches of Socs3 cKO skin induced KC and MCP-1 production, but not IL-12p40 production (**Fig. 6A**). We further injected small amounts of IL-6 and IL-19 (10 ng/mouse) intradermally into Socs3 deficient skin, and pathological signatures were assessed by histological analysis with K5 and MPO staining 14 days after the injection (**Fig. 6B**). This amount of IL-6 and IL-19 is not sufficient to induce skin diseases in wild type mice. However, in Socs3 cKO mice, both IL-6 and IL-19 independently caused epidermal hyperplasia and massive neutrophil migration, while control treatment (PBS) showed no pathological changes (**Fig. 6B**); an indication that IL-19 expression in the keratin layer led to the skin inflammation through the attraction of neutrophils.

We further investigated whether IL-20R related cytokines are required for the IL-6 induced epidermal hyperplasia. We first tested the inhibitory properties of two independent reagents, IL-20Rβ-Fc fusion protein and anti-IL-20Rα antibody. The inhibitory activity was assessed by IL-6 production from IL-19 activated keratinocytes, and the inhibition was observed with the IL-20Rβ-Fc fusion protein (**Fig. S3**). Next, Socs3 deficient mice were injected intradermally with IL-6 (20 ng/mouse) along with either control Ig or the IL-20Rβ-Fc fusion protein, and pathological signatures were assessed as epidermal hyperplasia at fourteen days after treatments. Treatment with the IL-20Rβ-Fc fusion protein completely abrogated the IL-6 induced epidermal hyperplasia (**Fig. 6C**). The same inhibition also observed in the mice treated with anti-IL-20 antibody (**Fig. S4**). These results demonstrated that IL-6-induced pathogenesis in the skin disease occurs though the induction of expression of IL-20R related cytokines.

Physical stimuli induced expression of IL-20R related cytokines and hyperplasia in Socs3 cKO mice

Skin lesions of Socs3 cKO mice were consistently observed on the head and face, where mice were able to scratch by themselves, suggesting that physical stimulation by scratching might be a key event responsible for the disrupted skin barrier. To examine this possibility, artificial stimulation was provided by shaving hair on the dorsal skin where mice are unable to directly scratch. Five days after shaving, Socs3 cKO mice, but not control mice, exhibited scaly skin and scabs at the shaved site, and the level of IL-19, IL-20 and IL-24 expression was comparably increased (**Fig. 7A**). Socs3 KO skin showed signs of epidermal hyperplasia on day 4 (**Fig. 7B&C**), and this symptom completely resolved by day 14. Therefore, in the absence of SOCS3, shaving is sufficient for the induction of hyperplasia. The hyperplasia was only partially resolved in Socs3 KO mice crossed with Il6$^{+/-}$ mice, but was completely resolved in Socs3 KO mice crossed with Il6 KO mice. Il6 KO skin exhibited very weak expression of IL-19 in the shaved area (**Fig. 7B**). These results clearly demonstrated that IL-6 is a critical cytokine in the initiation of the epidermal hyperplasia induced by physical stimulation.

The shaving-induced epidermal thickening was inhibited by Tetracyclic Pyridone 6 (P6), a pan-JAK inhibitor that has a higher sensitivity in the JAK1-STAT3 activation pathway [23]. A low dose of P6 (1 mg) showed no effect, while high dose (2 mg) treatment almost totally inhibited the shaving-induced epidermal thickening (**Fig. 7D**). These results indicate that the epidermal hyperplasia induced by physical stimulation is exacerbated through hyperactivation of the JAK-STAT pathway.

Discussion

Recently, accumulating evidence has pointed to a crucial role for cytokines in chronic skin inflammation. The present study proposed that negative regulator for cytokine signaling SOCS3 plays a crucial role to maintain the keratinocyte homeostasis, and showed that defective SOCS3 expression causes inflammatory skin disease. We also found that the disruption of SOCS3 leads to excess activation of the IL-6-STAT3-IL-20R related cytokine signaling pathway. It is suggested that the balance among IL-6, STAT3 and SOCS3 controls normal skin homeostasis and maintains normal keratinocyte growth and proliferation. Imbalance of this skin homeostasis caused increased expression of IL-20R-related cytokines, eventually leading to the psoriatic inflammation in skin. Keratinocyte-specific Socs3 deficient mice provided us with a quite useful window on the disease process explained by the combined initiation of STAT3 activation and the

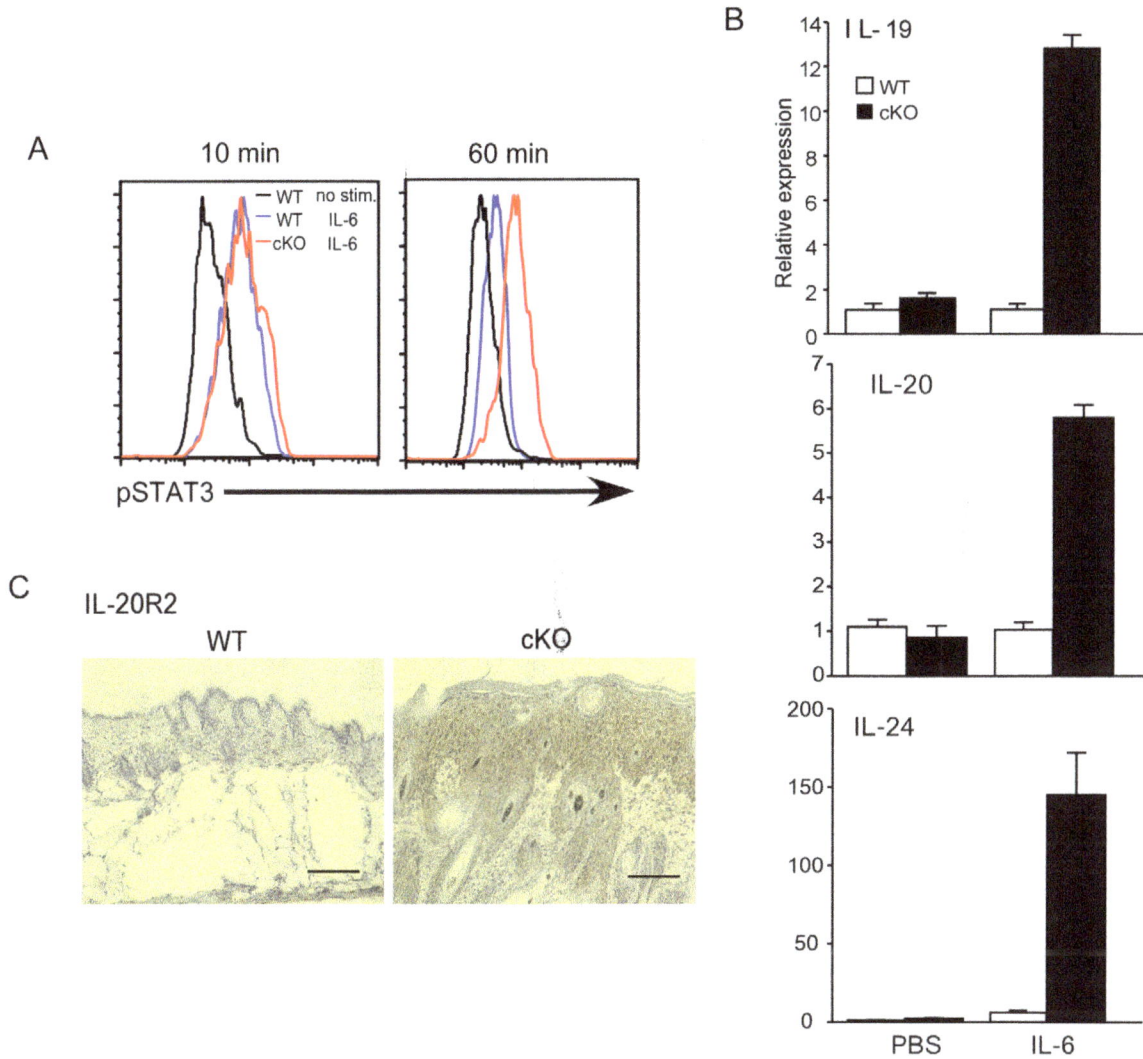

Figure 5. The effect of IL-6 on primary keratinocytes derived from Socs3 cKO mice. A) Mouse primary keratinocytes were stimulated with 10 ng/ml of IL-6 for 10 or 60 min and pSTAT3 was analyzed by flow cytometry. Black lines show the PBS control, blue lines show the keratinocytes from normal C57BL/6 mice, and red lines show the keratinocytes from *Socs3* cKO mice. Data are representative of 3 separate experiments. B) mRNA expression of IL-20R related cytokines in the keratinoyctes. Mouse primary keratinocytes were stimulated with or without IL-6 for 24 hrs and the expression of IL-19, IL-20 and IL-24 mRNA was investigated by quantitative RT-PCR. Open bars show the keratinocytes from C57BL/6 mice (WT), and closed bars show those of *Socs3* cKO mice. Data are relative expression to PBS-treated C57BL/6 keratinocytes. Data are mean ± SEM, n = 3. C) Increased expression of IL-20R2 protein in the diseased skin of *Socs3* cKO mice. Protein levels of IL-20R2 in the frozen skin sections from K5-Cre (WT) and the diseased *Socs3* cKO mice were analyzed by immunohistochemical staining (x200). Scale bar in each section indicates 150 υm.

IL-20R-related cytokine mediated psoriatic skin inflammation, and the understanding of the entire disease process.

Many skin diseases such as seborrheic dermatitis, atopic dermatitis and psoriasis involve inflammation, and in these skin disorders, T cells or T cell-derived cytokines are thought to associate with disease development and aggravation. However, our observations revealed that the dysregulation of cytokine signaling only in the keratinocytes is enough to induce severe inflammation. In *Socs3* cKO mice, the serum IgE level is up-regulated but this seems not to play a critical role in the disease development, suggesting that the up-regulation of IgE may be a secondary event in this skin disease.

In our study, IL-6 seems to be a trigger for the spiral of inflammation in *Socs3* KO skin. Regarding the source of IL-6 in the skin, neuropeptides are possible triggers. Several substances, including Substance P (SP) and vasoactive intestinal peptide (VIP)

which is released from dermal nerve endings, are known to stimulate keratinocytes to produce cytokines including IL-6 [24]. These neuropeptides like VIP can be induced under various stressful conditions including mental stress, alcohol consumption, and smoking. Bacterial infection could be another case for IL-6 induction, because we found plaque of streptococcus in the inflamed skin area of some, but not all, *Socs3* cKO mice (data not shown). Bacterial infections cause an acute form of inflammatory response leading to elevation of IL-6 production in the skin.

In the diseased *Socs3* cKO mouse skin, STAT3 is highly activated but other STAT family members are not (data not shown), indicating that SOCS3 in keratinocytes specifically regulates STAT3 activity. Furthermore, improvement of the skin disease by treatment with the P6 pan-JAK inhibitor confirmed that key cytokine signaling here utilizes the JAK/STAT pathway. SOCS3 specifically inhibits IL-6-induced STAT3 activation by

A

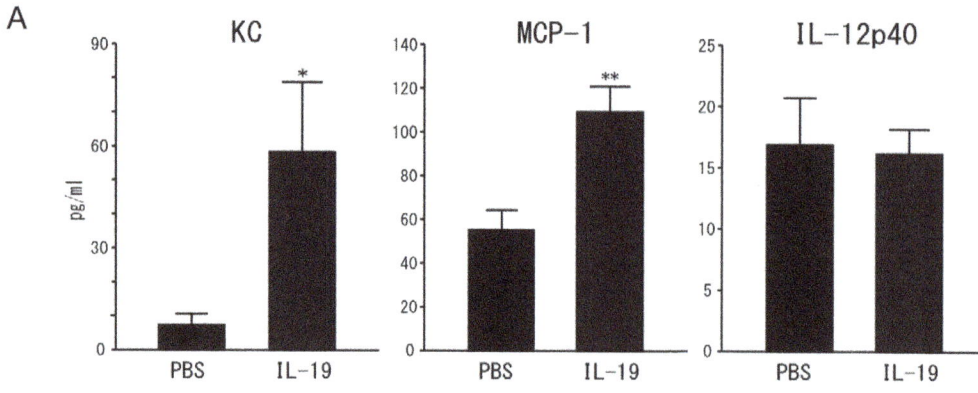

B

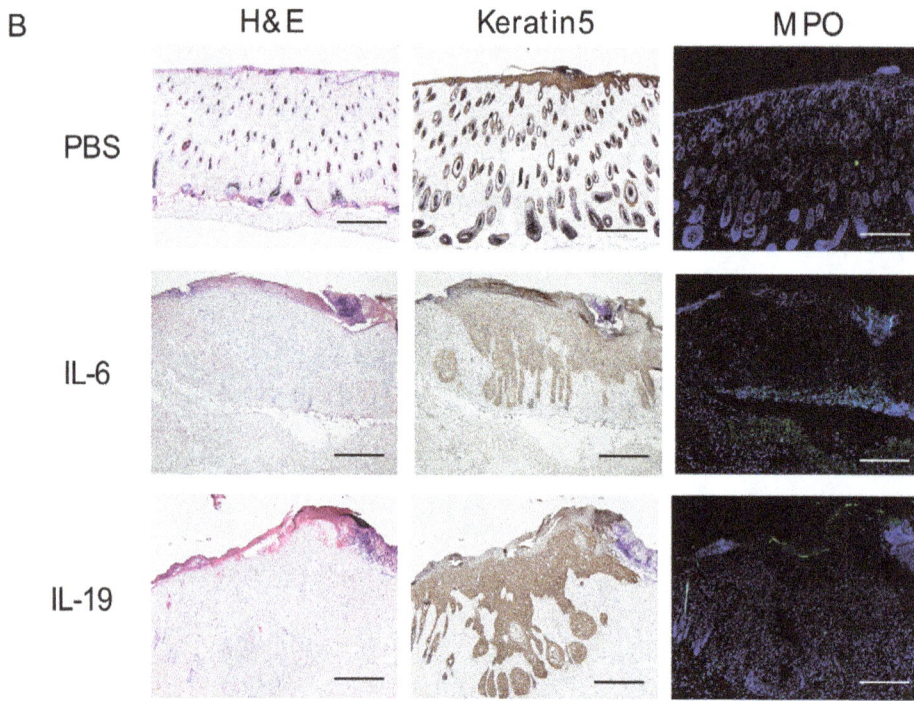

C

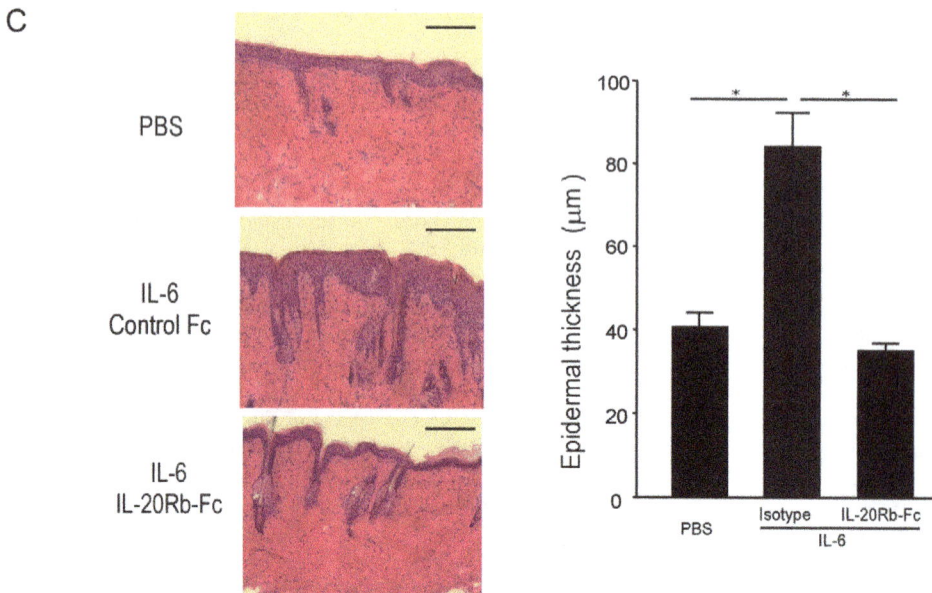

Figure 6. Effect of IL-19 on skin inflammation in the Socs3 cKO mice. A) Amounts of KC, MCP-1 and IL12p40 in the air pouches after IL-19 injection into C57BL/6 mice. IL-19 or PBS was injected into mouse air pouches, and chemokine concentration in the pouch lavage was measured after 5 hrs. Data are mean ± SEM, n = 5–6. B) IL-6 and IL-19 induced skin inflammation in the *Socs3* cKO mice. *Socs3* cKO mice were injected with PBS (upper rows), 10 ng of IL-6 (middle rows) or 10 ng of IL-19 (bottom rows) was injected intradermally and skin sections were obtained two weeks later. Left panels show the H&E staining, middle panels show K5 immunostaining, and right panels show MPO⁺ neutrophils (x40). Scale bar in each section indicates 750 υm. C) *Socs3* cKO mice were injected with PBS (upper rows) or 20 ng of IL-6 (middle and bottom rows) intradermally with 5 υg of control Fc or IL-20Rβ fusion Fc (IL-20Rβ-Fc). After two weeks, skin sections were stained with H&E and epidermal thickness was measured at the injection site (x200). Scale bar in each section indicates 150 υm. Bar graph (right panel) indicates the mean and SEM (n = 3) of epidermal thickness (υm).

binding to the STAT3 docking site (Tyr759) in one of the components of the IL-6 receptor, gp130 [25,26]. This pivotal role for SOCS3 in skin inflammation is supported by recent reports showing that a specific microRNA, miR203, is highly expressed in human psoriatic skin and inhibits the expression of SOCS3 [27]. IL-20R-related cytokines, IL-19, IL-20 and IL-24, transmit their signal through IL-20Rα/IL-20Rβ receptor complex. These cytokines have been reported to play important roles in the skin, and are often thought to be pro-inflammatory cytokines [28]. Here we report that IL-6 induced higher levels of IL-19, IL-20 and IL-24 mRNA in SOCS3 deficient keratinocytes than in the WT keratinocytes, consistent with IL-6 mediated IL-20 induction in human keratinocytes [29]. Together, these findings indicate that in the healthy condition, SOCS3 is required for inhibition of the IL-6 induced increases in pro-inflammatory IL-20R-related cytokines. The up-regulation of these cytokines leads to neutrophil accumulation directly or indirectly through the induction of neutrophil chemoattractants, S100A8/S100A9.

In conclusion, we have demonstrated that skin homeostasis is maintained by a balance among IL-6, STAT3 and SOCS3 in keratinocytes. Furthermore, when this balance is broken and STAT3 activation is out of control, inflammatory skin disease is induced without any abnormalities in the immune cells. This SOCS3 mediated homeostatic function plays a key role in negatively regulating STAT3 activity. The relation among IL-6, STAT3, and SOCS3 provides a useful tool for understanding the mechanism of chronic skin inflammation in humans.

Materials and Methods

Reagents

Polylactide-glycoside (PLGA) nanospheres have been reported as useful pulmonary drug delivery carriers for improving the pharmacological effect of drugs [30]. The pan-JAK inhibitor Tetracyclic Pyridone 2-tert- butyl- 9-fliro- 3,6-dihydro- 7H-benz[h]-imidaz[4,5-f]isoquinoline-7-one (P6) [23] was packaged with PLGA nanospheres by Hosokawa Powder Technology Research Institute (Osaka). P6 was dissolved in PBS when applied onto the skin of mice. The dorsal skin area of *Socs3*cKO was shaved with depilatory cream, and P6 (1 mg or 2 mg) or PBS was injected intradermally into the shaved area. Five days after shaving, skin samples were prepared and frozen for sectioning and H&E staining.

Mice

K5 Cre Tg [31], *Socs1*^f/f [32], Socs3^f/f [33], Il23⁻/⁻ [34], Il4r⁻/⁻ [35], Rag1⁻/⁻ [36] and Il6⁻/⁻ [37] mice are described elsewhere. All mice used in this study except *Il4r*⁻/⁻ were backcrossed into C57BL/6 mice, and *Il4r*⁻/⁻ mice were maintained on a BALB/c background. C57BL/6 and BALB/c mice were purchased from CLEA Japan, Inc. (Tokyo, Japan). All mice were maintained in SPF conditions.

Monitoring disease incidences

The clinical scoring was assessed with the incidence number of regions: 0, no lesion; 1, lesion in ear; 2, lesion in half of face; 3, lesion in whole face. The scoring was done until week 50.

Antibodies and Cytokines

Immunohistochemistry was carried out with the following antibodies. Biotinylated rat anti-mouse CD4 (H129.19), biotinylated mouse anti-ClassII (I-A^b) (KH74), rat-anti-IL-17A (TC11-18H10)-PE, mouse anti-pSTAT3 (4/P-STAT3)-Alexa 488 and rat anti-IFNγ (XMG1.2)-PE antibodies were purchased from BD Biosciences (San Diego, CA). Biotinylated rat anti-CD8 (53–6.7), biotinylated hamster anti-CD11c (N418), rat-anti-Langerin (eBioL31), biotinylated rat anti-FcεRIα (MAR-1) and rat anti-IL-20R2 (20RNTC) were purchased from e-Biosciences (San Diego, CA). Goat anti-IL-6 (AF-406-NA), rat anti-IL-19 (350105), recombinant murine IL-23R Fc chimera (1686-MR), rat anti-IL-24 (303308), rat anti-IL-20 (380605) antibodies and recombinant murine IL-20Rβ Fc chimera (4388-MR) were purchased from R&D Systems, Inc. (Minneapolis, MN). Rabbit anti-pSTAT1 (9171), anti-pSTAT5 (9351) and anti-pSTAT6 (9361) were purchased from Cell Signaling Technology (Massachusetts, MA). Rabbit anti-K5 (PRB-160P) was obtained from Covance Research Products Inc. (Denver, PA). Goat anti-PAR2 (sc-8205) was purchased from Santa Cruz Biotechnology, Inc. (Santa Cruz, CA). Rabbit MPO polyclonal antibody (PA1-28215) was obtained from Pierce Biotechnology (Rockford, IL). Rat anti-MCP-8 (TUG8) was purchased from BioLegend (San Diego, CA). Rabbit anti-IL-20Rα antibody (ab25922) was obtained from abcam (Cambridge, UK). Murine anti-rat and goat antibodies (Histofine MAX-PO), Histo-fine streptavidin, anti-rat IgG Alexa Fluor 488 and streptavidin Alexa Fluor 546 (Invitrogen), anti-human IgG HRP (Jackson immune research, Pennsylvania, PA) were used for 2nd antibodies for Immunohistochemistry. Recombinant murine IL-6 and IL-19 were purchased from Peprotech Inc. and R&D Systems, Inc., respectively.

In vitro keratinocyte culture

Primary keratinocytes were obtained from epidermis isolated from mouse ears. The epidermis was separated from the dermis following 1 hour incubation at 37°C in 0.25% trypsin/EDTA (Nacalai Tesque, Kyoto Japan) followed by filtration through 70 υm nylon mesh cell strainers (BD). Keratinocytes were suspended in the keratinocyte growth media (KGM-2, Lonza, Basel, Switzerland) containing 4 ng/ml mouse epidermal growth factor (EGF) and seeded at 5×10^5 cells/ml. Before cytokine stimulation, keratinocytes were deprived of growth factors for 4 hours, then stimulated with recombinant IL-6 (10 ng/ml). After 10 or 60 min stimulation, cells were harvested and intracellular staining of pSTAT3 was performed. The flow cytometric analysis was done with a FACS Calibur (BD). For the detection of mRNA expression, after 24 hours stimulation, cells were harvested and

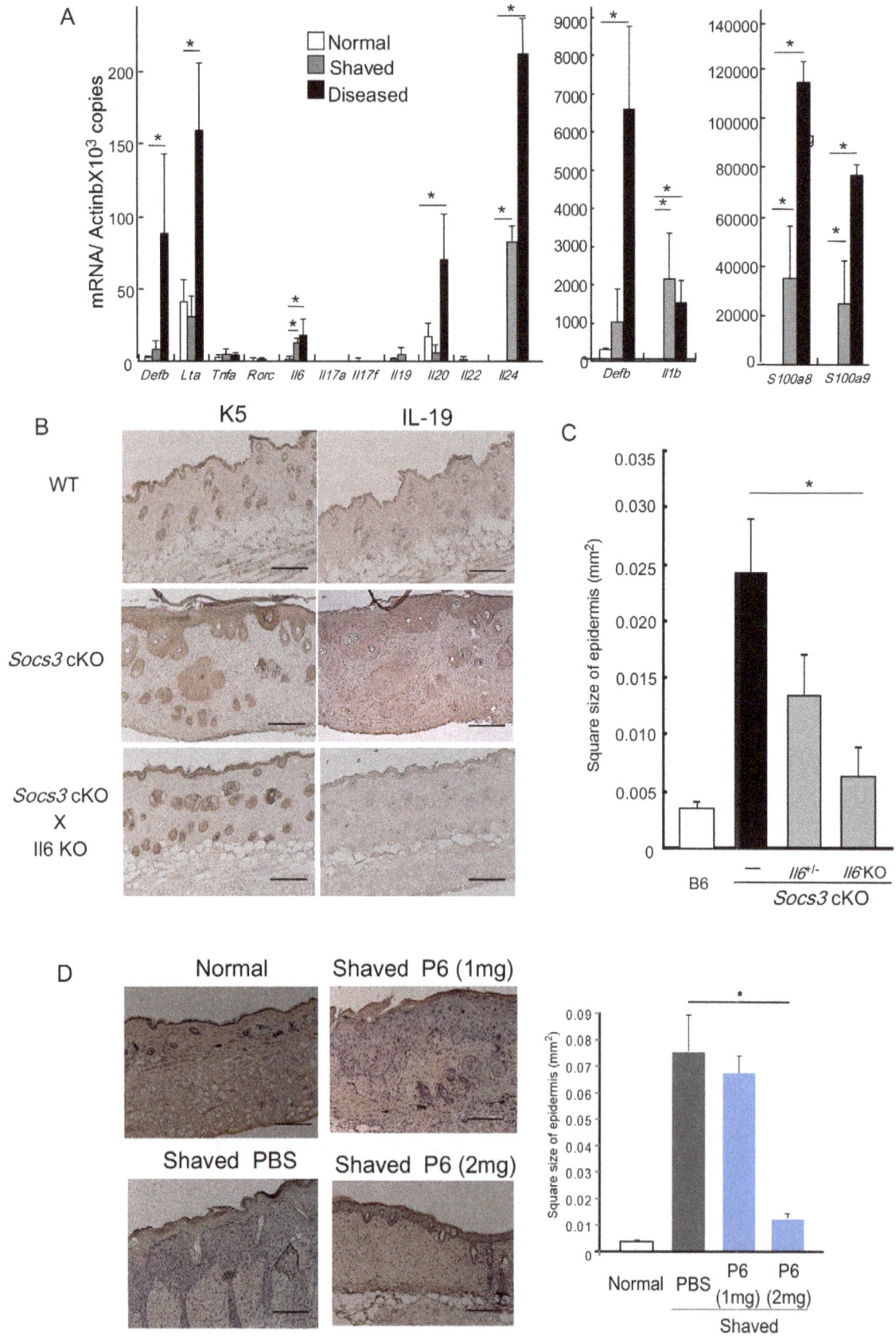

Figure 7. Physical stimulation initiates epidermal hyperplasia. A) mRNA was prepared from the skin of healthy K5-Cre (Normal), the shaved *Socs3* cKO mice (Shaved) and the diseased *Socs3* cKO mice (Diseased), and analyzed for the expression of the indicated genes by SYBR green real-time qPCR analysis. B) Immunohistochemical staining of keratinocytes (K5, left panels) and IL-19 positive cells (IL-19, left panels) in epidermis and dermis of

K5-Cre (WT), *Socs3* cKO mice and *Socs3* cKO mice crossed with *Il6* KO mice (*Socs3* cKO X *Il6* KO) (x40). Scale bar in each section indicates 750 υm. C) The role of IL-6 on the development of epidermal hyperplasia in *Socs3* cKO mice. B6, *Socs3* cKO mice, *Socs3* cKO mice crossed with *Il6*[+/−] or *Il6* KO mice were studied. The square area of epidermis (0.25 mm²) in the section was measured at day 5 after shaving and is indicated on the Y-axis. Data are mean of the square size and error bars indicate SEM (n = 3). D) Effect of PLGA-P6 on physical stimulation-induced epidermal hyperplasia in *Socs3* cKO mice. Left; The dorsal skin area of *Socs3* cKO was shaved with depilatory cream and PLGA-P6 (1 mg or 2 mg) or PBS was injected intradermally into the shaved area. The shaved area (Shaved) was then compared to the non-treated area (Normal). At day 5 after shaving, skin sections were examined by H&E staining to assess the appearance of hyperplasia. The images are representative of three independent experiments (x40). Scale bar in each section indicates 750 υm. Right; the square size of the epidermis (0.25 mm²) in the sections shown in the left image was measured at day 5 after shaving and is indicated on the Y-axis. Data are mean of the square size and error bars indicate SEM (n = 3).

RNA was extracted with RNAeasy mini kit (Qiagen). RT-PCR was done with SYBR green real-time quantitative PCR assay.

Histology and immunohistochemistry

The frozen skin sections were fixed with acetone and then stained with H&E. After blocking the sections with 3% BSA/PBS for 30 min, they were treated with primary abs in 1% BSA/PBS and were incubated for 30 min at room temperature. When the secondly abs were labeled with HRP, sections were then visualized by using DAB for 5 to 15 minutes. After washing the sections with water for 10 mins, sections were treated with EtOH and xylene and observed under light microscopy. When the secondly antibodies were fluorescently labeled, the sections were washed with PBS(−)-0.05% Tween20 after secondly antibody treatment. After washing the sections with water for 10 mins they were mounted with VECTA SHIELD/Prolong Gold reagent and imaged using an LSM 510 confocal microscopy system (Carl Zeiss, Germany). For the quantification of mast cells, basophils and neutrophils, toluidine blue, MCP-8 and MPO were used as cell markers respectively. We randomly picked four fields on the sections from each mouse for analysis.

Gene expression analysis

For gene expression analysis, total RNA was isolated using RNA STAT-60 (Tel-Test, Friendswood, TX, USA). Total RNA (5 υg) was subjected to treatment with DNase (Roche). DNase-treated total RNA was reverse-transcribed using Superscript II (Gibco/BRL). Primers were designed using Primer Express (PE Biosystems), or obtained commercially from Applied Biosystems. Real-time quantitative PCR on 10 ng of cDNA from each sample was performed using either of two methods. In the first method, two gene-specific unlabelled primers were utilized at 400 nM in a Perkin Elmer SYBR green real-time quantitative PCR assay utilizing an ABI 5700 instrument. In the second method, two unlabelled primers at 900 nM each were used with 250 nM of FAM-labeled probe (Applied Biosystems) in a TAQMAN™ real-time quantitative PCR reaction on an ABI 7700 sequence detection system. The absence of genomic DNA contamination was confirmed using primers that recognize the genomic region of the CD4 promoter – samples with detectable DNA contamination by real-time PCR were excluded from the study. Ubiquitin levels were measured in a separate reaction and used to normalize the data by the $\Delta - \Delta$ Ct method, using the mean cycle threshold (Ct) value for ubiquitin and the gene of interests for each sample; the equation 1.8 e (Ct ubiquitin − Ct gene of interest) x 10⁴ was used to obtain the normalized values.

Air pouch

C57BL/6 mice (8–9 wks) were injected with 5 ml of sterile air into the subcutaneous tissue of the back, followed by a second injection of 3 ml of sterile air into the pouch 3 days later. IL-19 (1 mg) in 1 ml of sterile PBS, or sterile PBS as a control were injected into the pouch 7 days after the first injection of air. After 5 hrs, mice were killed and pouch fluids were harvested by injecting 0.5 ml of PBS. After centrifugation, the supernatant were analyzed for cytokines/chemokines concentrations with Bioplex Cytokine assay kit (Bio-Rad Laboratories, Hercules, CA, USA) according to the manufacturer's protocol.

Supporting Information

Figure S1 Skin sections from the diseased *Socs3* cKO mice were stained with anti-pSTAT1, anti-pSTAT5, or anti-pSTAT6, and the sections were further probed with HRP labeled secondary antibody. Control indicates secondary antibody alone.

Figure S2 Expression of IL-17A and IL-23 protein in frozen sections of K5-Cre control (WT) and the diseased skin from *Socs3* cKO (cKO) mice was analyzed by immunohistochemical staining. The images are representative of five independent experiments (x40).

Figure S3 Isolated keratinocytes were cultured with IL-19 in the presence of IL-20Rβ-Fc fusion protein or anti-IL-20Rα antibody. After 6 hrs, IL-6 production in culture supernatant was measured by ELISA. Data are mean and SEM of three independent cultures.

Figure S4 *Socs3* deficient mice were injected intradermally with IL-6 (10 ng/mouse) with either control Ig (isotype) or anti-IL-20 antibody (100 υg). After two weeks, skin sections were stained with H&E and epidermal thickness was measured at the injection site (x200). Scale bar in each section indicates 150 υm. Bar graph (right panel) indicates the mean and SEM (n = 3) of epidermal thickness (υm).

Acknowledgments

The authors thank Dr. Shigetoshi Sano, Dr. Hiromitsu Hara, Dr. Douglas Osei-Hyiaman and Dr. Peter Barrows, for critical review and comments on the manuscript and Y. Sato, H. Dohi, Uno, T., Natsume, M., Miura, E., Ohmori, A., and Hayashi, E., for technical assistance.

Author Contributions

Conceived and designed the experiments: AU SS MK. Performed the experiments: AU KM NO YM YS DC. Analyzed the data: AU KM SS DC MK. Contributed reagents/materials/analysis tools: AY DC. Wrote the paper: AU KM SS MK.

Reference

1. Kubo M, Hanada T, Yoshimura A (2003) Suppressors of cytokine signaling and immunity. Nat Immunol 4: 1169–1176.
2. Yoshimura A, Naka T, Kubo M (2007) SOCS proteins, cytokine signalling and immune regulation. Nat Rev Immunol 7: 454–465.
3. Zhu BM, Ishida Y, Robinson GW, Pacher-Zavisin M, Yoshimura A, et al. (2008) SOCS3 negatively regulates the gp130-STAT3 pathway in mouse skin wound healing. J Invest Dermatol 128: 1821–1829.
4. Margadant C, Charafeddine RA, Sonnenberg A (2010) Unique and redundant functions of integrins in the epidermis. FASEB J 24: 4133–4152.
5. Wullaert A, Bonnet MC, Pasparakis M (2011) NF-kappaB in the regulation of epithelial homeostasis and inflammation. Cell Res 21: 146–158.
6. Jensen JM, Schutze S, Forl M, Kronke M, Proksch E (1999) Roles for tumor necrosis factor receptor p55 and sphingomyelinase in repairing the cutaneous permeability barrier. J Clin Invest 104: 1761–1770.
7. Shornick LP, De Togni P, Mariathasan S, Goellner J, Strauss-Schoenberger J, et al. (1996) Mice deficient in IL-1beta manifest impaired contact hypersensitivity to trinitrochlorobenzone. J Exp Med 183: 1427–1436.
8. Wang XP, Schunck M, Kallen KJ, Neumann C, Trautwein C, et al. (2004) The interleukin-6 cytokine system regulates epidermal permeability barrier homeostasis. J Invest Dermatol 123: 124–131.
9. Sano S, Chan KS, DiGiovanni J (2008) Impact of Stat3 activation upon skin biology: a dichotomy of its role between homeostasis and diseases. J Dermatol Sci 50: 1–14.
10. Sano S, Chan KS, Carbajal S, Clifford J, Peavey M, et al. (2005) Stat3 links activated keratinocytes and immunocytes required for development of psoriasis in a novel transgenic mouse model. Nat Med 11: 43–49.
11. Kataoka K, Kim DJ, Carbajal S, Clifford JL, DiGiovanni J (2008) Stage-specific disruption of Stat3 demonstrates a direct requirement during both the initiation and promotion stages of mouse skin tumorigenesis. Carcinogenesis 29: 1108–1114.
12. Pestka S, Krause CD, Sarkar D, Walter MR, Shi Y, et al. (2004) Interleukin-10 and related cytokines and receptors. Annu Rev Immunol 22: 929–979.
13. Kunz S, Wolk K, Witte E, Witte K, Doecke WD, et al. (2006) Interleukin (IL)-19, IL-20 and IL-24 are produced by and act on keratinocytes and are distinct from classical ILs. Exp Dermatol 15: 991–1004.
14. Stenderup K, Rosada C, Worsaae A, Clausen JT, Norman Dam T (2007) Interleukin-20 as a target in psoriasis treatment. Ann N Y Acad Sci 1110: 368–381.
15. Kingo K, Koks S, Nikopensius T, Silm H, Vasar E (2004) Polymorphisms in the interleukin-20 gene: relationships to plaque-type psoriasis. Genes Immun 5: 117–121.
16. Sa SM, Valdez PA, Wu J, Jung K, Zhong F, et al. (2007) The effects of IL-20 subfamily cytokines on reconstituted human epidermis suggest potential roles in cutaneous innate defense and pathogenic adaptive immunity in psoriasis. J Immunol 178: 2229–2240.
17. Leng RX, Pan HF, Tao JH, Ye DQ IL-19, IL-20 and IL-24: potential therapeutic targets for autoimmune diseases. Expert Opin Ther Targets 15: 119–126.
18. Sabat R, Philipp S, Hoflich C, Kreutzer S, Wallace E, et al. (2007) Immunopathogenesis of psoriasis. Exp Dermatol 16: 779–798.
19. Chan JR, Blumenschein W, Murphy E, Diveu C, Wiekowski M, et al. (2006) IL-23 stimulates epidermal hyperplasia via TNF and IL-20R2-dependent mechanisms with implications for psoriasis pathogenesis. J Exp Med 203: 2577–2587.
20. Lee E, Trepicchio WL, Oestreicher JL, Pittman D, Wang F, et al. (2004) Increased expression of interleukin 23 p19 and p40 in lesional skin of patients with psoriasis vulgaris. J Exp Med 199: 125–130.
21. Nair RP, Duffin KC, Helms C, Ding J, Stuart PE, et al. (2009) Genome-wide scan reveals association of psoriasis with IL-23 and NF-kappaB pathways. Nat Genet 41: 199–204.
22. Ouyang W, Rutz S, Crellin NK, Valdez PA, Hymowitz SG (2011) Regulation and functions of the IL-10 family of cytokines in inflammation and disease. Annu Rev Immunol 29: 71–109.
23. Pedranzini L, Dechow T, Berishaj M, Comenzo R, Zhou P, et al. (2006) Pyridone 6, a pan-Janus-activated kinase inhibitor, induces growth inhibition of multiple myeloma cells. Cancer Res 66: 9714–9721.
24. Park YM, Kim CW (1999) The effects of substance P and vasoactive intestinal peptide on interleukin-6 synthesis in cultured human keratinocytes. J Dermatol Sci 22: 17–23.
25. Schmitz J, Weissenbach M, Haan S, Heinrich PC, Schaper F (2000) SOCS3 exerts its inhibitory function on interleukin-6 signal transduction through the SHP2 recruitment site of gp130. J Biol Chem 275: 12848–12856.
26. Lehmann U, Schmitz J, Weissenbach M, Sobota RM, Hortner M, et al. (2003) SHP2 and SOCS3 contribute to Tyr-759-dependent attenuation of interleukin-6 signaling through gp130. J Biol Chem 278: 661–671.
27. Bostjancic E, Glavac D (2008) Importance of microRNAs in skin morphogenesis and diseases. Acta Dermatovenerol Alp Panonica Adriat 17: 95–102.
28. Boniface K, Lecron JC, Bernard FX, Dagregorio G, Guillet G, et al. (2005) Keratinocytes as targets for interleukin-10-related cytokines: a putative role in the pathogenesis of psoriasis. Eur Cytokine Netw 16: 309–319.
29. Otkjaer K, Kragballe K, Johansen C, Funding AT, Just H, et al. (2007) IL-20 gene expression is induced by IL-1beta through mitogen-activated protein kinase and NF-kappaB-dependent mechanisms. J Invest Dermatol 127: 1326–1336.
30. Hara K, Tsujimoto H, Tsukada Y, Huang CC, Kawashima Y, et al. (2008) Histological examination of PLGA nanospheres for intratracheal drug administration. Int J Pharm 356: 267–273.
31. Tarutani M, Itami S, Okabe M, Ikawa M, Tezuka T, et al. (1997) Tissue-specific knockout of the mouse Pig-a gene reveals important roles for GPI-anchored proteins in skin development. Proc Natl Acad Sci U S A 94: 7400–7405.
32. Tanaka K, Ichiyama K, Hashimoto M, Yoshida H, Takimoto T, et al. (2008) Loss of suppressor of cytokine signaling 1 in helper T cells leads to defective Th17 differentiation by enhancing antagonistic effects of IFN-gamma on STAT3 and Smads. J Immunol 180: 3746–3756.
33. Yasukawa H, Ohishi M, Mori H, Murakami M, Chinen T, et al. (2003) IL-6 induces an anti-inflammatory response in the absence of SOCS3 in macrophages. Nat Immunol 4: 551–556.
34. Cua DJ, Sherlock J, Chen Y, Murphy CA, Joyce B, et al. (2003) Interleukin-23 rather than interleukin-12 is the critical cytokine for autoimmune inflammation of the brain. Nature 421: 744–748.
35. Mohrs M, Ledermann B, Kohler G, Dorfmuller A, Gessner A, et al. (1999) Differences between IL-4- and IL-4 receptor alpha-deficient mice in chronic leishmaniasis reveal a protective role for IL-13 receptor signaling. J Immunol 162: 7302–7308.
36. Mombaerts P, Iacomini J, Johnson R, Herrup K, Tonegawa S, et al. (1992) RAG-1-deficient mice have no mature B and T lymphocytes. Cell 68: 869–877.
37. Kopf M, Baumann H, Freer G, Freudenberg M, Lamers M, et al. (1994) Impaired immune and acute-phase responses in interleukin-6-deficient mice. Nature 368: 339–342.

Filaggrin Genotype Determines Functional and Molecular Alterations in Skin of Patients with Atopic Dermatitis and Ichthyosis Vulgaris

Mårten C. G. Winge[1,3]*, **Torborg Hoppe**[2], **Berit Berne**[2], **Anders Vahlquist**[2], **Magnus Nordenskjöld**[3], **Maria Bradley**[1,3], **Hans Törmä**[2]

1 Dermatology Unit, Department of Medicine Solna and Center for Molecular Medicine, Karolinska Institutet, Karolinska University Hospital Solna, Stockholm, Sweden, **2** Department of Medical Sciences, Dermatology and Venereology, Uppsala University, Uppsala, Sweden, **3** Department of Molecular Medicine & Surgery and Center for Molecular Medicine, Karolinska Institutet, Karolinska University Hospital Solna, Stockholm, Sweden

Abstract

Background: Several common genetic and environmental disease mechanisms are important for the pathophysiology behind atopic dermatitis (AD). Filaggrin (FLG) loss-of-function is of great significance for barrier impairment in AD and ichthyosis vulgaris (IV), which is commonly associated with AD. The molecular background is, however, complex and various clusters of genes are altered, including inflammatory and epidermal-differentiation genes.

Objective: The objective was to study whether the functional and molecular alterations in AD and IV skin depend directly on FLG loss-of-function, and whether *FLG* genotype determines the type of downstream molecular pathway affected.

Methods and Findings: Patients with AD/IV (n = 43) and controls (n = 15) were recruited from two Swedish outpatient clinics and a Swedish AD family material with known *FLG* genotype. They were clinically examined and their medical history recorded using a standardized questionnaire. Blood samples and punch biopsies were taken and trans-epidermal water loss (TEWL) and skin pH was assessed with standard techniques. In addition to *FLG* genotyping, the *STS* gene was analyzed to exclude X-linked recessive ichthyosis (XLI). Microarrays and quantitative real-time PCR were used to compare differences in gene expression depending on *FLG* genotype. Several different signalling pathways were altered depending on *FLG* genotype in patients suffering from AD or AD/IV. Disease severity, TEWL and pH follow FLG deficiency in the skin; and the number of altered genes and pathways are correlated to FLG mRNA expression.

Conclusions: We emphasize further the role of FLG in skin-barrier integrity and the complex compensatory activation of signalling pathways. This involves inflammation, epidermal differentiation, lipid metabolism, cell signalling and adhesion in response to FLG-dependent skin-barrier dysfunction.

Editor: Johanna M. Brandner, University Hospital Hamburg-Eppendorf, Germany

Funding: The study was performed with grants from Welander and Finsen foundations, the Centre of Allergy Research (CFA) and through the regional agreement on medical training and clinical research (ALF) between Stockholm County Council and Karolinska Institutet and Uppsala County Council and Uppsala University. The funders had no role in study design, data collection and analysis, decision to publish, or preparation of the manuscript.

Competing Interests: The authors have declared that no competing interests exist.

* E-mail: marten.winge@ki.se

Introduction

Atopic dermatitis (AD; OMIM #605803) is a common chronic, non-contagious, inflammatory skin disorder. Clinical manifestations include early onset of dry skin, pruritus, eczema with typical age-dependent distribution, and personal or family history of atopic disease [1]. Knowledge of the pathophysiology behind the disease is emerging, several common genetic, environmental disease mechanisms and individual trigger factors being of importance [2]. Central in the pathogenesis are combinations of inherited and acquired insults thought to alter epidermal structure. These changes in the physiological skin barrier predispose to increased allergen presentation and are followed by immune activation, which in turn has negative consequences for skin-barrier homeostasis [3]. Impaired homeostasis of the skin leads to increased trans-epidermal water loss (TEWL) and changes in gene expression patterns [4] and enzymatic activity [5].

The most common monogenic disorder of keratinisation, ichthyosis vulgaris (IV; OMIM # 146700), is associated with AD and related atopic manifestations in up to 50% [6]. This contrasts with X-linked recessive ichthyosis (XLI; OMIM # 308100), which is due to mutations in the *STS* gene leading to accumulation of cholesterol sulphate in the stratum corneum. XLI occurs almost exclusively in males and may look almost indistinguishable from IV. However, skin histology and surface pH differ in the two conditions [7] and no association to AD has been reported in XLI. In 2006, it was found that mutations in the *FLG* gene resulting in filaggrin (FLG) dysfunction are the causative genetic factor for IV [8]. Following the frequent co-existence of IV and AD it was also discovered that 20–40% of European and

Asian patients with moderate-to-severe AD carry *FLG* mutations. This is so far the most significant genetic finding associated with AD [9]. FLG is important for the structural integrity of the skin, and other functions are attributed to acidic degradation products of FLG, e.g. urocanic acid (UCA) and pyrrolidone carboxylic acid (PCA). These are components of natural moisturizing factors (NMFs) [10] and contributes to maintaining a low pH in the stratum corneum (SC) [11].

In addition to FLG dysfunction, it has previously been demonstrated that the molecular background to the pathogenesis of AD is complex, and that several clusters of genes, including inflammatory and epidermal differentiation [4,12] are altered in lesional AD skin. We set out to study whether the functional and molecular alterations in AD and IV skin depend directly on FLG loss-of-function variants, and whether the *FLG* genotype determine the type of downstream molecular pathways affected.

Materials and Methods

Patient material

Patients (n = 43) with AD (n = 35), AD and IV (n = 5) and IV (n = 3) together with controls (n = 15; subjects without past or present history of AD, dry skin or other atopic manifestations) were identified at the dermatology outpatient clinics at Karolinska University Hospital Solna, Sophiahemmet Stockholm and Uppsala University Hospital; or recruited from a Swedish family material with known *FLG* genotype as described previously [13]. All patients were investigated by a dermatologist performing clinical examination and recording medical history with a standardized questionnaire. Inclusion criteria were: age 18–65 years and diagnosed AD and/or IV. Exclusion criteria were pregnancy; other concomitant skin disease; recent UV-treatment; or recent use of topical or systemic corticosteroids, systemic immunosuppressives or systemic retinoids (<4 weeks). AD was diagnosed according to the UK Working Party's diagnostic criteria and the disease severity for AD was assessed using the scoring atopic dermatitis index (SCORAD) [14]. IV was diagnosed by clinical examination and genetic testing of the *FLG* gene, and in male patients with ichthyosis genetic testing of the steroid sulphatase (*STS*) gene to rule out XLI. Other atopic manifestations such as allergic asthma and allergic rhinoconjunctivitis were assessed through the questionnaire. Blood samples and punch biopsies were taken from all patients and controls. Two 3 mm punch biopsies were obtained from a non-lesional area on each patients forearm, after local anaesthetic with lidocain hydrochloride with adrenalin (Astra Zeneca, Södertälje, Sweden). TEWL was assessed using a Tewameter TM 300 Multi Probe Adapter (Courage+Khazaka electronic GmbH, Köln, Germany) and skin pH was measured using a skin-pH-Meter PH 905 Multi Probe Adapter (Courage+Khazaka electronic GmbH). TEWL and pH were measured from the forearms of patients and controls. The patients were divided into three groups (AD *FLG*+/+; AD *FLG*+/− and AD/IV *FLG*−/−) depending on genotype of the four most prevalent European *FLG*-mutations [6].

Subjects for microarray analysis. Five patients from each patient group (AD *FLG*+/+, AD *FLG*+/− and AD/IV *FLG*−/−) were randomly selected for microarray analysis after removing outliers in TEWL and pH. In the AD *FLG*+/− group four were heterozygous carriers of the 2282del4 mutation and one was a heterozygous carrier of the R501X mutation. In the AD/IV *FLG*−/− group four were homozygous carriers of the 2282del4 mutation and one was a homozygous carrier of the R501X mutation. All selected patients had AD. The groups were compared to five healthy controls randomly selected after removing outliers compared to the rest of the control group regarding TEWL or pH. They carried no tested *FLG* mutations.

Ethics. The study was conducted according to Declaration of Helsinki principles and was approved by the regional ethics committees at Uppsala University and at Karolinska Institute. All study participants gave written informed consent.

Genotyping

Genomic DNA was isolated from peripheral blood using QIAamp® DNA mini kit (Qiagen, Hilden, Germany).

FLG genotyping. *FLG* genotyping was performed with allelic discrimination in patients and controls for the prevalent European *FLG* mutations R501X, S3247X and R2447X. Genomic DNA was PCR-amplified in 384-well plates. Each well contained 5 ng genomic DNA, 2.5 μl TaqMan Universal PCR Master Mix, 0.125 μl specific Taqman assay solution and 2.375 μl H$_2$O. Allelic discrimination was carried out with the ABI PRISM® 7900HT Sequence Detection System and the SDS 2.2.1 sequence detection system program (Applied Biosystems, Stockholm, Sweden). Primers and PCR conditions for tested *FLG* mutations were as described previously [6].

FLG mutation 2282del4 was screened for by direct sequencing using an overlapping PCR fragment covering this region [8]. In brief, 50 ng DNA was amplified with 1.25 μl 10 mM dNTPmix (2.5 mM of each), 2.5 μl 10×Rxn buffer - MgCl$_2$, 2 μl 50 mM MgCl$_2$, 2.5 μl PCR Enhancer, 0.3 μl PlatinumTaq DNA Polymerase (Invitrogen, Lidingö, Sweden), 10.45 μl H$_2$0 and 2.5 μl each of forward and reverse primer. Sequencing was analyzed using an ABI® 3730 DNA Analyzer instrument.

STS genotyping. Multiplex Ligation-dependent Probe Amplification (MLPA) analysis was run for the *STS* gene using the P160 A2 kit (MRC-Holland, Amsterdam, the Netherlands), as previously described [15] with minor modifications. Typically 100 ng genomic DNA was amplified. The sample was analyzed on the ABI 3130xl Genetic Analyzer. In addition, exon 1–10 of the STS gene was sequenced using primers and PCR conditions previously described in male patients where no deletion was detected [16].

All primer pairs were confirmed specific by database queries (using BLAST and BLAT). The polyphen [17] and the Alamut mutation interpretation software (Interactive Biosoftware, Rouen, France) was used to predict pathogenicity of single nucleotide polymorphisms (SNPs) compared to reference sequence.

RNA extraction

Skin biopsies were trimmed of subcutaneous fat prior to homogenization. The biopsies were placed in 1 ml Trizol (Invitrogen) and subsequently homogenized using a Polytron homogenizer. Total RNA was isolated as described elsewhere [18]. Total RNA concentration was determined with spectrophotometric analysis and purity was analyzed by the 260:280 absorbance ratios.

Microarray analysis

Microarray hybridization and scanning. Trizol-extracted total RNA was purified using the RNeasy MiniKit (Qiagen, Valencia, CA). Samples were re-quantified with spectroscopy, and purity was re-analyzed through the 260:280 absorbance ratios. RNA quality and integrity were assessed and ensured using Bioanalyzer 2100 (Agilent Technologies, Santa Clara, CA) and RNA 6000 NanoAssay. Hybridization was performed with Human Gene 1.0 ST arrays (Affymetrix, Inc, Santa Clara, CA). Briefly, 100 ng of total RNA from each sample was reverse-transcribed to complementary DNA (cDNA) using the Ambion

WT Expression kit. The cDNA was subsequently converted to complementary RNA using in vitro transcription with an amplification kit. 10 μg purified complementary RNA was used as a template for another cycle of first-strand cDNA synthesis. Single-stranded cDNA samples were fragmented and end-labeled with the Gene Chip WT cDNA Synthesis Kit (Affymetrix). Approximately 25 ng/μl cDNA was added to the hybridization cocktail, followed by hybridization with the Human Gene 1.0 ST Array GeneChip at 45°C for 16 hours. This was then washed using the Affymetrix Fluidics Station 450. A final step was to measure probe intensities using the GeneChip Scanner 3000. The raw intensity data was normalized using Command Console Software (Affymetrix). The average fluorescence intensity of all annotated genes was calculated using the Robust Multiarray Analysis (RMA) algorithm [19], including a quartile normalization (all arrays are considered to have an equal intensity distribution) and using a background correction for GC-content.

Microarray gene expression, data processing, quality control and statistical analysis. The values of individual probes belonging to one probe set were averaged and normalized using Partek Genomics Suite 6.4 (Partek Inc., St. Louis, MO, USA, www.partek.com), from which probes with lowest available p-value and a known GenBank accession ID correspondence were selected for functional analysis. The distribution of the intensity values on the individual arrays was visualized in a signal histogram. One sample was removed due to deviating intensity values compared to the other samples. No other obvious outliers were detected. The intensity values of probe sets specific for the pre-labeled hybridization controls were analyzed and corresponded with the expected values. To check overall data quality, the array contained probe sets for exonic and intronic regions of reference genes (genes thought to be constitutively expressed in many different samples). Their probe set intensities were used to calculate the difference between the area under the curve of the positive and negative probe sets according to the manufacturer's instructions [20].

Genes of interest, all over two-fold up/down-regulated genes (p<0.0005), were analyzed using the Database for Annotation, Visualization and Integrated Discovery functional annotation tool [21] with KEGG pathway analysis.

Functional annotations were also carried out using the Ingenuity Pathway Analysis (IPA; Ingenuity Systems, Redwood City, CA, http://www.ingenuity.com/), in which gene symbols and fold changes of the up- and down-regulated genes were imported.

All microarray data comply with MIAME guidelines and are deposited in ArrayExpress.

Identification of enriched cytobands. 2292 induced genes and 2076 repressed genes in the AD groups (Table 1) were analyzed for their enrichment in human cytoband regions and gene ontology (GO) terms as defined using the DAVID bioinformatics resources [21], with an individual cutoff for each gene of p<0.0005.

Quantitative Real-Time PCR

First strand cDNA was synthesized from 1.5 μg total RNA by combining oligo(d)T15, random hexamers, buffer and MMLV-reverse transcriptase (Invitrogen) as previously described [18]. cDNA (5–10 ng total RNA) was subsequently amplified by qPCR using TaqMan® Gene Expression Assays (Applied Biosystems) and TaqMan® Fast Universal PCR Master Mix (2×) in a ABI7500Fast PCR machine (Applied Biosystems). TaqMan gene expression assays used were *FLG* (Hs00856927_g1), ITGA3 (Hs00233722_m1), CD28 (Hs0174796_m1), LAMB3 (Hs00165078_m1),

Table 1. Number of up- and down-regulated genes in relation to *FLG* genotype in AD and AD/IV patients.

Phenotype and genotype	Upregulated	Downregulated
AD *FLG+/+*	131	181
AD *FLG+/−*	328	429
AD/IV *FLG−/−*	1833	1466
Total # genes	**2292**	**2076**

Genes with a minimum two-fold change and p-values<0.0005 were included. Top up- and down-regulated genes for included patients depending on *FLG* genotype. Genes with minimum 2-fold change and p-value<0.0005 were included.

CTNNA1 (Hs00944792_mH), WAS (Hs00166001_m1), JAM2 (Hs01022013_m1), ITGAE (Hs00559580_m1), PTK2B (Hs00169444_m1), TLR2 (Hs00152932_m1), STAT2 (Hs01013123_m1), with ubiquitination factor E4A (Hs01083625_m1), 18S ribosomal RNA 1 (Hs03928985_g1) and GAPDH (Hs02758991_g1) used as endogenous controls. Expression levels were measured in duplicate. For genes with expression below the C_T fluorescence threshold, C_T was set at 40 to calculate the relative expression. Analysis was performed using an ABI PRISM 7500Fast sequence detection system (Applied Biosystems).

Statistical analysis

To identify differentially expressed genes between the different experimental groups in the microarray analysis, a two-way analysis of variance (*ANOVA*) was performed for each patient group compared to the healthy control group using Partek Genomics Suite 6.4. For each comparison between two experimental groups the fold change of every annotated gene, together with their corresponding p-value, was exported to Microsoft Office Excel. For quantitative Real-Time PCR, the relative mRNA expression and statistical significance were calculated using the REST 2009 software (available at www.qiagen.com) using *Fisher's exact test*. For genes chosen for pathway analysis, significance was corrected with *Bonferroni multiple testing*. Statistical significance for SCORAD was calculated using *student's t -test*. P-values<0.05 were considered as significant.

Results

Genotyping and clinical presentation

Among the included patients (n = 43) fourteen carried none of the prevalent *FLG* mutations tested and were included in the AD *FLG+/+* group. Fourteen AD patients carried one prevalent heterozygous FLG mutation (one R501X; thirteen 2282del4) and were included in the AD *FLG+/−* group. Fifteen AD/IV patients carried either a homozygous or a compound heterozygous *FLG* mutation (two R501X; nine 2282del4; one S3247X; two 2282del4/S3247X and one 2282del4/R501X) and were included in the AD/IV *FLG−/−* group (of these fifteen patients, three had IV phenotype without AD at the time of examination). One patient was excluded from the AD/IV FLG−/−group after no *FLG* mutations were detected, and subsequent *STS* genotyping revealed a point mutation, recently published elsewhere [16]. In the AD *FLG+/+* group 78.6% were females, the average age was 56 (range 28–78) and the mean SCORAD was 7.6 (range 0–14.7). In the AD *FLG+/−* group, 64.3% were female, the average age was 54 (range 28–71) and the mean SCORAD was 15.4 (range 6.2–25.8). For the AD/IV *FLG−/−* group 46.7% were female, the average age was 59 (range 44–70) and the mean SCORAD for AD patients in this group was 14.1 (range 7–44.5). The AD *FLG+/+* had significantly lower SCORAD than the AD *FLG+/−* and the AD patients in the AD/IV *FLG−/−* group (p = 0.02). The control group consisted 43% females and the average age was 52 (range 24–75).

TEWL and pH

Significantly higher TEWL was observed in the AD/IV *FLG−/−* and AD *FLG+/−* than in the healthy control group. The mean TEWL was higher also in the AD *FLG+/+* group, although this did not reach statistical significance. pH was significantly higher in the AD/IV *FLG−/−* group than in the healthy control group. Mean pH was higher also for the AD *FLG+/−* and *FLG+/+* groups, although this did not reach statistical significance (Fig. 1a).

FLG mRNA expression depending on genotype

All patient -groups showed lower mRNA expression of *FLG* than the control group, both with microarray analysis and with quantitative real-time PCR (qPCR). The mRNA expression levels were lowest in the *FLG−/−* group (array p = 0.000008; qPCR p = 0.001), but significantly reduced also in the *FLG+/−* (array p = 0.04; qPCR p = 0.001) and with qPCR also in the *FLG+/+* group (array p = 0.59; qPCR p = 0.04) than in the healthy control group (Fig. 1b).

Altered expression profiles in AD

The microarrays representing 28869 annotated genes with 764885 distinct probes were used to identify and compare the gene expression of AD skin compared to healthy skin, and the difference in expression pattern depending on *FLG* genotype. The design of the Human Gene 1.0 ST array was based on the March 2006 (UCSC hg18, NCBI Build 36) human sequence assembly, containing over 99 percent coverage of sequences present in the RefSeq database. A full list of significantly altered genes is provided as Table S1. Among these, the Partek Genomics suite 6.4 was used to detect 4368 differentially expressed genes (minimum 2-fold change and p-value<0.0005) (Table 1). These differentially expressed genes were distributed according to the chromosomal enrichment illustrated in Table S2.

Distribution of differentially expressed genes

The distribution of differentially expressed genes in all patient groups depends on their *FLG* genotype (Fig. 2a). Hierarchical clustering was used to group these differentially expressed genes, based on similarity in expression across the samples and to group individuals on the basis of similarities in gene-expression patterns (Fig. 2b). Each column represents a single array experiment and clusters from Fig. 2a are marked I–VII, respectively.

Altered pathways for cellular development and differentiation, inflammatory response and cell-to-cell signaling in AD/IV skin compared to healthy controls, regardless of FLG status. Ingenuity Pathway Analysis of differentially expressed genes for all patient groups reveals a pathway mapped to inflammatory response that was significantly induced compared to the control group (Fig. 3). In addition, there were several altered pathways mapped to cellular development and differentiation compared to healthy controls (Fig. 3).

Significantly altered pathways depending on FLG genotype status. In AD/IV skin with *FLG−/−* genotype, several pathways were significantly altered compared to the healthy control group. Focal adhesion, extracellular matrix receptor interaction, regulation of actin cytoskeleton and calcium signaling pathways showed significantly altered expression (Table 2).

In AD skin with *FLG+/−* genotype, focal adhesion and extracellular matrix receptor interaction pathways displayed, similarly to the *FLG−/−* group, a significant deviation compared to the healthy controls, together with ABC transporting pathway and actin cytoskeleton regulation (Table 2).

For AD skin without *FLG* mutations focal adhesion, ECM receptor interaction and regulation of actin cytoskeleton show a deviating trend (Table 2), but this was not statistically significant. For a list of candidate genes mapped to altered pathways depending on *FLG* genotype see Table S3.

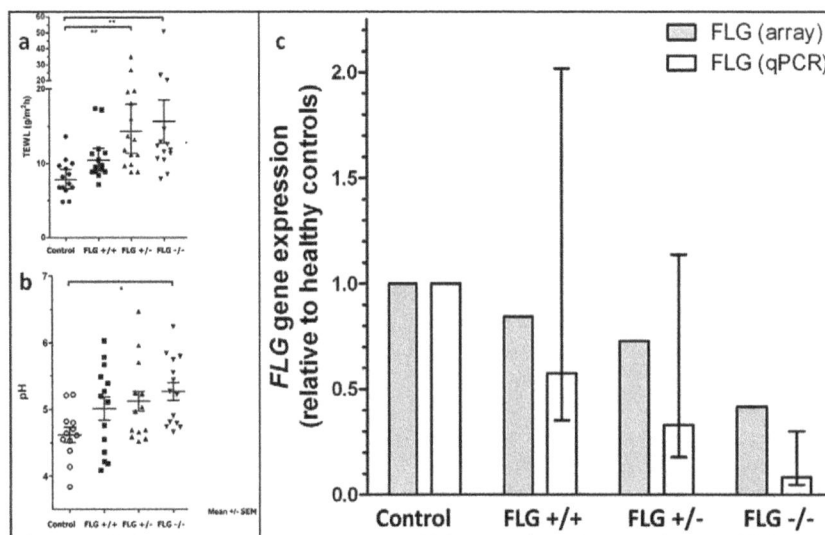

Figure 1. Mean trans-epidermal water loss (TEWL) (a) and pH (b) and decrease in mRNA expression (c) in the AD *FLG+/+*, AD *FLG+/−* and the AD/IV *FLG−/−* group. All groups compared to a healthy control group. Significant changes are denoted with * and ** (p<0.05 and p<0.01), respectively. All groups had significantly altered FLG expression compared to the healthy control group with qPCR; for the *FLG+/+* p = 0.04, the *FLG+/−* p = 0.001 and the *FLG−/−* group p = 0.001. From the array expression results the *FLG+/+* group was lower but not significant (p = 0.59) whereas the expression was significantly lower in the *FLG+/−* (p = 0.04) and *FLG−/−* groups (p = 0.000008).

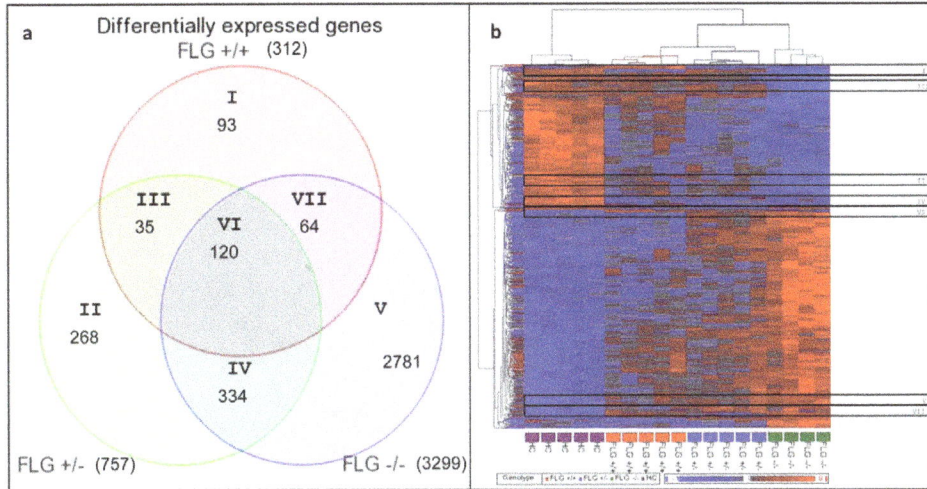

Figure 2. Top overlapping differentially expressed genes in AD skin (a) and heat map of transcriptional levels of genes in AD skin and controls (b). Genes with altered expression in patients with *FLG* wild type genotype *(FLG+/+)*, heterozygote *FLG* mutation genotype *(FLG+/−)*, and homozygote *FLG* mutation genotype *(FLG−/−)*. Clusters containing differentially expressed genes in marked regions I–VII are corresponding regions in a) and b). A list of p-values and fold changes for all differentially expressed genes are described in Table S1. Hierarchal clustering analysis was performed in both the gene (row) and experiment (column) dimension. Contrast value for each gene is shown, e.g. the standardized mean difference between the gene's expression in the group versus overall expression.

Quantitative Real-Time PCR

Identification of candidate genes. For complimentary testing of selected significantly differentially expressed genes mapped in the pathway analysis qPCR was performed from genes in cytobands previously associated to AD (Table S2 and Table S3) and with fold changes close to two-fold up- or down-regulation. Of significantly altered pathways, *ITGA3* and *CTNNA1* were mapped to focal adhesion, *LAMB3* to extracellular matrix receptor interaction, *ITGAE* to actin cytoskeleton, *JAM2* to tight junction pathway, *VAV1* and *CD28* to T cell receptor signaling pathway, and, *PTK2B4* was mapped to calcium signaling pathway; all mapped using DAVID bioinformatics resources [21] with the KEGG pathway analysis option. *TLR2* and *STAT2* represent genes associated with immunological response mapped using Ingenuity Pathways Analysis (Fig. 3).

Results of Quantitative Real-Time PCR. To study the relative expression of candidate genes, qPCR was performed in 40

patients and 13 controls. FLG was significantly down-regulated in all patient groups *(FLG+/+* p = 0.043; *FLG+/−* p = 0.001; *FLG−/−* p = 0.001) (Fig. 2). *CD28* (p = 0.007), *CTNNA1* (p = 0.003) and *LAMB3* (p = 0.01) were all significantly altered in the AD *FLG+/+* group. *STAT2* (p = 0.001) was significantly altered in the AD *FLG+/−* whereas *STAT2* (p = 0.01), *CTNNA1* (p = 0.001), *JAM2* (p = 0.001) and *CD28* (p = 0.001) all were significantly altered in the AD/IV *FLG−/−* group. Further details regarding qPCR expression for these genes are given in Table S4.

Discussion

FLG was shown to be down-regulated both by microarray analysis and qPCR in all AD/IV groups compared to the healthy controls. Although there was a gradient of down-regulation depending on *FLG* genotype with the lowest FLG expression in patients with *FLG−/−* genotype followed by the *FLG+/−*

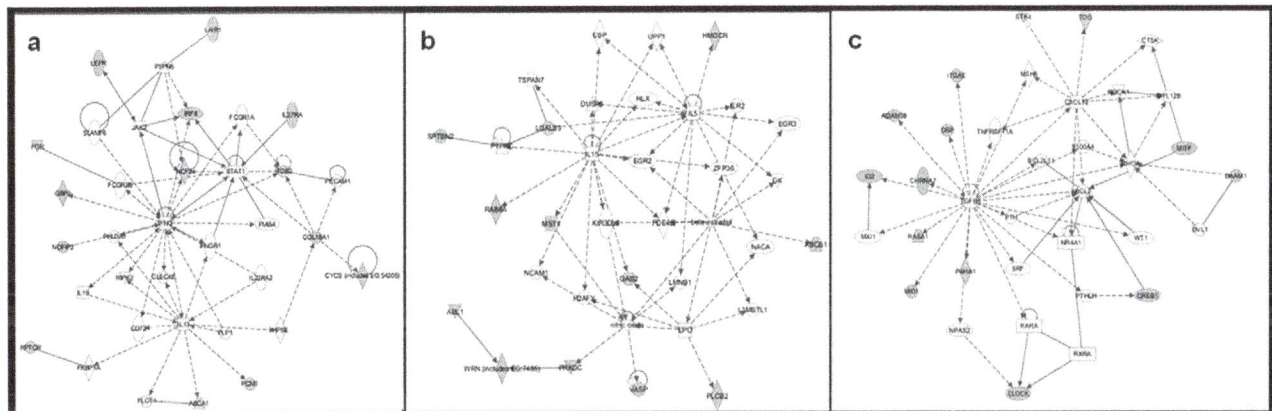

Figure 3. Ingenuity Pathways Analysis showing differentially expressed genes mapped to pathway for inflammatory response (a) and cellular development and differentiation (b and c) for all patient groups. Each gene mapped to this pathway (marked in grey) show significant altered expression to this pathway (p-value<0.0005).

Table 2. Top altered molecular pathways depending on *FLG* genotype.

AD *FLG+/+*	# genes	p-value
hsa04510:Focal adhesion	30	0.001
hsa04810:Regulation of actin cytoskeleton	29	0.006
hsa04512:ECM-receptor interaction	14	0.02
AD *FLG+/−*	**# genes**	**p-value**
hsa04512:ECM-receptor interaction	29	0.000005**
hsa04510:Focal adhesion	52	0.000009**
hsa02010:ABC transporters	19	0.00001**
hsa04810:Regulation of actin cytoskeleton	47	0.002*
hsa04020:Calcium signaling pathway	37	0.01
hsa04660:T cell receptor signaling pathway	23	0.04
hsa04520:Adherens junction	17	0.07
AD/IV *FLG−/−*	**# genes**	**p-value**
hsa04070:Phosphatidylinositol signaling system	54	0.0000008**
hsa04510:Focal adhesion	118	0.0000008**
hsa04512:ECM-receptor interaction	57	0.000002**
hsa04810:Regulation of actin cytoskeleton	123	0.000003**
hsa04020:Calcium signaling pathway	100	0.00004*
hsa04660:T cell receptor signaling pathway	64	0.0003
hsa02010:ABC transporters	31	0.0003
hsa04530:Tight junction	71	0.007

All included molecules were selected from Table S1 with matching inclusion criteria and mapped using KEGG Pathway analysis. Bonferroni corrected p-values<0.05 are indicated by * and Bonferroni corrected p-values<0.005 are indicated by **. Candidate genes mapped to each pathway are outlined in Table S3.

genotype, the *FLG+/+* group also displayed down-regulation compared to healthy control skin. Recent studies have shown that pro-inflammatory cytokines may modulate the expression of FLG, even in patients without *FLG* mutations, which might be one of the underlying explanations of our finding [22,23].

Many of the potential AD candidate genes significantly altered in our study were located in chromosomal regions previously linked to AD [24] (Table S2), further highlighting these regions as interesting loci for potential candidate genes involved in AD susceptibility. The distributions of these differentially expressed genes in our study depended on *FLG* genotype, where several clusters were unique for each group, and others overlapped (Fig. 2). Genes from these groups are mapped to significantly altered pathways in each patient group. The functional alterations evident from the significantly higher TEWL and pH (Fig. 1) in the FLG-deficient groups may influence the number of induced or repressed genes involved in tightly regulated processes such as inflammatory response following a more permeable barrier, as well as enzymatic activity where the pH level is important [11].

The importance of changes in TEWL and pH has recently been highlighted in FLG deficient skin; where reduced levels of FLG degradation products are proposed to increase TEWL and pH; decreasing stratum corneum hydration and altering enzymatic activity [25,26]. This may account for alterations in corneocyte and lipid organization within the SC [26]. Given the frequent phenotypic overlap between dry skin, IV and AD (evident in our *FLG−/−* group as well); it is proposed that these functional alterations are important for the pathogenesis in both IV and AD skin with FLG deficiency. In support of this hypothesis, our AD patients without *FLG* mutations displayed lower functional barrier

impairment measured by TEWL, lower pH and significantly lower mean SCORAD than AD patients with *FLG* mutations (*FLG*-repeat variation may also influence the phenotype [27]. However, we did not investigate this). In addition, the lowest number of significantly altered genes was detected in our AD *FLG+/+* group. This suggests a correlation between number of affected genes, barrier impairment and disease severity among included AD patients.

Of the many genes previously associated to AD [24] several were also dysregulated in our array data, such as serine protease inhibitor kazal-type 5 (*SPINK-5*), mast cell chymase (*CMA1* and interleukin 4 *(IL-4)* (Table S1). Any discrepancies regarding expression of inflammatory mediators commonly found in AD may at least in part be due to lower expression of these genes in non-lesional skin. *CD28* and *STAT2* are two inflammatory markers that were confirmed to be altered also by qPCR. *CD28* has been suggested to be involved in the inflammatory response in AD [28] and *STAT2* has been described as a candidate gene involved in mediating pro-inflammatory cytokines [29]. In addition, genes mapped to adhesion such as *CTNNA1*, *JAM2* and *LAMB3* were also confirmed to be significantly altered. Defects in cell adhesion have recently been highlighted as important in AD pathogenesis, with the finding of impairment in tight junctions contributing to the barrier dysfunction and immune dysregulation [30]. Down-regulation of tight-junction proteins such as occludin and ZO-1 has also been demonstrated in IV skin recently [26] and tallies with our gene-expression pattern in FLG-deficient skin (Table S1). The *LAMB3* gene encodes laminin-5, a glycoprotein that anchors basal cells to the underlying basal membrane [31], whereas *CTNNA1* and *JAM2*, in addition to their cell adhesion function, have been suggested to be involved in cell differentiation [32] and lymphocyte homing [33], respectively. Interestingly *CTNNA1* and *LAMB3* were significantly altered in the AD group without *FLG* mutations. The underlying explanation could in part be the effects of putative down-regulation of FLG also in this group, but as the expression of *LAMB3* did not reach significance in the AD *FLG−/−* group and neither did *CTNNA1* or *LAMB3* in the AD *FLG+/−* group, other explanations are plausible, including that these genes are candidates for the primary pathogenesis in AD in addition to FLG deficiency.

The molecular mechanisms involved in the phenotype of AD following the functional barrier impairment in our material involve altered pathways such as cytoskeleton structure, calcium- and phospatidylinositol signaling and ATP binding cassette (ABC) transport system (Table 2). It has been suggested that FLG is of importance for cytoskeleton organization by aggregating keratin intermediate filaments (KIFs); and that FLG deficiency may cause cytoskeleton abnormalities such as perinuclear keratin retraction in granular cells [26]. KIF polymerization is actin-dependent [34] and subsequently actin-cytoskeleton aberrations may contribute to the peripheral KIF retraction previously demonstrated in FLG-deficient skin [26]. However, the role of FLG in impaired intermediate filament aggregation has been challenged [35] and other factors than FLG deficiency may explain the alterations in the pathway for the regulation of the actin cytoskeleton. Our findings support this, as pathways for actin-cytoskeleton regulation were altered in all our patient groups including the group without *FLG* mutations. In addition, several keratins (including *KRT1* and *KRT10*) were significantly down-regulated in AD patients both with and without *FLG* mutations (Table S1). As the actin filament system has been suggested to be involved in KIF transport [34], it is possible that increased actin cytoskeleton regulation is a compensatory mechanism following a lower keratin expression. Altogether, our data suggests that both keratin expression and KIF regulation are subject to modulation in AD skin independently of *FLG* mutations.

FLG may be involved in calcium metabolism in the skin [36], and the calcium gradient is important for epidermal differentiation - a loss of this gradient increases keratinocyte proliferation and decreases differentiation [37]. Impaired calcium metabolism has been demonstrated in other conditions where the skin barrier is disrupted, such as Hailey-Hailey disease [38] and in psoriatic skin [39]. Further, defective lipid transportation and defects in lamellar body extrusion have previously been reported in AD [40,41] and mutations in this pathway may cause severe ichthyotic conditions such as Harlequin Ichthyosis [42]. Our FLG-deficient groups show alterations both in the pathway for calcium signaling and for ABC transport system, indicating that alterations in these pathways are involved in the pathogenesis of IV and AD with FLG deficiency.

In conclusion, we have demonstrated that several functional and molecular mechanisms *in vivo* in patients suffering from AD and IV depend on *FLG* genotype. Disease severity of AD, the gradient of TEWL and pH follow loss of FLG expression in the skin; and the number of altered genes and pathways may be correlated to FLG mRNA expression. We here emphasize further the role of FLG for the functional integrity of the skin barrier and the complex subsequent signaling systems involving inflammation, epidermal differentiation, lipid metabolism, cell signalling and adhesion that are affected in response to FLG deficiency.

Supporting Information

Table S1   Human Gene 1.0 ST array mRNA expression. P-values and fold change of each annotated gene are mean values of five subjects from each patient group (*FLG+/+*, *FLG+/−* and *FLG−/−*) compared to a five subjects from the healthy control group (using the March 2006: UCSC hg18, NCBI Build 36).

Table S2   Enrichment of chromosomal regions in all AD patients. Chromosomal regions (cytobands) enriched in 2292 induced genes and 2076 repressed genes using DAVID bioinformatics resource. Cytobands are sorted by p-value and previously described genetic association to AD is marked yellow.

Table S3   Candidate genes mapped to altered pathways depending on *FLG* genotype. Each annotated gene with corresponding p-value and fold change depending on *FLG* genotype and corresponding cytoband. Cytobands with previously reported AD association marked with yellow.

Table S4   Quantitative Real-Time PCR mRNA expression depending on *FLG* genotype. Selected genes with corresponding p-values and ratio of up- or down regulation in patient groups depending on *FLG* genotype compared to a healthy control group.

Acknowledgments

The cooperation of all participating patients and controls is gratefully acknowledged. Some of the MLPA analyses of the *STS* gene were kindly performed by Dr. Maritta Hellström Pigg at the Department of Clinical Genetics, Uppsala University Hospital, and Anna Hammarsjö at the Department of Clinical Genetics, Karolinska University Hospital, Solna.

Author Contributions

Conceived and designed the experiments: BB AV MN MB HT. Performed the experiments: MCGW TH HT. Analyzed the data: MCGW TH HT. Contributed reagents/materials/analysis tools: MCGW TH BB AV MN MB HT. Wrote the paper: MCGW TH BB AV MN MB HT.

References

1. Williams HC, Burney PG, Pembroke AC, Hay RJ (1994) The U.K. Working Party's Diagnostic Criteria for Atopic Dermatitis. III. Independent hospital validation. Br J Dermatol 131(3): 406–16.
2. Novak N, Simon D (2011) Atopic dermatitis – from new pathophysiologic insights to individualized therapy. Allergy 66(7): 830–839.
3. Elias PM, Steinhoff M (2008) "Outside-to-Inside" (and Now Back to "Outside") Pathogenic Mechanisms in Atopic Dermatitis. J Invest Dermatol 128(5): 1067–1070.
4. Sääf AM, Tengvall-Linder M, Chang HY, Adler AS, Wahlgren CF, et al. (2008) Global expression profiling in atopic eczema reveals reciprocal expression of inflammatory and lipid genes. PLoS One 3(12): e4017.
5. Voegeli R, Rawlings AV, Breternitz M, Doppler S, Schreier T, et al. (2009) Increased stratum corneum serine protease activity in acute eczematous atopic skin. British Journal of Dermatology 161(1): 70–77.
6. Sandilands A, Terron-Kwiatkowski A, Hull PR, O'Regan GM, Clayton TH, et al. (2007) Comprehensive analysis of the gene encoding filaggrin uncovers prevalent and rare mutations in ichthyosis vulgaris and atopic eczema. Nat Genet 39(5): 650–654.
7. Öhman H, Vahlquist A (1998) The pH gradient over the stratum corneum differs in X-linked recessive and autosomal dominant ichthyosis: a clue to the molecular origin of the "acid skin mantle". J Invest Dermatol 111(4): 674–7.

8. Smith FJ, Irvine AD, Terron-Kwiatkowski A, Sandilands A, Campbell LE, et al. (2006) Loss-of-function mutations in the gene encoding filaggrin cause ichthyosis vulgaris. Nat Genet 38(3): 337–42.

9. Sandilands A, Sutherland C, Irvine AD, McLean WHI (2009) Filaggrin in the frontline: role in skin barrier function and disease. Journal of Cell Science 122: 1285–1294.

10. Kezic S, O'Regan GM, Yau N, Sandilands A, Chen H, et al. (2011) Levels of filaggrin degradation products are influenced by both filaggrin genotype and atopic dermatitis severity. Allergy. pp 934–940.

11. Cork MJ, Danby SG, Vasilopoulos Y, Hadgraft J, Lane ME, et al. (2009) Epidermal Barrier Dysfunction in Atopic Dermatitis. J Invest Dermatol. pp 1892–908.

12. Toulza E, Mattiuzzo NR, Galliano MF, Jonca N, Dossat C, et al. (2007) Large-scale identification of human genes implicated in epidermal barrier function. Genome Biol 8(6): R107.

13. Ekelund E, Lieden A, Link J, Lee SP, D'Amato M, et al. (2008) Loss-of-function variants of the filaggrin gene are associated with atopic eczema and associated phenotypes in Swedish families. Acta Derm Venereol 88(1): 15–9.

14. Kunz B, Oranje AP, Labrèze L, Stalder JF, Ring J, et al. (1997) Clinical Validation and Guidelines for the SCORAD Index: Consensus Report of the European Task Force on Atopic Dermatitis. Dermatology 195(1): 10–19.

15. Nardi A, Pomari E, Zambon D, Belvedere P, Colombo L, et al. (2009) Transcriptional control of human steroid sulfatase. The Journal of Steroid Biochemistry and Molecular Biology 115(1–2): 68–74.

16. Winge MC, Hoppe T, Lieden A, Nordenskjöld M, Vahlquist A, et al. (2011) Novel point mutation in the STS gene in a patient with X-linked recessive ichthyosis. J Dermatol Sci 63(1): 62–4.

17. Ramensky V, Bork P, Sunyaev S (2002) Human non-synonymous SNPs: server and survey. Nucleic Acids Res 30(17): 3894–900.

18. Törmä H, Lindberg M, Berne B (2007) Skin Barrier Disruption by Sodium Lauryl Sulfate-Exposure Alters the Expressions of Involucrin, Transglutaminase 1, Profilaggrin, and Kallikreins during the Repair Phase in Human Skin In Vivo. J Invest Dermatol 128(5): 1212–1219.

19. Irizarry RA, Hobbs B, Collin F, Beazer-Barclay YD, Antonellis KJ, et al. (2003) Exploration, normalization, and summaries of high density oligonucleotide array probe level data. Biostatistics 4(2): 249–264.

20. Affymetrix Inc (2007) Quality Assessment of exon and gene arrays. Affymetrix whitepaper. Available:http://media.affymetrix.com/support/technical/white-papers/exon_gene_arrays_qa_whitepaper.pdf. Accessed 15th October 2010.

21. HuanG DW, Sherman BT, Lempicki RA (2008) Systematic and integrative analysis of large gene lists using DAVID bioinformatics resources. Nat Protocols 4(1): 44–57.

22. Howell MD, Kim BE, Gao P, Grant AV, Boguniewicz M, et al. (2009) Cytokine modulation of atopic dermatitis filaggrin skin expression. J Allergy Clin Immunol 124(3 Suppl 2): R7–R12.

23. Kim BE, Howell MD, Guttman E, Gilleaudeau PM, Cardinale R, et al. (2011) TNF-[alpha] Downregulates Filaggrin and Loricrin through c-Jun N-terminal Kinase: Role for TNF-[alpha] Antagonists to Improve Skin Barrier. J Invest Dermatol 131(6): 1272–1279.

24. Barnes KC (2010) An update on the genetics of atopic dermatitis: scratching the surface in 2009. J Allergy Clin Immunol 125(1): 16–29.e11.

25. Jungersted JM, Scheer H, Mempel M, Baurecht H, Cifuentes L, et al. (2010) Stratum corneum lipids, skin barrier function and filaggrin mutations in patients with atopic eczema. Allergy 65(7): 911–8.

26. Gruber R, Elias PM, Crumrine D, Lin TK, Brandner JM, et al. (2011) Filaggrin genotype in ichthyosis vulgaris predicts abnormalities in epidermal structure and function. Am J Pathol 178(5): 2252–63.

27. Ginger R, Blachford S, Rowland J, Rowson M, Harding C (2005) Filaggrin repeat number polymorphism is associated with a dry skin phenotype. Archives of Dermatological Research 297(6): 235–241.

28. Neuber K, Mähnss B, Hübner C, Gergely H, Weichenthal M (2006) Autoantibodies against CD28 are associated with atopic diseases. Clinical & Experimental Immunology 146(2): 262–269.

29. Gamero AM, Young MR, Mentor-Marcel R, Bobe G, Scarzello AJ, et al. (2010) STAT2 contributes to promotion of colorectal and skin carcinogenesis. Cancer Prev Res (Phila) 3(4): 495–504.

30. De Benedetto A, Rafaels NM, McGirt LY, Ivanov AI, Georas SN, et al. (2011) Tight junction defects in patients with atopic dermatitis. Journal of Allergy and Clinical Immunology 127(3): 773–786.e7.

31. Posteraro P, Sorvillo S, Gagnoux-Palacios L, Angelo C, Paradisi M, et al. (1998) Compound Heterozygosity for an Out-of-Frame Deletion and a Splice Site Mutation in the LAMB3 Gene Causes Nonlethal Junctional Epidermolysis Bullosa. Biochemical and Biophysical Research Communications 243(3): 758–764.

32. Zhu AJ, Watt FM (1996) Expression of a dominant negative cadherin mutant inhibits proliferation and stimulates terminal differentiation of human epidermal keratinocytes. J Cell Sci 109(Pt 13): 3013–23.

33. Palmeri D, van Zante A, Huang CC, Hemmerich S, Rosen SD (2000) Vascular Endothelial Junction-associated Molecule, a Novel Member of the Immuno-globulin Superfamily, Is Localized to Intercellular Boundaries of Endothelial Cells. Journal of Biological Chemistry 275(25): 19139–19145.

34. Kolsch A, Windoffer R, Leube RE (2009) Actin-dependent dynamics of keratin filament precursors. Cell Motil Cytoskeleton 66(11): 976–85.

35. Mildner M, Jin J, Eckhart L, Kezic S, Gruber F, et al. (2010) Knockdown of filaggrin impairs diffusion barrier function and increases UV sensitivity in a human skin model. J Invest Dermatol 130(9): 2286–94.

36. Brown SJ, McLean WHI (2009) Eczema genetics: current state of knowledge and future goals. J Invest Dermatol 129(3): 543–52.

37. Elias PM, Ahn SK, Denda M, Brown BE, Crumrine D, et al. (2002) Modulations in Epidermal Calcium Regulate the Expression of Differentia-tion-Specific Markers. 119(5): 1128–1136.

38. Proksch E, Brandner JM, Jensen JM (2008) The skin: an indispensable barrier. Experimental Dermatology 17(12): 1063–1072.

39. Menon GK, Elias PM (1991) Ultrastructural localization of calcium in psoriatic and normal human epidermis. Arch Dermatol 127(1): 57–63.

40. Mathay C, Pierre M, Pittelkow MR, Depiereux E, Nikkels AF, et al. (2011) Transcriptional Profiling after Lipid Raft Disruption in Keratinocytes Identifies Critical Mediators of Atopic Dermatitis Pathways. J Invest Dermatol 131(1): 46–58.

41. Elias PM, Hatano Y, Williams ML (2008) Basis for the barrier abnormality in atopic dermatitis: Outside-inside-outside pathogenic mechanisms. Journal of Allergy and Clinical Immunology 121(6): 1337–1343.

42. Akiyama M (2010) ABCA12 mutations and autosomal recessive congenital ichthyosis: A review of genotype/phenotype correlations and of pathogenetic conceptsa. Human Mutation 31(10): 1090–1096.

Targeting the Neurokinin Receptor 1 with Aprepitant: A Novel Antipruritic Strategy

Sonja Ständer*, Dorothee Siepmann, Ilka Herrgott, Cord Sunderkötter, Thomas A. Luger

Department of Dermatology, Neurodermatology and Competence Center Pruritus, University of Münster, Münster, Germany

Abstract

Background: Chronic pruritus is a global clinical problem with a high impact on the quality of life and lack of specific therapies. It is an excruciating and frequent symptom of e.g. uncurable renal, liver and skin diseases which often does not respond to conventional treatment with e.g. antihistamines. Therefore antipruritic therapies which target physiological mechanisms of pruritus need to be developed. Substance P (SP) is a major mediator of pruritus. As it binds to the neurokinin receptor 1 (NKR1), we evaluated if the application of a NKR1 antagonist would significantly decrease chronic pruritus.

Methods and Findings: Twenty hitherto untreatable patients with chronic pruritus (12 female, 8 male; mean age, 66.7 years) were treated with the NKR1 antagonist aprepitant 80 mg for one week. 16 of 20 patients (80%) experienced a considerable reduction of itch intensity, as assessed by the visual analog scale (VAS, range 0 to 10). Considering all patients, the mean value of pruritus intensity was significantly reduced from 8.4 VAS points (SD +/−1.7) before treatment to 4.9 VAS points (SD +/−3.2) ($p < 0.001$, CI 1.913–5.187). Patients with dermatological diseases (e.g. atopic diathesis, prurigo nodularis) had the best profit from the treatment. Side-effects were mild (nausea, vertigo, and drowsiness) and only occurred in three patients.

Conclusions: The high response rate in patients with therapy refractory pruritus suggests that the NKR1 antagonist aprepitant may indeed exhibit antipruritic effects and may present a novel, effective treatment strategy based on pathophysiology of chronic pruritus. The results are promising enough to warrant confirming the efficacy of NKR1 antagonists in a randomized, controlled clinical trial.

Editor: H. Peter Soyer, The University of Queensland, Australia

Funding: The authors thank MDS Sharp and Dohme Company for providing part of the medications. MDS Sharp and Dohme Company had no role in study design, data collection and analysis, decision to publish, or preparation of the manuscript.

Competing Interests: On behalf of all authors, Dr. Stander declares that the authors received a part (around 25%) of the medication (aprepitant) from MDS Sharp and Dohme Company. The authors received the samples o n demand, for free, without contract or involvement of anybody of the company in in study design, data collection and analysis, decision to publish, or preparation of the manuscript. No author has any other financial or personal relationship to the company such as ownership of stocks or shares, employment or consultancy, board membership, or patent applications. No author received research grants, travel grants for conferences, honoraria for speaking or participation at meetings or any other gifts.

* E-mail: sonja.staender@uni-muenster.de

Introduction

Chronic pruritus is a frequent and globally occurring symptom of systemic, dermatologic, neurological and psychiatric diseases [1–3]. It is currently estimated that 20 to 27% of all adults worldwide endure chronic pruritus [4–6]. Since the symptom is regularly characterized by a high intensity and long duration as well as by cutaneous self-injury due to scratching, it has a high impact on the quality of life and may lead to depression or even suicide of the sufferers [4,7,8]. Given that pruritus was regarded for a long time as subquality of pain [1], not much attention was paid to the neurobiological basis of the symptom in the past. A second reason for the lack of pursuit of specific treatment strategies was owed to the assumption that treatment of underlying disease would automatically relieve pruritus [2]. Therefore the mainstays of treatment for chronic pruritus until to date are still antihistamines, topical and systemic corticosteroids, or certain antidepressants [2]. However, their efficacy is limited and systemic application of corticosteroids and antidepressants may be associated with severe side-effects.

Recent studies have provided evidence that pruritus has a different pathophysiology than pain and that it does not parallel the course of the underlying disease [1,2]. Therefore we [9] and others [10] have pursued the concept to develop target-specific treatments targeting pathophysiological mechanism specific for pruritus. For example, in 2009, nalfurafine (which functions by activation of the spinal kappa-opioid-receptor) was licensed in Japan as the first oral drug against pruritus in hemodialysis patients [10]. Still, the development of new and targeted antipruritic therapies against this excruciating and frequent symptom not only in hemodialysis patients and for the benefit of patients worldwide is mandatory.

Substance P (SP) is an important mediator in the induction and maintenance of pruritus [11–13] and therefore represents an interesting target for antipruritic treatment. SP is a tachykinin which binds with different affinities to three neurokinin receptors (NKR 1–3), but mainly to NKR1, which is expressed in the central nervous system (CNS) and the skin [11]. We therefore investigated in chronic pruritus patients the possible antipruritic potency of the recently developed oral NKR1-antagonist aprepitant.

Methods

Twenty patients (12 female, 8 male; age range: 36–85 years; mean, 66.7 years; SD +/−13.7; median 68.5 years) with therapy refractory chronic pruritus (duration, 4 months to 20 years; mean, 61.3 months) were randomly selected for the treatment with the selective high-affinity NKR1-antagonist aprepitant. Previous to application of aprepitant, patients underwent clinical investigation to determine the underlying origin of pruritus [3]. All patients had been refractory to at least two (2 to 7) previous antipruritic treatments with topical, intralesional or systemic corticosteroids, antihistamines, and/or UV-irradiation. In 8 patients the origin of chronic pruritus was unclear despite extensive laboratory and radiological investigations (Table 1). In 12 patients underlying diseases were found: chronic kidney disease (uraemic pruritus, n = 5), and a combination of multiple causal factors (chronic kidney disease, diabetes mellitus, hyperuricaemia, and iron deficiency, n = 7). 10/20 patients had additionally an atopic diathesis (four with pruritus of unknown origin and six with pruritus of multifactorial origin). Clinically, 13/20 patients suffered from severe scratch lesions (prurigo nodularis), while seven patients reported chronic pruritus on clinically normal skin. Patients received a monotherapy with aprepitant 80 mg once daily for 3–13 days (mean, 6.6 days) without any other concomitant antipruritic therapy. Patients recorded on a daily base the average pruritus intensity on the visual analog scale (VAS) ranging from 0 (no pruritus) to 10 (severe pruritus). In addition, at the end of treatment, patients were interviewed on the total percentage of change in pruritus (100% reduction = complete relief of pruritus).

Patients' data were anonymously statistically analysed with the SPSS software package (Version 14.0, SPSS Inc., Chicago, Illinois, USA). Paired T-test was applied and p values less than 0.05 were considered statistically significant. Patients were treated individually with aprepitant and gave written informed consent to the off-label application of the drug. The data were encoded in our multidisciplinary pruritus database and retrospective analysis of the study was authorized by the local ethics committee (ethics committee of the medical association of Westphalia and medical faculty of the Westphalian Wilhelms University Münster).

Results

Sixteen out of 20 patients (80%) responded to short-term aprepitant monotherapy. Four patients experienced complete (100% reduction) or nearly complete (70–90%) cessation of pruritus, eight patients reported on partial reduction (40–60%) and four patients experienced weak reduction (10–30%) of pruritus within the treatment period (mean, 50.6% pruritus reduction). Four patients did not respond to the treatment. Pruritus intensity on the VAS before treatment ranged from 5 to 10 (mean, 8.4 points; SD +/−1.7; median VAS 8). After treatment with aprepitant, pruritus intensity was reduced to a mean of 4.9 points (SD +/−3.2; $p<0.001$; CI 1.913–5.187, Fig. 1). Patients with dermatological diseases appeared to respond best to therapy with aprepitant. Patients with atopic diathesis (n = 10) or prurigo

Table 1. Collective of patients: demographic, clinical and response parameters.

No.	Age (years), Gender	Diagnosis*, Origin of pruritus	Atopic diathesis[+]	Initial pruritus intensity on VAS (ranging 0 (best) to 10 (worst))	Response: reduction of pruritus in percent
1	68, f	CP*, renal	−	6	0
2	82, m	CP, renal	−	10	0
3	69, m	PN*, renal	−	7	30
4	72, m	CP, renal	+	7	40
5	78, m	CP, renal	+	8	50
6	82, f	PN, multifactorial (renal, hyperuricaemia)	−	10	20
7	66, f	PN, multifactorial (renal, dry skin)	+	5	40
8	55, f	CP, multifactorial (cholestatic, dry skin, psychosomatic factors)	+	10	50
9	73, f	PN, multifactorial (renal, diabetes)	+	10	60
10	59, m	PN, multifactorial (metabolic syndrome)	−	10	70
11	42, m	PN, multifactorial (thyreoid dysfunction, neurogenic)	−	8	90
12	66, f	PN, multifactorial (hyperuricaemia, iron deficiency)	+	8	100
13	68, f	PN, unknown	+	10	0
14	77, f	CP, unknown	−	10	0
15	81, f	PN, unknown	−	7	10
16	85, f	PN, unknown	−	10	10
17	36, m	CP, unknown	−	8	40
18	52, f	PN, unknown	+	10	50
19	72, m	PN, unknown	+	6	50
20	50, f	PN, unknown	+	8	100

*CP, chronic pruritus; PN, prurigo nodularis.
[+]Atopic diathesis; +, present; −, not present.

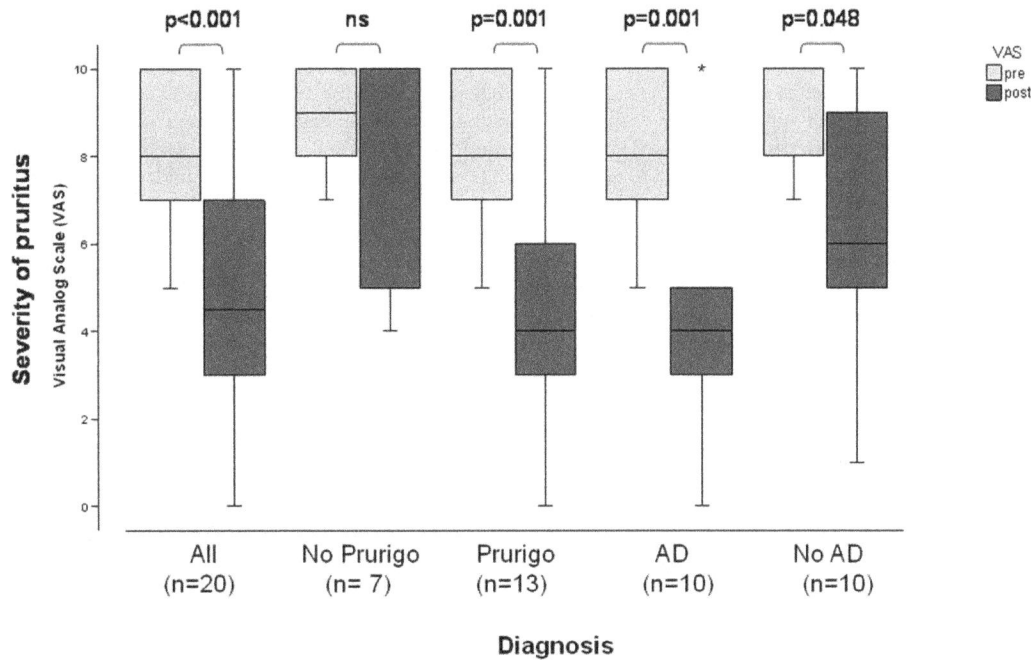

Figure 1. Distribution of values for pruritus intensity as scored on the visual analog scale (VAS) from 0 to 10 before (pre) and after (post) aprepitant. Response is shown for all patients (All, n = 20) as well as for several diagnostic subgroups: patients without (*No Prurigo*) or with (*Prurigo*) clinical presence of chronic scratch lesions as well as patients with (*AD*) and without (*No AD*) atopic predisposition. Best antipruritic effects were observed in patients with atopic predisposition and prurigo nodularis. Bar: median response in each group.

nodularis showed (n = 13) significant reduction of pruritus (p = 0.001; Table 2). The mean reduction of pruritus in atopic patients was 54% (p = 0.001; CI 2.144–6.656, Fig. 1). Patients without atopic diathesis (n = 10) experienced weak reduction of pruritus of 27% (p = 0.048; CI 0.025–5.086, Fig. 1). In the group of patients with prurigo nodularis, mean VAS reduction was 48.5% (p = 0.001; CI 1.863–6.137, Fig. 1) ultimately also leading to clinical improvement of scratch lesions. Patients without scratch lesions showed pruritus reduction of 25.7% (p = 0.094; CI-0.554–5.554, Fig. 1). Patients with systemic origin of pruritus such as chronic kidney disease (uraemic pruritus) responded only weakly to aprepitant (mean reduction, 24.0%). However, patients with uraemic pruritus and additional atopic diathesis showed a much better response, reporting a mean reduction of pruritus of 50%. Moreover, also prurigo nodularis patients responded better than patients without scratch lesions in patient subgroups with the same origin of pruritus (e.g., pruritus of unknown origin).

Interestingly, patients aged between 36 and 60 years (n = 6) responded significantly better (mean pruritus reduction, 66.7±24.2%; median 60%) than elderly patients aged over 65 years (n = 14; mean pruritus reduction, 29.3±29.5%; median 25%; p = 0.012). Gender analysis did not reveal a significant

difference in the response though men tend to respond better (n = 8; mean pruritus reduction, 46.3±26.7%; median 45%) than women (n = 12; mean pruritus reduction, 36.7±36.5%; median 30%; p = 0.507).

In sum, therapy with aprepitant leads to pruritus reduction mainly in dermatological diseases such as atopic diathesis and prurigo nodularis. Side-effects remained mild (nausea, vertigo, and drowsiness) and occurred in three patients. In none of these patients cessation of aprepitant therapy was required.

Discussion

Our patients with chronic, yet therapy refractory pruritus, experienced a significant, antipruritic effect (p<0.001) upon monotherapy with the NKR1-antagonist aprepitant within one week. This is the first clinical case series demonstrating that targeting the neuropeptide SP via applying the NKR1-antagonist aprepitant is an effective approach for the treatment of chronic pruritus in patients who all had not responded to previous therapies with topical, intralesional or systemic corticosteroids, antihistamines, and/or UV-irradiation. Those patients who had responded were extremely satisfied, gained new hope and

Table 2. Antipruritic effects in patients with or without atopic diathesis.

Atopic diathesis	Pruritus in chronic kidney disease number of patients/patients with response	Multifactorial origin of pruritus number of patients/patients with response	Pruritus of unknown origin number of patients/patients with response	Total Response
Present	2/2	4/4	4/3	9/10
Not present	3/0	3/2	4/1	3/10

confirmed a positive change in their quality of life since they had a long history of vexing pruritus and documentation of several futile therapies. The most significant response rate was observed in patients with atopic diathesis or clinical presentation of chronic scratch lesions of prurigo nodularis. This is further supported by previous findings of increased SP serum levels in patients with atopic dermatitis, which correlated with the pruritus intensity [14]. Moreover, atopic dermatitis and prurigo nodularis were reported to be characterized by increased SP-positive skin nerve fibers [15,16], which might explain the high response rate in our patients with these disorders. The observation of aprepitant exhibiting a significant antipruritic activity particularly in inflammatory and pruritic skin diseases was confirmed by a recent report. Accordingly, upon treatment with aprepitant a rapid and pronounced improvement was observed in three patients suffering from cutaneous T-cell lymphoma [17]. The results in our patients are promising enough to warrant assessing the efficacy of this novel effect of aprepitant in a randomized, controlled clinical trial.

Most importantly, the antipruritic effect was already observed as early as two days after initiating treatment. This rapid cessation of chronic pruritus in patients with a long history of pruritus (mean, 61.3 months) argues against a placebo effect or spontaneous remission in chronic pruritus patients who had not responded to multiple pre-treatments. The early onset of action suggests that aprepitant acts as a target-specific therapy. Experimental studies clearly showed that SP is involved in pruritus induction in animals and man [12,18]. Injected into the skin, SP rapidly induced pruritus in both normal and experimentally-evoked inflamed skin in non-atopic healthy volunteers [18]. In mice, SP injections resulted in a dose-dependent increase in scratching of the injected site [12]. The induction of pruritus is due to the SP-induced production of pro-inflammatory cytokines and release of pruritogenic mediators from mast cells such as histamine, tumor necrosis factor (TNF)-α, prostaglandin D2, and leukotriene B4 via binding of SP to NKR1 on keratinocytes and mast cells [13,19,20]. The neutralization of these effects by aprepitant most likely suppresses the release of pruritogenic mediators involved in induction and maintenance of chronic pruritus. Moreover, previous experimental studies demonstrated that SP-antagonists may be beneficial substrates for the treatment of inflammatory skin diseases in animal models [21,22].

Aprepitant is a selective high-affinity NKR1-antagonist with little or no affinity for other neurokinin receptors. It was developed and approved in 2003 for the prevention of chemotherapy-induced emesis and is usually administered for three days only [23,24]. However, long-term application of the compound for up to six or eight weeks was reported to be safe in a previous studies [25]. Since in long-term studies usually 80 mg were applied, we also decided to use this dosage. Thus, it needs to be investigated whether increasing the dosage and/or the therapeutic interval may increase the antipruritic effect. Aprepitant crosses the blood-brain barrier to mediate antiemetic effects in the CNS, most likely in the chemoreceptor trigger zone in area postrema at the base of the fourth ventricle [23]. Although pruritus can be induced by SP injection into the CNS in animals [26], recent central imaging studies in humans showed that major cerebral areas for pruriception are the somatosensory cortex, midcingulate gyrus, and prefrontal area [27] but not the fourth ventricle. Therefore, it may be speculated that the antipruritic effect of aprepitant is mainly mediated in the skin but not in the CNS. This speculation is underlined by the failure of pruritus relief in systemic diseases such as chronic kidney disease upon application of aprepitant. Due to a potential role of SP in depression and pain including mediation of neurogenic dural inflammation, it was speculated that aprepitant is effective in central and peripheral pain syndromes [28]. However, aprepitant failed to relieve pain in clinical and experimental studies such as the electrical hyperalgesia model [29]. Clinical trials investigating the efficacy of aprepitant in depression did not show significant benefit in safe, non-toxic doses leading to interruption of development and approval of NKR1-antagonists for this indication [26]. Recent studies clearly showed separate pathways for itch and pain [1]. SP plays an important role in both pain and pruritus pathways [1]. Interestingly, animal studies suggest that the neuropeptides SP and calcitonin gene-related peptide (CGRP) play an opposite role in pain and pruritus. While enhanced SP levels have been demonstrated to be related to reduced CGRP levels in an atopic dermatitis mouse model [30], pain studies showed a correlation to CGRP levels [31]. It might therefore be speculated that SP has a differential role in pain and pruritus possibly explaining opposite response in pain (failure of aprepitant) and pruritus (high response to aprepitant). It therefore seems likely that application of an NKR1 antagonist in SP-mediated pruritogenic diseases targets specific pruritus-related neuronal pathways different from pain pathways.

In conclusion our findings outline that aprepitant presents a novel, promising therapeutic approach of pruritus which is especially effective in patients with chronic pruritus due to atopic predisposition/dermatitis or prurigo nodularis. The tendency towards better response in young (male) patients suggest aprepitant to be a novel therapeutic option in adult but not elderly patients with atopic dermatitis.

Acknowledgments

We thank Rajam Csordas for assistance in preparation of the manuscript.

Author Contributions

Conceived and designed the experiments: SS TAL. Performed the experiments: SS. Analyzed the data: SS DS IH CS TAL. Wrote the paper: SS DS IH CS TAL.

References

1. Ikoma A, Steinhoff M, Ständer S, Yosipovitch G, Schmelz M (2006) Neurobiology of Pruritus. Nature Reviews Neuroscience 7: 535–547.
2. Ständer S, Weisshaar E, Luger TA (2008) Neurophysiological and neurochemical basis of modern pruritus treatment. Experimental Dermatology 17: 161–169.
3. Ständer S, Weisshaar E, Mettang T, Szepietowski JC, Carstens E (2007) Clinical classification of itch: a position paper of the International Forum for the Study of Itch. Acta Dermato-Venereologica 87: 291–294.
4. Dalgard F, Lien L, Dalen I (2007) Itch in the community: associations with psychosocial factors among adults. J Eur Acad Dermatol Venereol 21: 1215–1219.
5. Matterne U, Strassner T, Apfelbacher CJ, Diepgen TL, Weisshaar E (2009) Measuring the prevalence of chronic itch in the general population: development and validation of a questionnaire for use in large sale studies. Acta Derm Venereol 89: 250–256.
6. Weisshaar E, Dalgard F (2009) Epidemiology of itch: adding to the burden of skin morbidity. Acta Derm Venereol 89: 339–350.
7. Tessari G, Dalle Vedove C, Loschiavo C, Tessitore N, Rugiu C, et al. (2009) The impact of pruritus on the quality of life of patients undergoing dialysis: a single centre cohort study. J Nephrol 22: 241–248.
8. Weisshaar E, Diepgen TL, Bruckner T, Fartasch M, Kupfer J, et al. (2008) Itch intensity evaluated in the German Atopic Dermatitis Intervention Study (GADIS): correlations with quality of life, coping behaviour and SCORAD severity in 823 children. Acta Derm Venereol 88: 234–239.
9. Pogatzki-Zahn E, Marziniak M, Schneider G, Luger TA, Ständer S (2008) Chronic pruritus: targets, mechanisms and future therapies. Drug News Perspect 21: 541–551.
10. Kumagai H, Ebata T, Takamori K, Muramatsu T, Nakamoto H, et al. (2010) Effect of a novel kappa-receptor agonist, nalfurafine hydrochloride, on severe itch in 337 haemodialysis patients: a Phase III, randomized,

double-blind, placebo-controlled study. Nephrol Dial Transplant 25: 1251–1257.

11. Almeida TA, Rojo J, Nieto PM, Pinto FM, Hernandez M, et al. (2004) Tachykinins and tachykinin receptors: structure and activity relationships. Current Medicinal Chemistry 11: 2045–2081.

12. Andoh T, Nagasawa T, Satoh M, Kuraishi Y (1998) Substance P induction of itch-associated response mediated by cutaneous NK1 tachykinin receptors in mice. J Pharmacol Exp Ther 286: 1140–1145.

13. Kulka M, Sheen CH, Tancowny BP, Grammer LC, Schleimer RP (2008) Neuropeptides activate human mast cell degranulation and chemokine production. Immunology 123: 398–410.

14. Salomon J, Baran E (2008) The role of selected neuropeptides in pathogenesis of atopic dermatitis. J Europ Acad Dermatol 22: 223–228.

15. Abadia Molina F, Burrows NP, Jones RR, Terenghi G, Polak JM (1992) Increased sensory neuropeptides in nodular prurigo: a quantitative immunohistochemical analysis. Br J Dermatol 127: 344–351.

16. Jarvikallio A, Harvima IT, Naukkarinen A (2003) Mast cells, nerves and neuropeptides in atopic dermatitis and nummular eczema. Arch Dermatol Res 295: 2–7.

17. Duval A, Dubertret L (2009) Aprepitant as an antipruritic agent? N Engl J Med 361: 1415–1416.

18. Thomsen JS, Sonne M, Benfeldt E, Jensen SB, Serup J, et al. (2002) Experimental itch in sodium lauryl sulphate-inflamed and normal skin in humans: a randomized, double-blind, placebo-controlled study of histamine and other inducers of itch. Br J Dermatol 146: 792–800.

19. Furutani K, Koro O, Hide M, Yamamoto S (1999) Substance P- and antigen-induced release of leukotriene B4, prostaglandin D2 and histamine from guinea pig skin by different mechanisms in vitro. Arch Dermatol Res 291: 466–473.

20. Song IS, Bunnett NW, Olerud JE, Harten B, Steinhoff M, et al. (2000) Substance P induction of murine keratinocyte PAM 212 interleukin 1 production is mediated by the neurokinin 2 receptor (NK-2R). Exp Dermatol 9: 42–52.

21. Lofgren O, Qi Y, Lundeberg T (1999) Inhibitory effects of tachykinin receptor antagonists on thermally induced inflammatory reactions in a rat model. Burns 25: 125–129.

22. Palframan RT, Costa SK, Wilsoncroft P, Antunes E, de Nucci G, et al. (1996) The effect of a tachykinin NK1 receptor antagonist, SR140333, on oedema formation induced in rat skin by venom from the Phoneutria nigriventer spider. Br J Pharmacol 118: 295–298.

23. Dando TM, Perry C (2004) Aprepitant: a review of its use in the prevention of chemotherapy-induced nausea and vomiting. Drugs 64: 777–794.

24. Hesketh PJ, Grunberg SM, Gralla RJ, Warr DG, Roila F, et al. (2003) The oral neurokinin-1 antagonist aprepitant for the prevention of chemotherapy-induced nausea and vomiting: a multinational, randomized, double-blind, placebo-controlled trial in patients receiving high-dose cisplatin–the Aprepitant Protocol 052 Study Group. J Clin Oncol 21: 4077–4080.

25. Keller M, Montgomery S, Ball W, Morrison M, Snavely D, et al. (2006) Lack of efficacy of the substance p (neurokinin1 receptor) antagonist aprepitant in the treatment of major depressive disorder. Biol Psychiatry 59: 216–223.

26. Piercey MF, Dobry PJ, Schröder LA, Einspahr FJ (1981) Behavioral evidence that substance P may be a spinal cord sensory neurotransmitter. Brain Res 210: 407–412.

27. Schneider G, Ständer S, Burgmer M, Driesch G, Heuft G, et al. (2008) Significant differences in central imaging of histamine-induced itch between atopic dermatitis and healthy subjects. Eur J Pain 12: 834–841.

28. DeVane CL (2001) Substance P: a new era, a new role. Pharmacotherapy 21: 1061–1069.

29. Chizh BA, Göhring M, Tröster A, Quartey GK, Schmelz M, et al. (2007) Effects of oral pregabalin and aprepitant on pain and central sensitization in the electrical hyperalgesia model in human volunteers. Br J Anaesth 98: 246–254.

30. Katsuno M, Aihara M, Kojima M, Osuna H, Hosoi J J, et al. (2003) Neuropeptides concentrations in the skin of a murine (NC/Nga mice) model of atopic dermatitis. J Dermatol Sci 33: 55–65.

31. Mogil JS, Miermeister F, Seifert F, Strasburg K, Zimmermann K, et al. (2005) Variable sensitivity to noxious heat is mediated by differential expression of the CGRP gene. Proc Natl Acad Sci U S A 102: 12938–12943.

Differences between the Glycosylation Patterns of Haptoglobin Isolated from Skin Scales and Plasma of Psoriatic Patients

Bernardetta Maresca[1], **Luisa Cigliano**[1]*, **Maria Stefania Spagnuolo**[2], **Fabrizio Dal Piaz**[3], **Maria M. Corsaro**[4], **Nicola Balato**[5], **Massimiliano Nino**[5], **Anna Balato**[5], **Fabio Ayala**[5], **Paolo Abrescia**[1]

1 Dipartimento delle Scienze Biologiche, Università di Napoli Federico II, Napoli, Italia, 2 Istituto per il Sistema Produzione Animale in Ambiente Mediterraneo, Consiglio Nazionale delle Ricerche, Napoli, Italia, 3 Dipartimento di Scienze Farmaceutiche e Biomediche, Università degli Studi di Salerno, Fisciano (Salerno), Italia, 4 Dipartimento di Chimica Organica e Biochimica, Università di Napoli Federico II, Complesso Universitario M. S. Angelo, Napoli, Italia, 5 Dipartimento di Patologia Sistematica - Sezione di Dermatologia, Università di Napoli Federico II, Napoli, Italia

Abstract

Improved diagnosis of psoriasis, by new biomarkers, is required for evaluating the progression rate of the disease and the response to treatment. Haptoglobin (Hpt), a glycoprotein secreted by hepatocytes and other types of cells including keratinocytes, was found with glycan changes in psoriasis and other diseases. We previously reported that Hpt isolated from plasma of psoriatic patients is more fucosylated than Hpt of healthy subjects. The aim of this study was to compare the glycosylation pattern of Hpt isolated from skin scales or plasma of patients with psoriasis with that of Hpt from cornified epidermal layer or plasma of healthy subjects. High performance liquid chromatography analysis of the glycans isolated from the protein backbone revealed that glycan patterns from skin and plasma of patients were similar, and mostly displayed quantitative rather than qualitative differences from normal pattern. Biotin-labeled lectins were used to evaluate quantitative differences in the glycoforms of Hpt from plasma and psoriatic skin scales. Hpt from skin and plasma of patients showed more fucosylated and branched glycans than Hpt from plasma of healthy subjects. Tryptic glycopeptides of Hpt were also analyzed by mass spectrometry, and a decreased amount of sialylated glycan chains was found in glycopeptides of skin Hpt, as compared with Hpt from plasma. High levels of glycans with fucosylated and tetra-antennary chains were detected on the peptide NLFLNHSENATAK from Hpt of psoriatic patients. Our data demonstrate that specific changes in glycan structures of Hpt, such as enhanced glycan branching and fucose content, are associated with psoriasis, and that differences between circulating and skin Hpt do exist. A lower extent of glycan fucosylation and branching was found in Hpt from plasma of patients in disease remission. Altered glycoforms might reflect changes of Hpt function in the skin, and could be used as markers of the disease.

Editor: Roger Chammas, Faculdade de Medicina, Universidade de São Paulo, Brazil

Funding: This work was supported by a research grant from the University of Naples Federico II (Ric. Dip. 10112/2010). The funders had no role in study design, data collection and analysis, decision to publish, or preparation of the manuscript.

Competing Interests: The authors have declared that no competing interests exist.

* E-mail: luisa.cigliano@unina.it

Introduction

Haptoglobin (Hpt) is an acute-phase glycoprotein known to bind free haemoglobin (Hb) for degradation and iron recycling [1,2]. Hpt is produced mostly in liver by hepatocytes [3,4] and secreted into blood circulation. Its levels markedly increase during the acute phase of inflammation and in neoplastic disease in response to inflammatory cytokines [1]. In addition to binding Hb, a number of other physiological roles of Hpt were suggested. Hpt might play a role in angiogenesis and wound healing, as it inhibits gelatinases thus contributing to remodel the extracellular matrix [5]. Moreover, Hpt was recently reported to bind the apolipo-protein (Apo) A–I and ApoE, and impair their key function in stimulating the enzyme lecithin:cholesterol acyl transferase (LCAT) and mediating cholesterol delivery to hepatocytes [6,7]. Although the tissue-specific expression of Hpt in some peripheral organs was demonstrated [8–12], the role of Hpt in the skin or skin diseases like psoriasis has not yet been studied. Limited studies

provide evidence that Hpt might be synthesized and/or secreted into the skin [13], and demonstrate its inhibitory effect on the differentiation of immature epidermal Langerhans cells in antigen presenting cells [14]. Locally produced Hpt might have a modulatory role on skin cells and/or on cells of the immune system, recruited at the site of inflammation. We have previously demonstrated that, in Psoriasis vulgaris, plasma Hpt displays glycoforms with reduced affinity for both Hb and ApoA-I as compared with glycoforms isolated from plasma of healthy subjects, and inhibits the LCAT activity less than normal protein [15]. These glycoforms were suggested to be associated with skin disease and secreted at enhanced levels during inflammation [15,16]. Actually, abnormal glycosylation of glycoproteins has been correlated with cancer, inflammatory diseases, and congenital disorders [17]. Four asparagine residues of the Hpt subunit β are known to link glycans (N23, N46, N50, and N80) [18], and tri- or tetra-antennary glycans were found on this subunit from patients with rheumatoid arthritis [19], endometriosis [20], or ovarian cancer [21]. In addition, the levels of N-acetylneuraminic acid (NeuAc, also called sialic acid and indicated by the acronym S) and/or fucose (Fuc) were found associated with prostate cancer [22], pancreatic cancer [23], carbohydrate-deficient glycoprotein syndrome [24], or liver disease [25]. We recently reported that the glycan pattern of Hpt isolated from plasma of patients with acute coronary syndrome displays more branched and fucosylated structures as compared to that of Hpt from healthy subjects [26]. We also found higher number of different fucosylated and tri-antennary or tetra-antennary glycans in Hpt from plasma of patients with psoriasis than in controls [16].

Our objective was to study whether the Hpt glycan changes found in the plasma of patients with psoriasis are a consequence of systemic inflammation or can be also found in Hpt isolated from skin lesions. Moreover we compared glycan structures associated with Hpt isolated from skin scales of patients and epidermal layers of healthy subjects, in order to investigate whether specific glycoforms in the skin of patients do exist.

Results

HPLC analysis of Hpt glycans

Hpt was purified from plasma (pHpt-P) and skin scales (sHpt-P) of patients with psoriasis, or plasma of healthy donors (pHpt-N). Purified pHpt-P, sHpt-P, and pHpt-N were treated with N-glycosidase to separate N-linked glycans from the polypeptide backbone. The released glycans were labelled with the fluorophore 2-AB and analyzed by HPLC, as previously reported [27]. The elution patterns of the glycans from pHpt-P and sHpt-P were similar to that of glycans from pHpt-N. Six major (namely peaks a to f) and a number of minor peaks were present on chromatograms of glycans from pHpt-N (Figure 1, panel A). The pattern of pHpt-P glycans was similar to that of pHpt-N glycans, but peak b was missing (Figure 1, panel B), whereas only peaks c and f could be clearly detected in the glycan pattern from sHpt-P (Figure 1, panel C). Differences in maximum and area were found for peaks with the same migration (expressed in GU value). Quantitative measurements of the relative amount of the major peaks were done by integrating their areas on the chromatograms, and arbitrarily expressing the obtained values as ratios with the peak c area, which was given the value 1 (Table 1). The data suggest that the relative areas of peaks were different in patients when compared to controls. Peak f was found markedly increased in glycan patterns of pHpt-P and sHpt-P (see also Figure 1, panels B and C versus panel A). A relational database was used to sort out the structures of Hpt major glycans, on the basis of their GU ±0.1. A number of possible structures could correspond to the values of GU we found. Thus, for example, ten different tri- and tetra-antennary glycans (with or without Fuc) are all reported to migrate as peak c. These data confirm previous information on multiple structures of glycans of pHpt-P and pHpt-N, and indicate that also sHpt-P is glycosylated. In particular, the finding of higher amounts of peak f in the glycan pattern of sHpt-P, as compared with that of pHpt-P, suggests that sHpt-P diffuses from skin to blood, and comparative HPLC analysis of pHpt-P and pHpt-N might be a useful tool to monitor sHpt-P secretion into the skin.

Analysis of Hpt glycans by lectins

ELISA with biotin-labeled lectins is a widely used technique for analysing the amounts of different structures of complex N-linked glycans. The lectins Concanavalin A (ConA, binding the mannose core of glycans), Sambucus nigra (SNA, binding S α2,6-linked to galactose, from here on named G), Maackia amurensis (MAA,

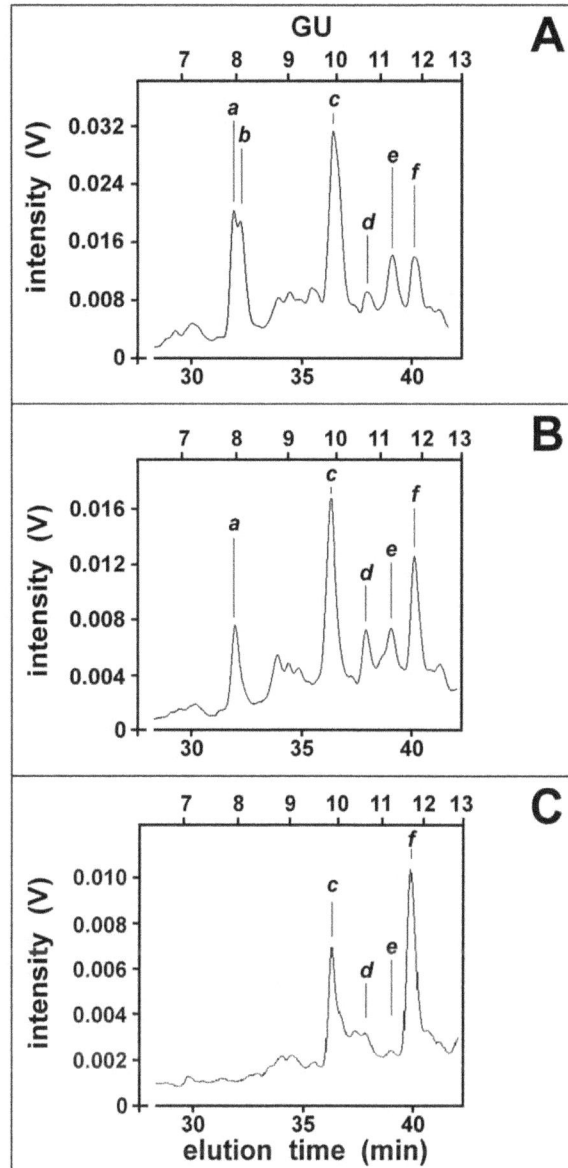

Figure 1. Normal phase HPLC pattern of 2AB-glycans from pHpt-N, pHpt-P and sHpt-P. Purified pHpt-N, pHpt-P, and sHpt-P were deglycosylated by treatment with PNGase F, and their glycans were labelled by 2 aminobenzamide. After solid phase extraction, the glycans were fractionated by HPLC using a TSK-gel Amide-80 column (4.6×250 mm) with a linear gradient of ammonium formate at pH 4.4 (87.5 to 162.5 mM) with CH_3CN (65 to 35%) in 75 min, at 0.4 ml/min flow rate. Elution was monitored by measuring the label fluorescence at 425 nm (λ_{EX} = 360 nm). Panel A: glycans from pHpt-N. Panel B: glycans from pHpt-P. Panel C: glycans from sHpt-P. The GU ladder represents the migration of labelled oligosaccharides with different units of glucose. The marked peaks were used for comparative analysis.

binding S α2,3-linked to G) and Lotus tetragonolobus agglutinin (LTA, binding Fuc), were used to evaluate quantitative differences in their reactivity to the glycoforms of Hpt from plasma of patients and controls, and psoriatic skin scales. On the basis of our preliminary HPLC analysis, which suggested the presence in pHpt-P and sHpt-P of highly branched tetra-antennary glycans, pHpt-P and sHpt-P were expected to display lower reactivity to ConA whereas higher reactivity to LTA than pHpt-N. In fact,

Table 1. Relative amounts of the glycan peaks eluted by HPLC of pHpt-N, pHpt-P and sHpt-P.

Peak	GU[1]	pHpt-N[2]	pHpt-P[2]	sHpt-P[2]
a	7.97	0.31	0.36	0
b	8.06	0.39	0	0
c	9.88	1.00	1.00	1.00
d	10.68	0.25	0.34	0.46
e	11.25	0.40	0.40	0.23
f	11.80	0.40	0.71	1.78

[1]GU value represents the peak elution as compared to that of 2-aminobenzamide-labelled oligomers of glucose. A mixture of standards (1 to 20 units of glucose) was used for the chromatography calibration.
[2]The HPLC pattern of Hpt glycans, shown in Figure 1, was analyzed. The relative area of each peak is expressed as ratio with peak c area. Data from one experiment are shown. Inter-assay CV of each peak, from three separate experiments, was less than 5%.

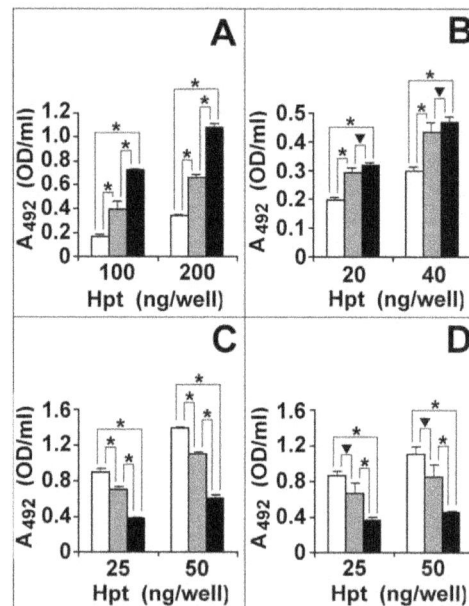

Figure 2. Binding of lectins to Hpt. The wells of a microtiter plate were coated with different amounts of pHpt-N (white bars), pHpt-P (grey bars), or sHpt-P (black bars). Solutions containing 1 μM biotinylated LTA (panel A), MAA (panel B), ConA (panel C), or SNA (panel D) were separately incubated into the wells. Avidin-HRP and hydrogen peroxide were used to develop color from OPD. Color intensity was determined by measuring the absorbance at 492 nm (A_{492}). Five equal aliquots of each sample were processed, and means ± SEM are shown. Asterisk: significant difference between the linked bars ($P < 0.0001$). Triangle: not significant difference ($P > 0.05$). Data from one experiment are shown. Inter-assay CV for each sample, from three separate experiments, was less than 5%.

glycoforms with more highly branched glycans (as supposed in pHpt-P and sHpt-P) should have the mannose core more hindered by the glycan arms and, consequently, should react to ConA with decreased affinity. Furthermore, the HPLC data also suggested that more Fuc residues might be harboured on pHpt-P and sHpt-P glycoforms, which were therefore thought more reactive to LTA than pHpt-N glycoforms. Equal amounts of pHpt-N, pHpt-P, or sHpt-P were separately loaded into the wells of a microtiter plate, and processed for the binding of biotinylated lectins. As shown in Figure 2, the three distinct populations of Hpt glycoforms displayed significant differences in their affinity for each of the used lectins. In detail, sHpt-P and pHpt-P reacted worse than pHpt-N with biotin labelled ConA (25 ng: 42.78±0.4 and 78.1±3.4% respectively; 50 ng: 42.69±3.23 and 74.60±1.25%; Figure 2, Panel C). Moreover, sHpt-P and pHpt-P bound LTA more than pHpt-N (100 ng: 389.60±1.50 and 288.89±14.3% respectively; 200 ng: 316.90±7.60 and 187.13±7.26% respectively; Figure 2, Panel A), and MAA as well (20 ng: 159.40±1.84 and 146.91±7.23% respectively; 40 ng: 157.04±5.94 and 145.86±12.20% respectively; Figure 2, Panel B). Conversely, pHpt-P and sHpt-P reacted to SNA worse than pHpt-N (25 ng: 41.20±3.34 and 76.15±13.88% respectively; 50 ng: 41.52±0.78 and 76.64±12.77% respectively). These results confirm that pHpt-P and sHpt-P have more fucosylated and branched glycans than pHpt-N, and indicate that they display increased ratio of α2,3-linked with α2,6-linked S as compared with normal glycoforms.

Mass spectrometry (MS) analysis of glycopeptides from trypsin treatment of Hpt

MS analysis demonstrated that, in patients with moderate psoriasis, circulating Hpt displays both quantitative and qualitative changes in its glycan structures [16]. Hpt, purified from skin scales of psoriatic patients (sHpt-P) and cornified epidermal layer of healthy subjects (sHpt-N), was analyzed by MS following trypsin digestion, in order to further characterize glycan structures associated to Hpt from skin lesions, and to verify whether specific glycoforms in the skin of patients do exist. The digestion was predicted to yield 3 glycopeptides namely P1 (m/z 2679.39) carrying a single glycosylation site on N184, P2 (m/z 1458.74) with 2 glycosylation sites on N207 and N211, and P3 (m/z 1795.01) with a single glycosylation site on N241. The peptide mixtures were purified by gel filtration and processed for both liquid chromatography (LC)/MS and LC/MS/MS analysis.

Many glycopeptides from both patients and controls were identified. MS spectra of the glycopeptides are reported in Figures 3–5, while Tables 2, 3, 4 report the observed masses, the corresponding predicted structures and the relative abundance of the established species. Peptides identification was based on the good agreement between experimental and theoretical mass values. Sialylated bi-antennary glycans were the major structures in Hpt from all sources. With regard to P1 (Figure 3), major glycans from sHpt-P were found to share structures with sHpt-N glycans (Table 2) or pHpt-P [16]. Most of the glycans found in the P2 repertoire (Figure 4; Table 3) from sHpt-P was also found in the previously reported glycan pattern of pHpt-P (18/29 signals found in pHpt-P) [16]. In particular, tetra-antennary N-glycans with one or two Fuc were observed in psoriatic Hpt (both skin and plasma), but not in control Hpt. Interestingly, the N-glycan repertoire of P2 from sHpt-P showed the presence of significant amounts of fucosylated structures and five glycan chains (harboured on species named as Lk, Lw, Lx, Ly and Lz) not detectable in the previously reported glycan pattern of pHpt-P [16]. These glycan structures were compatible with fucosylated but not fully sialylated glycan chain (Table 3). So, in agreement with the ELISA results shown above, the level of fucosylated glycans was found enhanced in sHpt-P (in particular in P2 glycoforms) compared to both pHpt-N and pHpt-P. Further, the Lw glycoform (not detectable in plasma) was also revealed in the P2 repertoire (Figure 4) from sHpt-N (Table 3), thus suggesting that these glycan structures are specifically associated with skin Hpt, and not with

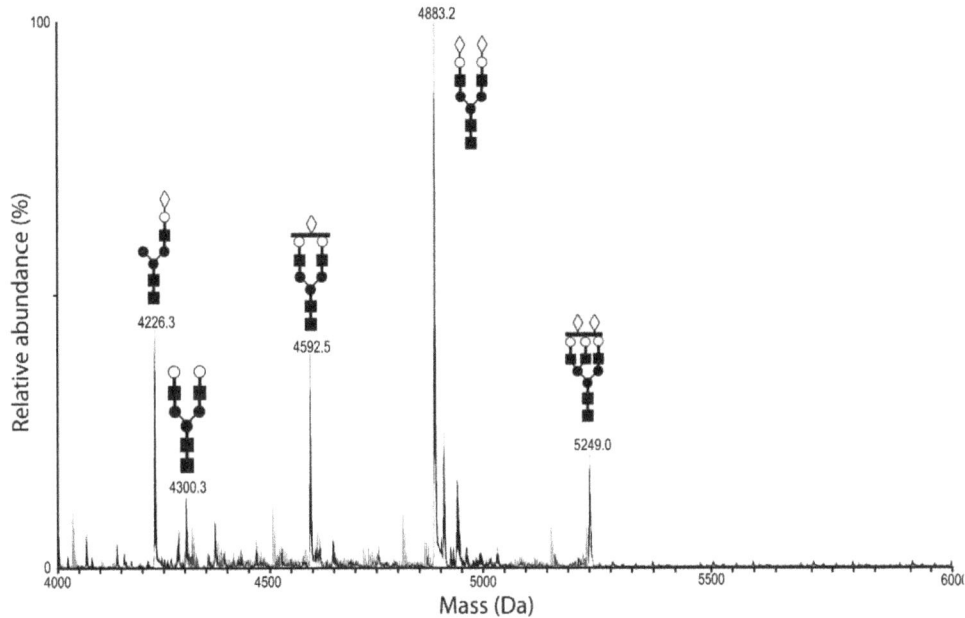

Figure 3. Mass spectrum of the P1 glycopeptide repertoire from skin of patients. Purified sHpt-P was digested by trypsin, and the resulting fragments were fractionated by UPLC and analyzed by ESI-MS. Positive ions of P1 (MVSHHNLTTGATLINEQWLLTTAK) glycopeptides from Hpt of skin of patients is shown. Glycopeptide peaks are indicated with their observed mass value (see Table 2) and chain structure. Peaks with mass attributable to non-glycosylated species were ignored.

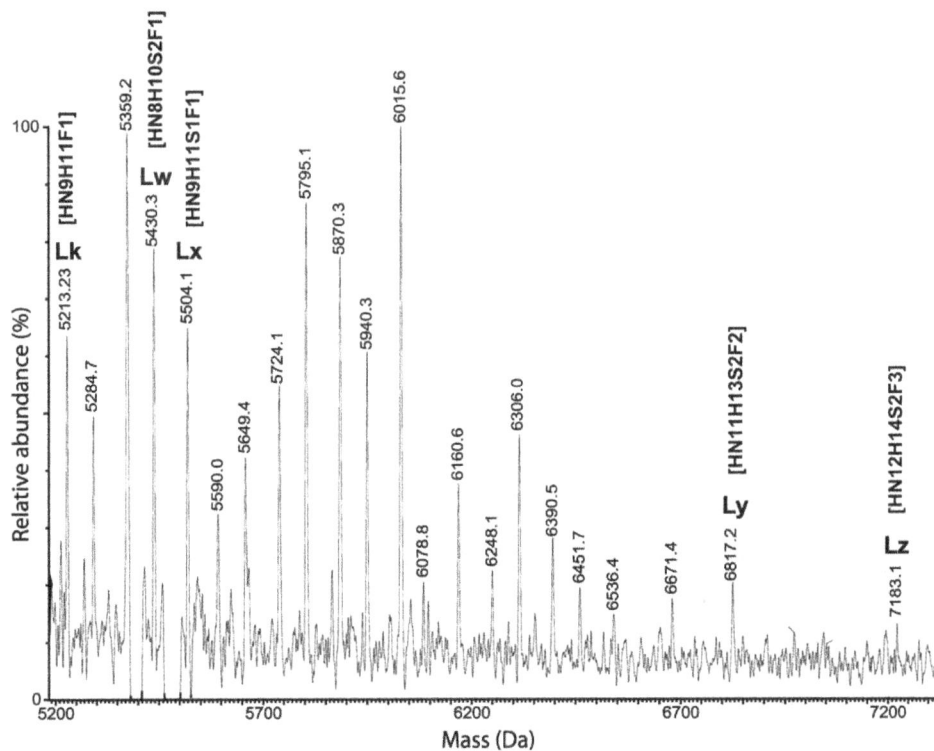

Figure 4. Mass spectrum of the P2 glycopeptide repertoire from skin of patients. Purified sHpt-P was digested by trypsin, and the resulting fragments were fractionated by UPLC and analyzed by ESI-MS. Positive ions of P2 (NLFLN HSENATAK) glycopeptides from Hpt of skin of patients is shown. Glycopeptide peaks are indicated with their observed mass value (see Table 3). The glycoforms found only in sHpt-P and not in pHpt-N and in pHpt-P are indicated. Peaks with mass attributable to non-glycosylated species were ignored.

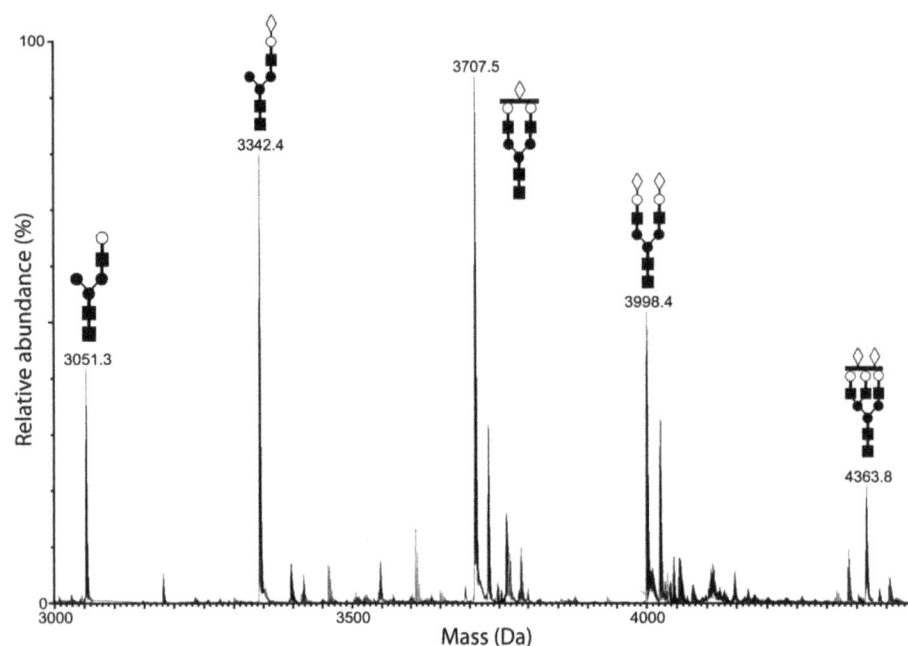

Figure 5. Mass spectrum of the P3 glycopeptide repertoire from skin of patients. Purified sHpt-P was digested by trypsin, and the resulting fragments were fractionated by UPLC and analyzed by ESI-MS. Positive ions of P3 (VVLHPNYSQVDIGLIK) glycopeptides from Hpt of skin of patients is shown. Glycopeptide peaks are indicated with their observed mass value (see Table 4) and chain structure. Peaks with mass attributable to non-glycosylated species were ignored.

the pathology. Moreover, the overall level of fucosylated residues in sHpt-N was found lower than that from sHpt-P.

In the P3 repertoire (Figure 5), the glycoform population of sHpt-P (5 species) was less heterogeneous than that previously found in pHpt-P (14 species) [16]. Minor differences in relative abundance for some glycans or in glycan structures, between sHpt-P and sHpt-N, are shown in Table 4.

The glycan structures were also analyzed in Hpt purified from a pool of plasma of patients (pHpt-R) that, after treatment with the anti-TNF- α drug Adalimumab for 16 weeks, displayed disease remission (PASI = 3.9±1.2). No significant differences were found in the P1 repertoire from pHpt-R (Table 5), in comparison with that previously reported in pHpt-P [16], while fucosylated and highly branched glycans were found in significantly lower amounts

in the P2 and P3 repertoire from pHpt-R (Table 6 and 7, respectively). As TNF-α was shown to induce the expression of α2,6-sialyl transferase and fucosyl transferase [28,29], our results suggest a potential inhibitory effect of Adalimumab on these enzyme activities.

Discussion

Identification of clinically important protein biomarkers with possible glycosylation alteration is an expanding area of research that can improve diagnosis of psoriasis. Our previous results showed that Hpt from psoriatic patients contains quantitative and qualitative glycoform variants from those circulating in normal conditions [16]. In this study, we provide the first evidence of

Table 2. Glycopeptides in the P1 repertoire of Hpt tryptic digest from skin of patients and controls, and their relative abundance.

Species	Observed Mass (Da)	Calculated Mass (Da)	Glycopeptide P1 (MVSHHNLTTGATLINEQWLLTTAK)[a]	Relative peak intensity[b]	
				Skin control	Skin scale Patients
M1	4227.02	4226.93	[NeuAc$_1$Hex$_1$HexNAc$_1$+Man$_3$GlcNAc$_2$]	31.2±1.2	21.1±1.8
M2	4300.51	4300.97	[Hex$_2$HexNAc$_2$+Man$_3$GlcNAc$_2$]	4.8±0.3	2.9±0.9
M3	4591.56	4592.06	[NeuAc$_1$Hex$_2$HexNAc$_2$+Man$_3$GlcNAc$_2$]	18.6±1.4	21.1±1.6
M4	4883.61	4883.16	[NeuAc$_2$Hex$_2$HexNAc$_2$+Man$_3$GlcNAc$_2$]	46.4±1.8	47.8±3.1
M6	5248.66	5248.29	[NeuAc$_2$Hex$_3$HexNAc$_3$+Man$_3$GlcNAc$_2$]	ND[c]	7.2±1.3

[a]The asparagine residue harbouring the glycan is underlined.
[b]Quantitative analysis for relative abundance of species was obtained taking into account all the observed multicharged ions. The values are expressed as means (from three technical replicates) ± standard deviations.
[c]ND = not detected. The ratio signal-to-noise = 3 was used as detection threshold.
Glycan species are indicated with the same nomenclature previously used for pHpt-P and pHpt-N [16].

Table 3. Glycopeptides in the P2 repertoire of Hpt tryptic digest from skin of patients and controls, and their relative abundance.

Species	Observed Mass (Da)	Calculated Mass (Da)	Glycopeptide P2 (NLFLNHSENATAK)[a]	Relative peak intensity[bc]	
				Skin Control	Skin scale Patients
L2	4993.82	4993.99	[NeuAc$_1$Hex$_2$HexNAc$_2$+Man$_3$GlcNAc$_2$] + [Hex$_2$HexNAc$_2$+Man$_3$GlcNAc$_2$]	ND	ND
L3	5067.96	5068.03	[Hex$_3$HexNAc$_3$+Man$_3$GlcNAc$_2$] + [Hex$_2$HexNAc$_2$+Man$_3$GlcNAc$_2$]	7.6±1.0	ND
Lk	5213.23	5214.08	[Hex$_3$HexNAc$_3$+Man$_3$GlcNAc$_2$+Fuc$_1$] + [Hex$_2$HexNAc$_2$+Man$_3$GlcNAc$_2$]	ND	4.9±0.8
L4	5284.93	5285.08	[NeuAc$_1$Hex$_1$HexNAc$_1$+Man$_3$GlcNAc$_2$] + [NeuAc$_1$Hex$_2$HexNAc$_2$+Man$_3$GlcNAc$_2$]	14.2±0.7	6.6±1.1
L5	5358.97	5359.12	[Hex$_2$HexNAc$_2$+Man$_3$GlcNAc$_2$] + [NeuAc$_1$Hex$_3$HexNAc$_3$+Man$_3$GlcNAc$_2$]	13.4±1.3	5.6±1.1
Lw	5430.03	5431.14	[NeuAc$_1$Hex$_2$HexNAc$_2$+Man$_3$GlcNAc$_2$+Fuc$_1$] + [NeuAc$_1$Hex$_2$HexNAc$_2$+Man$_3$GlcNAc$_2$]	5.4±0.9	13.3±1.2
Lx	5504.09	5505.18	[NeuAc$_1$Hex$_3$HexNAc$_3$+Man$_3$GlcNAc$_2$+Fuc$_1$] + [Hex$_2$HexNAc$_2$+Man$_3$GlcNAc$_2$]	ND	5.7±0.6
L6	5575.88	5576.18	[NeuAc$_2$Hex$_2$HexNAc$_2$+Man$_3$GlcNAc$_2$] + [NeuAc$_1$Hex$_2$HexNAc$_2$+Man$_3$GlcNAc$_2$]	19.7±1.5	ND
L7	5650.08	5650.21	[NeuAc$_1$Hex$_2$HexNAc$_2$+Man$_3$GlcNAc$_2$] + [NeuAc$_1$Hex$_3$HexNAc$_3$+Man$_3$GlcNAc$_2$]	6.8±0.3	5.6±1.2
L8	5722.18	5722.23	[NeuAc$_2$Hex$_2$HexNAc$_2$+Man$_3$GlcNAc$_2$+Fuc$_1$] + [NeuAc$_1$Hex$_2$HexNAc$_2$+Man$_3$GlcNAc$_2$]	ND	3.5±0.4
L9	5796.11	5796.27	[NeuAc$_1$Hex$_3$HexNAc$_3$+Man$_3$GlcNAc$_2$+Fuc$_1$] + [NeuAc$_1$Hex$_2$HexNAc$_2$+Man$_3$GlcNAc$_2$]	3.9±0.4	8.7±0.7
L10	5866.80	5867.27	[NeuAc$_2$Hex$_2$HexNAc$_2$+Man$_3$GlcNAc$_2$] + [NeuAc$_2$Hex$_2$HexNAc$_2$+Man$_3$GlcNAc$_2$]	9.9±0.9	4.9±0.8
L11	5941.74	5941.31	[NeuAc$_2$Hex$_3$HexNAc$_3$+Man$_3$GlcNAc$_2$] + [NeuAc$_1$Hex$_2$HexNAc$_2$+Man$_3$GlcNAc$_2$]	4.7±0.3	7.6±0.5
L12	6015.27	6015.35	[NeuAc$_1$Hex$_3$HexNAc$_3$+Man$_3$GlcNAc$_2$] + [NeuAc$_1$Hex$_3$HexNAc$_3$+Man$_3$GlcNAc$_2$]	6.5±0.2	9.1±0.8
L14	6161.34	6161.40	[NeuAc$_1$Hex$_3$HexNAc$_3$+Man$_3$GlcNAc$_2$+Fuc$_1$] + [NeuAc$_1$Hex$_3$HexNAc$_3$+Man$_3$GlcNAc$_2$]	7.9±0.5	3.5±0.4
L16	6307.41	6307.46	[NeuAc$_1$Hex$_3$HexNAc$_3$+Man$_3$GlcNAc$_2$+Fuc$_1$] + [NeuAc$_1$Hex$_3$HexNAc$_3$+Man$_3$GlcNAc$_2$+Fuc$_1$]	ND	4.9±0.6
L18	6452.43	6452.49	[NeuAc$_2$Hex$_3$HexNAc$_3$+Man$_3$GlcNAc$_2$+Fuc$_1$] + [NeuAc$_1$Hex$_3$HexNAc$_3$+Man$_3$GlcNAc$_2$]	ND	2.1±0.8
L21	6672.36	6672.60	[NeuAc$_1$Hex$_4$HexNAc$_4$+Man$_3$GlcNAc$_2$+Fuc$_1$] + [NeuAc$_1$Hex$_3$HexNAc$_3$+Man$_3$GlcNAc$_2$+Fuc$_1$]	ND	6.6±0.1
Ly	6817.23	6818.65	[NeuAc$_1$Hex$_4$HexNAc$_4$+Man$_3$GlcNAc$_2$+Fuc$_2$] + [NeuAc$_1$Hex$_3$HexNAc$_3$+Man$_3$GlcNAc$_2$+Fuc$_1$]	ND	6.0±0.6
Lz	7183.13	7183.79	[NeuAc$_1$Hex$_4$HexNAc$_4$+Man$_3$GlcNAc$_2$+Fuc$_2$] + [NeuAc$_1$Hex$_4$HexNAc$_4$+Man$_3$GlcNAc$_2$+Fuc$_1$]	ND	0.7±0.2
L29	7329.44	7329.85	[NeuAc$_1$Hex$_4$HexNAc$_4$+Man$_3$GlcNAc$_2$+Fuc$_2$] + [NeuAc$_1$Hex$_4$HexNAc$_4$+Man$_3$GlcNAc$_2$+Fuc$_2$]	ND	0.4±0.2

[a]The asparagine residue harbouring the glycan is underlined.
[b]Quantitative analysis for relative abundance of species was obtained taking into account all the observed multicharged ions. The values are expressed as means (from three technical replicates) ± standard deviations.
[c]ND = not detected. The ratio signal-to-noise = 3 was used as detection threshold.
Glycan species are indicated with the same nomenclature previously used for pHpt-P and pHpt-N [16].

Table 4. Glycopeptides in the P3 repertoire of Hpt tryptic digest from skin of patients and controls, and their relative abundance.

Species	Observed Mass (Da)	Calculated Mass (Da)	Glycopeptide P3 (VVLHPNYSQVDIGLIK)[a]	Relative peak intensity[b]	
				Skin Control	Skin scale Patients
N1	3051.15	3051.45	[Hex$_1$HexNAc$_1$+Man$_3$GlcNAc$_2$]	10.8±0.6	15.4±1.6
N2	3342.20	3342.55	[NeuAc$_1$Hex$_1$HexNAc$_1$+Man$_3$GlcNAc$_2$]	19.9±1.8	26.9±2.8
N4	3707.26	3707.68	[NeuAc$_1$Hex$_2$HexNAc$_2$+Man$_3$GlcNAc$_2$]	26.3±1.1	29.9±2.2
N7	3998.28	3998.78	[NeuAc$_2$Hex$_2$HexNAc$_2$+Man$_3$GlcNAc$_2$]	33.6±1.9	19.2±2.0
N10	4363.30	4363.91	[NeuAc$_2$Hex$_3$HexNAc$_3$+Man$_3$GlcNAc$_2$]	9.4±1.0	8.5±1.3

[a]The asparagine residue harbouring the glycan is underlined.
[b]Quantitative analysis for relative abundance of species was obtained taking into account all the observed multicharged ions. The values are expressed as means (from three technical replicates) ± standard deviations.
Glycan species are indicated with the same nomenclature previously used for pHpt-P and pHpt-N [16].

Table 5. Glycopeptides in the P1 repertoire of Hpt tryptic digest from plasma of patients in disease remission.

Species	Observed Mass (Da)	Calculated Mass (Da)	Glycopeptide P1 (MVSHHNLTTGATLINEQWLLTTAK)[a]	Relative peak intensity[b]
M1	4227.02	4226.93	[NeuAc$_1$Hex$_1$HexNAc$_1$+Man$_3$GlcNAc$_2$]	25.8±1.5
M2	4300.51	4300.97	[Hex$_2$HexNAc$_2$+Man$_3$GlcNAc$_2$]	5.4±0.8
M3	4591.56	4592.06	[NeuAc$_1$Hex$_2$HexNAc$_2$+Man$_3$GlcNAc$_2$]	23.3±1.3
M4	4883.61	4883.16	[NeuAc$_2$Hex$_2$HexNAc$_2$+Man$_3$GlcNAc$_2$]	41.3±2.6
M6	5248.66	5248.29	[NeuAc$_2$Hex$_3$HexNAc$_3$+Man$_3$GlcNAc$_2$]	5.2±0.8

[a]The asparagine residue harbouring the glycan is underlined.
[b]Quantitative analysis for relative abundance of species was obtained taking into account all the observed multicharged ions. The values are expressed as means (from three technical replicates) ± standard deviations.
Glycan species are indicated with the same nomenclature previously used for pHpt-P and pHpt-N [16].

differences between circulating and skin Hpt. Here we report that the HPLC patterns of glycans from pHpt-P and sHpt-P were different from that of glycans from pHpt-N. In particular, some pHpt-P glycans, as compared with pHpt-N glycans displaying the same GU value, were present at lower level, or missing whereas other glycans were more abundant. The observed quantitative differences were enhanced in the pattern from skin Hpt. In this pattern we detected greater amounts of two major peaks, and material containing highly branched glycans. These data provide evidence on changes in glycan structures linked to Hpt of patients with psoriasis, and suggest that disease condition enhances glycan branching and Fuc content. In this frame, the finding that quantitatively rather than qualitatively changes increase in glycans of skin Hpt, as compared with those of pHpt-P, led us to argue that glycoforms of the former protein population might diffuse from epidermis to blood thus modifying the glycoform composition of circulating Hpt. Hpt with altered glycosylation pattern might be produced by keratinocytes [13] in the skin at the site of

inflammation and secreted into the plasma. Our hypothesis on changes and source of psoriasis-associated Hpt glycoforms was strengthened by results from experiments with lectins. In fact, besides the HPLC experiments, also the assays of Hpt reactivity to specific lectins indicate that pHpt-P contains more highly branched glycans and higher Fuc level than pHpt-N, and such a difference increases with skin Hpt. The MS analysis of skin Hpt confirmed that clear differences in the N-glycan repertoire do exist between psoriatic and healthy subjects. Actually P2 glycoforms with fucosylated tri- or tetra-antennary N-glycans (Lk, Lw, Lx, Ly, and Lz), that were not previously detected in pHpt-P and pHpt-N [16], were detected in sHpt-P. The finding of the glycoform Lw also in the glycan repertoire of sHpt-N suggests that its glycan structure is specifically associated with skin Hpt, and not with the disease. Moreover, the amount of fucosylated residues was higher in sHpt-P than in sHpt-N. Significant increases in Fuc levels and glycan branching in Hpt have been found to be associated with ovarian cancer [21,30], lung cancer [31], pancreatic cancer [23],

Table 6. Glycopeptides in the P2 repertoire of Hpt tryptic digest from plasma of patients in disease remission.

Species	Observed Mass (Da)	Calculated Mass (Da)	Glycopeptide P2 (NLFLNHSENATAK)[a]	Relative peak intensity[b]
L2	4993.82	4993.99	[NeuAc$_1$Hex$_2$HexNAc$_2$+Man$_3$GlcNAc$_2$] + [Hex$_2$HexNAc$_2$+Man$_3$GlcNAc$_2$]	3.5±0.7
L3	5067.96	5068.03	[Hex$_3$HexNAc$_3$+Man$_3$GlcNAc$_2$] + [Hex$_2$HexNAc$_2$+Man$_3$GlcNAc$_2$]	3.9±0.5
L4	5284.93	5285.08	[NeuAc$_1$Hex$_1$HexNAc$_1$+Man$_3$GlcNAc$_2$] + [NeuAc$_1$Hex$_2$HexNAc$_2$+Man$_3$GlcNAc$_2$]	8.4±1.0
L5	5358.97	5359.12	[Hex$_2$HexNAc$_2$+Man$_3$GlcNAc$_2$] + [NeuAc$_1$Hex$_3$HexNAc$_3$+Man$_3$GlcNAc$_2$]	8.8±0.7
Lw	5430.03	5431.14	[NeuAc$_1$Hex$_2$HexNAc$_2$+Man$_3$GlcNAc$_2$+Fuc$_1$] + [NeuAc$_1$Hex$_2$HexNAc$_2$+Man$_3$GlcNAc$_2$]	12.2±0.8
Lx	5504.09	5505.18	[NeuAc$_1$Hex$_3$HexNAc$_3$+Man$_3$GlcNAc$_2$+Fuc$_1$] + [Hex$_2$HexNAc$_2$+Man$_3$GlcNAc$_2$]	6.5±0.6
L6	5575.88	5576.18	[NeuAc$_2$Hex$_2$HexNAc$_2$+Man$_3$GlcNAc$_2$] + [NeuAc$_1$Hex$_2$HexNAc$_2$+Man$_3$GlcNAc$_2$]	7.6±0.2
L7	5650.08	5650.21	[NeuAc$_1$Hex$_2$HexNAc$_2$+Man$_3$GlcNAc$_2$] + [NeuAc$_1$Hex$_3$HexNAc$_3$+Man$_3$GlcNAc$_2$]	4.2±0.3
L9	5796.11	5796.27	[NeuAc$_1$Hex$_3$HexNAc$_3$+Man$_3$GlcNAc$_2$+Fuc$_1$] + [NeuAc$_1$Hex$_2$HexNAc$_2$+Man$_3$GlcNAc$_2$]	6.1±0.5
L10	5866.80	5867.27	[NeuAc$_2$Hex$_2$HexNAc$_2$+Man$_3$GlcNAc$_2$] + [NeuAc$_2$Hex$_2$HexNAc$_2$+Man$_3$GlcNAc$_2$]	9.4±0.5
L11	5941.74	5941.31	[NeuAc$_2$Hex$_3$HexNAc$_3$+Man$_3$GlcNAc$_2$] + [NeuAc$_1$Hex$_2$HexNAc$_2$+Man$_3$GlcNAc$_2$]	10.2±1.0
L14	6161.34	6161.40	[NeuAc$_1$Hex$_3$HexNAc$_3$+Man$_3$GlcNAc$_2$+Fuc$_1$] + [NeuAc$_1$Hex$_3$HexNAc$_3$+Man$_3$GlcNAc$_2$]	9.3±1.5
L16	6307.41	6307.46	[NeuAc$_1$Hex$_3$HexNAc$_3$+Man$_3$GlcNAc$_2$+Fuc$_1$] + [NeuAc$_1$Hex$_3$HexNAc$_3$+Man$_3$GlcNAc$_2$+Fuc$_1$]	4.8±0.5
L21	6672.36	6672.60	[NeuAc$_1$Hex$_4$HexNAc$_4$+Man$_3$GlcNAc$_2$+Fuc$_1$] + [NeuAc$_1$Hex$_3$HexNAc$_3$+Man$_3$GlcNAc$_2$+Fuc$_1$]	5.1±0.8

[a]The asparagine residue harbouring the glycan is underlined.
[b]Quantitative analysis for relative abundance of species was obtained taking into account all the observed multicharged ions. The values are expressed as means (from three technical replicates) ± standard deviations. Glycan species are indicated with the same nomenclature previously used for pHpt-P and pHpt-N [16].

Table 7. Glycopeptides in the P3 repertoire of Hpt tryptic digest from patients in disease remission.

Species	Observed Mass (Da)	Calculated Mass (Da)	Glycopeptide P3 (VVLHP<u>N</u>YSQVDIGLIK)[a]	Relative peak intensity[b]
N1	3051.15	3051.45	$[Hex_1HexNAc_1+Man_3GlcNAc_2]$	14.7 ± 1.6
N2	3342.20	3342.55	$[NeuAc_1Hex_1HexNAc_1+Man_3GlcNAc_2]$	27.0 ± 2.3
N4	3707.26	3707.68	$[NeuAc_1Hex_2HexNAc_2+Man_3GlcNAc_2]$	28.9 ± 1.6
N7	3998.28	3998.78	$[NeuAc_2Hex_2HexNAc_2+Man_3GlcNAc_2]$	22.1 ± 1.6
N10	4363.30	4363.91	$[NeuAc_2Hex_3HexNAc_3+Man_3GlcNAc_2]$	7.3 ± 0.9

[a]The asparagine residue harbouring the glycan is underlined.
[b]Quantitative analysis for relative abundance of species was obtained taking into account all the observed multicharged ions. The values are expressed as means (from three technical replicates) ± standard deviations.
Glycan species are indicated with the same nomenclature previously used for pHpt-P and pHpt-N [16].

colon cancer [32] and hepatocellular carcinoma [33]. A body of information is available about highly branched glycans and increased Fuc level in other acute phase glycoproteins in several diseases. Therefore, it is conceivable that such glycans might play a role during inflammation. On the other side, changes in normal glycan structures might be associated with loss of normal function. These two consequences of glycan modification might not be alternative, and both might occur in disease. As a matter of fact, glycans of Hpt are known to be engaged in binding haemoglobin [34], but pHpt-P was found displaying lower binding activity than pHpt-N [15].

Our results also show that Hpt from patients contains lower amount in sialic acid residues $\alpha 2,6$-linked to galactose than normal Hpt. This type of glycosidic bond is required for immunosuppression of lymphocytes B [35]. Conversely, in psoriasis, Hpt contains higher amount in sialic acid residues $\alpha 2,3$-linked to galactose than normal Hpt. This change in the type of glycosidic bond likely occurs on tri-antennary chains because $\alpha 2,3$-sialyltrasferase shows a much higher affinity than $\alpha 2,6$-sialyltransferase for arms growing on branched glycans [36]. Therefore increase in the amount of $\alpha 2,3$-linked sialic acid well agrees with increase in branching of Hpt from patients. These features are both known to promote the binding of glycoproteins to Galectin-3 [37,38]. Hpt glycoforms which binds Galectin-3 were actually detected [39,40]. Galectins is known to play regulatory roles in inflammation, immunity and cancer [41–44]. In particular, Galectin-3 plays a number of roles on lymphocytes T such as modulation of cell adhesion and induction of apoptosis [45], and secretion of IL-6 [46]. Galectin-3 is abundantly expressed also by keratinocytes and other epithelial cell, and was suggested to inhibit ERK and stimulate Akt [47]. It is therefore conceivable that Hpt, in the skin of patients with psoriasis, might participate to mechanisms regulating the immune response. Also Galectin-1 was found bound to Hpt glycoforms, that were present at increased levels in sera of patients with breast cancer [48]. These glycoforms, containing N-linked glycans with less terminal sialic acids and more arms than normal glycoforms, had different trafficking, as compared to non-bound glycoforms, after their endocytosis into macrophages [48]. Further analyses are needed to evaluate whether skin Hpt interacts with Galectin-1 or Galectin-3 in the skin, or targets cells involved in the autoimmune response in psoriasis, and to disclose molecular mechanisms in which the specific glycoforms we detected might participate (o fail to participate).

The analysis of glycan structures of pHpt-R showed the presence of a lower amount of fucosylated and highly branched structures, when compared with the previously reported N-glycan repertoire of pHpt-P [16]. Furthermore, the N-glycan repertoire of

pHpt-R revealed the presence of two glycoforms (namely Lw and Lx). Since these glycan structures were present in sHpt-P and sHpt-N, but not in pHpt-N and pHpt-P [16], this result suggests that the anti-TNF-α treatment might support Lw and Lx production in the anti-inflammatory response.

In conclusion, three glycoforms (Lk, Ly and Lx) were specifically detected only in psoriatic skin, and might be used as markers of the pathology, although it remains to clarify whether these glycoforms are specific for psoriasis or are also associated with skin diseases different from psoriasis. However, a more detailed analysis of changes in the glycan structures of Hpt from both plasma and skin is required to assess whether these changes are associated with disease progression and/or relapse.

Materials and Methods

Materials

Chemicals of the highest purity, bovine serum albumin (BSA), human Hpt (mixed phenotypes: Hpt 1-1, Hpt 1–2, Hpt 2–2), rabbit anti-human Hpt IgG, goat anti-rabbit horseradish peroxidase-conjugated (GAR-HRP) IgG, o-phenylenediamine (OPD), 2-aminobenzamide, N-glycosidase from *Flavobacterium meningosepticum* (PNGase F, E.C. 3.5.1.52), phenylmethanesulfonyl fluoride (PMSF), and Avidin conjugated with horseradish peroxidase (Avidin-HRP), were purchased from Sigma-Aldrich (St. Louis, MO, USA). Organic solvents were purchased from Romil (Cambridge, UK), and polystyrene 96-wells microtiter plates from Nunc (Roskilde, Denmark). 2-aminobenzamide-labelled glycans, and glucose oligomers for HPLC calibration were obtained from Ludger (Culham Science Center, Oxfordshire, UK). Discovery DPA-6S solid-phase extraction columns were purchased from Supelco (Bellefonte, PA, USA), and the TSK-gel Amide-80 column was from Tosoh Bioscience (Stuttgart, Germany). Sephacryl S-200, HiTrap Blue HP polypropylene column, and CNBr-activated Sepharose CL-4B of GE Healthcare (Uppsala, Sweden) were used. The Biotin-labelled lectins LTA, MAA, SNA, and ConA were purchased from EY laboratories (San Mateo, CA, USA).

Ethic statements

The present investigation conforms to the principles outlined in the declaration of Helsinki, and it was approved by the Ethics Committee of the University of Naples Federico II. Patients and healthy subjects were enrolled in the study after their informed consent.

Patients

Patients (n = 5) with psoriasis vulgaris and control subjects (n = 9), matched for age (range: 30-40 years) and cardiovascular risk factors were enrolled after their written informed consent. In particular patients with PASI>15 (disease of moderate entity), not taking anti-inflammatory drugs, were included in the study. Patients in disease remission (average PASI = 3.9±1.2; n = 7), after anti-TNF-α treatment with adalimumab for 16 weeks, were also enrolled. The treatment produced a decrease of PASI of 82.0±4.3%. No subject had any symptom or laboratory finding of kidney, liver or thyroid dysfunction, infection, diabetes, cardiovascular disease, or malignancy.

Hpt purification

Hpt was purified from pooled plasma (each sample contributing in the pool with equal volume) of patients with moderate psoriasis (n = 5), patients under remission (n = 7), or controls (n = 9) as previously reported [16]. Hpt was also isolated from pooled skin scales (2.2 g, each sample contributing in the pool with equal weight) of psoriatic patients (n = 6) or from cornified epidermal layer (4.4 g) of healthy subjects (n = 14) as follows. The scales were cut into small pieces, and ground in liquid nitrogen by a mortar. The powder was recovered in 10 volumes of ice-cold solution containing 0.5% (w/v) deoxycholate, 250 mM NaCl, 2 mM EDTA, and 1 mM PMSF in 50 mM Tris-HCl at pH 8.0. The resulting homogenate was centrifuged (30 min; 20,000 g; 0°C), and the supernatant was applied onto anti-Hpt IgG affinity column chromatography (1.5×5 cm) according to manufacturer's instructions. After sample loading, the column was extensively washed by 50 mM sodium phosphate at pH 7.4 to remove unbound material. Column-bound Hpt was eluted with 20 ml of 0.1 M glycine-HCl at pH 3.0 neutralized with 10 µl of 1 M Tris, and then subjected to SDS-PAGE analysis for purity check, as previously reported [7], before further experiments.

PNGase F digestion of Hpt and preparation of fluorescent glycans

PNGase F digestion was carried out on Hpt purified from plasma and skin of patients or plasma of controls (pHpt-P, sHpt-P, and pHpt-N respectively). Hpt samples (50 µg), in 45 µl of 10 mM sodium phosphate at pH 7.4, were mixed with 2 µl of 5% SDS and 3 µl of 1.6 M β-mercaptoethanol, and then heated at 100°C for 5 min. The solution was supplemented with 5 µl of 15% Triton X-100 and 10 µl of 500 units/ml PNGase F. Following incubation overnight at 37°C, the samples were heated at 100°C for 5 min, and then analyzed by SDS-PAGE to control effective deglycosylation. SDS-PAGE analysis of glycosylated and deglycosylated Hpt showed that the protein purification procedure and the β subunit deglycosylation were effective, and provided evidence that only such a subunit harbours.

N-linked glycans. The free oligosaccharides were labelled by conjugating the fluorescent probe 2-aminobenzamide to their reducing end through reductive amination reaction. The reagent mixture for fluorescent labelling was prepared by dissolving 2-aminobenzamide and sodium cyanoborohydride (0.24 and 0.68 M final concentration, respectively) in a solution containing 3.5 ml of DMSO and 2 ml of glacial acetic acid. An aliquot of 5 µl from this mixture was added to the solution containing glycans with deglycosylated Hpt. After 3 h at 70°C, the labelled oligosaccharides were purified using a Discovery DPA-6S column for solid-phase extraction. This column, equilibrated with 2 ml of CH_3CN, was loaded with the sample under gravity at room temperature, and washed with 4 ml of 99% CH_3CN, and then 0.5 ml of 97%

CH_3CN. The labelled glycans were eluted with 1 ml of 0.5 M formic acid. The glycan solution was dried under vacuum, and re-dissolved by 40 µl of 87.5 mM ammonium formate in CH_3CN. Aliquots of 20 µl were used for HPLC analysis.

HPLC

Purified labelled glycans were fractionated by normal phase HPLC using a TSK-gel Amide-80 column (4.6×250 mm) essentially according to He et al., 2006 [27]. The fluorescence detector was set at $\lambda_{EX} = 360$ nm and $\lambda_{EM} = 425$ nm. The chromatography was performed at 30°C. CH_3CN and 250 mM ammonium formate at pH 4.4 were used for the mobile phase. Elution was carried out at 0.4 ml/min, by simultaneous linear gradients of CH_3CN (65 to 35%) and formate (35 to 65%) in 75 min. A mixture of labelled glucose and glucose oligomers (1 to 20 glucose units, namely GU) was used for calibration. The GU ladder was used as a scale for elution of the glycans from Hpt. Standard labelled glycans ($NeuAc_2Hex_2HexNAc_2+Man_3GlcNAc_2$; $NeuAc_1Hex_2HexNAc_2+Man_3GlcNAc_2$; $NeuAc_2Hex_2HexNAc_2+Man_3GlcNAc_2+Fuc_1$; $NeuAc_3Hex_3HexNAc_3+Man_3GlcNAc_2$) served as chromatography controls. The database used in this work was GlycoBase (http://glycobase.ucd.ie).

Glycan assay by Lectins

Purified Hpt was analyzed for its reactivity to different lectins, by ELISA. Four lectins (LTA, MAA, SNA and ConA) were used to detect glycan specific structures. LTA actually binds Fuc α1,6- or α1,3-linked to N-acetylglucosamine in arm or dichitobiose respectively. MAA can detect glycans containing S α2,3-linked to G, whereas SNA binds S α2,6-linked to G. ConA is commonly used to detect the mannose core of N-linked complex glycans, and such a detection is recognized to be negatively correlated with the number of arms (i.e. substitutions of mannose residues) because more arms more steric hindrance shields the mannose core. Microtiter wells were incubated with different amount of Hpt in coating buffer (7 mM Na_2CO_3, 17 mM $NaHCO_3$, 1.5 mM NaN_3, pH 9.6) for 2 h at room temperature. In detail, 100 and 200 ng/well of Hpt were used for LTA binding, 20 and 40 ng/well for MAA, and 25 and 50 ng/well for ConA or SNA. Wells not coated with Hpt were used as control. Unbound Hpt was removed by three washes with 130 mM NaCl and 0.05% (w/v) Tween-20 in 20 mM Tris-HCl at pH 7.3, and further three washes with 500 mM NaCl in 20 mM Tris-HCl at pH 7.3. The possible sites of protein absorption were then blocked by incubation (1 h, 37°C) with 130 mM NaCl, 20 mM Tris-HCl, pH 7.4 (TBS) containing 2% (w/v) Tween 20. After extensive washing, as above, the wells were loaded with either biotin-labelled lectin (1 µM in binding buffer, that was TBS containing 1 mM $CaCl_2$, 1 mM $MgCl_2$, and 0.05% Tween-20), and incubated overnight at 4°C. After extensive washing, the wells were loaded with Avidin-HRP (1:12,000 dilution in binding buffer) and incubated for 1 h at 37°C. The lectin binding was detected by measuring at 492 nm the colour developed from OPD in the presence of hydrogen peroxide. Wells, coated with the same aliquots of Hpt used for lectin binding, were incubated with rabbit anti-Hpt IgG and GAR-HRP according to a published procedure [49], as controls of protein amounts used for assaying comparative reactivity of pHpt-N, pHpt-P, and sHpt-P for any lectin used.

Mass spectrometry

MS analysis of Hpt, purified from skin scales of patients, or from cornified epidermal layer of healthy donors, or plasma of patients in remission, was carried out. In particular, purified Hpt was analyzed by MS, after trypsin digestion and fragments fractionation by UPLC, as previously reported [16].

Decoding of sugar composition into structure of complex N-linked glycans

Three N-linked glycopeptides were expected to result from Hpt (accession number: P00738) digestion by trypsin, namely glycosylated fragments P1, P2, and P3 (containing the amino acid sequences 179–202, 203–215, and 236–251, respectively). The data on the carbohydrate composition were obtained as follows. The mass of a given glycopeptide was considered to be the sum of glycan mass plus peptide mass. Therefore, the masses of P1 (2679.39), P2 (1458.74), and P3 (1795.01) were subtracted from each glycopeptides mass, and the three resulting values were analyzed separately for their content in units of hexose (Hex, H for acronym), N-acetylhexosamine (HexNAc, HN for acronym), deoxyhexose (dHex), and N-acetylneuraminic acid (NeuAc, or S for acronym as already mentioned).

Composition decoding was done by a step-to-step building up procedure starting from the reducing end of the glycan, according to current information and nomenclature for structures of N-linked complex glycans. Thus, for example, the composition unit HexNAc2Hex3 was considered to account for dichitobiose (two residues of N-acetylglucosamine joined by a β1–4 glycosidic bond), followed by a mannose core (β1–4 linked mannose, which is 3-O- and 6-O-substituted with two α mannose), and named Man3-GlcNAc2. Further steps were substitutions of the mannose core with HexNAc, which is named antenna, or bisecting if linked to terminal or dichitobiose-linked mannose, respectively. Each arm was elongated with Hex (galactose). NeuAc, when present, was considered to be at the terminal end of the arm. Substitution of dichitobiose or arm(s) with Fuc accounted for dHex units. Where Fuc is linked (on dichitobiose or antenna) and whether NeuAc is

α2,3 or α2,6 linked to Hex was not assessed in this study. Thus, a mass compatible with, for example, Hex5HexNAc4NeuAc1 was expressed as (NeuAc1Hex2HexAc2+Man3GlcNAc2) in MS analysis or HN4H5S1 for brevity. Similarly, the carbohydrate composition from two glycans of P2, e.g. (NeuAc1Hex1HexNAc1+Man3GlcNAc2) together with (NeuAc1Hex2HexNAc2+Man3GlcNAc2) was also expressed as HN7H9S2.

Statistics

In the HPLC experiments, at least three separate preparations of Hpt glycans were used, and inter-assay CV for homologous peaks of pHpt-N, pHpt-P, or sHpt-P was calculated. In assays of lectin binding, experiments with three separate preparations of pHpt-N, pHpt-P, and sHpt-P were carried out, and five equal aliquots of each preparation were analyzed. In these assays, data from each experiment were expressed as means ± SEM. Statistical differences were determined using t-test or, where appropriate, one-way ANOVA, followed by Tukey's test for multiple comparisons (GraphPad Software Inc., San Diego, CA). Differences were considered statistically significant when the two-sided P value was less than 0.05.

Acknowledgments

The skilful technical assistance of Dr. C.R. Pugliese in ELISA experiments is acknowledged.

Author Contributions

Conceived and designed the experiments: BM LC PA MMC FA. Performed the experiments: LC BM MSS FDP AB. Analyzed the data: LC BM MSS MMC FDP PA. Contributed reagents/materials/analysis tools: LC MSS FDP FA NB MN PA. Wrote the paper: LC BM MSS PA.

References

1. Langlois MR, Delange JR (1996) Biological and clinical significance of haptoglobin polymorphism in humans. Clin Chem 4: 1589–1600.
2. Wada T, Oara H, Watanabe K, Kinoshita H, Yachi A (1970) Autoradiographic study on the site of uptake of the haptoglobin-hemoglobin complex. J Reticuloendothel Soc 8: 185–193.
3. Bowman BH, Kurosky A (1982) Haptoglobin: the evolutionary product of duplication, unequal crossing over, and point mutation. Adv Hum Genet 12: 189–261, 453–454.
4. Kalmovarin N, Friedrichs WE, O'Brien HV, Linehan LA, Bowman BH, et al. (1991) Extrahepatic expression of plasma protein genes during inflammation. Inflammation 15: 369–379.
5. de Kleijn DP, Smeets MB, Kemmeren PP, Lim SK, Van Middelaar BJ, et al. (2002) Acute-phase protein Haptoglobin is a cell migration factor involved in arterial restructuring. FASEB J 16: 1123–1125.
6. Spagnuolo MS, Cigliano L, D'Andrea LD, Pedone C, Abrescia P (2005) Assignment of the binding site for haptoglobin on apolipoprotein A-I. J Biol Chem 280: 1193–1198.
7. Cigliano L, Pugliese CR, Spagnuolo MS, Palumbo R, Abrescia P (2009) Haptoglobin binds the anti-atherogenic protein Apolipoprotein E: impairment of the apolipoprotein E stimulation on both the enzyme lecithin-cholesterol acyltransferase activity and cholesterol uptake by hepatocytes. FEBS J 276: 6158–6171.
8. Dobrotina NA, Ezhova GP (1977) Glycoprotein components of the skin under normal conditions and in several types of pathology (in Russian). Vopr Med Khim 23: 215–219.
9. Dobryszycka W (1997) Biological functions of haptoglobin-new pieces to an old puzzle. Eur J Clin Chem Clin Biochem 35: 647–654.
10. Lim SK, Kim H, Lim SK, bin Ali A, Lim YK, et al. (1998) Increased susceptibility in Hp knockout mice during acute hemolysis. Blood 92: 1870–1877.
11. Yang F, Haile DJ, Berger FG, Herbert DC, Van Beveren E, et al. (2003) Haptoglobin reduces lung injury associated with exposure to blood. Am J Physiol Lung Cell Mol Physiol 284: L402–L409.
12. D'Armiento J, Dalal SS, Chada K (1997) Tissue, temporal and inducible expression pattern of haptoglobin in mice. Gene 195: 19–27.
13. Wang H, Gao XH, Wang YK, Li P, He CD, et al. (2005) Expression of haptoglobin in human keratinocytes and Langerhans cells. Br J Dermatol 153: 894–899.
14. Xie Y, Li Y, Zhang Q, Stiller MJ, Wang CL, et al (2000) Haptoglobin is a natural regulator of Langerhans cell function in the skin. J Dermatol Sci 24: 25–37.
15. Cigliano L, Maresca B, Salvatore A, Nino M, Monfrecola G, et al. (2008) Haptoglobin from psoriatic patients exhibits decreased activity in binding haemoglobin and inhibiting lecithin-cholesterol acyltransferase activity. J Eur Acad Dermatol 22: 417–425.
16. Maresca B, Cigliano L, Corsaro MM, Pieretti G, Natale M, et al. (2010) Quantitative determination of haptoglobin glycoform variants in psoriasis. Biol Chem 391: 1429–1439.
17. Varki A, Freeze HH (2009) Essentials of Glycobiology. Cold Spring Harbor (NY). p 784.
18. Kurosky A, Barnett DR, Lee TH, Touchstone B, Hay RE, et al. (1980) Covalent structure of human haptoglobin: a serine protease homolog. Proc Natl Acad Sci USA 77: 3388–3392.
19. Thompson S, Dargan E, Griffiths ID, Kelly CA, Turner GA (1993) The glycosylation of haptoglobin in rheumatoid arthritis. Clin Chim Acta 220: 107–114.
20. Piva M, Moreno JI, Sharpe-Timms KL (2002) Glycosylation and over-expression of endometriosis-associated peritoneal haptoglobin. Glycoconj J 19: 33–41.
21. Thompson S, Dargan E, Turner GA (1992) Increased fucosylation and other carbohydrate changes in Haptoglobin in ovarian cancer. Cancer Lett 66: 43–48.
22. Fujimura T, Shinohara Y, Tissot B, Pang PC, Kurogochi M, et al. (2008) Glycosylation status of Haptoglobin in sera of patients with prostate cancer vs benign prostate disease or normal subject. Int J Cancer 122: 39–49.
23. Nakano M, Nakagawa T, Ito T, Kitada T, Hijioka T, et al. (2008) Site-specific analysis of N-glycans on haptoglobin in sera of patients with pancreatic cancer: a novel approach for the development of tumor markers. Int J Cancer 122: 2301–2309.
24. Ferens-Sieczkowska M, Midro A, Mierzejewska-Iwanowska B, Zwierz K, Katnik-Prastowska I (1999) Haptoglobin glycoforms in a case of carbohydrate-deficient glycoprotein syndrome. Glycoconj J 16: 573–577.

25. Mann AC, Record CO, Self CH, Turner GA (1994) Monosaccharide composition of haptoglobin in liver diseases and alcohol abuse: large changes in glycosylation associated with alcoholic liver disease. Clin Chim Acta 227: 69–78.

26. Spagnuolo MS, Cigliano L, Maresca B, Pugliese CR, Abrescia P (2011) Identification of plasma haptoglobin forms which loosely bind hemoglobin. Biol Chem 392: 371–376.

27. He Z, Aristoteli LP, Kritharides L, Garner B (2006) HPLC analysis of discrete haptoglobin isoform N-linked oligosaccharides following 2D-PAGE isolation. Biochem Bioph Res Com 343: 496–503.

28. Azuma Y, Murata M, Matsumoto K (2000) Alteration of sugar chains on alpha(1)-acid glycoprotein secreted following cytokine stimulation of HuH-7 cells in vitro. Clin Chim Acta 294: 93–103.

29. Ishibashi Y, Inouye Y, Okano T, Taniguchi A (2005) Regulation of sialyl-lewis x epitope expression by TNF-alpha and EGF in an airway carcinoma cell line, Glycoconj J 22: 53–62.

30. Saldova R, Royle L, Radcliffe CM, Abd Hamid UM, Evans R, et al. (2007) Ovarian cancer is associated with changes in glycosylation in both acute-phase proteins and IgG. Glycobiology 17: 1344–1356.

31. Kossowska B, Ferens-Sieczkowska M, Gancarz R, Passowicz-Muszyńska E, Jankowska R (2005) Fucosylation of serum glycoproteins in lung cancer patients. Clin Chem Lab Med 43: 361–369.

32. Park SY, Lee SH, Kawasaki N, Itoh S, Kang K, et al. (2011) α1-3/ fucosylation at Asn 241 of β-haptoglobin is a novel marker for colon cancer: A combinatorial approach for development of glycan biomarkers. Int J Cancer 130 (10): 2366–2376.

33. Comunale MA, Lowman M, Long RE, Krakover J, Philip R, et al. (2006) Proteomic analysis of serum associated fucosylated glycoproteins in the development of primary hepatocellular carcinoma. J Proteome Res 5: 308–315.

34. Kaartinen V, Mononen I (1998) Hemoglobin binding to deglycosylated haptoglobin. Biochem Biophys Acta 14: 345–352.

35. Hanasaki K, Powell LD, Varki A (1995) Binding of human plasma sialoglycoproteins by the B-cell specific lectin CD-22. Selective recognition of immunoglobulin M and haptoglobin. J Biol Chem 270: 7543–7550.

36. Nemansky M, Schiphorst WE, Van den Eijnden DH (1995) Branching and elongation with lactosaminoglycan chains of N-linked oligosaccharides result in a shift toward termination with alpha 2–>3-linked rather than with alpha 2–>6-linked sialic acid residues. FEBS Lett 363: 280–284.

37. Leffler H, Carlsson S, Hedlund M, Qian Y, Poirier F (2004) Introduction to galectins. Glycoconj J 19: 433–440.

38. Stowell SR, Arthur CM, Mehta P, Slanina KA, Blixt O, et al. (2008) Galectin-1, −2, and −3 exhibit differential recognition of sialylated glycans and blood group antigens. J Biol Chem 283: 10109–10123.

39. Cederfur C, Salomonsson E, Nilsson J, Halim A, Öberg CT, et al. (2008) Different affinity of galectins for human serum glycoproteins: Galectin-3 binds many protease inhibitors and acute phase proteins. Glycobiology 18: 384–394.

40. Bresalier RS, Bryd JC, Tessler D, Lebel J, Koomen J, et al. (2004) A circulating ligand for galectin-3 is a haptoglobin-related glycoprotein elevated in individuals with colon cancer. Gastroenterology 127: 741–748.

41. Almkvist J, Karlsson A (2004) Galectins as inflammatory mediators. Glycoconj J 19: 575–581.

42. Dumic J, Dabelic S, Flögel M (2006) Galectin-3: an open-ended story. Biochim Biophys Acta 1760: 616–635.

43. Ideo H, Seko A, Yamashita K (2005) Galectin-4 binds to sulfated glycosphin-golipids and carcinoembryonic antigen in patches on the cell surface of human colon adenocarcinoma cells. J Biol Chem 280: 4730–4737.

44. Rabinovich GA, Liu FT, Hirashima M, Anderson A (2007) An emerging role for galectins in tuning the immune response: lessons from experimental models of inflammatory disease, autoimmunity and cancer. Scand J Immunol 66: 143–158.

45. Chen IJ, Chen HL, Demetriou M (2007) Lateral compartmentalization of T cell receptor versus CD45 by Galectin-N-glycan binding and microfilaments coordinate basal and activation signalling. J Biol Chem 282: 35361–35372.

46. Fukaya Y, Shimada H, Wang LC, Zandi E, DeClerck YA (2008) Identification of galectin-3-binding protein as a factor secreted by tumor cells that stimulates interleukin-6 expression in the bone marrow stroma. J Biol Chem 283: 18573–18581.

47. Saegusa J, Hsu DK, Liu W, Kuwabara I, Kuwabara Y (2008) Galectin-3 protects keratinocytes from UVB-induced apoptosis by enhancing AKT activation and suppressing ERK activation. J Invest Dermatol 128: 2403–2411.

48. Carlsson MC, Cederfur C, Schaar V, Balog CIA, Lepur A (2011) Galectin-1-Binding Glycoforms of Haptoglobin with Altered Intracellular Trafficking, and Increase in Metastatic Breast Cancer Patients. PLoS ONE 6: e26560.

49. Cigliano L, Spagnuolo MS, Abrescia P (2003) Quantitative variations of the isoforms in haptoglobin 1–2 and 2–2 individual phenotypes. Arch Biochem Biophys 416: 227–237.

Skin-Targeted Inhibition of PPAR β/δ by Selective Antagonists to Treat PPAR β/δ – Mediated Psoriasis-Like Skin Disease *In Vivo*

Katrin Hack[1], Louise Reilly[1], Colin Palmer[1], Kevin D. Read[5], Suzanne Norval[5], Robert Kime[5], Kally Booth[4], John Foerster[2,3]*

1 Medical Research Institute, College of Medicine, Dentistry, and Nursing, University of Dundee, Dundee, Scotland, 2 Department of Dermatology, College of Medicine, Dentistry, and Nursing, University of Dundee, Dundee, Scotland, 3 Education Division, College of Medicine, Dentistry, and Nursing, University of Dundee, Dundee, Scotland, 4 Medical School Biological Resource Unit, College of Medicine, Dentistry, and Nursing, 5 Biological Chemistry and Drug Discovery Unit, College of Life Sciences, University of Dundee, Dundee, Scotland

Abstract

We have previously shown that peroxisome proliferator activating receptor ß/δ (PPAR β/δ is overexpressed in psoriasis. PPAR β/δ is not present in adult epidermis of mice. Targeted expression of PPAR β/δ and activation by a selective synthetic agonist is sufficient to induce an inflammatory skin disease resembling psoriasis. Several signalling pathways dysregulated in psoriasis are replicated in this model, suggesting that PPAR β/δ activation contributes to psoriasis pathogenesis. Thus, inhibition of PPAR β/δ might harbour therapeutical potential. Since PPAR β/δ has pleiotropic functions in metabolism, skin-targeted inhibition offer the potential of reducing systemic adverse effects. Here, we report that three selective PPAR β/δ antagonists, GSK0660, compound 3 h, and GSK3787 can be formulated for topical application to the skin and that their skin concentration can be accurately quantified using ultra-high performance liquid chromatography (UPLC)/mass spectrometry. These antagonists show efficacy in our transgenic mouse model in reducing psoriasis – like changes triggered by activation of PPAR β/δ. PPAR β/δ antagonists GSK0660 and compound 3 do not exhibit systemic drug accumulation after prolonged application to the skin, nor do they induce inflammatory or irritant changes. Significantly, the irreversible PPAR β/δ antagonist (GSK3787) retains efficacy when applied topically only three times per week which could be of practical clinical usefulness. Our data suggest that topical inhibition of PPAR β/δ to treat psoriasis may warrant further exploration.

Editor: Johanna M. Brandner, University Hospital Hamburg-Eppendorf, Germany

Funding: This work was supported by the Medical Research Council UK (MRC DPFS award ref. no. G900864). The funders had no role in study design, data collection and analysis, decision to publish, or preparation of the manuscript.

Competing Interests: The authors have read the journal's policy and have the following conflicts: JF and CP have filed patent for the use of PPAR delta antagonists in the treatment of inflammatory skin disease. Patent title: Psoriasis Mouse model, Inventors, Professor Colin Palmer, Dr. Nainamalai Sitheswaran, Dr. John Foerster, Patent application no. GB01814094; PCT/GB2009/050967, priority date: 1 August 2008. JF and CP are employed by the University of Dundee and are not paid consultants for any third party relevant to this patent or the present patent.

* E-mail: j.foerster@dundee.ac.uk

Introduction

One prominent clinical aspect of psoriasis is the clinical overlap with metabolic syndrome [1] and its association with increased body mass index [2], indicative of overlapping signalling pathways in psoriasis and other disorders of metabolism and chronic inflammation. Peroxisome proliferator activated receptors (PPAR) beta/delta (PPAR β/δ), one of three PPAR isoforms, is a key regulator of glucose and lipid metabolism [3]. In psoriasis plaques, PPAR β/δ is up-regulated, while the other PPAR isoforms, alpha, and gamma, are down-regulated [4]. PPARs act as regulators of transcription, being activated by lipid ligands to bind cognate cis-acting elements in target promoters upon heterodimerization with retinoic x receptor (RXR) alpha.

In the skin, PPAR β/δ is involved in keratinocyte differentiation and the wound response [5]. It is induced (among other factors) by TNFα [6,7], stimulates proliferation and blocks apoptosis in keratinocytes [8], and induces angiogenesis [9]. In psoriasis lesions,

PPAR β/δ exhibits prominent nuclear localisation in the upper spinous layer [4]. While not expressed in adult inter-follicular skin in mice, its activation in the spinous layer is sufficient to elicit an inflammatory skin disease harbouring major elements of psoriasis. Thus, PPAR β/δ transgenic mice exhibit psoriasis-typical immunological changes, STAT3 activation, as well as psoriasis – specific gene dysregulation [4]. Moreover, the gene dysregulation profile induced by epidermal PPAR β/δ activation significantly overlaps with that characteristic of psoriasis, including faithful replication of well recognised functional clusters such as the entire Il1-module or the cholesterol biosynthesis program, suggesting that the subsets of genes dysregulated by PPAR β/δ activation are also regulated by PPAR β/δ in psoriasis. Collectively, these observations indicate that PPAR β/δ signalling may contribute to the overlap between psoriasis and metabolic, as well as cardiovascular disease [10], since it is up-regulated in chronic inflammation and regulated by caloric intake [11,12]. TNFα, obesity, chronic inflammation, and dyslipidemia all may increase the penetrance of psoriasis by inducing PPAR β/δ expression and/or activation. Taken together, several lines of evidence suggest that PPAR β/δ activation contributes to psoriasis pathogenesis and that blocking its activation may reduce disease activity.

In light of the complex role PPAR β/δ exerts in metabolism, a topical ointment approach would seem an attractive targeting strategy in order to minimise the chance of adverse systemic effects. However, isoform – selective PPAR β/δ antagonists have only recently become available [13–16], and have not yet been evaluated for their activity in vivo via transdermal application. A major limitation in assessing the latter aspect is the availability of a validated and robust method to quantify the active compounds in the skin.

Here we describe the formulation of three selective PPAR β/δ antagonist into ointments and the quantification of their concentration in murine skin. In order to assess their ability to inhibit PPAR β/δ in vivo, we employ a previously described transgenic model [4]. In this model, human PPAR β/δ is constitutively expressed in sebaceous glands. Addition of the PPAR β/δ selective synthetic agonist GW501516 triggers both epidermis-specific transcriptional induction and ligand-mediated activation of PPAR β/δ, causing the development of an inflammatory skin disease with similarity to psoriasis. We show that PPAR β/δ antagonists in ointment formulation can deliver pharmacologically active concentrations in the skin, show very little systemic absorption, that prolonged administration does not cause inflammatory changes, and that they inhibit PPAR β/δ mediated psoriasis-like pathogenesis in vivo.

Results

Choice of PPAR β/δ selective antagonists

PPAR β/δ isoform-selective antagonists have only recently been described [13–17]. For the present work we used the first one to be reported, GSK0660, based on high antagonist potential, high affinity, its documented anti-inflammatory effect [18], and a reported lack of bioavailability upon systemic administration [17], thus potentially increasing its usefulness as a skin specific targeting compound. In order to ensure that any effects seen in vivo are indeed due to PPAR β/δ antagonism and not caused by off-target effects related to the chemical structure of GSK0660, we also included an alternative antagonist, compound 3 h [13], in a subset of experiments. Compound 3 h was chosen because of its low reported Ki (11 nM), high competitive antagonist potency, as well as lack of activity on other PPAR isoforms [13], The structure and key properties of these antagonists are shown in figure 1. An alternative reported compound appears to be less isoform selective [14]. Finally, one additional PPAR β/δ antagonist irreversibly inactivates the receptor by forming a covalent bond (GSK3787) [15,16]. This compound was included to address the feasibility of achieving treatment effects with less frequent dosing.

Ointment formulation

A variety of vehicles, additives, and procedures were screened as vehicles for the incorporation for GSK0660 and compound 3 h. These included drug incorporation into liquified vehicle at 70°C, pre-disolvement in DMSO, ethanol, isopropanol, polyethyene glycol 300, and olive oil followed by vehicle incorporation, as well as a variety of vehicles (liquid paraffin, Hydromol ointment, aqueous ointment BP). Drug solubility was assessed using a previously reported method relying on the absence of crystals detectable by polarised microscopy [19]. It was furthermore found that GSK0660 underwent a visible colour change from yellow to

green after storage at room temperature and light exposure, indicating instability possibly due to oxidation, which would be predicted given its chemical structure (fig. 1). Thus, alpha-tocopherol was added to GSK0660 preparations to increase stability. The optimised formulation of both compounds is detailed in Methods, was found to be devoid of drug crystals up to 2% (w/w) for both compounds, and exhibited functional activity, as described below.

Lack of systemic absorption of PPAR β/δ antagonists

Targeting PPAR β/δ is potentially fraught with serious adverse effects, since PPAR β/δ impacts on a wide variety of metabolic processes. We developed a robust quantitative assay based on ULPC/mass spectrometry to allow quantification of GSK0660, as well as compound 3 h, in skin samples subjected to ointment treatment (see Methods). Using this technology, we investigated whether the topical application of PPAR β/δ antagonists to murine skin results in significant systemic drug accumulation. As shown in figure 2, peak systemic concentration of GSK0660, measured 1 h after topical application, remained well below reported EC50 and IC50 values while that of compound 3 h was slightly above the in vitro determined EC50 value at this time point (figure 1). The total amount of detectable compound was less than 0.01% of total drug applied. By contrast, the PPAR β/δ agonist used in this study, GW501516, exhibited 100-fold higher systemic absorption, achieving peak serum concentrations of 400 nM at 1 h post application, despite being concentrated 10-fold less (0.1% ointment). This concentration of GW501516 is well within the range of its expected pharmacological activity [20]. Pharmacokinetic measurements of GSK0660 in blood for 24 h after drug application showed no evidence of drug accumulation. Systemic concentration remained well below the predictive active concentration, and amounted to less than 0.01% of total drug applied being detectable (figure 2b). By contrast, the same amount of drug was able to achieve a high local concentration in skin, exhibiting a half life of approximately. 90 min (figure 3). These data demonstrate that topical administration of PPAR β/δ antagonists achieves skin specific drug application, thereby avoiding potential hazards associated with PPAR β/δ inhibition in other organ systems. Of note, since application of even 10-fold less concentrated agonist ointment (GW501516) achieves significant serum levels, only partial biological activity would be expected for the antagonists in this in vivo model.

Lack of inflammatory changes in skin after topical application of PPAR β/δ antagonists

We next determined the local concentrations in skin at steady state after prolonged topical application. GSK0660 or compound 3 h were administered to shaven dorsal skin twice daily for seven days. Skin samples were then extracted and analysed by mass spectrometry for concentration determination as well as processed for histology. As shown in figure 4a, both compounds achieved high local concentrations even for the lower dose used (0.2%), suggesting active concentrations are present locally for prolonged time periods at the twice-daily dosing regimen, assuming a half life of approximately. 90 min (cf. fig. 2b). Under these conditions, neither antagonist produced notable epidermal hyperplasia (fig. 4, panels on right). The number of dermal nuclei counted per high power field was also unchanged as compared to vehicle-only treated skin (not shown). This was also found for the alternative PPAR β/δ antagonist GSK3787 (figure 4b). Infrequently, we noted apoptotic epidermal keratinocytes (inset, middle row of H&E sections). Since these cells were also found in transgenic PPAR β/δ mice treated with the agonist only (figure S1), the exact

	GSK0660[1]	Compound 3h[2]	GSK3787[3]
IC50 PPARβ/δ binding (nmol / l)	155	10	6.7
EC50 PPARβ/δ competitive antagonism (nmol / l)	300	11	100
Functional effects on inflammatory pathways	Blocks PPARβ/δ mediated IL1β and IL8 induction[4]		
Activity on other PPAR isoforms	Not active at 10 μM	Not active at 1 μM	Active on PPARγ at 1 μM[5]

[1]Shearer et al, Mol Endocrinol 2008, [2]Kasuga et al, Bioorg Medic Chem Lett 2010, [3]Shearer et al, J Medic Chem 2010, [4]Hall and McDonnel, Mol Endocrinol 2007, [5]Palkar et al, Mol Pharmacol 2010

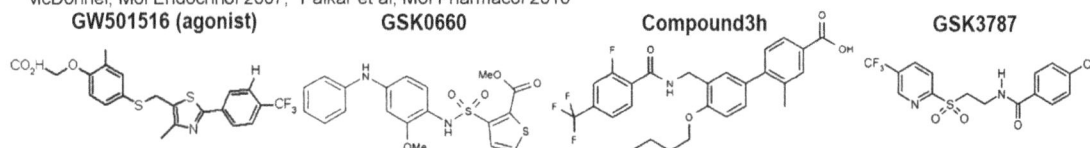

Figure 1. PPAR β/δ selective antagonists used in this study. Chemical structures and in vitro pharmacodynamic data shown are taken from the references listed. The structure of the PPAR β/δ selective agonist GW501516 used in this study is given for comparison.

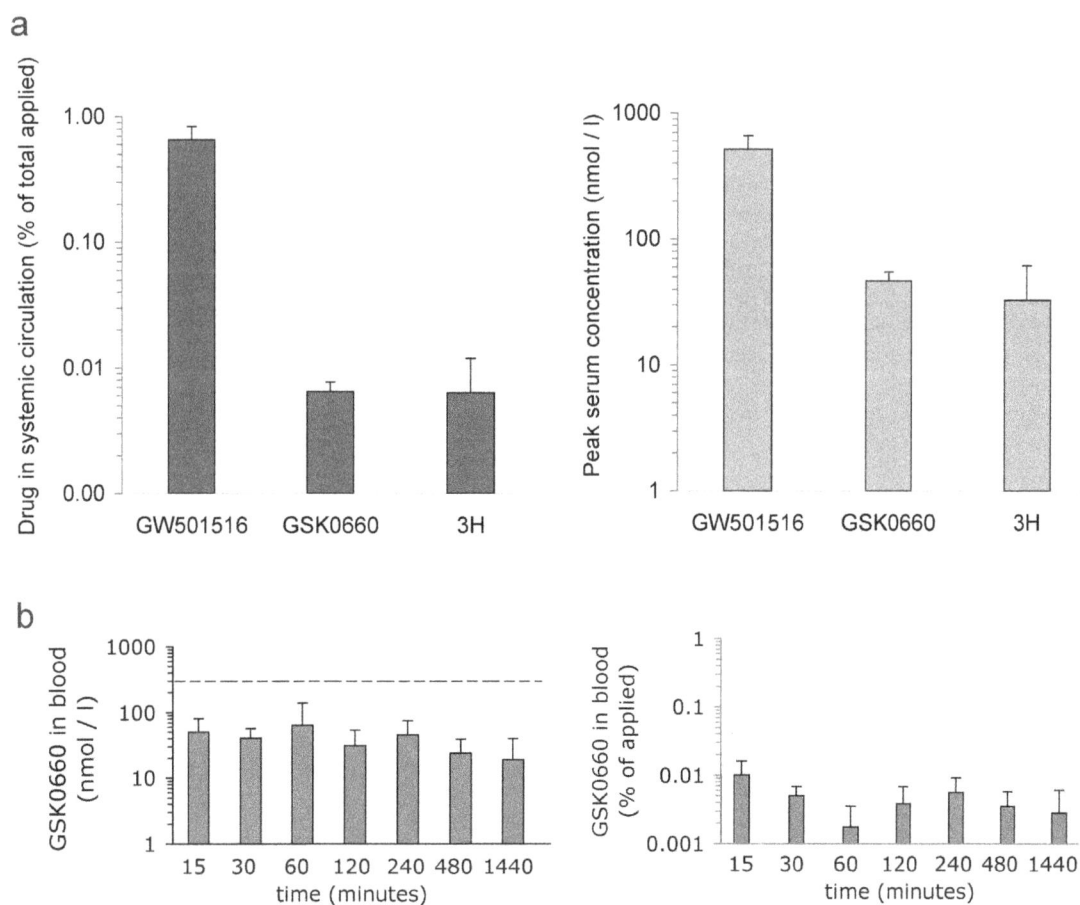

Figure 2. Low systemic absorption of topically applied PPAR β/δ antagonists. A. Peak blood concentrations of PPAR β/δ agonist GW501516, and antagonists GSK0660 and compound 3 h, respectively, at 1 h after topical application to skin. Left: Amount of drugs detected in systemic circulation, expressed as fraction of total amount applied, was calculated as detailed in methods. Right: Drug concentration expressed as molar concentration. **B**. GSK0660 concentration in blood (left) and total amount of circulating drug as fraction of amount applied (right, calculated as described in Methods) at the indicated time points after drug application. The horizontal dashed line represents the reported IC50 for GSK0660 acting on PPAR β/δ reported previously (300 nmol/L). Data shown represent average ± s.d. of n = 3 mice per data point.

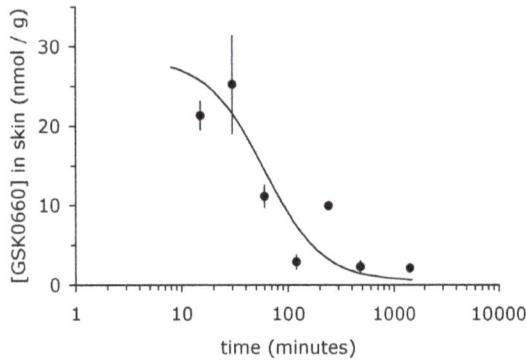

Figure 3. Half – life of GSK0660 after topical application to skin. 42 mg of GSK0660 ointment was applied to dorsal skin of C57Bl/6j wild type mice. Mice were sacrificed at the time after drug application indicated in the figure and drug concentration determined by mass spectrometry, as detailed in Methods. Data shown represent average ± s.d. of n = 3 mice per data point.

underlying cause is unclear but unlikely to underlie the treatment effect of the antagonist creams.

Inhibition of PPAR β/δ mediated psoriasis-like skin disease

We next sought to determine whether skin-targeted administration of PPAR β/δ antagonists would be sufficient to inhibit PPAR β/δ agonist-driven development of skin disease. In a first set of experiments we applied both the agonist (GW501516), as well as either antagonist (GSK0660 or compound 3 h) directly to the skin in order to minimise pharmacokinetic differences associated with alternative routes of drug administration (i.e. oral verus transdermal) between the competing chemicals. GW501516 was formulated as an 0.1% ointment and applied five times per week to shaved dorsal skin of PPAR β/δ transgenic mice. This agonist concentration was chosen because (a) lower agonist concentrations had resulted in significantly prolonged time-to-onset of the phenotype in pilot experiments and (b) higher concentrations

would not achieve a molar excess of the antagonist (using 1% ointments for the antagonists), which was important since the available *in vitro* data suggested that competitive antagonism at the receptor might not be achieved at equimolar concentrations of both agonist and antagonist. Antagonist-containing ointments were applied once per day six hours apart from the agonist in order to minimise any influence of penetration of both chemicals. Mice receiving GW501516 ointment and vehicle-only served as positive control, while mice receiving only vehicle ointments for both the antagonist as well as the agonist served as negative control. After 20 days of treatment, mice were sacrificed and skin samples processed for H&E histology. As shown in figure 5, both GSK0660 and compound 3 h, respectively, significantly attenuated the psoriasis – like epidermal hyperplasia induced by GW501516-mediated activation of PPAR β/δ. These data suggest that bioavailability of both antagonists is sufficient upon transdermal delivery to compete for agonist-binding to the receptor *in vivo*. MS-based quantification of GSK0660 in PPAR β/δ mice 12 h after the last cream application showed a concentration of 48 ± 18 ng/g of tissue while no GSK was detectable in blood (threshold of detection: 25 nmol/l), showing that penetration through inflamed skin with altered permeability properties does not lead to increased local or systemic accumulation of GSK0660 after prolonged administration.

We next investigated whether PPAR β/δ antagonists are able to reverse established skin disease. For this experiment, we administered the agonist GW501516 orally in order to allow twice – daily topical application of the antagonist without possible interference with drug penetration. We thus induced skin disease by oral dosing of GW501516, using a modified dosing regimen to that previously described as detailed in Methods. Three weeks after initiation of treatment with antagonists, mice were sacrificed and skin samples analysed. As shown in figure 6a, both PPAR β/δ antagonists were able to partially reverse epidermal hyperplasia. The influx of both CD4+ and CD8+ T lymphocyte subsets was also reduced, as shown in figure 6b. (cell numbers were too low to allow quantification of IL17+ T cell subsets). Finally, we also quantified expression levels of genes previously shown to be induced by PPAR β/δ in the skin [21], HB-EGF, a direct target gene of PPAR β/δ [22], as well as two strongly induced indirect

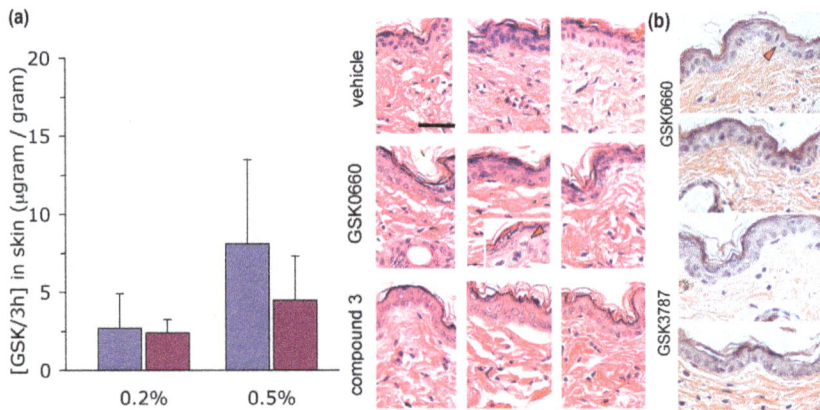

Figure 4. Absence of inflammatory changes induced by PPAR β/δ antagonists in skin after topical application. (a) C57Bl/6j wild type mice were treated with ointments containing GSK0660 or compound 3 h applied twice daily to shaved dorsal skin for one week. Mice were sacrificed 1 h after the last ointment application and skin tissue processed for H&E based histology and mass spectrometry, as described in Methods. Data shown represent average ± s.d. of n = 3 mice per data point (left) treated with GSK (blue columns) or compound 3 h (red). Representative histology sections of all treated mice are shown on right. The inset in the middle panel shows a section of GSK0660-treated epidermis showing apoptotic looking cells (marked by red arrow head). Horizontal bar represents 5 μm. (b) Representative H&E sections of C57Bl/6j wild type mice treated for one week with either GSK0660 (top) or GSK3787 (bottom). Red arrow-heads denoting apoptotic looking cells.

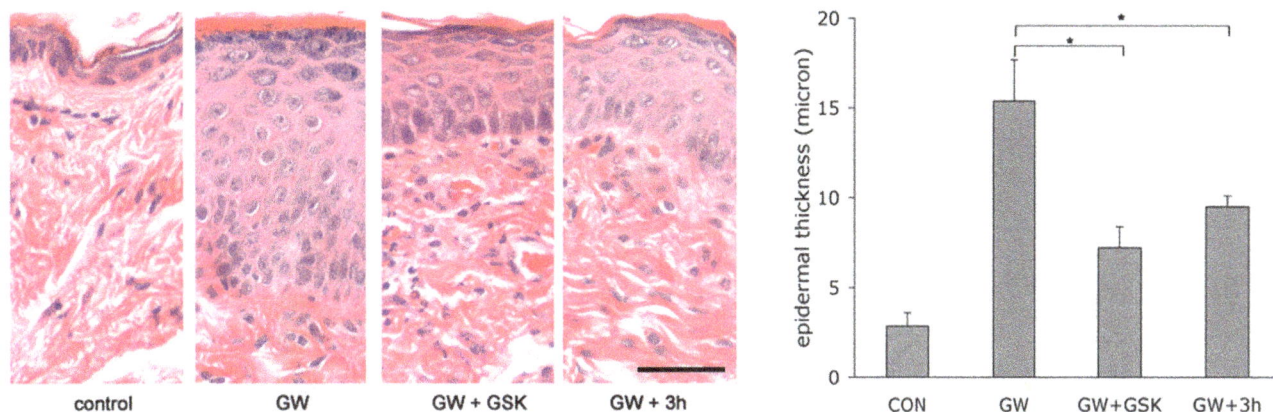

Figure 5. Prevention of epidermal hyperplasia by transdermal application of selective PPAR β/δ antagonists. Both the PPAR β/δ agonist GW501516 (GW) and the antagonists GSK0660 (GSK) or compound 3 h were applied topically to the skin, as described in the text. Left: representative H&E-stained paraffin-sections of dorsal skin from PPAR β/δ transgenic mice after treatment with ointments containing the indicated drugs for twenty days, as detailed in Methods. Horizontal bar represents 5 μm. Right: quantification of H&E-based epidermal thickness observed in n = 4 mice per group, performed as detailed in Methods. * p<0.05 in a two-sided independent t-test.

target genes, IL1b and LCE3e. As shown in figure 6c, the upregulation of both HB-EGF and LCE3e was partially reversed by treatment with both PPAR β/δ antagonists, although this reached statistical significance only for LCE3e. Reversal of IL1b expression was only observed using the ointment containing GSK0660. Taken together, these data show that transdermal application of PPAR β/δ antagonists is able to reverse established psoriasis-like disease in PPAR β/δ transgenic mice.

Reduced-frequency PPAR β/δ antagonist ointment application may be feasible using an irreversible antagonist

The half-life of GSK0660 suggested that the frequency of cream application might be limiting for treatment efficacy. Indeed, we found that twice-daily ointment application was required for full efficacy (fig. S1). The PPAR β/δ antagonist GSK3787 has been shown to covalently bind to its target, causing permanent inactivation. Since this property may be extremely useful clinically by offering the potential of less frequent cream application, we explored the effect of GSK3787 in the present system. As shown in figure 7, treatment using GSK3787-containing ointment proved to be as effective as GSK0660 in preventing epidermal hyperplasia (fig. 7a), as well as reducing the amount of dermal infiltrate (fig. 7b), even when applied only 3× per week. The tissue level of unmodified GSK3787 in lesional skin (GSK3787 covalently attached to PPAR β/δ could not be quantified) did not differ significantly between the three treatment groups 16 h after the final application and was found overall slightly higher than that found for GSK0660 (240 ± 116 nmol/g of tissue vs. 91 ± 21 nmol/g for GSK0660), indicating that slightly better tissue penetration may contribute to treatment efficacy. Efficacy of GSK3787 at reduced frequency application was further confirmed in an additional experiment testing the effect of twice-daily versus three times weekly application of GSK3787 (figure 8). This experiment also verified suppression of the PPAR β/δ target genes LCE3f, IL1-beta, and HBEGF (fig. 8b). Quantification of GSK3787 in blood of at the end of the experiment (16 h after last cream application) yielded a concentration of 445 ± 429 nmol/l, suggesting higher systemic resorption than GSK0660. Systemic resorption appears to be facilitated through inflamed skin since GSK3787 blood concentration in healthy mice

after 20 days of twice-daily treatment was only 50.2 ± 25.7 nmol/l (n = 3 mice). Nonetheless, the therapeutic activity is mediated locally, since efficacy was limited to the area of cream application (figure S2). Taken together, the data show that irreversible covalent modification of PPAR β/δ may harbour the potential of less frequent ointment application.

Discussion

The treatment of psoriasis with PPAR ligands has been previously explored. Since PPAR β/δ may act as a direct antagonist to PPARγ [23] and PPARγ activation inhibits STAT3 [24], activation of PPARγ unsurprisingly has a mild inhibitory effect on psoriasis [25,26]. Systemic administration of the PPARγ agonist pioglitazone to psoriasis arthritis patients, while showing signs of anti-arthritic acitivity, produced no marked reduction of PASI scores [27]. Topical application of the preferential PPARγ agonist rosiglitazone and the pan-PPAR agonist tetradecylthioacetic acid (TTA) showed no effect [26], possibly since concurrent activation of both PPARγ and PPARß/δ produces mutually neutralising effects (contrary to a commonly held view, rosiglitazone not only activates PPARγ but can also activate PPAR β/δ [18]). As selective PPAR β/δ antagonists have only recently become available, they have not yet been tested clinically. Our current data clearly support the notion that these may act anti-inflammatory in psoriasis.

The observation of therapeutic efficacy using three alternative PPAR β/δ antagonists confirms that the effects seen are mediated through PPAR β/δ binding rather than ideosyncratic off-target effects. The results presented here show some variation between the compounds tested (figs 5, 6b,c, 7, 8). GSK3787 stands out both by allowing reduced frequency application, as well as by exhbiting appreciable systemic concentrations in blood after prolonged application. More detailed kinetic follow-up studies on human skin will be required to ascertain whether this finding represents a potential safety issue. In this regard, the establishment of an ultra-sensitive quantitative mass-spectrometry assay will be instrumental.

The effect of the PPAR β/δ antagonists on the phenotype in the present model were only partial. Thus, it is possible that alternative PPAR β/δ antagonists would be more potent. More likely, however, limited efficacy is inherent to the model used here, as the

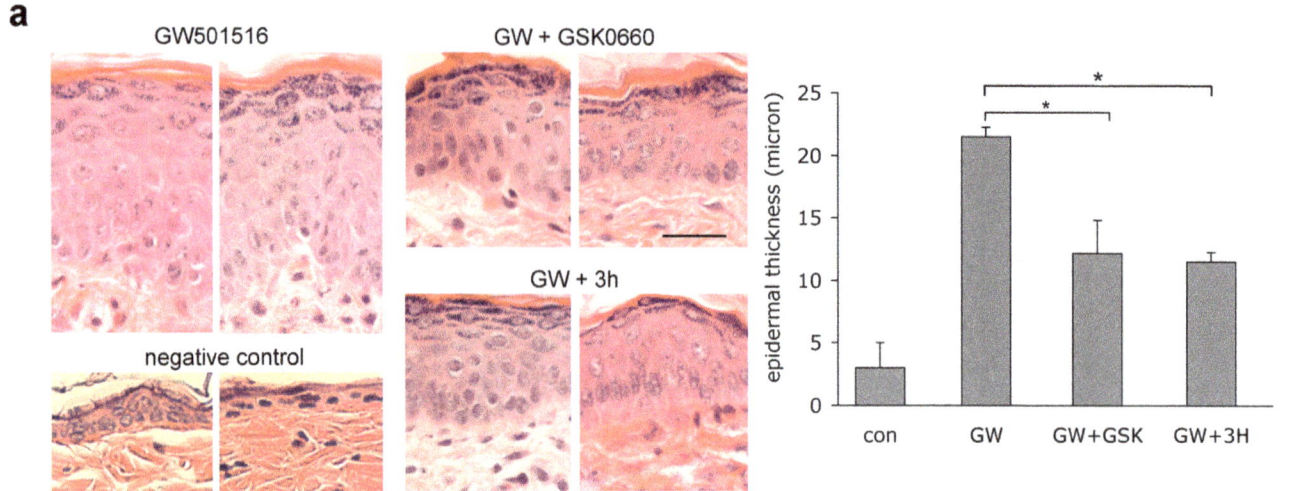

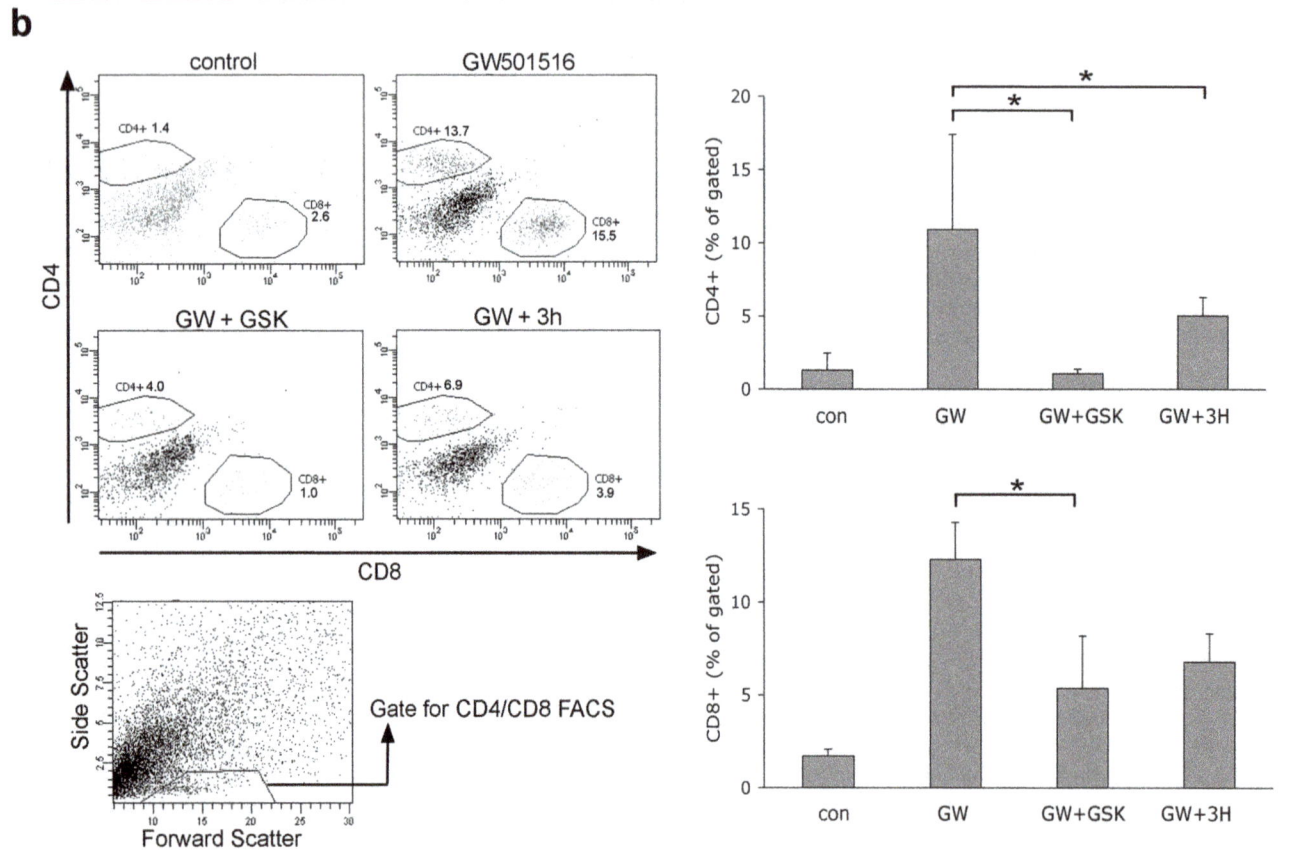

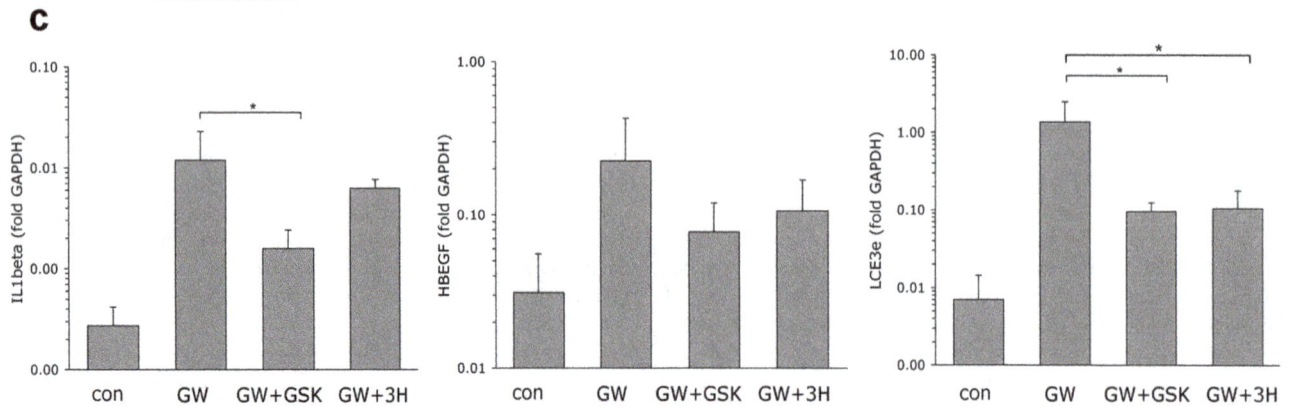

Figure 6. Reversal of psoriasis-like skin disease in PPAR β/δ mice by PPAR β/δ antagonists. Skin disease was induced by systemic oral administration of the PPAR β/δ agonist GW501516. (Control mice received standard chow). Subsequently, GW501516 dose was lowered to allow maintenance of phenotype as described in the text and mice were treated twice daily with either vehicle only (GW501516 group) or antagonist-containing ointments, as indicated. **A**. Reversal of epidermal hyperplasia, performed as described in the legend for figure 5. Horizontal bar represents 5 μm. **B**. Reduction of T cell infiltration. Skin samples of the treated skin regions were processed and stained for FACS analysis as described in Methods. Scatter plots shown on left show representative data, column diagrams on right show quantification of FACS data in n = 4 mice per group. The scatter plot shown at the bottom indicates the lympocyte gate used for quantification of CD4/CD8 cells, as previously described [21]. **C**. Quantification of target genes previously been shown to be induced in PPAR β/δ transgenic mice by qPCR, as detailed in Methods. * p<0.05 in a two-sided independent t-test.

antagonists need to compete with the highly potent agonist GW501516 to induce and maintain the phenotype. In psoriasis patients, such a synthetic ligand is not at work. Conversely, it is worth pointing out that oral administration of GW501516, currently explored to treat metabolic syndrome, may trigger

psoriasis flares in susceptible individuals. Endogenous activation of PPAR β/δ occurs by unknown natural ligand(s). A variety of arachidonic acid species have been described as candidates. One very plausible candidate would be 12-(R)-HETE which accumulates in psoriasis [28], particularly because the enzyme catalysing

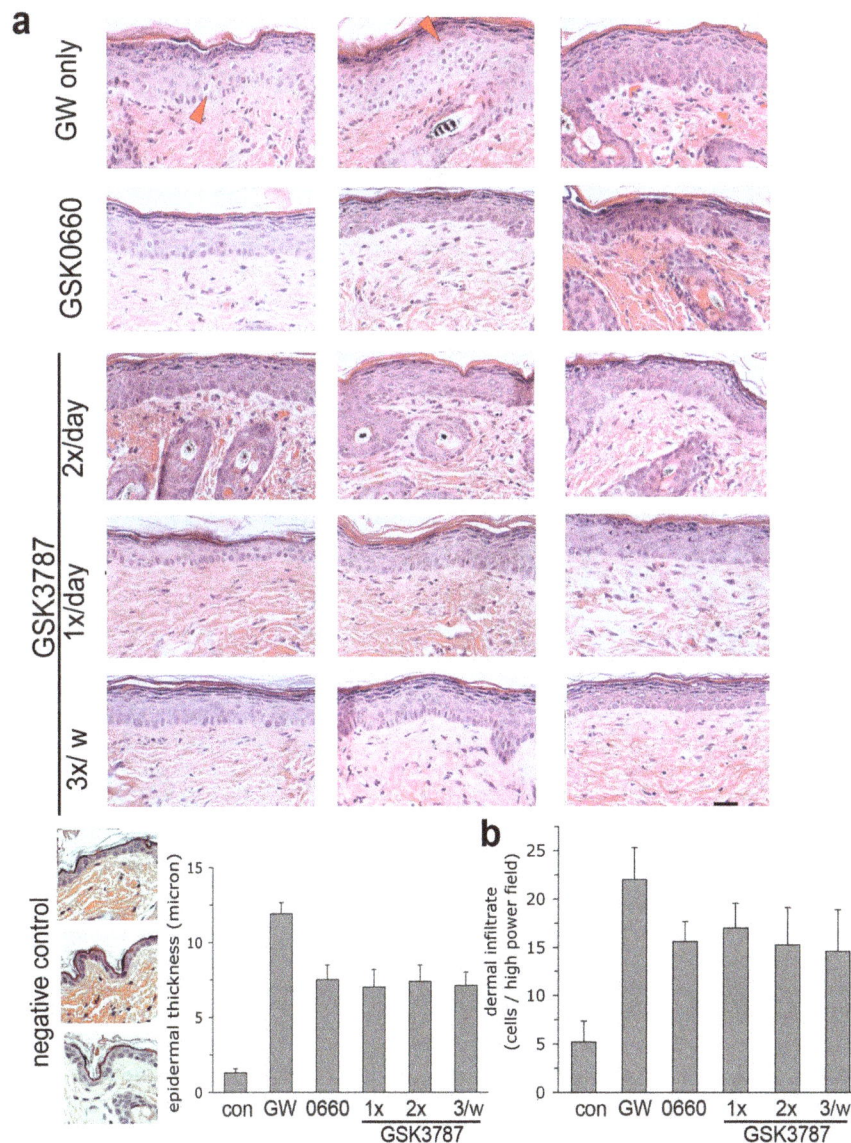

Figure 7. Control of PPAR β/δ – mediated skin disease using reduced-frequency application of ointment containing an irreversible PPAR β/δ antagonist. Skin disease in PPAR β/δ transgenic mice was induced by i.p. injection of the agonist GW501516. Additionally, mice were shaved on their abdomen and were treated with vehicle-ointment or ointment containing either GSK0660 (twice daily) or GSK3787 at the indicated frequencies. Red arrow denotes apoptotic cells noted in the GW-only treatment group. **A**. Top: Representative H&E stains from 3 different mice in each treatment group. Horizontal bar represents 5 μm. Bottom: Quantification of epidermal thickness (p<0.01 in all treatment groups vs. GW-only). **B**. Quantification of dermal infiltrate. Data shown represent average ± s.d. of five mice per group.

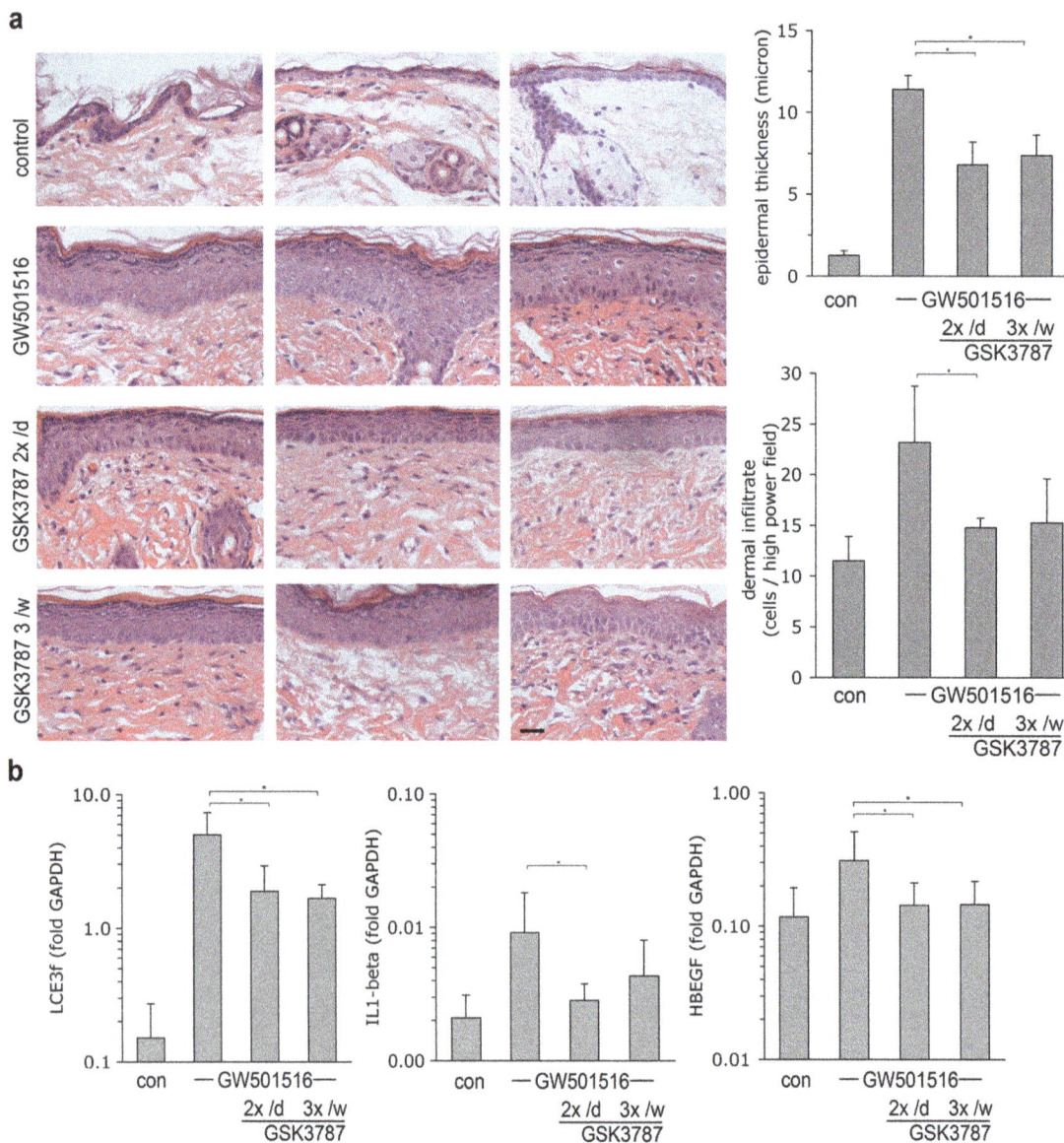

Figure 8. Effect of GSK3787 on PPAR β/δ -mediated skin disease applied either twice daily or three times per week (once per day). A. Left: representative H&E stains from 3 different mice in each treatment group. Horizontal bar represents 5 μm. Right: Quantification of epidermal thickness and dermal nuclei, respectively. * p<0.05 vs. GW501516 only. B. Q-PCR based quantification of the PPAR β/δ target genes LCE3f, IL1β, and HBEGF, as in figure 6c. Data shown represent n = 5 mice per treatment group.

its synthesis is also selectively upregulated in psoriasis [29] and localised to the same sub-epidermal compartment as PPAR β/δ, i.e. the upper spinous layer. However, none of the naturally occurring PPAR β/δ ligands display a potency comparable to GW501516. Thus, it is quite possible that application of PPAR β/δ antagonists may be more efficient than in the transgenic model.

The role of PPAR β/δ in inflammation is complex. On the one hand, some reports suggest anti-inflammatory properties (e.g. [30]). However, PPAR β/δ deficient mice do not show phenotypes indicative of increased systemic inflammatory signalling. On the other hand, PPAR β/δ activation causes pro-inflammatory changes in a number of systems, including IL-8 and IL1β induction in macrophages [18], and massive inflammatory changes in gastric tumors caused by PPAR β/δ activation, including IL1, IL6, IL24 induction [31]. When activated in the epidermis in mice, PPAR β/δ also induces the complete IL-1

signalling "module" characteristic of psoriasis including pro-inflammatory (IL1β, IL1F8), as well as anti-inflammatory cytokines (IL-1F5, IL1RA). As noted by others, the effect of PPAR β/δ activation on inflammatory signalling appears dependent on the tissue studied [31]. In the epidermis of PPAR β/δ transgenic mice harbouring PPAR β/δ expression comparable to human epidermis, it clearly acts pro-inflammatory [4]. The present data provide no evidence for pro-inflammatory changes caused by PPAR β/δ inhibition, confirming a previous report that failed to identify inflammatory changes upon systemic administration of a PPAR β/δ antagonist *in vivo* [16].

The obvious limitation of the current results is that only one model is being tested. Although widening the scope two alternative models may be desirable, this is hampered by practical considerations. The SCID model, hailed as "gold standard" by many authors, has inherent limitations: first, each data point generated requires a patient biopsy, second, biopsy grafts are fragile and not robust enough to withstand the mechanical challenge of cream treatment. It may be feasible to use this model at least to test systemic application of PPAR β/δ antagonist which is currently being explored. Of many other models propagated [32], all are limited in their modelling capacity of psoriasis for a variety of reasons [33], thereby curtailing predictive power for the human system. In addition to psoriasis-specific limitations, murine skin harbours penetration properties quite different from human skin. Thus, further preclinical testing will benefit most from porcine skin for penetration aspects as well as preclinical testing of GMP-grade products on human skin. Thus, short term ex-vivo treatment of human skin obtained from surgical procedures can be used not only to further investigate the presence of keratinocyte apoptosis but also the formation of PPAR β/δ -GSK3787 adducts.

In conclusion, we here show that selective antagonists of PPAR β/δ can be transdermally delivered, achieve pharmacologically active concentrations, and are able to antagonise PPAR β/δ activation by a potent agonist delivered orally, thereby partially inhibiting the development of an inflammatory skin disease. Their potential to treat psoriasis or related conditions remains to be explored in clinical trials.

Methods

Ointment formulation

All PPAR β/δ antagonists were custom-synthesized by AF-Chempharm (UK). Purity was >98% (GSK0660) and 97% (3 h, GSK3787), respectively, as determined by mass spectrometry. GSK0660 and alpha-tocopherol were predissolved in DMSO, vortexed, and incorporated into Hydromol ointment at room temperature using a melamin bowl and pestle to yield final concentrations of 0.5% (w/w) GSK0660, 0.1% (w/w) alpha-tocopherol, and 5% (w/w) of DMSO, respectively. Compound 3 h was pre-dissolved in DMSO, left at room temperature for 20 min at low agitation and then incorporated into Hydromol ointment using a melamin bowl to yield final concentrations of 0.5% (w/w) 3 h, and 5% (w/w) of DMSO, respectively. GSK3787 ointment (containing 0.5% final w/w) was made exactly analogous to GSK0660 ointment. Vehicle-only contro ointment was prepared exactly as GSK0660 ointment while omitting the chemical itself. Ointments were stored in airtight containers at 4°C in the dark and made fresh once a week.

Chow formulation

All GW chow concentrations were made up by diluting a stock of powdered chow containing 0.3% GW501516 with standard powdered chow and by mixing thoroughly. GW chow was stored at 4°C and replaced approx. once a week.

Evaluation of peak serum concentration and GSK0660 pharmacokinetics

GSK0660 ointment was prepared fresh, loaded into a 1 mL syringe allowing variability of drug to remain less than 10% CV, and 42 ± 5 mg of ointment was applied to 2×2 cm of shaven dorsal skin of C57Bl/6j wild type mice. Mice were sacrificed 1 h post application in a CO_2 chamber (for peak blood concentrations determined for GW501516, GSK0660, compound 3 h), or at the time points indicated in the figure. 50 μL of cardiac blood were diluted 1:2 (v:v) with milipore water and snap frozen immediately. Previously treated skin segments were shaved, tape-stripped three times to remove residual hair and non-absorbed ointment on the surface, and then snap frozen in liquid nitrogen. Frozen skin was ground and ten times the volume of methanol-water (1:1 v/v) was

added per weight unit of skin. A minimum of 20 mg of skin was used per each sample. Samples were homogenized with a Covaris S2 acoustic homogeniser. For both cardiac blood and skin homogenate, proteins were precipitated by adding 3 volumes of acetonitrile containing a suitable internal standard. All samples were then centrifuged for 10 minutes at 2800 rpm before transfer of 200 μL of supernatant into a 96 well plate and 100 μL of milliQ water added. Calibration curves were constructed in either untreated homogenised skin or blood to cover at least 3 orders of magnitude (1–2000 ng/mL) and extracted as for aforementioned study samples. All cardiac blood, skin samples and standards were then investigated by mass spectrometry as described below. For calculation of total blood volume, mice were weighed and an average blood volume of 7% (mL/g) of body mass was assumed.

UPLC and mass spectrometry

An Acquity ultra high performance liquid chromatography (UPLC) system; consisting of an autosampler, the Acquity UPLC Sample Manager with Sample Organiser, a pump, the Acquity UPLC Binary Solvent Manager, an in-built column oven, a UV detector, the Acquity UPLC Photo Diode Array) and a Quattro Premier XE triple quadrupole mass spectrometer (Waters, UK). Masslynx version.4.1 data acquisition software, was used in the determination of GW501516, GSK0660, compound 3 h, and GSK3787 in blood and skin samples using positive electrospray ionization. The analytical column was an Acquity UPLC BEH C18, 2.1 mm i.d. ×50 mm length, 1.7 μm particle size (Waters, UK). No guard column was used, but a vanguard 0.2°C.

Mobile phase A was Milli-Q reverse phase de-ionised water with formic acid (0.1%, v:v), mobile phase B was acetonitrile with formic acid (0.1%, v:v). Mobile phase was delivered at a flow rate of 0.6 mL/min. Gradient elution was used, for MRM analysis mobile phase B was set initially at 5% for 0.5 min was then linearly increased to 95% over 1.5 min and kept at 95% for 0.5 min. Finally mobile phase B was returned to 5% over 0.1 min and maintained at this composition for 0.4 min. Total run time 3 min.

The entire flow was introduced into the Mass spectrometer. The autosampler was set at 4°C and an injection voloume of 5 μL was used (partial loop). Mass spectrometric detection was performed using Multiple reaction monitoring (MRM) using the following mass transitions; GW501516, m/z 454.21 to 257.13, cone voltage (CV) 15 V, collision energy (CE) 33 V; GSK0660, m/z 419.20 to 214.17, (CV) 25 V, (CE) 19 V; compound 3 h, m/z 504.33 to 297.19 (CV) 5 V, (CE) 12 V. Desolvation temperature was 500°C and gas flow 1000 L/h (Nitrogen). An in-house proprietary internal standard was used for determination of all 3 analytes. Example chromatograms of standard, QC, Sample and blank are presented as well as the calibration curves are shown for GW501516 (Methods S1), as well as GSK0660 and compound 3H (Methods S2).

Animal handling and dosing

All animal studies reported here were subject to approval of Tayside Research Ethics Committee, and are conducted in accordance with UK Home Office procedures (project licence 60/3800, licence holder JF). Breeding of PPAR β/δ transgenic mice and genotyping were all carried out as described previously [21]. For the experiments described in Figure 6, GW501516 was administered at a concentration 0.002% in powder chow for 48 h to induce transgene induction, followed by reducing concentration to 0.0025%. Application of antagonists in ointment was initiated after 20 days and continued twice daily for 3 weeks. For the experiment described in figure 7, skin disease was induced by 3× weekly i.p. injection of 150 μg GW501516 dissolved in 5% DMSO/PEG 700 after additional pilot studies had shown that this route of dosing allowed for tighter control of GW501516 serum concentration, reduced inter-individual variability in phenotype severity, as well as reduced overall consumption of GW501516.

Quantification of acanthosis

Mice were sacrificed, skin samples obtained and processed for H&E based histology as described [21]. All samples were photographed at 200× magnification. Epidermal thickness was measured for all slides by a blinded observer at perpendicular angle to the basement membrane. The absence of variable planes of tissue sectioning as a confounder for apparent epidermal thickness was ruled out by verifying visible perpendicular insertion of hair follicles into the epidermis. For each sample, two measurements were taken in two separately photographed non-adjacent sections of the H&E stained skin sample.

Flow-cytometry of skin-resident T cells

Skin was shaven and cut to appr. 10–15 mm^3 size using scissors. Skin-associated fatty and vascular tissue was thoroughly scraped off using a scalpel to reduce the presence of T cells located in blood and lymphatic vessels. Samples were incubated for 30 min at 37°C in 2 mL of RPMI incl. Pen/Strep and 10% FCS, 2 mg/mL collagenase IV (Roche, cat-nr. 110880855001) and 1.1 U/mL dispase I (Roche, cat-nr. 04942086001) reconstituted in HBSS. Skin was washed with PBS over a cell strainer (100 μm Falcon) and subsequently incubated in 2 mL of RPMI incl. Pen/Strep and 10% FCS, 0.5 μg/mL PMA, 0.5 μg/mL ionomycin for 2 h. In modification of the previously described procedure 0.61 U/μL of DNase (Invitrogen) was to minimise clumping of cells. This addition significantly increased the yield of cells. The following antibodies served for surface staining: CD4-FITC (BD, Clone RM4-4), CD8-PerCP-Cy5.5b (BD, 53–6.7). Flow cytometry analysis was performed using a BD LSR Fortessa flow cytometer and data was analysed by means of BD FACSDiva Software.

Real-time PCR

Skin was processed by removing subcutaneous tissue and small skin pieces were snap frozen in liquid nitrogen. Frozen skin was ground and RNA was extracted using the NucleoSpin RNA/Protein kit from Macherey-Nagel. cDNA synthesis was done with the SuperScript Vilo cDNA synthesis kit from Invitrogen. Gene

expression levels were quantified using TaqMan-based real-time PCR using Assays-on-Demand kits obtained from Applied biosystems according to the manufacturer's instruction and quantification performed as calibrated to the internal housekeeping gene GAPDH (LCE3f: Mm02605425, Il1β: Mm01336189, Hb-EGF: Mm00439305).

Supporting Information

Methods S1 Example chromatograms of standard, QC, Sample and blank are presented as well as the calibration curves for GW501516.

Methods S2 Example chromatograms of standard, QC, Sample and blank are presented as well as the calibration curves for GSK0660 and compound 3H.

Figure S1 Inhibition of PPAR β/δ -induced skin disease by topically administered antagonist GSK0660 requires twice-daily application for full efficacy. PPAR β/δ – transgenic mice were dosed with GW501516 by 3× weekly i.p. injection of the agonist GW501516 as detailed in Methods, and additionally treated with vehicle or GSK0660 ointment once or twice daily. (a) Representative H&E stains for each of the treatment groups (left) as well as quantification of acanthosis, as well as dermal infiltrate (cells per high power field, right). Red arrow head denotes apoptotic cell observed in the GW-only group. (b) Expression analysis of target genes known to be induced in lesional skin of PPAR β/δ mice, as analysed by qPCR. Data shown represent average ± s.d. of four individual mice per group. * p<0.01 in a two-sided t-test.

Figure S2 Limited range of PPAR β/δ antagonist ointment activity. H&E samples from the abdominal area treated with antagonist ointment were obtained in the experiment described in figure 7 and images obtained from the treated area (left) as well as the edge of the treated area (right), indicating that the effect of treatment is limited to the area treated.

Author Contributions

Conceived and designed the experiments: JF KDR CP. Performed the experiments: KH LR SN RK KB. Analyzed the data: KH LR JF. Wrote the paper: JF.

References

1. Sommer DM, Jenisch S, Suchan M, Christophers E, Weichenthal M (2006) Increased prevalence of the metabolic syndrome in patients with moderate to severe psoriasis. Arch Dermatol Res 298: 321–328.

2. Naldi L, Chatenoud L, Linder D, Belloni Fortina A, Peserico A, et al. (2005) Cigarette smoking, body mass index, and stressful life events as risk factors for psoriasis: results from an Italian case-control study. J Invest Dermatol 125: 61–67.

3. de Lange P, Lombardi A, Silvestri E, Goglia F, Lanni A, et al. (2008) Peroxisome Proliferator-Activated Receptor Delta: A Conserved Director of Lipid Homeostasis through Regulation of the Oxidative Capacity of Muscle. PPAR Res 2008: 172676. 172676 p.

4. Romanowska M, Reilly L, Palmer CN, Gustafsson MC, Foerster J (2010) Activation of PPARbeta/delta causes a psoriasis-like skin disease in vivo. PLoS One 5: e9701.

5. Icre G, Wahli W, Michalik L (2006) Functions of the peroxisome proliferator-activated receptor (PPAR) alpha and beta in skin homeostasis, epithelial repair, and morphogenesis. J Investig Dermatol Symp Proc 11: 30–35.

6. Tan NS, Michalik L, Noy N, Yasmin R, Pacot C, et al. (2001) Critical roles of PPAR beta/delta in keratinocyte response to inflammation. Genes Dev 15: 3263–3277.

7. Di-Poi N, Michalik L, Tan NS, Desvergne B, Wahli W (2003) The anti-apoptotic role of PPARbeta contributes to efficient skin wound healing. J Steroid Biochem Mol Biol 85: 257–265.

8. Icre G, Wahli W, Michalik L (2006) Functions of the Peroxisome Proliferator-Activated Receptor (PPAR) alpha and beta in Skin Homeostasis, Epithelial Repair, and Morphogenesis. J Invest Dermatol 126 Suppl. pp 30–35.

9. Piqueras L, Reynolds AR, Hodivala-Dilke KM, Alfranca A, Redondo JM, et al. (2006) Activation of PPAR{beta}/{delta} Induces Endothelial Cell Proliferation and Angiogenesis. Arterioscler Thromb Vasc Biol.

10. Azfar RS, Gelfand JM (2008) Psoriasis and metabolic disease: epidemiology and pathophysiology. Curr Opin Rheumatol 20: 416–422.

11. Sun L, Ke Y, Zhu CY, Tang N, Tian DK, et al. (2008) Inflammatory reaction versus endogenous peroxisome proliferator-activated receptors expression, re-exploring secondary organ complications of spontaneously hypertensive rats. Chin Med J (Engl) 121: 2305–2311.

12. Masternak MM, Al-Regaiey KA, Del Rosario Lim MM, Bonkowski MS, Panici JA, et al. (2005) Caloric restriction results in decreased expression of peroxisome proliferator-activated receptor superfamily in muscle of normal and long-lived growth hormone receptor/binding protein knockout mice. J Gerontol A Biol Sci Med Sci 60: 1238–1245.

13. Kasuga J, Ishida S, Yamasaki D, Makishima M, Doi T, et al. (2009) Novel biphenylcarboxylic acid peroxisome proliferator-activated receptor (PPAR) delta selective antagonists. Bioorg Med Chem Lett 19: 6595–6599.

14. Zaveri NT, Sato BG, Jiang F, Calaoagan J, Laderoute KR, et al. (2009) A novel peroxisome proliferator-activated receptor delta antagonist, SR13904, has anti-proliferative activity in human cancer cells. Cancer Biol Ther 8: 1252–1261.

15. Shearer BG, Wiethe RW, Ashe A, Billin AN, Way JM, et al. (2010) Identification and characterization of 4-chloro-N-(2-{[5-trifluoromethyl)-2-pyridyl]sulfonyl}ethyl)benzamide (GSK3787), a selective and irreversible peroxisome proliferator-activated receptor delta (PPARdelta) antagonist. J Med Chem 53: 1857–1861.

16. Palkar PS, Borland MG, Naruhn S, Ferry CH, Lee C, et al. (2010) Cellular and pharmacological selectivity of the peroxisome proliferator-activated receptor-beta/delta antagonist GSK3787. Mol Pharmacol 78: 419–430.

17. Shearer BG, Steger DJ, Way JM, Stanley TB, Lobe DC, et al. (2008) Identification and characterization of a selective peroxisome proliferator-activated receptor beta/delta (NR1C2) antagonist. Mol Endocrinol 22: 523–529.

18. Hall JM, McDonnell DP (2007) The molecular mechanisms underlying the proinflammatory actions of thiazolidinediones in human macrophages. Mol Endocrinol 21: 1756–1768.

19. Kobayashi N, Saitoh I (1998) A method to measure the solubility of drugs in ointment bases. Chem Pharm Bull (Tokyo) 46: 1833–1835.

20. Oliver WR, Jr., Shenk JL, Snaith MR, Russell CS, Plunket KD, et al. (2001) A selective peroxisome proliferator-activated receptor delta agonist promotes reverse cholesterol transport. Proc Natl Acad Sci U S A 98: 5306–5311.

21. Romanowska M, Reilly L, Palmer CN, Gustafsson MC, Foerster J (2010) Activation of PPARbeta/delta causes a psoriasis-like skin disease in vivo. PLoS One 5: e9701.

22. Romanowska M, al Yacoub N, Seidel H, Donandt S, Gerken H, et al. (2008) PPARdelta enhances keratinocyte proliferation in psoriasis and induces heparin-binding EGF-like growth factor. J Invest Dermatol 128: 110–124.

23. Zuo X, Wu Y, Morris JS, Stimmel JB, Leesnitzer LM, et al. (2006) Oxidative metabolism of linoleic acid modulates PPAR-beta/delta suppression of PPAR-gamma activity. Oncogene 25: 1225–1241.

24. Wang LH, Yang XY, Zhang X, Huang J, Hou J, et al. (2004) Transcriptional inactivation of STAT3 by PPARgamma suppresses IL-6-responsive multiple myeloma cells. Immunity 20: 205–218.

25. Malhotra S, Bansal D, Shafiq N, Pandhi P, Kumar B (2005) Potential therapeutic role of peroxisome proliferator activated receptor-gamma agonists in psoriasis. Expert Opin Pharmacother 6: 1455–1461.

26. Kuenzli S, Saurat JH (2003) Effect of topical PPARbeta/delta and PPARgamma agonists on plaque psoriasis. A pilot study. Dermatology 206: 252–256.

27. Bongartz T, Coras B, Vogt T, Scholmerich J, Muller-Ladner U (2005) Treatment of active psoriatic arthritis with the PPARgamma ligand pioglitazone: an open-label pilot study. Rheumatology (Oxford) 44: 126–129.

28. Woollard PM (1986) Stereochemical difference between 12-hydroxy-5,8,10,14-eicosatetraenoic acid in platelets and psoriatic lesions. Biochem Biophys Res Commun 136: 169–176.

29. Romanowska M, Al Yacoub N, Seidel H, Donandt S, Gerken H, et al. (2007) PPARdelta Enhances Keratinocyte Proliferation in Psoriasis and Induces Heparin-Binding EGF-Like Growth Factor. J Invest Dermatol.

30. Barish GD, Atkins AR, Downes M, Olson P, Chong LW, et al. (2008) PPARdelta regulates multiple proinflammatory pathways to suppress atherosclerosis. Proc Natl Acad Sci U S A 105: 4271–4276.

31. Pollock CB, Rodriguez O, Martin PL, Albanese C, Li X, et al. (2010) Induction of metastatic gastric cancer by peroxisome proliferator-activated receptordelta activation. PPAR Res 2010: 571783. 571783 p.

32. Wagner EF, Schonthaler HB, Guinea-Viniegra J, Tschachler E (2010) Psoriasis: what we have learned from mouse models. Nat Rev Rheumatol 6: 704–714.

33. Sterry W, Foerster J (2005) What must a model display for proof as a model of psoriasis? In Ernst Schering Res Found Workshop. pp 193–201.

Novel Sulfated Polysaccharides Disrupt Cathelicidins, Inhibit RAGE and Reduce Cutaneous Inflammation in a Mouse Model of Rosacea

Jianxing Zhang[1,2], Xiaoyu Xu[1,2], Narayanam V. Rao[3], Brian Argyle[1], Lindsi McCoard[1], William J. Rusho[4], Thomas P. Kennedy[3]*, Glenn D. Prestwich[1,2], Gerald Krueger[5]

1 Center for Therapeutic Biomaterials, University of Utah, Salt Lake City, Utah, United States of America, **2** Department of Medicinal Chemistry, University of Utah, Salt Lake City, Utah, United States of America, **3** Department of Internal Medicine, University of Utah, Salt Lake City, Utah, United States of America, **4** Department of Pharmaceutics and Pharmaceutical Chemistry, University of Utah, Salt Lake City, Utah, United States of America, **5** Department of Dermatology, University of Utah, Salt Lake City, Utah, United States of America

Abstract

Background: Rosacea is a common disfiguring skin disease of primarily Caucasians characterized by central erythema of the face, with telangiectatic blood vessels, papules and pustules, and can produce skin thickening, especially on the nose of men, creating rhinophyma. Rosacea can also produce dry, itchy eyes with irritation of the lids, keratitis and corneal scarring. The cause of rosacea has been proposed as over-production of the cationic cathelicidin peptide LL-37.

Methodology/Principal Findings: We tested a new class of non-anticoagulant sulfated anionic polysaccharides, semi-synthetic glycosaminoglycan ethers (SAGEs) on key elements of the pathogenic pathway leading to rosacea. SAGEs were anti-inflammatory at ng/ml, including inhibition of polymorphonuclear leukocyte (PMN) proteases, P-selectin, and interaction of the receptor for advanced glycation end-products (RAGE) with four representative ligands. SAGEs bound LL-37 and inhibited interleukin-8 production induced by LL-37 in cultured human keratinocytes. When mixed with LL-37 before injection, SAGEs prevented the erythema and PMN infiltration produced by direct intradermal injection of LL-37 into mouse skin. Topical application of a 1% (w/w) SAGE emollient to overlying injected skin also reduced erythema and PMN infiltration from intradermal LL-37.

Conclusions: Anionic polysaccharides, exemplified by SAGEs, offer potential as novel mechanism-based therapies for rosacea and by extension other LL-37-mediated and RAGE-ligand driven skin diseases.

Editor: H. Peter Soyer, The University of Queensland, Australia

Funding: This work was supported by a Centers of Excellence grant from the State of Utah to GlycoMira LLC, by the Center for Therapeutic Biomaterials, also a Utah Center of Excellence, and by NIH grant R43 AR057281 to Drs. Zhang, Prestwich and Kennedy. The funders had no role in study design, data collection and analysis, decision to publish, or preparation of the manuscript.

Competing Interests: Drs. Zhang, Rao, Krueger, Prestwich and Kennedy hold equity in GlycoMira, LLC, which licensed the SAGE technology from the University of Utah. Drs. Xu and Zhang, Ms. McCoard, and Mr. Argyle were employed in part by GlycoMira.

* E-mail: tkennedy@mail.mcg.edu

Introduction

Rosacea is a common skin disease afflicting primarily Caucasian women of Celtic descent [1]. Rosacea is characterized by central erythema of the face, with telangiectatic blood vessels, papules and pustules, and can produce skin thickening, especially on the nose of men, creating rhinophyma. Rosacea can also produce dry, itchy eyes with irritation of the lids, keratitis and corneal scarring. The disease disfigures in a prominent manner, and its treatment is empiric and imperfect [2]. The pathogenesis of rosacea has been attributed in part to cutaneous over-production of a cationic anti-microbial cathelicidin peptide produced by the processing serine proteinase stratum corneum tryptic enzyme (SCTE) [3,4]. Cathelicidins are highly cationic 18 kDa propeptides cleaved to an active 37-amino acid C-terminal anti-microbial peptide, LL-37 [5]. LL-37 induces interleukin-8 (IL-8) secretion by human keratinocytes, and injection of LL-37 into mouse skin recapitulates rosacea-like redness and PMN infiltration [3].

We have evaluated a family of sulfated and metabolically stabilized anionic polysaccharide derivatives known as semi-synthetic glycosaminoglycan ethers (SAGEs). We hypothesized that a topically-applied SAGE could be used as a novel therapy for rosacea by binding and inhibiting the inflammatory activity of excess cationic cathelicidins. We show that one SAGE, GM-1111, exhibits substantial anti-inflammatory activities at nanomolar concentrations, including inhibition of cationic PMN proteases, inhibition of the leukocyte adhesion receptor P-selectin, and inhibition of the interaction of the receptor for advanced glycation end-products (RAGE) with its disparate ligands. GM-1111 avidly bound LL-37 and inhibited IL-8 secretion in cultured human keratinocytes in response to LL-37 stimulation. When mixed with LL-37, SAGEs prevented the extensive erythema and PMN infiltration produced by direct intradermal injection of LL-37 into mouse skin [3]. More importantly, topical application of a 1% SAGE-containing emollient to overlying injected skin also substantially reduced the redness and cutaneous PMN infiltration induced by intradermal LL-37. Herein, data demonstrate anionic polysaccharides, exemplified by SAGEs, as the first mechanism-based therapy that targets the proposed molecular etiology of rosacea.

Results

SAGEs are non-animal derived

Twenty-five novel derivatives of hyaluronic acid (HA) were obtained from GlycoMira, LLC (Salt Lake City, UT). HA is an immunoneutral skin polysaccharide consisting of long polymers (up to 10 MDa) of the disaccharide N-acetylglucosamine (GlcNAc) and glucuronic acid (GlcA) linked GlcNacβ1-3GlcAβ1-4 in repeating units along the chain. Fermentation-derived HA was chemically alkylated to provide lipophilicity to both improve dermal penetration and reduce hydrolysis by hyaluronidases [6]. Subsequently, the HA ethers were sulfated to adjust polyanionic charge and anti-inflammatory properties. The HA used as a starting material varied from 50 kDa to 950 kDa. A representative SAGE structure is illustrated in Figure 1. For further study, we chose the SAGE GM-1111, which was produced from 53 kDa HA and had a final molecular weight of 5.5 kDa.

SAGEs bind P-selectin, Mac-1 and RAGE, and potently inhibit P-selectin, cationic PMN proteases and interaction of RAGE with its disparate ligands

The SAGE GM-1111 showed anti-inflammatory activities similar to those of heparin or its low anticoagulant analogs [6] in a number of in vitro assays.

First, SAGEs avidly bound to the adhesion molecule P-selectin, the Mac-1 integrin (CD11b/CD18) and the multi-ligand immunoglobulin superfamily receptor RAGE. Figure 2 shows that GM-1111 exhibited saturable binding to P-selectin with a K_D of 0.0036 nM (Figure 2A), to Mac-1 with a K_D of 0.175 nM (Figure 2B) and to RAGE with a K_D of 1.69 nM (Figure 2C).

Second, SAGEs were potent inhibitors of the leukocyte adhesion molecule P-selectin [7]. Competitor-mediated displacement of U937 human monocytes, which loosely adhere to P-selectin through P-selectin glycoprotein ligand-1 (PSGL-1), was studied using fluorescent-labeled U937 cells. Table 1 and Figure 3A show that the SAGE GM-1111 inhibited U937 binding

to P-selectin with a 50% inhibitory concentration (IC_{50}) of 24.9 nM, approximately three times higher than the IC_{50} for heparin (7.9 nM).

Third, as sulfated polyanions, SAGEs were potent inhibitors of cationic PMN proteases such as human leukocyte elastase [8]. GM-1111 inhibited the PMN protease human leukocyte elastase (HLE) with an IC_{50} of 44.7 nM (Table 1 and Figure 3B), approximately three times higher than the IC_{50} of 14.9 nM for heparin. Thus, the polyanionic nature of the SAGEs would be expected to reduce protease activity in part via electrostatic interactions. However, this simplistic explanation cannot account for the totality of observed SAGE pharmacology in vitro [6].

Fourth, SAGEs were found to be potent inhibitors of RAGE binding with its ligands. The advanced glycation end-product (AGE) carboxymethyl lysine-modified (CML) protein is prominently formed in the dermis as the consequence of sun exposure, and avidly ligates and activates RAGE inflammatory signaling [9]. RAGE binds to immobilized CML-bovine serum albumin (BSA) in a dose dependent manner with an equilibrium constant (K_D) of 0.43 nM [10]. GM-1111 potently inhibited interaction of CML-BSA with RAGE (Table 1 and Figure 3C) with an with an IC_{50} of 413 nM. Once PMNs have migrated into inflamed dermis, PMN secretion of S100 calgranulins provides an active RAGE ligand to perpetuate inflammatory signaling even in the absence of AGE products [11]. RAGE engages immobilized S100b in a dose-dependent manner with a K_D of 0.45 nM [10]. GM-1111 inhibited ligation of RAGE by S100b calgranulin with an IC_{50} of 275 nM, compared with IC_{50} of 92 nM for heparin (Table 1 and Figure 3D) Likewise, RAGE binds immobilized human high mobility box group protein-1 (HMGB-1) in a saturable fashion with a K_D of 0.64 nM [10]. HMGB-1 is secreted by monocytes and macrophages as an inflammation producing cytokine and is also released by necrotic cells into areas of injury [12]. GM-1111 inhibited ligation of RAGE by HMGB-1 with an IC_{50} of 80 nM, compared with an IC_{50} of 2.9 nM for heparin (Table 1 and Figure 3E). Finally, using the Mac-1 (CD11b/CD18) as a counter-ligand, leukocytes ligate RAGE on vascular endothelium as an adhesion molecule essential for exiting the circulation into areas of inflammation [13]. GM-1111 inhibited binding of U937 monocytes to RAGE with an IC_{50} of 7.6 nM, essentially equipotent with the IC_{50} of 7.9 nM for heparin (Table 1 and Figure 3F). Taken together, these results suggest that SAGEs may provide considerable anti-inflammatory activity in diseases mediated by RAGE-ligand interactions, including the skin, where RAGE likely plays a role in lymphocyte-mediated diseases such as atopic dermatitis and psoriasis, as well as photo-ageing.

SAGEs are safe when administered topically

When applied to cultured human dermal fibroblasts (nHDF) and keratinocytes (nHEK), GM-1111 did not inhibit proliferation or cause cell toxicity up to 1 mg/ml (data not shown). Furthermore, none of the SAGEs tested, including GM-1111, elicited any skin reaction in Draize tests up to 10 mg/ml [14] (data not shown). SAGEs are also effectively non-anticoagulant in nature; for example, GM-1111 has approximately 0.2–0.5% of the anticoagulant activity of heparin. Specifically GM-1111 shows values of 0.3 IU/mg anti-Xa activity and 0.8 IU/mg anti-IIa activity, compared to 150–160 IU/mg each for unfractionated heparin. Unlike heparin, many highly charged polyanionic polymers are potent activators of Factor XII (Hagemann factor), secondarily producing kinins [15]. GM-1111 failed to show any activation of Factor XII [16], even at concentrations 10 to 100-fold higher than needed to achieve pharmacologic inhibition of

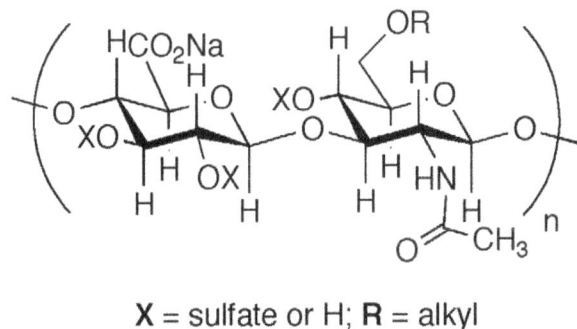

$X = $ sulfate or H; $R = $ alkyl

Figure 1. Structure of semi-synthetic glycosaminoglycan ethers (SAGEs). SAGEs can vary in molecular size, and in extent of alkylation and sulfation. GM-1111 is a low-molecular weight SAGE with an average molecular weight of 5.5 kDa.

A

Kd = 0.0036 nM

B

Kd = 0.175 nM

C

Kd = 1.69 nM

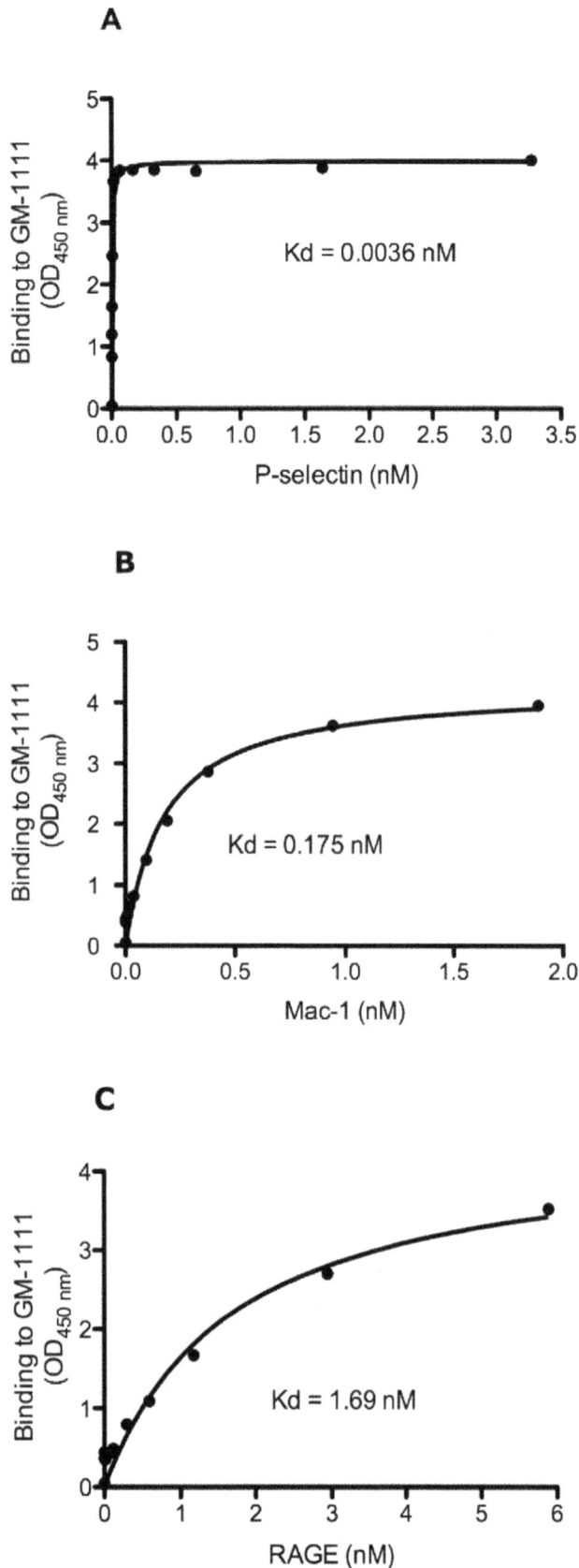

Figure 2. SAGEs bind to vascular adhesion proteins. GM-1111 was studied to determine binding affinity for P-selectin (**A**), Mac-1 (**B**), and RAGE (**C**). Binding affinity (K_D) values were 0.0036 nM for GM-1111

binding to P-selectin, 0.175 nM for GM-1111 binding to Mac-1 and 1.69 nM for GM-1111 binding to RAGE.

inflammation (data not shown). From these data, we concluded that the GM-1111 was safe as a lead candidate for topical use.

SAGEs bind to LL-37 and inhibit the biologic activity of LL-37 *in vitro*

The SAGE GM-1111 bound to the polycationic LL-37 peptide in a saturable fashion with a K_D of 0.225 nM (Figure 4A). This suggests that at least some of the biologic activity of the polyanionic SAGEs could be due to saturable, charge-neutralization of the cationic cathelicidins. However, electrostatic interactions alone cannot account for the overall SAGE pharmacology. For example, similar to previous reports [3], LL-37 induced IL-8 secretion by cultured human keratinocytes (Figure 4B). Addition of GM-1111 to the medium in addition to LL-37 significantly reduced IL-8 production by cultured keratinocytes (Figure 4B).

SAGEs inhibit cutaneous inflammation from intradermal LL-37

Intradermal injection of LL-37 into Balb/c mice at four 12-h intervals for 48 h produced cutaneous erythema with central necrosis (Figure 5A), prominent intradermal PMN infiltration (Figure 5C and Figure 6B), marked edema of the dermis (Figure 5C) and increased tissue myeloperoxidase (MPO) activity (Figure 5E). This reproduced the previously described murine model of rosacea [3]. The area of erythema (Figures 5B and F) and redness score (3.8 ± 0.5 after LL-37 alone vs 1.2 ± 0.5 after LL-37+ SAGE, $P<0.05$) were both significantly reduced by co-injection of GM-1111 with LL-37. Simultaneous injection of GM-1111 with LL-37 also significantly decreased PMN infiltration, as assessed by histology (Figure 5D) or tissue MPO activity (Figure 5E). Thus, at a minimum, charge neutralization of LL-37 by SAGE co-injection results in a significant reduction of LL-37-induced inflammation.

To determine if topical SAGEs were effective topical anti-inflammatory agents in this rosacea model, we formulated GM-1111 into a standard triglyceride-based transdermal emollient that contained 20% (w/w) water and 1% (w/w) of active drug. LL-37 was injected intradermally every 12 h for 48 h. In treated animals (n = 6 per group), the injected skin was gently rubbed with

Table 1. Anti-Inflammatory Activities of SAGE, GM-1111, *In Vitro*[1].

Anti-Inflammatory Assay	IC$_{50}$ values (nM)	
	SAGE*	Heparin*
[1]U937 monocyte binding to P-selectin	24.9	7.9
[2]Human Leukocyte Elastase activity	44.7	14.9
[3]CML-BSA binding to RAGE	412.7	27.8
[3]S100b binding to RAGE	274.5	92.1
[3]HMGB-1 binding to RAGE	79.6	2.9
[1]U937 monocyte binding to RAGE	7.6	7.9

*The average molecular mass of SAGE is 5.5 kDa and heparin is 14 kDa.
Details of [1]cell surface binding assays, [2] inhibition of human leukocyte elastase (HLE) and [3]solid phase binding assays are found in Methods. Detailed graphical plots of the results from cell surface binding assays, inhibition of HLE and solid phase binding assays are shown in Figure 3.

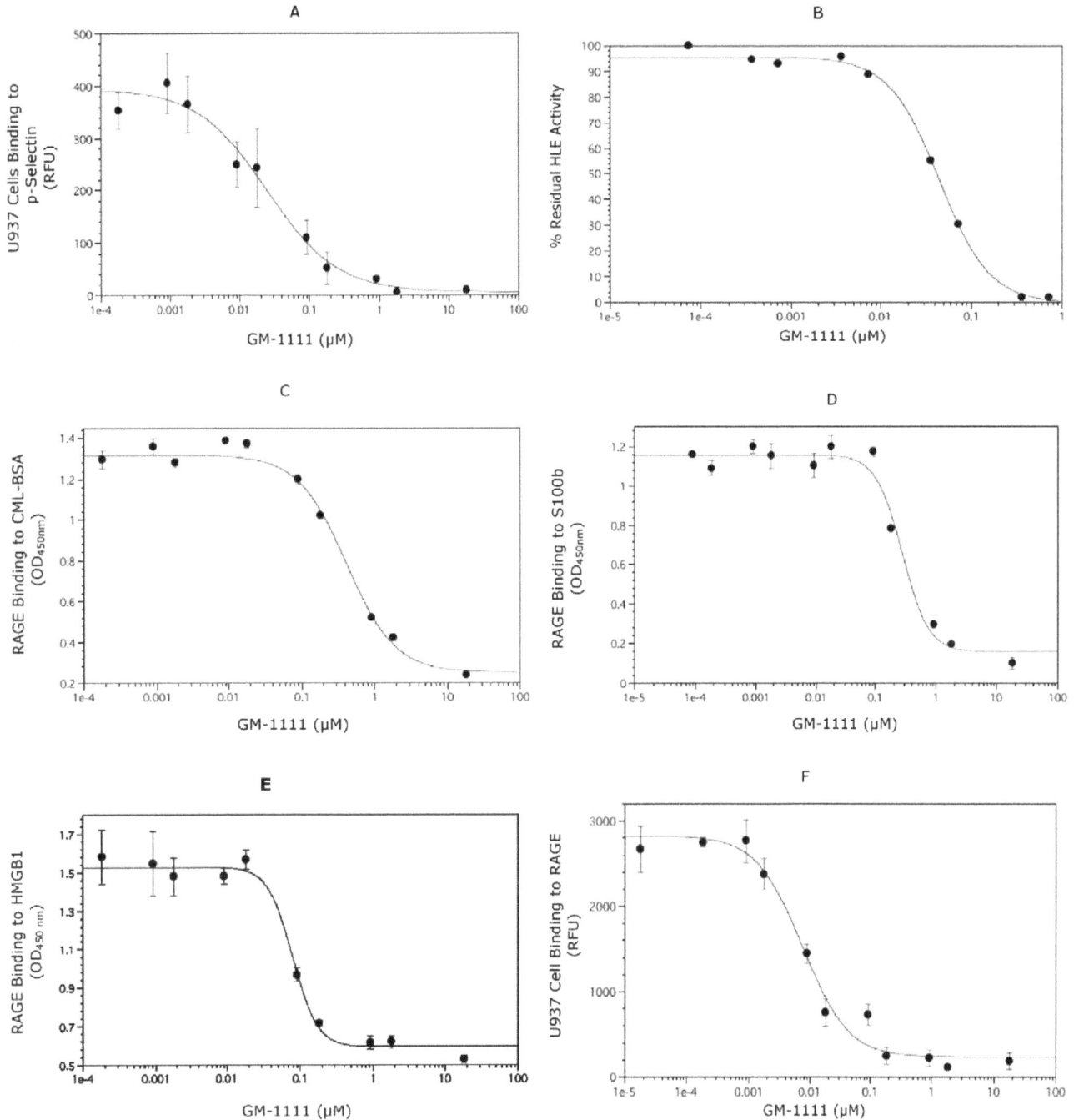

Figure 3. SAGEs inhibit P-selectin, HLE, interaction of RAGE with its many ligands. Data points in each figure represent the average value ± standard deviation of quadruplicate wells for each concentration of SAGE. **A.** SAGEs inhibit P-selectin. Inhibition of P-selectin glycoprotein ligand-1 (PSGL-1) binding to P-selectin by SAGEs was studied using calcein-labeled U937 cells incubated in microwells coated with P-selectin. After 1 h, plates were washed, bound cells were lysed with Triton-X100 buffer and bound cells were quantified using an excitation of 494 nm and emission of 517 nm. GM-1111 inhibits PSGL-1 attachment to P-selectin with an IC_{50} of 25 nM. **B.** SAGEs inhibit HLE. HLE (100 nM) was incubated with GM-1111 at 1–100 nm concentrations in 0.5 M HEPES buffer for 15 min. Following incubation, the elastase substrate, Suc-Ala-Ala-Val-pNA was added to the reaction mixture to the final concentration of 0.3 mM. Absorbance due to p-NA hydrolysis was monitored for 15 min at absorbance of 405 nm. GM-1111 inhibits HLE with an IC_{50} of 45 nM. **C–E.** SAGEs inhibit interaction of the AGE product CML-BSA, the calgranulin S100b and the alarmin HMGB-1 with RAGE. Microwell plates coated with CML-BSA (**C**), S100b calgranulin (**D**) or HMGB-1 (**E**) were incubated with RAGE-Fc chimera with or without GM-1111 for 2 h. Plates were washed, incubated with anti-RAGE antibody, incubated for 1 h, washed again four times and incubated with horse-radish peroxidase conjugated secondary for 1 h. A colorimetric reaction was produced by addition of tetramethyl benzidine chromogen (TMB) and quantified by absorbance at 450 nm. GM-1111 inhibits interaction of RAGE with CM-BSA, S100b and HMGB-1 with IC_{50} values of 413, 275 and 80 nM, respectively. **F.** SAGEs inhibit function of RAGE as an adhesion ligand. Inhibition of Mac-1-dependent ligation of RAGE by U937 cells was studied as in **A**, but using microwells coated with RAGE. GM-1111 inhibits Mac-1 attachment to RAGE with an IC_{50} of 7.6 nM.

A

B

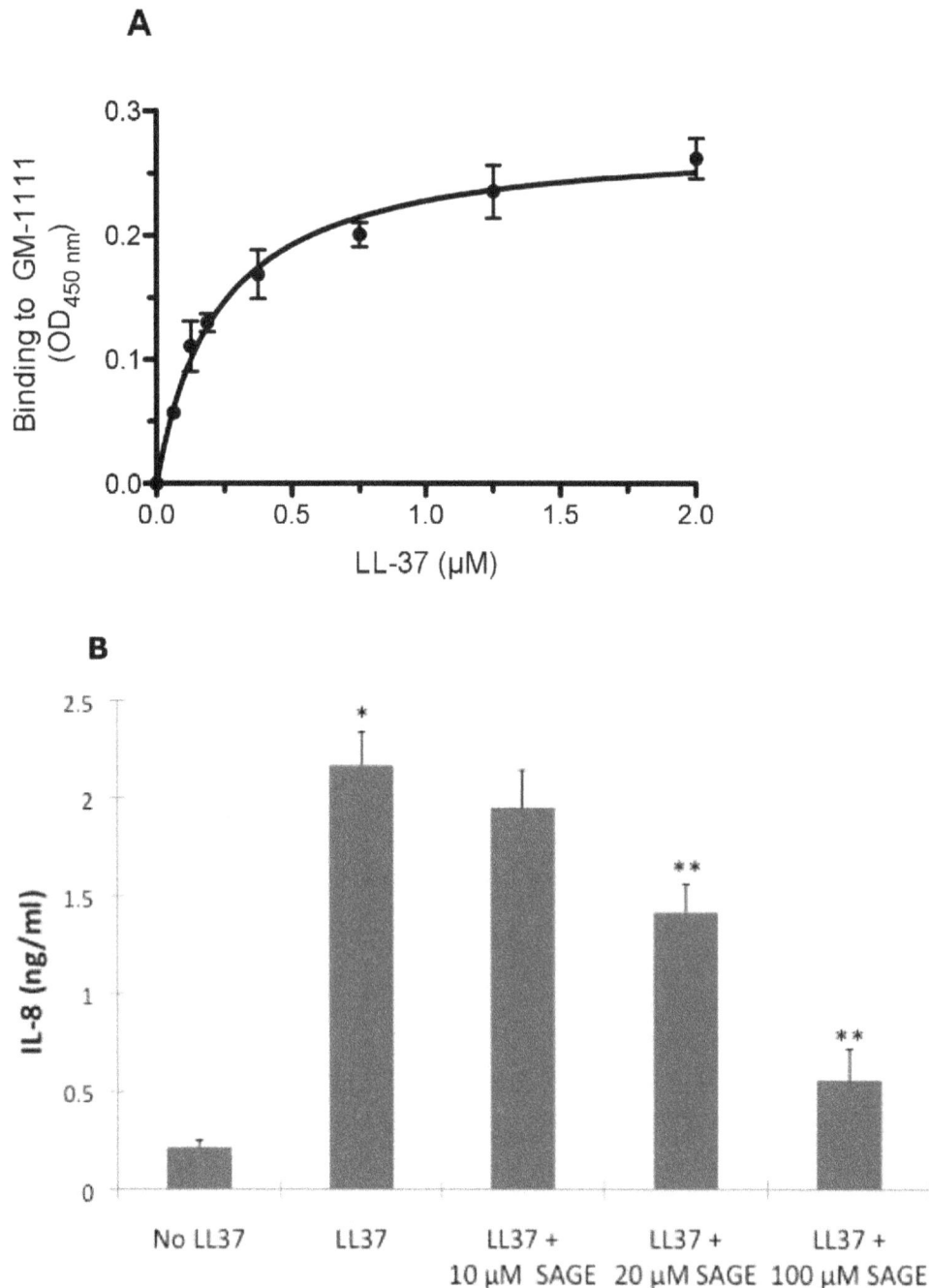

Figure 4. SAGE binds LL-37 and inhibits LL-37-induced interleukin-8 (IL-8) expression *in vitro.* **A.** SAGE binds LL-37. Microwell plates coated with GM-111 were incubated with LL-37 at 37°C for 2 h. Plates were washed, incubated with anti-LL-37 antibody, incubated for 1 h, washed again four times and incubated with peroxidase-conjugated secondary antibody for 1 h. A colorimetric reaction was produced by addition of TMB and quantified by absorbance at 450 nm. LL-37 binds to GM-1111 with a K_D of 0.225 nM. **B.** SAGE inhibits IL-8 production LL-37 stimulated keratinocytes. Human keratinocytes were grown to confluence and treated with 3.2 μM LL-37 or LL-37 and a 4x molar excess of GM-111101 for 6 h. Supernatants were collected and placed in a sterile 96-well plate. Production of IL-8 was determined by ELISA (R&D Systems, Minneapolis, MN) in accordance with manufacturer's instructions. Co-addition of GM-1111 significantly inhibited IL-8 release into medium. *P<0.01 as compared with negative control group without LL37; **P<0.05 as compared with positive control group without GM-111101 treatment.

drug-free emollient (control) or emollient with 1% GM-1111 either immediately (t = 0) or 12 h after the first injection (t = 12 h). Emollient application was repeated after each of the intradermal LL-37 injections. Cutaneous inflammation from intradermal LL-37 was significantly reduced by topical 1% GM-1111 (Figure 7). Whether applied at t = 0 or t = 12 h after the first LL-37 injection, topical GM-1111-containing emollient significantly reduced both

erythema (t = 0, Figure 7B; t = 12 h, Figure 7C) and PMN infiltration (t = 0, Figures 7E, 7G and Figure 6C; t = 12 h, Figures 7F, 7G and Figure 6D) relative to untreated or vehicle only animals receiving the intradermal LL-37. The SAGE-containing emollient also significantly reduced the area of erythema (Figure 7H) and redness score [4.6±0.3 after LL-37 alone, 1.6±0.4 after LL-37+ SAGE (t = 0) and 1.5±0.5 after LL-

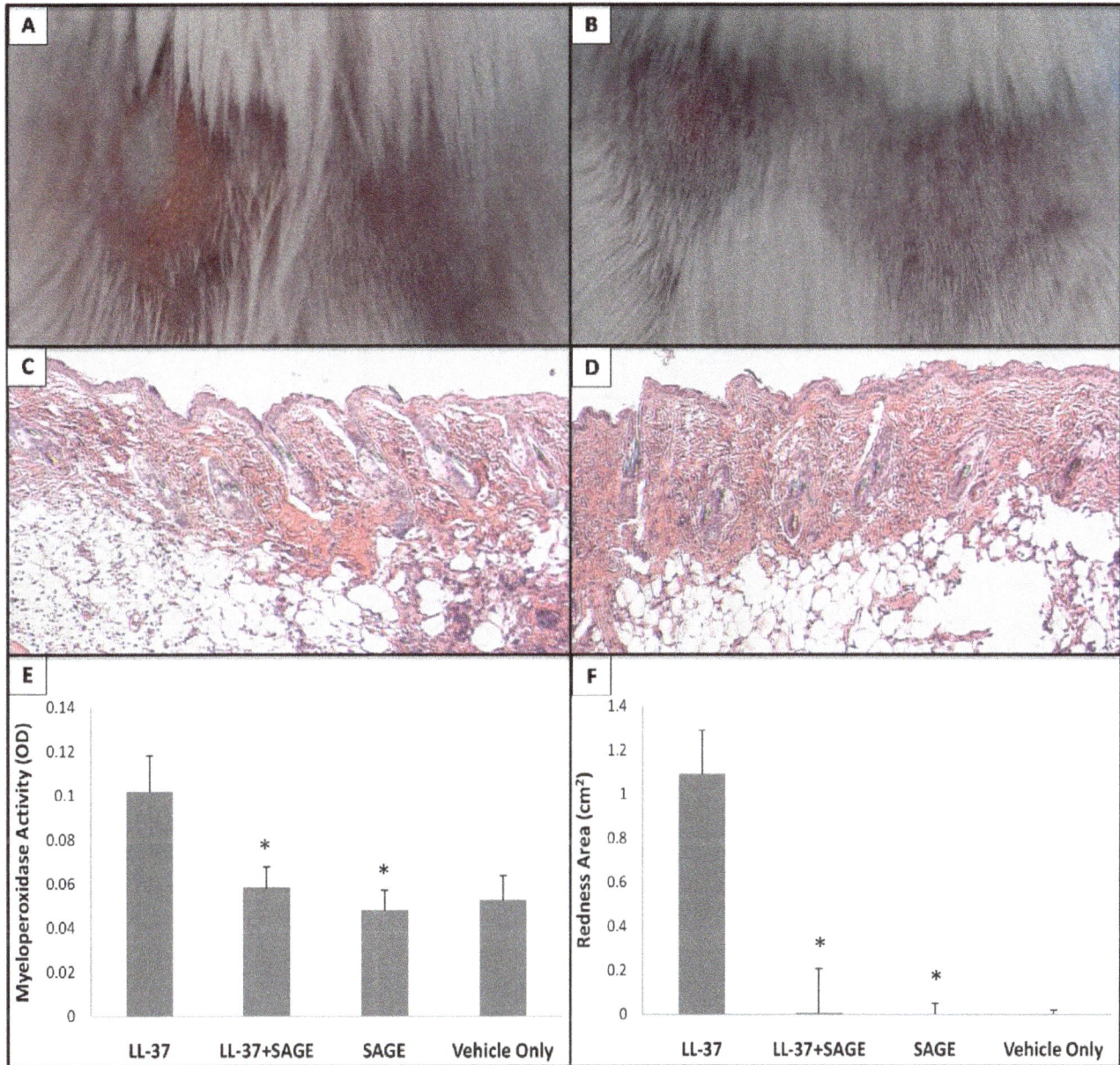

Figure 5. SAGE co-injection inhibits erythema and PMN infiltration from intradermal LL-37. Balb/c mice were shaved to expose an area of skin on the back. Twenty-four hours later, mice were intradermally injected with 40 µl of vehicle (nanopure water), LL-37 (at 320 µM concentration in water), SAGE GM-1111 (1,280 µM in water), or LL-37+ GM-1111 mix (peptide +4 molar equivalents of SAGE) placed intradermally into the shaved skin using a 31-gauge needle and 0.5 ml insulin syringe. Injections were repeated every 12 h thereafter. Forty-eight hours after the initial injection (four injections in total), animals were lightly anesthetized with isoflurane, the area of injected skin was photographed, the intensity of erythema was assessed as a redness score (from 1 to 5, with 5 as the most red), and the area of erythema was measured with micrometer calipers. The injected skin was then biopsied for histopathologic staining and to assess PMN infiltration through measurement of myeloperoxidase (MPO) activity. **A**. Gross picture of LL-37 injected skin region. **B**. Co-injection model of LL-37 and SAGE GM-1111. **C**. H&E-stained cross-sectional view of a LL-37 injected skin sample. **D**. H&E-stained cross-sectional view of a LL-37 mixed with GM-1111- injected skin region. **E**. MPO activity measurement of LL-37 injection with different treatments. **F**. Area of erythema from LL-37 injection. *P<0.05 vs intradermal LL-37 alone; n = 6 per group.

37+ SAGE (t = 12 h), both P<0.05 vs LL-37 alone], and decreased MPO activity within biopsies of injected skin (Figure 7G). Anti-inflammatory effects were not evident using 1% concentration of 53 kDa HA in the emollient in place of the GM-1111 (Figure 8). Confocal microscopy was performed on LL-37 injected mouse skin after topical treatment with emollient containing fluorescent-labeled GM-1111 (Figure 9). In the presence of irritant disruption of the stratum corneum, labeled SAGE penetrated deeply into inflamed skin. These results support

our hypothesis that the SAGE GM-1111, but not HA, would be topically effective in a pharmaceutically acceptable emollient to treat the cathelicidin peptide-mediated elements of inflammation associated with rosacea.

S100 calgranulins have not been previously reported as pathobiologically important in rosacea, but their presence would not be surprising in light of the prominent PMN infiltration in this disease [1]. Immunohistochemical staining for the RAGE ligand S100A8 confirmed the presence of this mouse homologue for the

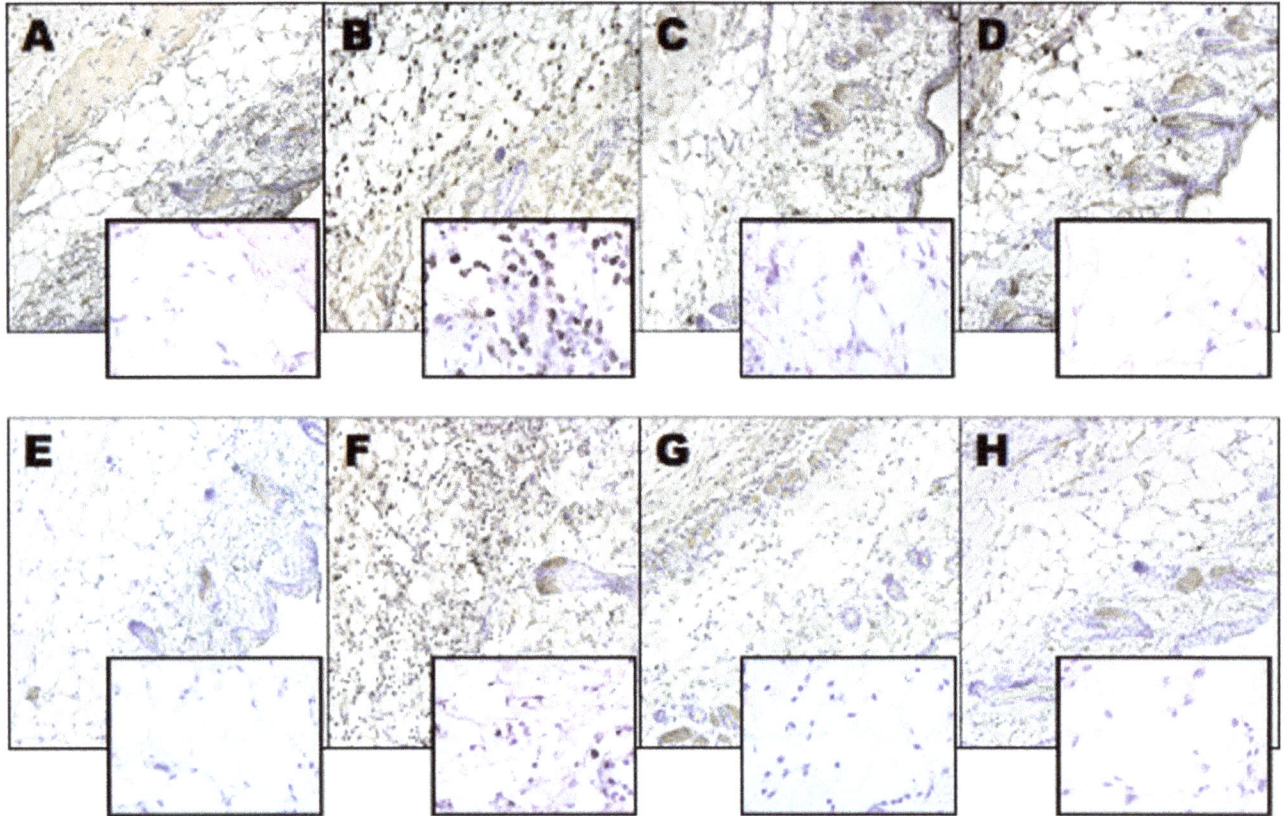

Figure 6. Topical SAGE reduces PMN infiltration and S100 calgranulin accumulation from intradermal LL-37. LL-37, PBS and LL-37 and SAGE-injected mouse skin was stained with antibody to mouse Gr-1 to examine neutrophil infiltration, and also for S100A8 calgranulin, the major RAGE-binding calgranulin present in murine PMNs [17] as described in Methods. **A.** Staining of normal control skin for the PMN antigen Gr-1. **B.** Staining of LL-37 injected skin for the PMN antigen Gr-1. **C.** Staining of skin injected with LL-37 plus GM-1111 (applied at t = 0) for the PMN antigen Gr-1. **D.** Staining of skin injected with LL-37 plus GM-1111 (applied at t = 12 h) for the PMN antigen Gr-1. **E.** Staining of normal control skin for the RAGE ligand S100A8. **F.** Staining of LL-37 injected skin for the RAGE ligand S100A8. **G.** Staining of skin injected with LL-37 plus GM-1111 (applied at t = 0) for the RAGE ligand S100A8. **H.** Staining of skin injected with LL-37 plus GM-1111 (applied at t = 12 h) for the RAGE ligand S100A8. Figures and insets are shown at 20x and 40x magnification, respectively.

human leukocyte S100 calgranulin S100A12 [17] in LL-37-injected skin (Figures 6E vs 6F). Importantly, topical GM-1111 treatment reduced S100A8 staining expression compared to LL-37 alone (Figures 6G and 6H vs 6F).

SAGEs inhibit cutaneous inflammation from croton oil

As another model, we employed croton oil, which is commonly used to study PMN-mediated skin inflammation in screening anti-inflammatory compounds for dermatologic use [18]. Croton oil contains the phorbol ester tetradecyl phorbol acetate (TPA), which activates protein kinase C in skin cells, producing abundant chemotaxins which can signal PMN influx. Cutaneous inflammation from croton oil has also recently been linked in part to recruitment of inflammatory cells by HMGB-1 released from TPA-exposed keratinocytes [19]. When painted on the ear, croton oil produces intense redness (Figure 10A bottom), accompanied by edema (Figure 10C) and intradermal increase in MPO activity (Figure 10E), indicative of PMN infiltration, compared to the control ear (Figures 10A top, B and E). Topical application of GM-1111 significantly decreased phorbol-induced ear edema (Figure 10D), MPO activity (Figure 10E), increase in erythema (Figure 10F), and increase in ear thickness (Figure 10G). This indicates that topical SAGEs may have utility in treating other dermatoses that are in part or completely mediated by PMNs.

Discussion

Herein we show that novel sulfated glycosaminoglycan ethers have broad anti-inflammatory activity. The SAGE GM-1111 avidly bound to the leukocyte adhesion molecule P-selectin, the Mac-1 integrin and the pro-inflammatory pattern recognition receptor RAGE. This SAGE also potently inhibited P-selectin, blocked catalytic activity of the cationic PMN protease HLE, and inhibited the interaction of RAGE with its disparate ligands, including the AGE product CML-BSA, the S100 calgranulin S100b and the nuclear alarmin HMGB-1. Furthermore, GM-1111 demonstrated the ability to block leukocytes from using RAGE as an alternative adhesion ligand. The activities exemplified by GM-1111 (Table 1 and Figures 2 and 3) are generally demonstrated by a wide range of SAGEs with distinct structures and distinctive structure-activity profiles [6]. In aggregate, these activities would be predicted to be broadly anti-inflammatory. We confirmed this to be the case using a recently reported model of human rosacea [3]. LL-37 avidly bound to SAGE (Figure 4A) and addition of GM-1111 to medium blocked the ability of LL-37 to induce IL-8 expression by cultured human keratinocytes (Figure 4B). Further, co-injection of GM-1111 with LL-37 inhibited development of erythema (Figures 5A vs B and F) and skin infiltration of PMNs (Figure 5C vs 5D and 5E) in response to intradermal LL-37 peptide. Topical GM-1111 was also effective at

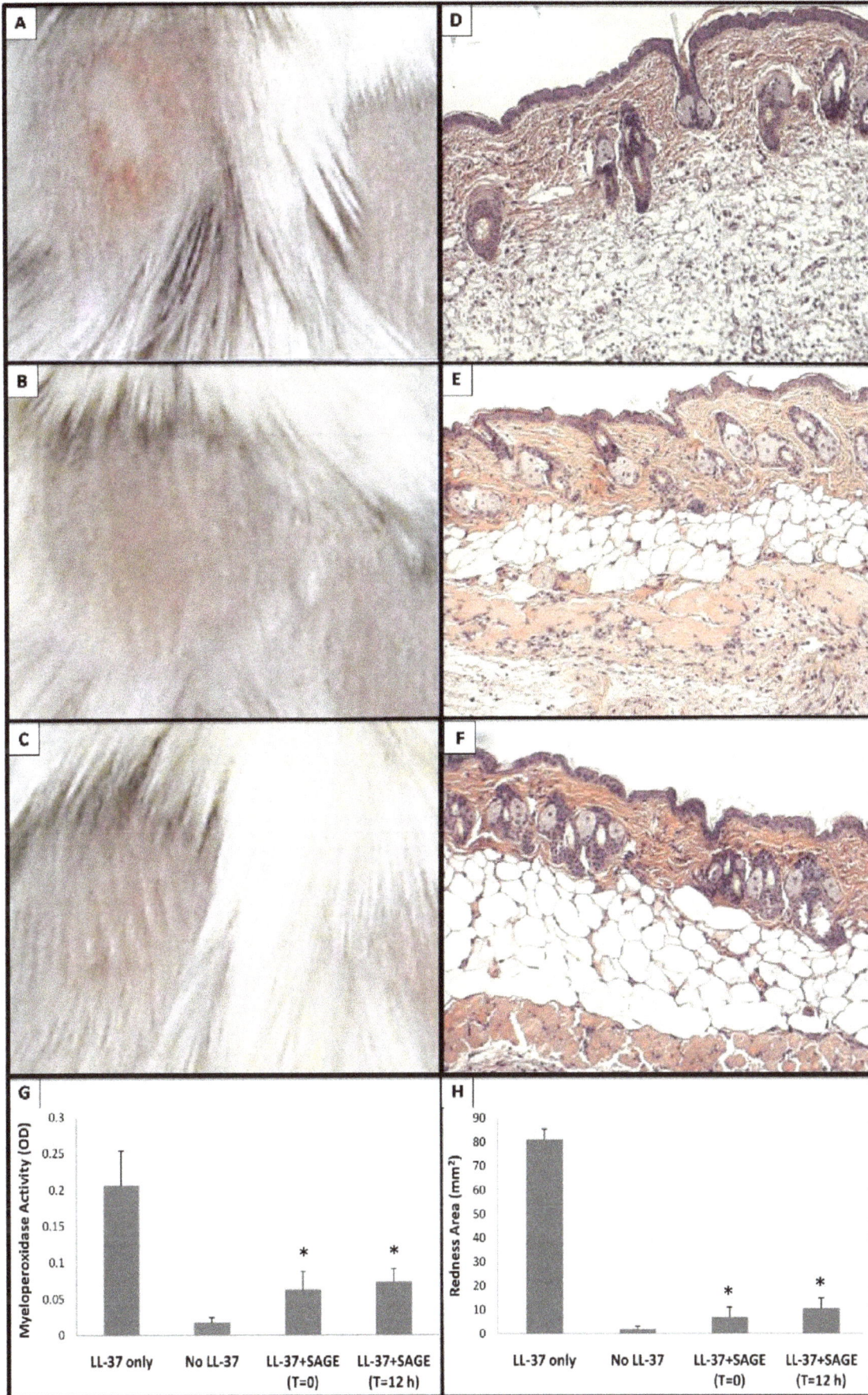

Figure 7. Topical SAGE reduces LL-37-induced inflammation. Balb/c mice were injected intradermally as described in Figure 5, and treated topically with GM-1111-1 (1% w/w) in a triglyceride-based emollient. **A–C**. Gross pictures of LL-37 injected skin region: **A**, no treatment; **B**, GM-1111 treatment immediately (t = 0) after LL-37 injection; **C**, GM-1111 treatment beginning at t = 12 h after LL-37 injection. **D**. H&E-stained cross-sectional view of a LL-37 injected skin sample. **E**. H&E-stained cross-sectional view of GM-1111 treatment at t = 0 in LL-37 injected skin region. **F**. H&E-stained cross-sectional view of GM-1111 at t = 12 h treatment in LL-37 injected skin region. **G**. MPO activity measurement of LL-37 injection with different treatments. **H**. Area of erythema from LL-37 injection. *P<0.05 vs intradermal LL-37 alone; n = 6 per group.

ameliorating LL-37 induced skin inflammation (Figure 7), and similarly reduced inflammatory edema and PMN infiltration in response to dermal application of croton oil (Figure 10). Thus, topical SAGEs are the first mechanistically based approach for treating rosacea that intersects with currently understood pathogenic mechanisms in this disease [3], and may also be therapeutic for other leukocyte mediated skin disorders.

Cathelicidin peptides are polycationic antimicrobial peptides important for innate immunity of skin and other organs [5]. In humans, the major cathelicidin peptide is LL-37, which is produced by proteolytic processing of its precursor hCAP18

(human cationic antimicrobial protein 18). In addition to being antimicrobial, antifungal and antiviral, LL-37 is chemoattractant through activation of the formyl peptide receptor-like 1 (FPRL1) receptor on leukocytes, and can induce keratinocyte IL-8 and IL-18 secretion through activation of the epidermal growth factor receptor or the p38 and ERK1/2 MAP kinase pathways, respectively [5]. Through FPRL1, LL-37 also activates endothelial cells, resulting in angiogenesis [20]. These activities account for the erythema, telangiectases and PMN infiltration of rosacea [3].

The polyanionic glycosaminoglycan heparin has been previously reported to inhibit LL-37 binding to lipopolysaccharide [21]

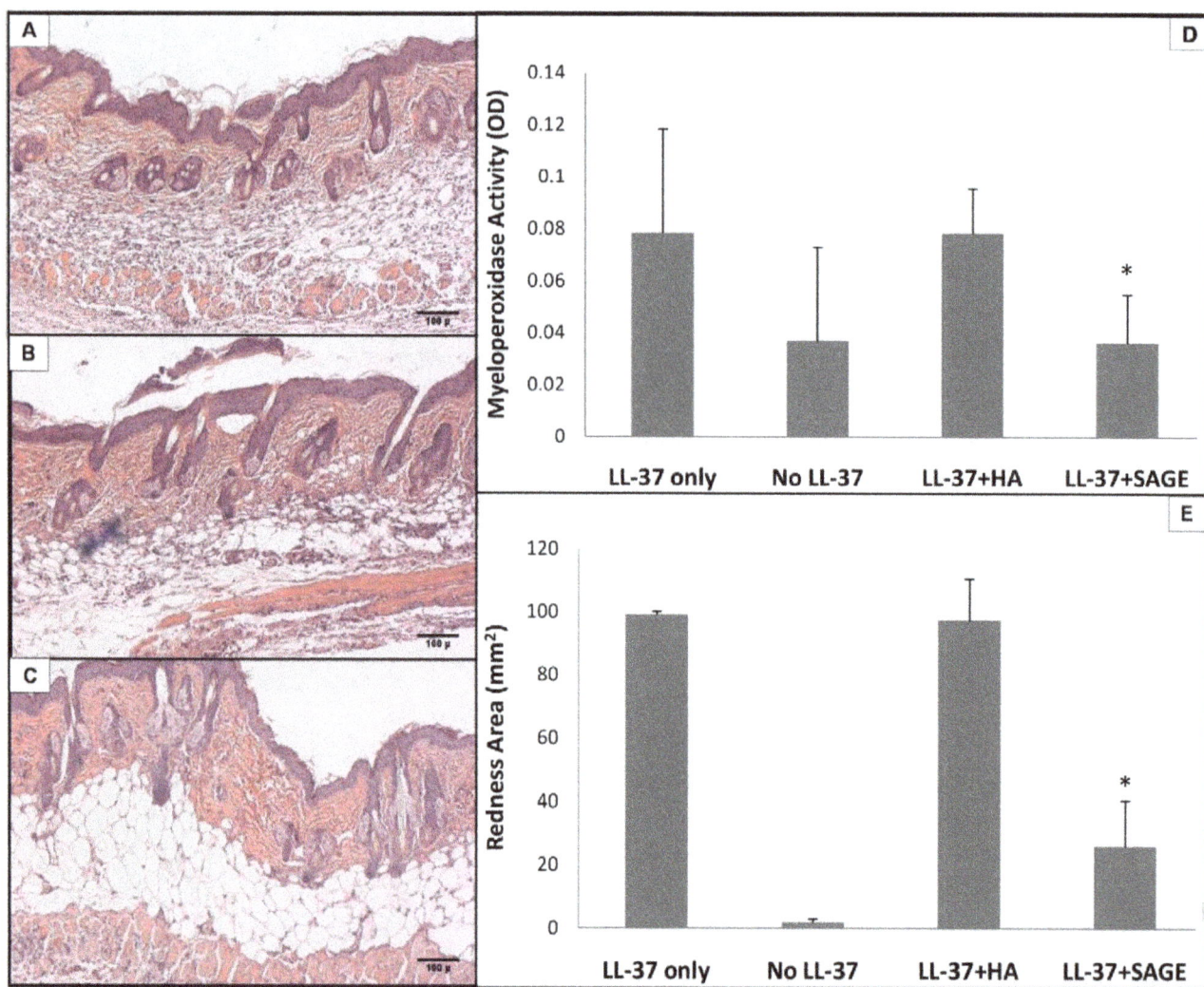

Figure 8. HA emollient does not reduce LL-37-induced inflammation. Experiments were performed as in Figure 7, but with immediate (t = 0) application of 1% w/w HA-containing emollient (53 kDa HA) or 1% w/w GM-1111 emollient. *P<0.05 vs LL-37 alone. **A**. H&E-stained cross-sectional view of LL-37 injected skin. **B**. H&E-stained section of LL-37 injected skin treated with topical HA emollient alone. **C**. H&E-stained section of LL-37 injected skin treated with topical emollient containing 1% SAGE GM-1111. **D**. MPO activity measurement of LL-37 injection with different treatments. **E**. Area of erythema from LL-37 injection. Erythema scores after LL-37 injection were: 5.1±0.1 after LL-37 alone; 4.9±0.44 after LL-37+ HA; 2.3±0.7 after LL-37+ SAGE (P<0.05 LL-37 alone vs LL-37+ SAGE). *P<0.05 vs intradermal LL-37 alone; n = 6 per group.

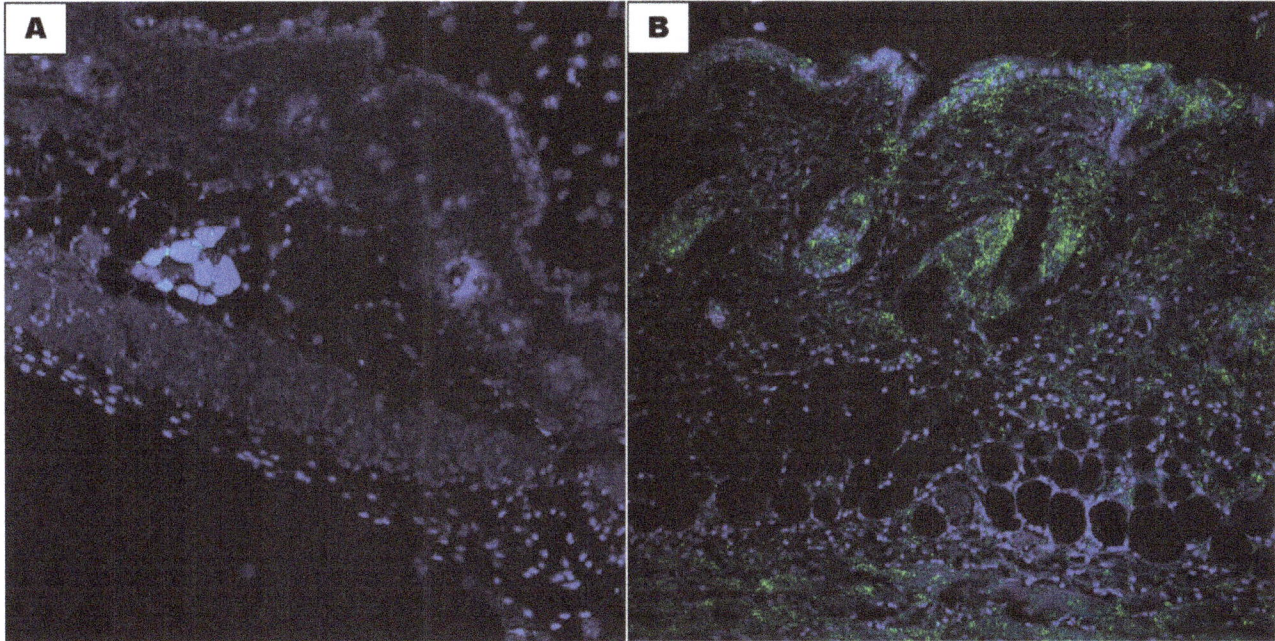

Figure 9. Topical SAGE penetrates into inflamed mouse skin. Balb/c mice were injected intradermally with LL-37 every 12 h for 48 h as in Figure 7. Control emollient [3% (w/w) methylcellulose] or emollient containing Alexa Fluor 633-labeled GM-1111 was applied topically to the injected skin after the last two LL-37 injections. Under low light conditions, skin was harvested 12 h after the last emollient application, fixed in paraformaldehyde and embedded in paraffin. Slides were deparaffinized with xylene, stained with DAPI (1:100 dilution in fluorescent mounting medium) and imaged using an FV1000 confocal microscope. The skin surface is oriented at the top of each image. **A**. Skin from controls demonstrates blue DAPI ($\lambda_{ex}=358$ nm; $\lambda_{em}=461$ nm) image but no SAGE fluorescence. **B.** Skin treated with Alexa Fluor 633-labeled GM-1111 demonstrates fluorescence ($\lambda_{ex}=633$ nm; $\lambda_{em}=647$ nm; false colored green in the image) consistent with SAGE penetration into LL-37-inflamed skin.

and thereby reduce the antibacterial effects of LL-37 [22]. Heparin also neutralizes the toxicity of other cationic peptides, including eosinophil major basic protein and eosinophil cationic protein [23,24]. This led us to hypothesize that the SAGEs could charge neutralize and reduce the biologic effects of exuberantly expressed LL-37 in humans with rosacea. The data from *in vitro* (Figure 4) and *in vivo* (Figures 5 and 7) experiments support this

hypothesis. GM-1111 not only bound LL-37 (Figure 4A) and inhibited LL-37 when co-mixed with it prior to intradermal injection (Figure 5), but also when applied topically to the skin (Figure 7). Because LL-37 is also overexpressed in psoriatic skin, where it has been proposed to form complexes with human self-DNA to activate plasmacytoid dendritic cells and the processes that lead to lesions of psoriasis [5,25], GM-1111 or other SAGEs

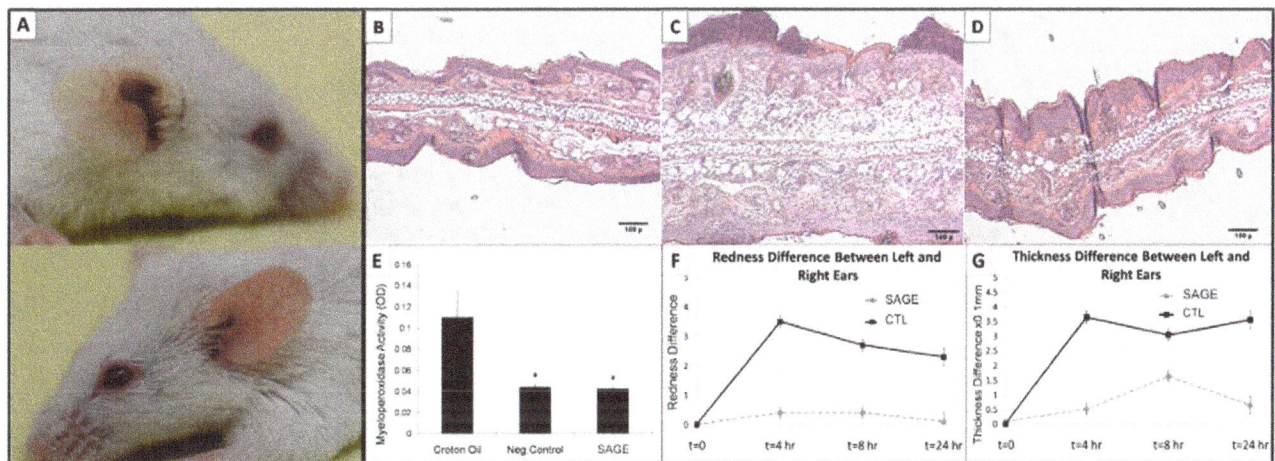

Figure 10. Topical SAGE reduces ear edema from croton oil. GM-1111 (1%) was applied topically in the croton oil model. **A**. Normal control right ear (top) and croton oil painted left ear (bottom). **B**. H&E section of control normal ear. **C**. H&E-stained cross-sectional view of a croton oil painted ear with vehicle treatment. **D**. H&E-stained cross-sectional view of croton oil painted ear with SAGE treatment. **E**. MPO activity measurement in ears. **F**. Ear thickness differences between left (croton oil) and right (normal) ears. **G**. Redness difference between right and left ears. *P<0.05 vs croton oil with vehicle emollient alone (negative control).

might also prove therapeutically useful in other common inflammatory skin diseases.

In addition to blocking cathelicidin peptides, SAGEs are also potent inhibitors of RAGE with at least four of its disparate ligands (Table 1 and Figure 3). The pathogenic role of RAGE in skin diseases has only recently been explored. However, RAGE is already known to be centrally important in photo-ageing [9], the S100 calgranulins S100A7 and S100A17 are highly upregulated in psoriatic skin [26], and HMGB-1 has been recently reported to mediate cutaneous inflammation from topical croton oil [19]. Our finding that S100A8, the mouse homologue for human S100A12 [17], is increased in LL-37-injected skin (Figure 6) suggests that S100 calgranulins also may have a prominent role in the cutaneous inflammation seen in patients with rosacea.

RAGE is a promiscuous pattern recognition receptor from the immunoglobulin superfamily and plays a prominent role in magnifying inflammation [27,28]. Once ligated, RAGE mediates post-receptor signaling including activation of nuclear factor-κB (NF-κB), leading to a profound inflammatory response [27,28]. Through a prominent NF-κB-responsive consensus sequence in its promoter, RAGE activation also leads to even greater RAGE expression [27,28]. Furthermore, RAGE interacts with the leukocyte Mac-1 integrin (CD11b/CD18) and p150,95 (CD11c/CD18) to facilitate leukocyte inflammatory cell recruitment [13]. Attraction of leukocytes to inflammation is additionally augmented by interaction of the RAGE ligands S100 calgranulins and HMGB-1 [13,27–29].

Structurally, RAGE is comprised of three immunoglobulin-like regions: a distal "V" type domain, followed by two "C" type domains, a short transmembrane domain and a cytoplasmic tail required for signaling [27,28]. The extracellular domain of RAGE has been used in detailed analyses of RAGE-ligand interactions [30] and the crystal structure of the receptor [31]. SAGEs likely inhibit RAGE-ligand interaction in part through interactions with the V domain, which consists of a large hydrophobic cavity rimed on its surface with basic amino acids to form a cationic center [30]. This is supported by a crystal structure for RAGE which reveals an elongated molecule with a large basic patch and a large hydrophobic patch, both highly conserved [31], which might offer attractive sites for binding of both acidic anionic and alkyl groups, respectively, of SAGEs. The dramatic differences among structurally similar SAGEs [6] and ligand specific structure-activity relationships strongly suggest that charge alone is only a small contributor to overall anti-inflammatory effects. Binding of polyanions such as SAGEs to this cationic region might be expected to not only inhibit binding of AGEs, which ligate RAGE at its V domain, but also, dependent upon the nature of substituent alkyl groups, to produce steric interference with the binding of other ligands such as S100/calgranulins and HMGB-1 which require adjacent C1 and/or C2 regions for full RAGE ligation [32].

A major issue with the use of sulfated polysaccharides such as SAGEs for topical treatment of skin diseases is their availability to the dermis. Literature on the bioavailability of sulfated polysaccharides across skin is conflicting, with some groups reporting little penetration but others suggesting transdermal absorption of heparin and unfractionated heparin as a result of their detergent properties [33–39]. In the most recently published work, fluorescent-labeled unfractionated heparin was found to adhere to keratinocytes in culture, and within 48 hours, almost half of topically applied labeled heparin was found to transcutaneously penetrate the skin of hairless rats mounted onto a Franz static diffusion cell [40]. Whereas SAGEs might permeate normal skin in humans less well than in mice, inflammation could serve to greatly increase SAGE penetration (Figure 9), as seen with other drugs used for serious skin diseases [41] and similar to the well-recognized enhancement of antibiotic penetration into cerebrospinal fluid in the presence of a disrupted blood-brain barrier in meningitis. Various techniques have been developed to enable transdermal delivery of low molecular weight (~5,000 Da) heparin, including penetration enhancers [42,43], liposomal formulation [43,44], iontophoresis [45,46] and low frequency ultrasound [45,47,48]. These strategies might also facilitate dermal penetration of similarly sized SAGEs to enable their effective topical use in skin disorders.

The chemistry and function of HA have been well explored in cutaneous biology, and bacterial and animal-derived HA continue to be an important component for the cosmetics, pharmaceutical and medical device industries. Our research suggests that simple chemical modifications of HA can generate novel anionic polysaccharides with broad anti-inflammatory activities. SAGEs have the additional advantage of being non-animal derived, thus circumventing the risks of adulteration and sourcing problems inherent in animal-derived sulfated polysaccharides [15]. Our observations suggest that SAGEs in topical application may prove to be a safe and useful treatment not only for rosacea, but also other inflammatory skin diseases.

Materials and Methods

Materials

Polyclonal goat anti-human RAGE (Cat# AF1145), recombinant HMGB-1, recombinant human P-selectin/Fc chimera, and recombinant human RAGE/Fc chimera were purchased from R&D Systems (Minneapolis, MN). Rabbit polyclonal IgG antibody to LL-37 (Cat# sc-50423) was from Santa Cruz Biotechnology (Santa Cruz, CA), and peroxidase-linked goat anti-rabbit polyclonal IgG (Cat# A0545) was from Sigma Aldrich (St. Louis, MO). Human S100b calgranulin was from Calbiochem (San Diego, CA). Alexa Fluor® 633 hydrazide was from Molecular Probes (Eugene, OR). The AGE product CML-BSA was from MBL International (Woburn, MA). Protein A, horse radish peroxidase (HRP)-conjugated rabbit polyclonal anti-goat IgG (Cat# 31402), carbonate-bicarbonate buffer and bovine serum albumin blocker (10x) were from Piercenet (Rockford, IL). Calcein AM, Dulbecco's modified Eagle's medium (DMEM), EpiLife medium, ethylenediamine tetraacetic acid (EDTA), fetal bovine serum (FBS), HEPES, non-essential amino acids, penicillin/streptomycin/L-glutamine solution, RPMI-1640 without L-glutamine, sodium bicarbonate, and tetramethyl benzidine chromogen (TMB) single solution chromogen were from Invitrogen (Carlsbad, CA). High-bind 96-well microplates were from Corning Life Sciences (Corning, NY), and heparin binding plates were from BD Biosciences (Bedford, MA). U937 monocytes and nHDF cells were purchased from American Type Culture Collection (Manassas, VA). nHEK cells were obtained from Invitrogen (Madison, WI). Antibodies for immunohistochemistry were sourced as identified in figure legends. All other chemicals not specified were from Sigma-Aldrich (St. Louis, MO). HA was obtained commercially from a recombinant *B. subtilis* expression system (Novozymes Biopolymers, Bagsvaerd, Denmark) or from streptococcal fermentation (LifeCore, Chaska, MN).

Animal Care and Use

All animal protocols were approved by the University of Utah institutional animal care and use committee (IACUC). Approved protocols include 08-06002, 08-06005 and 08-11008.

Characterization of SAGEs

A variety of SAGEs were prepared with four parameters varied: molecular weight, type of ether modification, substitution degree of ether modification, and degree of sulfation. These data are reported elsewhere [6]. Ether substitution degree (SD) of SAGE was determined by ^{1}H NMR, and for GM-1111 was estimated to be SD = 1, or ~1 alkyl group per disaccharide unit. After sulfation, GM-1111 was dissolved in water, dialyzed, and lyophilized to give a white powder shown by ^{1}H NMR to have a sulfation SD of 1.0–1.5. Fluorescent-labeled GM-1111 was synthesized by conjugation with Alexa Fluor 633 hydrazide.

Molecular weight was determined with gel permeation chromatography using a Waters 515 HPLC pump, Waters 410 differential refractometer, Waters 486 tunable absorbance detector, and Ultrahydrogel 250 or 1000 columns (7.8 mm i.d X 130 cm) (Milford, MA). Eluent was 200 mM phosphate buffer (pH 6.5): MeOH = 80:20 (v/v), and flow rate was 0.3 or 0.5 mL/min. The system was calibrated with standard HA samples from Dr. U. Wik (Pharmacia, Uppsala, Sweden). Average molecular weight of GM-1111 was ~5,000–6,000 Da.

Formulation of GM-1111 emollient

A 1% (w/w) emollient was prepared in Spectrum Transdermal Ointment (Lotioncrafters, Olga, WA), a commercially available proprietary ointment comprised of cetyl ricinoleate, carnuba wax, D-α-tocopheryl acetate, shea butter, caprylic triglyceride, lecithin and beeswax. GM-1111 (100 mg) was dissolved in 2.0 g of nanopure water, ointment was added to give 10.0 g, the mixture blended thoroughly and the emulsion processed through an ointment mill. Control emollient was made with 2 g water without active ingredient. Sodium hyaluronate emollient was prepared with 100 mg of 53 kDa HA (Novozymes, Bagsvaerd, Denmark) following an analogous protocol. Each formulation was stored at 4°C.

Cell culture

U937 monocytes were grown in suspension at 37°C in 5% CO_2-95% air in RPMI-1640 supplemented with 10% heat inactivated FBS, 2 mM L-glutamine, 1 mM sodium pyruvate, 0.1 mM MEM non-essential amino acids, 100 units/ml penicillin and 100 mg/ml streptomycin. nHDF cells were grown in DMEM supplemented with 10% FBS and penicillin-streptomycin. nHEK cells were grown in EpiLife medium supplemented with 0.06 mM Ca^{2+}, 1% EpiLife defined growth supplement and penicillin-streptomycin. Experiments were performed with cells from passages 1-5.

Factor XII activation assay

Five μl of pooled normal human plasma was incubated with 100 μl of GM-1111 ranging from 0.1-1000 μg/ml in 0.05M HEPES containing 0.05% TritonX-100 for 5 min at 25°C. Amidolytic activity was determined with 0.5 mM H-D-CHT-Gly-Arg-pNA by following the change of optical density (OD) for 30 min at 405 nm [16]. The OD obtained at 30 min was plotted against the concentrations of the activator.

Cell surface binding assays

The effect of GM-1111 on binding of U937 monocytes to P-selectin or RAGE was studied using calcein labeled cells incubated in micro plates coated with P-selectin-Fc or RAGE-Fc chimeras. These methods have been reported in detail [10].

Inhibition of human leukocyte elastase (HLE)

Inhibition of HLE by SAGEs was determined using the specific chromogenic substrate suc-Ala-Ala-Val-pNA, according to methods previously described [10].

Solid phase binding assays

Three types of ELISAs were performed: one to study the binding of vascular adhesion molecules and LL-37 to GM-1111, and another to study binding between RAGE and its ligands, including CML-BSA, HMGB-1 and S100b. A competitive ELISA was also performed to study the ability of GM-1111 to inhibit/compete RAGE binding to its ligands. These ELISAs have been reported in detail [10].

In vitro cytotoxicity and anticoagulant assays

nHDF cells were seeded (4,000/100 μl medium) in each well of 96-well flat-bottomed microplates, and incubated at 37°C in 5% CO_2 for 12 hours. Medium was changed with complete medium containing GM-1111 at final concentrations of 10 to 10^6 ng/ml to each well. At 48 hours, 20 μl MTS (CellTiter96® Aqueous One assay; Promega, Madison, WI) was added to each well, and cells were further incubated for 2 h. Absorbance of the samples was measured at 490 nm using a 96-well plate reader to determine cytotoxicity. Cytotoxicity was assessed similarly in nHEK cells. Automated amidolytic assays for anti-Xa and anti-IIa activity were performed by BioCascade, Arlington, WI.

Skin irritation tests in mice

SAGEs were tested *in vivo* to assess dermal irritation potential. GM-1111 was prepared at 0.1, 1 and 10 mg/ml. Formic acid (10%) and PBS were used as positive and negative control, respectively. Balb/c mice (n = 6 per group), free from skin irritation, trauma, or adverse clinical signs prior to study, were randomized and grouped for test conditions. Backs of animals were clipped free of fur. Each mouse received four parallel epidermal abrasions with a sterile needle at the bottom area of the test site, while the upper area of the test site remained intact. Under isofluorane anesthesia, two 0.5-ml samples of the test solution were applied to the entire test site under a double gauze layer to an area of skin approximately 2.5 cm^2. Patches were backed with plastic, covered with a non reactive tape and the test site wrapped with a bandage. After 24 h exposure to the agent, the bandage and soaked test gauze were removed and test sites were wiped with tap water to remove remaining test compound. At 24 and 72 h after application, test sites were examined for dermal reactions in accordance with the FHSA- recommended Draize scoring criteria [14]. Primary Irritation Index (P.I.I.) of test article was calculated following test completion. A material producing a P.I.I. score of greater than or equal to 5.00 would be considered positive and be classed as a primary irritant to skin.

Peptide synthesis

LL-37 was prepared by the core peptide facility at the University of Utah, containing the amino acid sequence: LLGDFFRKSKEKIGKEFKRIVQRIKDFLRNLVPRTES. Synthetic peptides were purified to >95% by HPCL and sequence was confirmed by mass spectrometry.

LL-37-mediated skin inflammation models

To study the effect of SAGE in rosacea, we used a previously reported disease model produced by intradermal injection of LL-37 [3]. Balb/c mice were shaved prior to study to expose skin on the back. Twenty-four hours later, 40 μl of vehicle (nanopure water), LL-37 (320 μM), SAGE (1,280 μM), or LL-37+ SAGE mix (peptide + 4x molar concentration of SAGE) was injected intradermally into the shaved skin using a 0.5 ml syringe and 31-gauge insulin needle in a manner to raise an intact dermal bleb, identifying that administration was at the lower epidermis or dermis. To standardize results, all intradermal injections were performed by a single investigator with experience performing intradermal injections on the human volar forearm with needle bevel facing upward. SAGE and LL-37 were mixed together in PBS and allowed to incubate 15 min at room temperature before injection. Injections were repeated every 12 h thereafter. Forty-eight hours after the initial injection (four injections in total), animals were anesthetized with isoflurane. Injected skin was photographed to record severity of erythema and edema. Mice were euthanized with CO_2, and injected skin was excised for hematoxylin and eosin staining and immunochemistry. From the center of excised skin, a 6 mm punch biopsy was obtained, weighed, snap frozen in liquid N_2 and stored at -80 C for measurement of tissue MPO.

To study topical SAGE in this model, mice were injected with LL-37 as described above. GM-1111 was then applied topically as a 1% concentration in 50 μl of emollient, either immediately after the first LL-37 injection or 12 h thereafter, with repeated application every 12 h after each LL-37 injection. After application, emollient was massaged into the affected area of skin with a gloved finger rubbed 32 consecutive times in a counter-clockwise direction. Control animals were treated similarly with emollient alone. To standardize treatment, all topical medication applications were performed by a single investigator after the individual performing intradermal injections had finished the injections and left the laboratory area. After four LL-37 intradermal injections, mice were photographed and biopsied as above.

Croton oil inflammation model

As another model of PMN-mediated skin inflammation, we employed croton oil [18]. Croton oil (0.8% solution in acetone) was painted (10 μl each side) on one ear of Balb/c mice, with the other ear as a control. Fifteen minutes later, GM-1111 was then dosed topically as a 1% concentration in 50 μl of emollient applied to each side of the croton-oil treated ear. After application, emollient was massaged into each side of the ear with a gloved finger rubbed 32 consecutive times in a counter-clockwise direction. Control animals were treated in a similar fashion with emollient alone. To standardize treatment, all topical medication applications were performed by a single investigator after the individual performing croton oil applications had left the laboratory area. After 4, 8 and 24 h, ear thickness was measured near the top of the ear distal to the cartilaginous ridges. Change in ear thickness from control was taken as an edema index. Following 24 h measurements, mice were euthanized with CO_2 and 6 mm ear punch biopsies taken, weighed, frozen and stored at $-80°C$ for determination of MPO activity. A single investigator performed all measurements and biopsies in order to standardize the procedure. Remaining ears were removed, embedded and frozen for hematoxylin and eosin stains and immunohistochemistry.

MPO assay

Tissue MPO activity was measured using the method of Suzuki et al. [49] modified by Young et al. [50]. Biopsies were placed in 0.75 ml of 80 mM PBS (pH 5.4) containing 0.5% hexadecyltri-methyl-ammonium bromide (HTAB). Each sample was homogenized for 45 s at 4°C with a Tissue Tearor Homogenizer (Model

985-370; Biospec Products, Bartlesville, OK). Homogenate was transferred to a microcentrifuge tube with an additional 0.75 ml HTAB in PBS. The 1.5 ml sample was centrifuged at $12,000 \times g$ for 15 min at 4°C. Triplicate 30 μl samples of the resulting supernatant were added to 96-well microtiter plates. For MPO assay, 200 μl of a mixture containing 100 μl of 80 mM PBS (pH 5.4), 85 μl of 0.22 M PBS (pH 5.4), and 15 μl of 0.017% hydrogen peroxide were added to each well. To this, 20 μl of 18.4 mM tetramethylbenzidine HCl in 8% aqueous dimethylformamide (DMF) was added to start the reaction. Microtiter plates were incubated at 37°C for 3 min, and placed on ice. The reaction was stopped with the addition of 30 μl of 1.46 M sodium acetate. MPO activity was assessed at 630 nm and expressed as optical density (OD)/biopsy.

Immunohistochemistry

LL-37, PBS and LL-37 and SAGE-injected mouse skin was stained with antibody to mouse Gr-1 to examine neutrophil infiltration, and also for S100A8 calgranulin, the major RAGE-binding calgranulin present in murine PMNs [17]. Slides were deparaffinized and hydrated through Citrisolv and graded ethanol washes. Endogenous peroxidase activity was blocked with 1% H_2O_2 in PBS with 0.1% Tween-20 (PBST) for 20 min. Antigen retrieval was performed by microwaving in 1% antigen unmasking solution (Vector Laboratories) for 20 min followed by incubation at room temperature for 30 min. Immunostaining was performed using the Vectastain Elite ABC peroxidase kit (Vector Laboratories). Briefly, non-specific antibody binding was minimized by incubating sections for 90 min in diluted normal blocking serum. Sections were incubated overnight at 4°C in a humidified chamber with primary goat anti-mouse calgranulin A antibodies (Santa Cruz #sc-8113) at a 1:200 dilution and rat anti-mouse Gr-1 (R&D Systems #RB6-8C5) at a 1:500 dilution. Following overnight incubation, slides were washed in PBST for 9 min, incubated 2 h with biotinylated secondary antibody diluted to 5 μg/ml in PBST, followed by Vectastain Elite ABC Reagent (Vector) diluted in PBST for 30 min. Between incubations, sections were washed for 12 min in PBST. Immunoreactivity was detected by incubating with the DAB peroxidase substrate kit (Vector Laboratories) for 1–2 min. Sections were then washed in nanopure water and counterstained with hematoxylin before dehydration and mounting with coverslips.

Statistical Analysis

All experiments were performed in triplicate or quadruplicate for *in vitro* tests. Results are expressed as means ± standard error of the mean (SEM). Significant differences between samples were calculated by comparison of means using the Aspin−Welch test. In experiments with multiple groups or treatments, a one-way analysis of variance (ANOVA) followed by Student-Newman-Keuls *post hoc* test was used to analyze for group differences. Significance was declared at $P<0.05$.

Author Contributions

Conceived and designed the experiments: GDP NVR TPK. Performed the experiments: JZ XX NVR BA LM WJR. Analyzed the data: XX LM. Contributed reagents/materials/analysis tools: JZ XX NVR. Wrote the paper: TPK NVR GDP GK.

References

1. Powell FC (2005) Rosacea. N Engl J Med 352: 793–803.
2. Elewski BE, Draelos Z, Breno B, Jansen T, Layton A, et al. (2010) Rosacea—global diversity and optimized outcome: proposed international consensus from the Rosacea International Expert Group. J Europ Academ Dermatol Venereology doi:10.1111/j.1468-3083.2010.03751.x.
3. Yamasaki K, Di Nardo A, Bardan A, Murakami M, Ohtake T, et al. (2007) Increased serine protease activity and cathelicidin promotes skin inflammation in rosacea. Nat Med 13: 975–980.
4. Bevins CL, Liu F-T (2007) Rosacea: skin innate immunity gone awry? Nat Med 13: 904–906.

5. Kenshi Y, Gallo RL (2008) Antimicrobial peptides in human skin disease. Eur J Dermatol 18: 11–21.

6. Prestwich G, Zhang J, Kennedy TP, Rao N, Xu X (2010) Alkylated semi-synthetic glycosaminoglycosan ethers, and methods for making and using thereof. U.S. Patent 7,855,187B1.

7. Wang L, Brown JR, Varki A, Esko JD (2002) Heparin's anti-inflammatory effects require glucosamine 6-O-sulfation and are mediated by blockade of L- and P-selectins. J Clin Invest 110: 127–136.

8. Fryer A, Huang Y-C, Rao G, Jacoby D, Mancilla E, et al. (1997) Selective O-desulfation produces nonanticoagulant heparin that retains pharmacologic activity in the lung. J Pharmacol Exp Ther 282: 208–219.

9. Lohwasser C, Neureiter D, Weigle B, Kirchner T, Schuppan D (2006) The receptor for advanced glycation end products is highly expressed in the skin and upregulated by advanced glycation end products and tumor necrosis factor-alpha. J Invest Dermatol 126: 291–299.

10. Rao NV, Argyle B, Xu X, Reynolds PR, Walenga JM, et al. (2010) Low anticoagulant heparin targets multiple sites of inflammation, suppresses heparin-induced thrombocytopenia, and inhibits interaction of RAGE with its ligands. Am J Physiol Cell Physiol 299: C97–C110.

11. Foell D, Wittkowski H, Vogl T, Roth J (2007) S100 proteins expressed in phagocytes: a novel group of damage-associated molecular pattern molecules. J Leukoc Biol 81: 28–37.

12. Klune JR, Dhupar R, Cardinal J, Billiar TR, Tsung A (2008) HMGB1: endogenous danger signaling. Mol Med 14: 476–484.

13. Chavakis T, Bierhaus A, Al-Fakhri N, Schneider D, Witte S, et al. (2003) The pattern recognition receptor (RAGE) is a counterreceptor for leukocyte integrins: a novel pathway for inflammatory cell recruitment. J Exp Med 10: 1507–1515.

14. Bosshard E (1985) Review on skin and mucous-membrane irritations tests and their application. Food Chem Toxicol 23: 149–154.

15. Kishimoto TK, Viswanathan K, Ganguly T, Elankumaran S, Smith S, et al. (2008) Contaminated heparin associated with adverse clinical events and activation of the contact system. N Engl J Med 358: 2457–2467.

16. Silverberg M, Dunn JT, Garen L, Kaplan AP (1980) Autoactivation of human Hageman factor. Demonstration using a synthetic substrate. J Biol Chem 255: 7281–7286.

17. Fuellen G, Foell D, Nacken W, Sorg C, Kerkhoff C (2003) Absence of S100A12 in mouse: implications of RAGE-S100A12 interaction. Trends Immunol 24: 622–624.

18. Bralley EE, Greenspan P, Hargrove JL, Wicker L, Hartle DK (2008) Topical anti-inflammatory activity of Polygonum cuspidatum extract in the TPA model of mouse ear inflammation. J Inflammation 5: 1–7. doi:10.1186/476-9255-5-1.

19. Mittal D, Saccheri F, Venereau E, Pusteria T, Bianchi ME, et al. (2010) TLR4-mediated skin carcinogenesis is dependent on immune and radioresistant cells. EMBO J 29: 2242–2252.

20. Koczulla R, von Degenfeld G, Kupatt C, Krotz F, Zahler S, et al. (2003) An angiogenic role for the human peptide antibiotic LL-37/hCAP-18. J Clin Invest 111: 1665–1672.

21. Ogata M, Fletcher MF, Kloczewiak M, Loiselle PM, Zanzot EM, et al. (1997) Effect of anticoagulants on binding and neutralization of lipopolysaccharide by the peptide immunoglobulin conjugate CAP18$_{106-138}$-immunoglobuin G in whole blood. Infect Immun 65: 2160–2167.

22. Baranska-Rybak W, Sonesson A, Nowicki R, Schmidtchen A (2006) Glycos-aminoglycans inhibit the antibacterial activity of LL-37 in biological fluids. J Antimicrob Chemotherapy 57: 260–265.

23. Barker RL, Gundel RH, Gleich GJ, Checkel JL, Loegering DA, et al. (1991) Acidic polyamino acids inhibit human eosinophil granule major basic protein toxicity. Evidence of a functional role for ProMBP. J Clin Invest 88: 798–805.

24. Fryer AD, Jacoby DB (1992) Function of pulmonary M_2 muscarinic receptors in antigen-challenged guinea pigs is restored by heparin and poly-L-glutamate. J Clin Invest 90: 2292–2298.

25. Nestle FO, Kaplan DH, Barker J (2009) Psoriasis. N Engl J Med 361: 496–590.

26. Wolf R, Howard OMZ, Dong H-F, Voscopoulos C, Boeshans K, et al. (2008) Chemotactic activity of S100A7 (psoriasin) is mediated by RAGE and potentiates inflammation with highly homologous but functionally distinct S100A15. J Immunol 181: 1499–1506.

27. Schmidt AM, Yan SD, Yan SF, Stern DM (2001) The multiligand receptor RAGE as a progression factor amplifying immune and inflammatory responses. J Clin Invest 108: 949–955.

28. Alexiou P, Chatzopoulou M, Pegklidou K, Demopoulos VJ (2010) RAGE: a multiland receptor unveiling novel insights in health and disease. Curr Med Chem 17: 2232–2252.

29. Orlova VV, Choi EY, Xie C, Chavakis E, Bierhaus A, et al. (2007) A novel pathway of HMGB1-mediated inflammatory cell recruitment that requires Mac-1 integrin. EMBO J 26: 1129–1139.

30. Matsumoto S, Yoshida T, Murata H, Harada S, Fujita N, et al. (2008) Solution structure of the variable-type domain of the receptor for advanced glycation end products: new insight into AGE-RAGE interaction. Biochem 47: 12299–12311.

31. Park H, Boyington JC (2010) The 1.5 Å crystal structure of human receptor for advanced glycation endproducts (RAGE) ectodomains reveals unique features determining ligand binding. J Biol Chem doi/10/1074/jbc.M110/169276.

32. Xie J, Reverdatta S, Frolov A, Hoffmann R, Burz DS, et al. (2008) Structural basis for pattern recognition by the receptor for advanced glycation end products (RAGE). J Biol Chem 282: 27255–27269.

33. Schraven E, Trottnow D (1973) Perkutane Resorption von Heparin-^{35}S aus einer speziell zubereiteten Öl-in-Wasser-Emulsion. Arzneim-Forsch/Drug Res 23: 274–275.

34. Schaefer H, Zesch A (1976) Die Penetration von Heparin in die menschliche Haut. Pharmazie 31: 251–254.

35. Zesch A, Schaefer H (1976) Penetration, Permeation und Resorption von Heparin in-vivo-Untersuchungen an der menschlichen Haut. Arzneim-Forsch/Drug Res 26: 1365–1368.

36. Zimmermann RE (1982) Untersuchungen zur transkutanen Heparinapplikation. Therapiewoche 32: 6157–6164.

37. Stuttgen G, Panse P, Bauer E (1990) Permeation of the human skin by heparin and mucopolysaccharide polysulfuric acid ester. Arzneim-Forsch/Drug Res 40: 484–489.

38. de Moerlosse P, Gavillet O, Salomon D, Minazio P, Reber G (1992) Heparin-related activity in peripheral venous blood after percutaneous application of various glycosaminoglycan containing creams. Blood Coag Fibrinol 3: 827–878.

39. Bonina FP, Montenegro L (1994) Vehicle effects on in vitro heparin release and skin penetration from different gels. Int J Pharm 102: 19–24.

40. Parisel C, Saffar L, Gattegno L, Andre V, Abdul-Malak N, et al. (2003) Interactions of heparin with human skin cells: Binding, location, and transdermal penetration. J Biomed Mater Res 67A: 517–523.

41. Meingassner JG, Aschauer H, Stuetz A, Biollich A (2005) Pimecrolimus permeates less than tacrolimus through normal, inflamed, or corticosteroid-pretreated skin. Exp Dermatol 14: 752–757.

42. Karande P, Jain A, Mitragotri S (2004) Discovery of transdermal penetration enhancers by high-throughput screening. Nat Biotech 22: 192–197.

43. Betz G, Nowbakht P, Imboden R Imanidis G (2001) Heparin penetration into and permeation through human skin from aqueous and liposomal fomulations in vitro. Int J Pharm 228: 147–159.

44. Song Y-K, Kim C-K (2006) Topical delivery of low-molecular-weight heparin with surface-charged flexible liposomes. Biomaterials 27: 271–280.

45. Lanke SSS, Kolli CS, Strom JG, Banga AK (2009) Enhanced transdermal delivery of low molecular weight heparin by barrier perturbation. Int J Pharm 365: 26–33.

46. Pacini S, Punzi T, Gulisano M, Cecchi F, Vannucchi S, Ruggiero M (2006) Transdermal delivery of heparin using pulsed current iontophoresis. Pharmaceutical Res 23: 114–120.

47. Mitragotri S, Kost J (2001) Transdermal delivery of heparin and low-molecular weight heparin using low-frequency ultrasound. Pharmaceutical Res 18: 1151–1156.

48. Ogura M, Paliwwal S, Mitragotri S (2008) Low-frequency sonophoresis: Current status and future prospects. Adv Drug Del Rev 60: 1218–1223.

49. Suzuki K, Ota H, Sasagawa S, Sakatani T, Fujikura T (1983) Assay method for myeloperoxidase in human polymorphonuclear leukocytes. Anal Biochem 132: 345–352.

50. Young JM, Spires DA, Bedord CJ, Wagner B, Ballaron SJ, et al. (1984) The mouse ear inflammatory response to topical arachidonic acid. J Invest Dermatol 82: 367–371.

13

L-selectin and Skin Damage in Systemic Sclerosis

James V. Dunne[1,2]*, Stephan F. van Eeden[1,3], Kevin J. Keen[4]

1 Department of Medicine, University of British Columbia, Vancouver, British Columbia, Canada, **2** British Columbia Scleroderma Clinic, Vancouver, British Columbia, Canada, **3** James Hogg Heart and Lung Institute, Vancouver, British Columbia, Canada, **4** Department of Mathematics and Statistics, University of Northern British Columbia, Prince George, British Columbia, Canada

Abstract

Background: L-selectin ligands are induced on the endothelium of inflammatory sites. L-selectin expression on neutrophils and monocytes may mediate the primary adhesion of these cells at sites of inflammation by mediating the leukocyte-leukocyte interactions that facilitate their recruitment. L-selectin retains functional activity in its soluble form. Levels of soluble L-selectin have been reported as both elevated and lowered in patients with systemic sclerosis (SSc). This preliminary study seeks to discern amongst these disparate results and to discover whether there is an association between L-selectin concentrations in plasma and skin damage in SSc patients.

Methodology and Principal Findings: Nineteen cases with limited systemic sclerosis (lSSc) and 11 cases with diffuse systemic sclerosis (dSSc) were compared on a pairwise basis to age- and sex-matched controls. Criteria of the American College of Rheumatology were used to diagnose SSc. Skin involvement was assessed using the modified Rodnan skin score (mRSS). We find no association between mRSS and plasma L-selectin concentration in lSSc cases ($p = 0.9944$) but a statistically significant negative correlation in dSSc cases ($R^2 = 73.11$ per cent, $p = 0.0008$). The interpretation of the slope for dSSc cases is that for each increase of 100 ng/ml in soluble L-selectin concentration, the mRSS drops 4.22 (95 per cent CI: 2.29, 6.16). There was also a highly statistically significant negative correlation between sL-selectin and disease activity ($p = 0.0007$) and severity ($p = 0.0007$) in dSSc cases but not in lSSc cases ($p = 0.2596$, $p = 0.7575$, respectively).

Conclusions and Significance: No effective treatments exist for skin damage in SSc patients. Nor is there a laboratory alternative to the modified Rodnan skin score as is the case for other organs within the body. Modulation of circulating L-selectin is a promising target for reducing skin damage in dSSc patients. Plasma levels of soluble L-selectin could serve as an outcome measure for dSSc patients in clinical trials.

Editor: Songtao Shi, University of Southern California, United States of America

Funding: This work was supported by research grants from the Scleroderma Association of British Columbia and the Heart and Stroke Foundation of Canada. Actelion Pharmaceuticals provides a grant-in-aid to the British Columbia Scleroderma Clinic. KJK received financial support from Merck Canada Inc. for an honorarium and travel. SvE is a Senior Scholar of the Michael Smith Foundation for Health Research, a Career Investigator of the American Lung Association and the Canadian Institutes of Health Research(CIHR/GSK) Professor in Chronic obstructive pulmonary disease. The funders had no role in study design, data collection and analysis, decision to publish, or preparation of the manuscript.

Competing Interests: The authors have declared that no competing interests exist.

* E-mail: James.Dunne@VCH.ca.

Introduction

Systemic sclerosis (SSc) is an inflammatory obliterative micro-vasculopathy disorder of unknown etiology characterized by excessive collagen deposition causing fibrosis predominantly in the dermis but also in internal organs. Systemic sclerosis is a very rare rheumatic disease that affects about 250 individuals per one million adults and carries the burden of a standardized mortality rate of 3.53 [95% CI: 3.03, 4.11], that is, a survival rate of 70 per cent at 10 years after onset [1]. A hallmark of the disorder is circulating auto-antibodies. It has been proposed that the primary insult is to the microvasculature with activation of the endothelium promoting the recruitment of leukocytes into the extravascular space.

Adhesion molecules borne by both endothelial cells and circulating leukocytes guide the process of extravasation. The selectin family of adhesion molecules is responsible for the early stages of leukocyte adhesion and recruitment involving initial endothelial-leukocyte contact with rolling of the leukocytes on the endothelium. L-selectin (CD62L) is expressed on leukocytes and P- and E-selectin on the endothelium [2]. It has been demonstrated using L-selectin deficient mice that defects in this initial adhesive interaction are responsible for the inability of T cells to home to and be sensitized within peripheral lymph nodes [3]. L-selectin appears to play a critical role in comparison to P- and E-selectin with L-selectin deficient mice essentially equivalent to normal mice treated with antibodies blocking P- and E-selectin [4]. In addition, L-selectin expression on circulating nonspecific effector cells (neutrophils and monocytes) has been suggested to be an important mediator of the primary adhesion of these cells at sites of inflammation [5]. It has been further suggested that L-selectin may exert its effect at inflammatory sites by mediating leukocyte-leukocyte interactions that facilitate the recruitment of neutrophils and lymphocytes [6,7]. Uniquely, L-selectin is shed after cellular activation, retains functional activity in its soluble form and is involved in the regulation of leukocyte attachment to an inflamed endothelium [8]. Circulating soluble L-selectin (sL-selectin) derives mostly from lymphocytes [7,9]. L-selectin ligands are induced on the endothelium of inflammatory sites and the cutaneous sites of chronic inflammation [10]. However, sL-selectin may inhibit the attachment of lymphocytes to cytokine-activated endothelium [8].

Decreased levels of sL-selectin have been found in patients with coronary artery disease or acute respiratory distress syndrome compared to controls and it has been postulated that this reflects ongoing endothelial and leukocyte activation [9,11]. We also report that sL-selectin concentration in plasma was found to be decreased in dSSc cases in comparison to controls but both lSSc cases and controls had similar levels. Levels of sL-selectin have been reported as elevated with concomitant decreased expression on CD8+ cells in SSc [12]. Blann *et al.* had found a lower mean plasma concentration of sL-selectin in 18 SSc patients compared to 42 controls but did not characterize SSc cases as limited (lSSc) or diffuse (dSSc) [13]. Shimada *et al.* reported higher mean sL-selectin levels in plasma in 25 lSSc patients and in 26 dSSc patients compared to their 30 controls [12]. In a murine contact hypersensitivity model, L-selectin was found to mediate infiltration of inflamed skin by CD8+ type 1 cytoxic T (Tc1) cells [14], suggesting that L-selectin is a possible target for therapeutic modulation of skin damage in diffuse cutaneous disease.

The purpose of this preliminary study was to determine in SSc patients, with limited or diffuse disease, whether sL-selectin concentration in plasma is associated with skin damage. The finding of a significant correlation would be a novel result not previously described [15].

Materials and Methods

Objectives

Hypothesis tests were conducted to assess whether sL-selectin in plasma was lower in lSSc and dSSc cases compared to their age- and sex-matched controls. Hypothesis tests were conducted to determine the strength of the linear association between plasma levels of sL-selectin and each of disease severity, disease activity and the modified Rodnan skin score (mRSS) in lSSc and dSSc patient groups.

Participants

Thirty cases with SSc and 30 age- and sex-matched controls participated in this study. All patients were seen at the British Columbia Scleroderma Clinic at St Paul's Hospital in Vancouver which serves the province of British Columbia which has a universal health care insurance system for its population of 4.4 million. Sequential patients, either new or follow up, from a population of 265 SSc patients were enrolled in the study. None approached refused to participate. Healthy controls were recruited from health care staff, hospital volunteers, or partners of patients. All gave informed written consent in compliance with the Declaration of Helsinki and the Research Ethics Boards of the University of British Columbia and the University of Northern British Columbia. All patients fulfilled the American College of Rheumatology Criteria for SSc and were classified as having limited or diffuse disease according to the criteria of LeRoy *et al.* [16]. None of the age- and sex-matched controls had hypertension, known coronary artery disease, diabetes or lung disease.

Each SSc case was age- and sex-matched with one healthy control. Upon statistical analysis, a mismatch with respect to sex was discovered for one male dSSc case so this case-control pair were dropped from any pairwise comparisons and the healthy control from any statistical analysis. For dSSc cases: one match had an age difference of 7 years, 90% of the other matches with controls were within 4 years. For lSSc cases: 100% were matched within 5 years, 89% of the other matches with controls were within

4 years. Age- and sex-matching were done to minimize as much as possible potentially confounding effects of age and gender in a small sample. The cases considered do form a cohort but in the context of this study, only a cross-sectional snapshot in time is considered.

Clinical Variables

Disease duration was measured from the onset of the first non-Raynaud's phenomenon. Skin involvement was assessed using the modified Rodnan skin score at 17 different body areas [17]. Disease severity for each patient was evaluated on the degree of involvement of nine organ systems using the Medsger scale [18] and then summed. Disease activity was scored by the indices developed by Valentini *et al.* in which ten clinical items are given weighted scores on a scale of zero (no activity) to ten (maximal activity) [19]. Active ulcers were documented at the time of phlebotomy and classified as previously described [20,21]. Pulmonary function was examined but only predicted forced vital capacity (FVC) and predicted diffusing level of carbon monoxide (DLCO) are reported. All clinical variables were recorded at time of plasma collection or within 2 months prior.

In the instance of variables relating to physical assessment by a rheumatologist, these were obtained from clinical record review by the rheumatologist who did the physical assessment. All imaging, lung function and blood test results were obtained from record review by the rheumatologist or pulmonologist who ordered the tests. The pulmonary function tests were conducted by respiratory technicians under the supervision of an MD specialist.

sL-selectin Concentration

All plasma samples from cases and controls were aliquoted and stored at −80 C until analysis. Plasma levels of sL-selectin were measured using a Searchlight Custom Array (Pierce Searchlight Products, Thermo Fisher Scientific Woburn, Massachusetts, USA) and analyzed using a 16-bit Searchlight CCD imaging and analysis system (Pierce Biotechnology, Rockford, Illinois, USA).

Ethics Statement

Research was carried out in compliance with the Helsinki Declaration of 1975, as revised in 1983, and approved by the Research Ethics Boards of The University of British Columbia and The University of Northern British Columbia. All participants signed informed consent forms approved by the Research Ethics Board of The University of British Columbia.

Statistical Analysis

Estimates of location are reported as a mean ± SE. Given small sample sizes, nonparametric methods were used for comparisons. Statistical calculations and graphing were done using release 2.11.1 of the R statistical software system [22]. Normality was assessed by the Shapiro-Wilk test. Welch's version of the two-sample *t* test was used when homoscedasticity (equal variances) was not assumed. The *stats* package in R was used to calculate the exact *P* values for the Wilcoxon test of no shift in location for matched case-control pairs. The *coin* package in R was used to calculate the exact *P* values for the Mann-Whitney test for location with two independent random samples [23].

Results

Demographics and Clinical Features of Patients

Blood samples were available for 19 patients diagnosed with lSSc and 11 with dSSc (Table 1). No gender difference in age was detected for lSSc patients (p = 0.9773) or for dSSc patients (p = 0.6970). Combining genders, patients diagnosed with lSSc had a mean (±SE) age of 58.53±2.50 years (range: 36–74 years) while patients diagnosed with dSSc had a mean age of 49.64±3.17 years (range: 30–65 years). The difference in median age between lSSc and dSSc is statistically significant (p = 0.0399).

No gender difference in disease duration was detected for lSSc (p = 0.6895) or for dSSc (p = 0.8485) patients. Combining genders, patients diagnosed with lSSc had a mean (±SE) disease duration of 10.68±2.68 years (range: 1–43 years) whilst patients diagnosed with dSSc had a mean disease duration of 2.91±0.48 years (range: 2–11 years). Disease duration is significantly shorter (p = 0.0381) in dSSc cases compared to lSSc as expected.

A gender difference in mRSS was detected between the 18 women and the sole man for lSSc (p = 0.0004) but not amongst men and women for dSSc (p = 0.7576). Mean (±SE) mRSS was 9.05±1.29 (range: 1–20) in lSSc cases and 22.82±2.82 (range: 4–36) in dSSc cases. Skin score is worse in dSSc cases compared to lSSc as expected (p = 0.0002).

There was no difference in location of the distribution of disease severity scores between women and the single man with lSSc (p = 0.2774) or amongst the female and male dSSc patients (p>0.9999). Combining genders, patients diagnosed with lSSc had

a mean (±SE) disease severity index of 7.00±0.78 (range: 2–16). Patients diagnosed with dSSc had a mean maximum disease severity index of 7.18±0.91 (range: 2–11).

There was a difference in location of the distribution of activity scores between the 18 women and the single man with lSSc (p = 0.0033) but not amongst the female and male dSSc patients (p = 0.7662). Combining genders, patients diagnosed with lSSc had a mean (±SE) activity index of 3.39±0.38 (range: 1–18). Patients diagnosed with dSSc had a mean activity index of 4.27±0.75 (range: 1–8).

There was no statistically significant difference between lSSc and dSSc cases with respect to the location of the distribution of the disease severity index ($p = 0.6638$). Likewise, there was no difference between lSSc and dSSc cases with respect to the location of the distribution of the disease activity index ($p = 0.7662$). It is speculated that the lack difference in disease severity and activity between the limited and diffuse forms of the disease are a consequence of either aggressive clinical management or referral bias, or both, in this population of patients being treated in a tertiary scleroderma clinic serving 4.4 million people in the province of British Columbia, Canada.

Table 1. Demographics, auto-antibodies and treatments.

Variable	lSSc Estimate	Count	dSSc Estimate	Count
Proportion Female:Male	18.0:1	18:1	1.2:1	6:5
Modified Rodnan Skin Score	9.05±1.29	19	22.82±2.82	11
Severity Index	7.00±0.78	18	7.18±0.91	11
Activity Index	3.39±0.38	18	4.27±0.75	11
Duration of Disease	10.68±2.68 yr	19	2.91±0.48 yr	11
Age				
Cases	58.53±2.50 yr	19	49.64±3.17 yr	11
Controls	59.42±2.53 yr	19	49.80±3.64 yr	10
Lung				
ILD	47.4±11.5%	19	63.6±14.5%	11
PAH	47.4±11.5%	19	36.4±14.5%	11
FVC Predicted	86.6±4.5%	16	73.4±6.5%	11
DLCO Predicted	63.1±4.9%	19	64.8±8.3%	10
Telangiectasia	17.6±9.2%	17	20.0±12.6%	10
Digits				
Raynaud's	100%	18	100%	11
Active digital ulcers	35.3±11.6%	17	30.0±14.5%	10
No. of digits with active digits ulcers	0.71±0.28	17	0.88±0.48	9
Contracture of phalanges	41.2±11.9%	17	63.6±14.5%	11
Autoantibodies				
ACA positive	15.8±8.4%	19	0%	11
ANA positive	84.2±8.4%	19	90.1±8.7%	11
Scl-70 positive	15.8±8.4%	19	72.7±13.4%	11
Treatment				
Methotrexate	0%	19	18.2±11.6%	11
Cyclophosphamide	0%	19	45.5±15.0%	11

Values given as mean ± SE or proportion ± SE if a percentage is indicated.

On the basis of the preceding statistical analyses, decisions were made to disregard gender but treat limited and diffuse forms of SSc as distinct.

With regard to autoantibodies and treatment modalities, dSSc and lSSc cases have distinctly different profiles (Table 1).

mRSS, Severity and Activity

The distribution of mRSS appears to be normal for both lSSc (p = 0.3300) and dSSc (p = 0.2318) cases. Assuming normality, the estimate of the mean for mRSS is 9.05 (95 per cent CI: 6.35, 11.76) and 22.82 (95 per cent CI: 16.52, 29.11) in lSSc and dSSc cases, respectively. As expected, the means for lSSc and dSSc cases are significantly different by Welch's two-sample t test (p = 0.0005, 95 per cent CI: 7.12, 20.41). In fact, mean mRSS is significantly lower in lSSc cases compared to dSSc cases (Figure 1 A).

The distribution of the disease severity index appears to be normal for both lSSc (p = 0.2490) and dSSc (p = 0.6222). Without

assuming equal variances, the means are not different by Welch's two-sample t test (p = 0.8812, 95 per cent CI: −2.31, 2.67).

The distribution of the disease activity index appears to be normal for both lSSc (p = 0.5294) and dSSc (p = 0.9512). Without assuming equal variances, the means are not different by Welch's two-sample t test (p = 0.3086, 95 per cent CI: −0.90, 2.67).

sL-selectin Concentration

The distribution of sL-selectin concentration appears to be normal for controls (p = 0.1329), lSSc (p = 0.4153) and dSSc (p = 0.3657) cases. The point estimate of the mean sL-selectin concentration is 906 (95 per cent CI: 834, 978) ng/ml in controls. The point estimate of the mean sL-selectin concentration is 961 (95 per cent CI: 833, 1090) ng/ml and 755 (95 per cent CI: 628, 882) ng/ml in lSSc and dSSc cases, respectively. Because sL-selectin concentration was measured in controls as well as cases, it is possible to test the null hypothesis of no location shift between cases with pairwise matched controls. One male dSSc case did not match a female control and so both were dropped from comparison for sL-selectin. Because the number of pairs is 19 for lSSc and only 10 for dSSc, it would be prudent to use the nonparametric Wilcoxon signed rank test instead of the matched pairs t test. There appears to be no shift of location for lSSc cases (p = 0.2753) but there does appear to be a shift for dSSc cases (p = 0.0273). Nevertheless, and consistently, a paired t test for the mean difference for lSSc cases compared to their matched controls is statistically insignificant (p = 0.2424, 95 per cent CI: −62, 229 ng/ml) while the mean difference for dSSc cases compared to their matched controls is statistically significant (p = 0.0369, 95 per cent CI: −362, −14 ng/ml). The mean sL-selectin concentrations for lSSc and dSSc cases are significantly different by Welch's two-sample t test (p = 0.0005, 95 per cent CI: 7, 20 ng/ml). So we can conclude that the mean sL-selectin concentration for dSSc is lower than that of either lSSc cases or controls (Figure 1 B).

Association between sL-selectin Concentration and mRSS

The standard test assuming normality for a linear relationship between mRSS and sL-selectin concentration in lSSc cases is statistically insignificant (0.9944). The point estimate of the simple correlation coefficient is 0.00172 with 95 per cent confidence interval (−0.45284, .45558). The point estimate of Spearman's rho, the nonparametric counterpart, is −0.0026 (p = 0.9914).

The standard test assuming normality for a linear relationship between mRSS and sL-selectin concentration in dSSc cases is highly statistically significant (p = 0.0008). The point estimate of the simple correlation coefficient is −0.855021 with 95 per cent confidence interval (−0.96166, -.52381). The point estimate of Spearman's rho, the nonparametric counterpart, is −0.72189 (p = 0.0121).

P-values for tests of normality for the residuals of the simple linear regression model for mRSS as a function of sL-selectin concentration are 0.3318 and 0.5165 for lSSc and dSSc cases, respectively. Thus there is no need to resort to the nonparametric alternative of Spearman's rho.

We conclude that the separate simple linear regression models for each of lSSc and dSSc cases fit the data well (Figure 2). The slope of the regression line for lSSc cases is not different from zero (p = 0.9944). The estimate of the slope of the regression line for dSSc is (−0.04224, 95 per cent CI: −0.06156, −0.02292 $(ng/ml)^{-1}$).

Cyclophosphamide (CYC) has been implicated in the reduction of CD34+ cells expressing L-selectin [24]. Likewise, the combination of CYC, methotrexate (MTX) and an infusion of CD62L+ T cells expressing L-selectin has been associated with improved disease-free and overall survival in patients receiving allogeneic

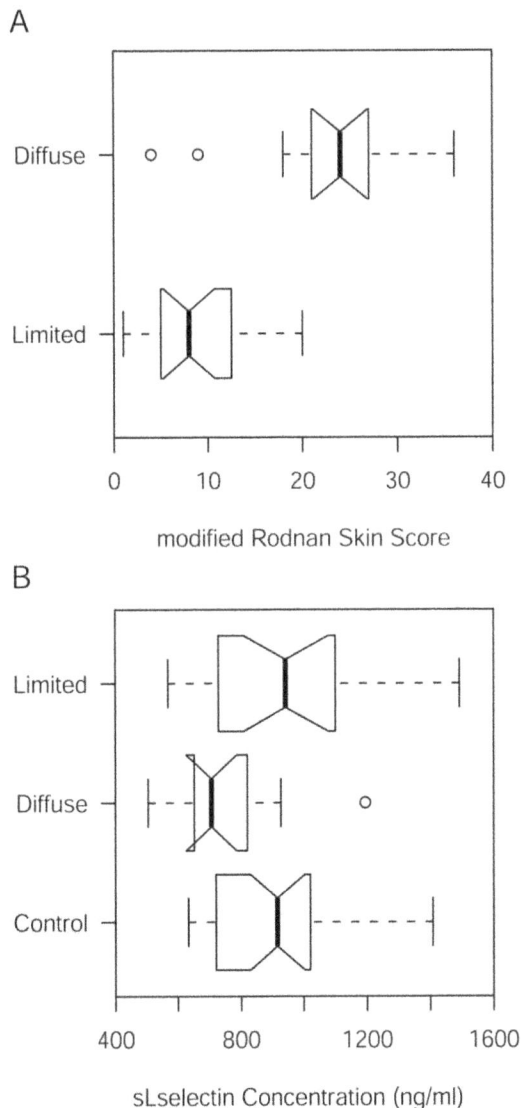

Figure 1. Notched boxplots of mRSS and sL-selectin. If the notches overlap in a pairwise comparison then the difference is significant at the 5% level for the individual test. (A) Notched boxplot of mRSS. (B) Notched boxplot of sL-selectin.

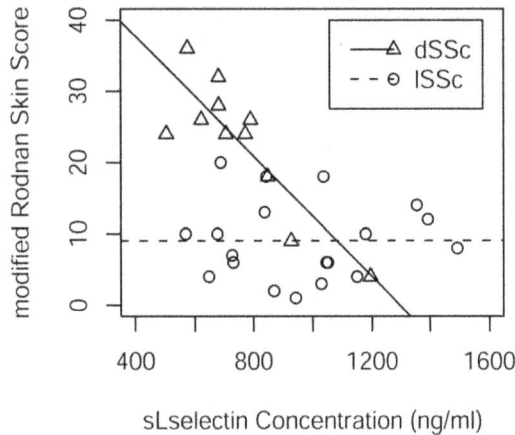

Figure 2. Scatterplot of mRSS and sL-selectin for lSSc and dSSc cases. There are separate least squares regression lines for each of lSSc and dSSc cases.

hematopoietic stem cell transplants [25]. As 6 of the 11 dSSc patients were receiving CYC and another 2 were receiving MTX, hypothesis tests were conducted separately for the inclusion of CYC status and MTX status with sL-selectin in the linear model for mRSS (Figure 3). The tests for CYC (p = 0.7652) and MTX (p = 0.6795) were negative for inclusion as was the test for inclusion of both (p = 0.8950).

To allay concerns about a dosage-duration effect, we did a chart review and found with one exception that all dSSc patients who had been on either cyclophosphamide or methotrexate were on it for 2 years or less and maintained high mRSS scores. The one exception was the patient in Figure 3 with the second lowest modified Rodnan skin score who had been on oral cyclosphosphamide for 4 years and maintained a low score for the two years prior to testing from an initial score of 30. Running a test whereby this patient is dropped from the simple linear regression analysis, we find the estimate of Pearson's correlation coefficient to be −0.85045 (P = 0.00182) and Spearman's rank correlation to be −0.62767 (p = 0.05198). With the patient included, the estimate of Pearson's correlation coefficient is −0.855021 (p = 0.0008) and

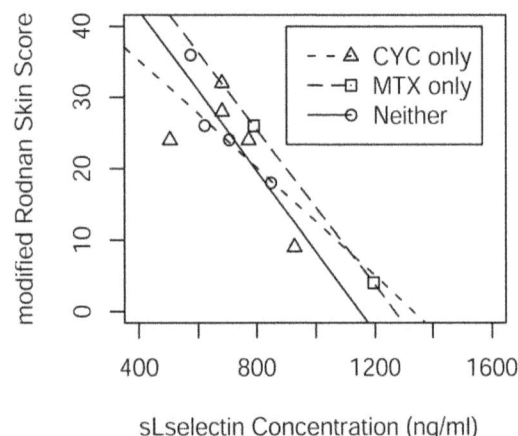

Figure 3. Scatterplot of mRSS and sL-selectin indicating drug prescribed for dSSc cases only. There are separate least squares regression lines for dSSc cases receiving cyclophosphamide (CYC) only, methotrexate (MTX) only, and neither.

Spearman's rank correlation is −0.72189 (p = 0.0121). In short, there is not much of a difference with or without the patient.

Association between sL-selectin Concentration and Disease Severity

The standard test assuming normality for a linear relationship between disease severity and sL-selectin concentration in lSSc cases is statistically insignificant (p = 0.2596). The point estimate of the simple correlation coefficient is −0.28048 with 95 per cent confidence interval (−0.66082, 0.21448). The point estimate of Spearman's rho, the nonparametric counterpart, is −0.3738 (p = 0.1265).

The standard test assuming normality for a linear relationship between disease severity and sL-selectin concentration in dSSc cases is highly statistically significant (p = 0.0007). The point estimate of the simple correlation coefficient is −0.85795 with 95 per cent confidence interval (−0.96247, −0.53174). The point estimate of Spearman's rho, the nonparametric counterpart, is −0.7717 (p = 0.0054).

P-values for tests of normality for the residuals of the simple linear regression model for disease severity as a function of sL-selectin concentration are 0.3396 and 0.5167 for lSSc and dSSc cases, respectively. Thus there is no need to resort to the nonparametric alternative of Spearman's rho.

We conclude that the separate simple linear regression models for each of lSSc and dSSc cases fit the data well. The slope of the regression line for lSSc cases is not different from zero (p = 0.2596). The estimate of the slope of the regression line for dSSc is (−0.01370, 95 per cent CI: −0.01988, −0.00751 (ng/ml)$^{-1}$).

Association between sL-selectin Concentration and Disease Activity

The standard test assuming normality for a linear relationship between disease activity and sL-selectin concentration in lSSc cases is statistically insignificant (p = 0.7575). The point estimate of the simple correlation coefficient is −0.07828 with 95 per cent confidence interval (−0.52593, 0.40333). The point estimate of Spearman's rho, the nonparametric counterpart, is −0.20313 (p = 0.4188).

The standard test assuming normality for a linear relationship between activity and sL-selectin concentration in dSSc cases is highly statistically significant (p = 0.0007). The point estimate of the simple correlation coefficient is −0.85897 with 95 per cent confidence interval (−0.96276, −0.53451). The point estimate of Spearman's rho, the nonparametric counterpart, is −0.87416 (p = 0.0004).

P-values for tests of normality for the residuals of the simple linear regression model for severity as a function of sL-selectin concentration are 0.5177 and 0.4891 for lSSc and dSSc cases, respectively. Thus there is no need to resort to the nonparametric alternative of Spearman's rho.

We conclude that the separate simple linear regression models for each of lSSc and dSSc cases fit the data well. The slope of the regression line for lSSc cases is not different from zero (p = 0.0071). The estimate of the slope of the regression line for dSSc is (−0.01125, 95 per cent CI: −0.01631, −0.00619 (ng/ml)$^{-1}$).

Discussion

We found no statistically significant linear association between sL-selectin concentration and either of disease severity (p = 0.2596), disease activity (p = 0.7575) or mRSS (p = 0.9944) in lSSc cases. But we did find statistically significant associations in dSSc cases between sL-selectin concentration and each of disease severity (p = 0.0007), activity (p = 0.0007) and mRSS (p = 0.0008). The amount of variation in dSSc cases for each of disease severity, disease activity, and mRSS explained by a linear relationship with sL-selectin is 73.61 per cent, 73.78 per cent and 73.11 per cent, respectively. The amount of variation explained by the linear association with sL-selectin is arguably the lowest for mRSS amongst the three variables but we have chosen to focus in this discussion on the skin score mRSS because in part the other two indices are functions of mRSS. The definition for disease activity adds 0.5 to a maximum score of 10 if mRSS exceeds 14 [19], whereas, that for disease severity has a graded approach with zero (mRSS = 0), 1 (1 ≤ mRSS ≤ 14), 2 (15 ≤ mRSS ≤ 29), 3 (30 ≤ mRSS ≤ 39) and 4 (mRSS ≥ 40) [18]. Moreover, it can be argued that either the disease activity index or disease severity score capture only an additional 0.67 and 0.5 per cent, respectively, of variation for all the other organs combined. Disease activity has additional variables for skin but also for the heart, lungs, muscles, kidneys, and vasculature. Disease severity assesses these and the gastrointestinal tract too. There is also the issue of no statistically significant difference in mean disease severity and mean disease activity between lSSc and dSSc cases (p = 0.8812, p = 0.3086, respectively) but a striking statistically significant difference in mean mRSS (p = 0.0005) in this group of patients from a tertiary referral facility for scleroderma patients.

We found that sL-selectin levels are low in dSSc cases compared to their controls and within the range of normal controls for lSSc cases. We showed a significant negative relationship between sL-selectin and the magnitude of skin involvement in dSSc. This suggests that sL-selectin could serve as a blood biomarker of the extent of skin involvement in dSSc. It also implicates a possible pathogenic role for L-selectin in the chronic inflammatory obliterative microvasculopathy of dSSc.

Blann et al. found a lower mean (±SE) plasma concentration of sL-selectin of 797±71 ng/ml in 18 SSc patients compared to 1 244±42 ng/ml in 42 controls (P ≤ 0.0001) but did not characterize SSc cases as limited or diffuse [13]. The results of Blann et al. are comparable to our estimates of the mean plasma concentration of soluble serum sL-selectin in dSSc cases (p = 0.6498) and for lSSc cases (p = 0.0890) but not our controls (p<0.0001) (Table 1). However, caution in interpreting these hypothesis tests must be exercised because of the difference in assay methods.

Shimada et al. reported higher mean (±SE) sL-selectin serum levels in 25 lSSc patients (1 280±130 ng/ml) and in 26 dSSc patients (1 830±324 ng/ml) compared to their 30 controls (990±450 ng/ml) [12]. The differences between Shimada et al. mean values and ours are unclear but may be due to different antibodies and techniques used to measure sL-selectin. Inaoki et al. also reported significantly (p<0.0100) higher mean (±SE) sL-selectin serum levels in 24 SSc patients (2 260±1590 ng/ml) compared to 20 age- and sex-matched controls (1 200±400 ng/ml) [26]. Sato et al. similarly reported significantly (0.0100<p<0.0500) higher mean (±SE) sL-selectin serum levels in 32 SSc patients (1 500±1300 ng/ml) compared to 20 age- and sex-matched controls (900±400 ng/ml) [15]. The articles by Shimada et al., Inaoki et al., and Sato et al. were all published in 2001 from the same laboratory at Kanazawa University in Japan using the same assay. As the counts of cases and controls are not equal in each of these three articles, it is not know how the matching was done. As it is possible that there is an overlap in cases for the three articles, a meta analysis is not possible. Spertini et al. showed no difference in the concentration of sL-selectin measured in serum as compared to plasma for the assay method of the three papers from the laboratory at Kanazawa University [27].

Differences in assay, however, has no bearing on the finding in these three articles of significantly higher levels of sL-selectin in serum in SSc cases compared to healthy controls. This is just the opposite of findings by Blann et al. and this study. Neither Sfikakis et al. [28] or Ates et al. [29] found a significant difference in the location of serum sL-selectin levels between cases and controls but neither study differentiated between lSSc and dSSc.

All studies are limited by being cross-sectional on a small number of patients. Clearly larger sample sizes are necessary.

A major point of departure for this study compared to its predecessors is the examination of the relationship between the concentration of soluble L-selectin and the modified Rodnan skin score in lSSc and dSSc cases, separately. Blann et al. [13], Shimada et al. [12], Inaoki et al. [26], Sfikakis et al. [28], and Ates et al. [29] did not examine the relationship between the concentration of soluble L-selectin and the modified Rodnan skin score. Incidental to their report of interleukin-6 and interleukin-10 correlating with mRSS, Sato et al. [15] stated: "Furthermore, multiple regression analysis showed that modified Rodnan TSS was significantly positively correlated with serum IL-6 levels (P<0.05) and IL-10 levels (P<0.005), but not with other soluble mediators." Presumably, Sato et al. did not estimate correlation coefficients for their 16 lSSc and 16 dSSc cases separately. Additionally, Sato et al. did not explicitly report an estimate of the correlation coefficient between mRSS and sL-selection serum concentrations in the pooled lSSc and dSSc patients.

This preliminary study has more lSSc cases than the number of SSc cases in Blann et al. [13]. It has more lSSc cases than either Sfikakis et al. [28], Shimada et al. [12], Inaoki et al. [26], or Sato et al. [15]. This study has as many SSc cases as Ates et al. [29] but this study differentiates between limited and diffuse forms of systemic sclerosis while Ates et al. [29] did not. There are more controls in this study than either Shimada et al. [12], Inaoki et al. [26], Sato et al. [15]. or Ates et al. [29].

In a contact-hypersensitivity murine model, L-selectin deficient mice exhibit a reduction of Tc1 infiltration in inflamed skin compared to wild type [14]. As well, a bleomycin-induced murine model of SSc demonstrated that Th2 and Th17 cell infiltration into skin and lungs was inhibited by L-selectin while L-selectin loss attenuated the development of fibrosis [30]. In a tight skin (L-selectin −/− TSK+) mouse model, however, skin thickness was similar to the skin thickness of TSK+ wild type mice [31]. DNA microarray studies of cutaneous gene expression in a murine sclerodermatous graft-versus-host disease model show mRNA for cell adhesion molecules are upregulated. L-selection, vascular adhesion molecule-1 and intercellular adhesion molecule-1 are upregulated during the early inflammatory phase of cutaneous fibrosis [32]. This suggests that interference with the selectins and their ligands may be useful candidates for treatment of SSc beginning with dSSc cases.

Soluble L-selectin is generated by the shedding of the L-selectin molecule from the surfaces of neutrophil granulocytes and lymphocytes. It has been reported in a study done in Japan that while the frequency of expression on L-selectin on $CD8^+$ T cells was insignificantly different (p>0.0500) in the peripheral blood of 14 SSc cases compared with to 18 health controls, the frequency of expression of L-selectin on the $CD161^+CD8^+$ subset of T cells was significantly increased (p<0.0100) in SSc cases compared to health controls [33]. But the frequency and total number of $CD161^+CD8^+$ T cells in SSc cases was decreased significantly (p<0.0500, p<0.0010, respectively) compared to healthy controls so it is unclear as to whether L-selectin concentration from T cell sources would increase or decrease in SSc cases compared to health controls based on this study from Japan.

Adverse outcomes and posttraumatic complications after surgical trauma have been associated with low levels of sL-selectin and decreased L-selectin expression. Stimulation with tumor necrosis factor alpha (TNF-α) has been shown to effect a significant decrease in L-selectin expression [34]. Taking the diffuse cutaneous form of SSc as a chronic inflammatory disease suggests a possible therapeutic role of a TNF-α blocker, or other biologics, or interference with the selectins or their ligands, in reducing skin damage in SSc patients through the effect of increased L-selectin expression, which can in turn be monitored by looking for increasing soluble L-selectin in the plasma of patients. Elevated serum levels of sL-selectin have been found in SSc patients after intravenous injection of lipo-postaglandin E_1 which is known to have anti-inflammatory effects on endothelial cells and subsets of leukocytes [26]. Candidates for TNF-α inhibitors include the circulating receptor fusion protein etanercept and the monoclonal antibodies rituximab, infliximab, adalimumab, certolizumab pegol, and golimumab. Although a systematic literature review has shown promising results in small-enrolment clinical trials with respect to histological skin changes for rituximab [35], systematic literature reviews have not revealed consistent statistically significant results for skin score for etanercept, rituximab or infliximab in small-enrolment clinical trials [35,36]. A clinical study of 72 SSc cases receiving rituximab that were recruited from 27 European centers showed significant improvements in mRSS ($p = 0.0002$) after 7 months on the drugs, total number of digital ulcers ($p = 0.0086$), creatine kinase levels ($p = 0.0300$) and the European SSc activity score ($p = 0.0100$) but not lung fibrosis, DAS-28, or S-HAQ [37]. This is promising but larger multi-center randomized controlled trials with adequate power are needed before the book is closed on TNF-α blockers, or other treatment modalities, in the context of skin damage in SSc [38].

We conclude that sL-selectin is decreased in subjects with dSSc and showed a negative correlation with the magnitude of skin disease (mRSS). Moreover in dSSc, for each increase of 100 ng/ml in sL-selectin concentration, the modified Rodnan skin score drops 4.22 (95 per cent CI: 2.29, 6.16). Disease severity and disease activity in dSSc cases drop 1.37 (95 per cent CI: 0.75, 1.99) and 1.13 (95 per cent CI: 0.062, 1.63), respectively, for each increase of 100 ng/ml in sL-selectin concentration. The theoretical range in values for disease severity, disease activity, and mRSS are [0, 36], [0, 10] and [0, 51], respectively, while the observed ranges of our sample of dSSc cases were [2,11], [0.5, 8] and [4,36], respectively. Thus the drops in disease severity, disease activity and mRSS in dSSc cases for an increase of 100 ng/ml in sL-selectin concentration for disease severity disease activity and mRSS are comparable to a good approximation and in concordance with the postulate that improvement in the skin score is the driving force.

Serum levels of sL-selectin have been shown to increase in acute inflammatory conditions while those with chronic disease have been shown to have low levels suggesting an important role for sL-selectin in modulating chronic inflammatory diseases [9]. The key significance of the finding of a significant negative correlation between mRSS and sL-selectin concentration in the plasma of dSSc patients is the suggestion that *in vivo* modulation of L-selectin, or its ligands, is a pathway for reducing collagen deposition, fibrosis, and avascularization in the skin (the body's largest organ) in the most desperate of patients with systemic sclerosis, that is, those patients with the diffuse form of the disease. Modulating sL-selectin thus presents a potential therapeutic target for addressing skin damage in dSSc patients.

Limitations

While comparable with the published literature for SSc, this study is limited by the small samples of lSSc and dSSc cases. There were two independent sets of multiple hypothesis tests for each of lSSc and dSSc. For an overall 0.05 level of significance, a conservative Bonferroni correction would thus be a level of $0.05 \div 26 = 0.0019$ for each individual test. This level was exceeded for the tests of linear association assuming normality between sL-selectin and each of mRSS ($p = 0.0008$), disease severity ($p = 0.0007$) and activity ($p = 0.0007$) for the dSSc cases only.

Future Research

While participant recruitment continues at the British Columbia Scleroderma Clinic to increase sample size for the purpose of improving the power of hypothesis tests used herein, a proposal for a prospective international multi-center study, with a protocol common to all centers, is being developed.

Acknowledgments

Thanks for laboratory work to Anna Meredith and Elizabeth Whalen with the James Hogg Heart and Lung Institute at St. Paul's Hospital and The University of British Columbia, Vancouver, British Columbia, Canada. Thanks also for assistance with statistical analysis to William Petrcich with the Department of Mathematics and Statistics at The University of Northern British Columbia, Prince George, British Columbia, Canada.

Author Contributions

Conceived and designed the experiments: JVD. Performed the experiments: JVD SvE. Analyzed the data: JVD SvE KJK. Contributed reagents/materials/analysis tools: JVD SvE KJK. Wrote the paper: JVD SvE KJK.

References

1. Elhai M, Meune C, Avouac J, Kahan A, Allanore Y (2012) Trends in mortality in patients with systemic sclerosis over 40 years: a systematic review and meta-analysis of cohort studies. Rheumatology 51: 1017–1026.

2. Kansas GS (1996) Selectins and their ligands-current concepts and controversies (review). Blood 88: 3259–3287.

3. Catalina MD, Carroll MC, Arizpe H, Takashima A, Estess P, et al. (1996) The route of antigen entry determines the requirement for L-selectin in immune responses. J Exp Med 184: 2341–2351.

4. Catalina MD, Estess P, Siegelman MH (1999) Selective requirements for leukocyte adhesion molecules in models of acute and chronic cutaneous inflammation: participation of E- and P- but not L-selectin. Blood 93: 580–589.

5. Arbones ML, Ord DC, Ley K, Ratech H, Maynard CC, et al. (1994) Lymphocyte homing and leucocyte rolling and migration are impaired in L-selectin-deficient mice. Immunity 1: 247–260.

6. Bargatze RF, Kurk S, Butcher EC, Jutila MA (1994) Neutrophils roll on adherent neutrophils bound to cytokine-induced endothelial cells via L-selectin on the rolling cells. J Exp Med 180: 1785–1792.

7. Tang MLK, Steeber DA, Zhang X-Q, Tedder TF (1998) Intrinsic differences in L-selectin expression levels affect T and B lymphocyte subset-specific recirculation pathways. J Immunol 160: 5113–5121.

8. Schleiffenbaum B, Spertini O, Tedder TF (1992) Soluble L-selectin is present in human plasma at high levels and maintains functional activity. J Cell Biol 199: 229–238.

9. Haught WH, Mansour M, Rothlein R, Kishimoto TK, Mainolfli EA, et al. (1996) Alterations in circulating intracellular adhesion molecule-1 and L-selectin: further evidence for chronic inflammation in ischemic heart disease. Am Heart J 132: 1–8.

10. Michie SA, Streeter PR, Bolt PA, Butcher EC, Picker LJ (1993) The human peripheral lymph node vascular addressin. An inducible endothelial antigen involved in lymphocyte homing. Am J Pathol 143: 1688–1698.

11. Donnelly SC, Haslett C, Dransfield I, Robertson CE, Carter DC, et al. (1994) Role of selectins in development of adult respiratory distress syndrome. Lancet 344: 215–219.

12. Shimada Y, Hasegawa K, Takehara K, Sato S (2001) Elevated serum L-selectin levels and decreased L-selectin expression on CD8+ lymphocytes in systemic sclerosis. Clin Exp Immunol 124: 474–479.

13. Blann AD, Sanders PA, Herrick A, Jayson MIV (1996) Soluble L-selectin in the connective tissue diseases. Br J Haematol 95: 192–194.

14. Hirata T, Furie BC, Furie B (2002) P-, E-, and L-selectin mediate migration of activated CD8+ T lymphocytes into inflamed skin. J Immunol 169: 4307–4313.

15. Sato S, Hasegawa M, Takehara K (2001) Serum levels of interleukin-6 and interleukin-10 correlate with total skin thickness score in patients with systemic sclerosis. Journal of Dermatological Science 27: 140–146.

16. LeRoy EC, Black C, Fleischmajer R, Jablonska S, Krieg T, et al. (1988) Scleroderma (systemic sclerosis): classification, subsets and pathogenesis. J Rheumatol 15: 202–205.

17. Clements P LP, Siebold J, White B, Weiner S, et al. (1995) Inter and intraobserver variability of total skin score (modified Rodnan TSS) in systemic sclerosis. J Rheumatol 22: 1281–1285.

18. Medsger Jr TA, Bombardieri S, Czirjak L, Scorza R, Della Rossa A, et al. (2003) Assessment of disease severity and prognosis. Clin Exp Rheumatol 21: S42–S46.

19. Valentini G, Silman AJ, Veale D (2003) Assessment of disease activity. Clin Exp Rheumatol 21: S39–S41.

20. Keen KJ, van Eeden SF, Dunne JV (2012) Limited cutaneous and diffuse cutaneous scleroderma: circulating biomarkers differentiate lung involvement. Rheumatology: Current Research S:1. Available: http://www.omicsonline.org/2161-1149/2161-1149-S1-006.pdf. Accessed 16 August 2012.

21. Dunne JV, Keen KJ, van Eeden SF (2012) Circulating angiopoietin and Tie-2 levels in systemic sclerosis. Rheumatology International: In press. DOI: 10.1007/s00296-012-2378-4. Accessed 16 August 2012.

22. R Development Core Team (2010) R: A language and environment for statistical computing Vienna, Austria: R Foundation for Statistical Computing.

23. Hothorn T, Hornik K, van de Wiel MA, Zeileis A (2008) Implementing a class of permutation tests: the coin package. Journal of Statistical Software 28: 1–23.

24. Gazitt Y, Shaugnessy P, Liu Q (2001) Expression of adhesion molecules on CD34+ cells in peripheral blood of Non-Hodgkin's lymphoma patients mobilized with different growth factors. Stem Cells 19: 134–143.

25. Vela-Ojeda J, Montiel-Cervantes L, Granados-Lara P, Reyes-Maldonado E, Garcia-Latorre E, et al. (2010) Role of CD4+ CD25+ highFoxp3+ CD62L+ regulatory T cells and invariant NKT cells in human allogenic hematopoietic stem cell transplantation. Stem Cells Dev 19: 333–340.

26. Inaoki M, Sato S, Shimada Y, Takehara K (2001) Elevated serum levels of soluable L-selectin in patients with systemic sclerosis declined after intravenous injection of lipo-postaglandin E$_1$. Journal of Dermatological Science 25: 78–82.

27. Spertini O, Schleiffenbaum B, White-Owen C, Philip Ruiz J, Tedder TT (1992) ELISA for quantification of L-selectin shed from leukocytes in vivo. Journal of Immunological Methods 156: 115–123.

28. Sfikakis PP, Charalambopoulos D, Vaiopoulos G, Mavrikakis M (1999) Circulating P- and L-Selectin and T-Lymphocyte Activation in Patients with Autoimmune Rheumatic Diseases. Clin Rheum 18: 28–32.

29. Ates A, Kinikli G, Turgay M, Duman M (2004) Serum-Soluble Selectin Levels in Patients with Rheumatoid Arthritis and Systemic Scleroris. Scand J Immunol 59: 315–320.

30. Yoshizaki A, Yanaba K, Iwata Y, Komura K, Ogawa A, et al. (2010) Cell Adhesion Molecules Regulate Fibrotic Process via Th1/Th2/Th17 Cell Balance in a Bleomycin-Induced Scleroderma Model. J Immunol 185: 2502–2515.

31. Matsushita T, Hasegawa M, Hamaguchi Y, Takehara K, Sato S (2006) Longitudinal analysis of serum cytokine concentrations in systemic sclerosis: association of interleukin 12 elevation with spontaneous regression of skin sclerosis. Journal of Rheumatology 33: 275–284.

32. Zhou L, Askew D, Wu C, Gilliam AC (2007) Cutaneous gene expression by DNA microarray in murine sclerodermatous graft-versus-host disease, a model for human scleroderma. Journal of Investigative Dermatology 127: 281–292.

33. Mitsuo A, Morimoto S, Nakiri Y, Suzuki J, Kaneko H, et al. (2006) Decreased CD161+CD8+ T cells in the peripheral blood of patients suffering from rheumatic diseases. Rheumatology 45: 1477–1484.

34. Mommsen P, Bakhausen T, Hildebrand F, Zeckey C, Krettek C, et al. (2011) Regulation of L-selectin expression by trauma-relevant cytokines. Pathol Res Pract 207: 142–147.

35. Daoussis D, Liossis S-NC, Yiannopoulos G, Andonopoulos AP (2011) B-cell depletion therapy in systemic sclerosis: experimental rationale and update on clinical evidence. International Journal of Rheumatology 2011. Available: http://www.hindawi.com/journals/ijr/2011/214013. Accessed 16 August 2012.

36. Phumethum V, Jamal S, Johnson SR (2011) Biologic therapy for systemic sclerosis: a systematic review. J Rheumatol 38: 289–296.

37. Jordan S, Distler J, Maurer B, Allanore Y, Laar JV, et al. (2012) Safety and efficacy of rituximab in SSc: an analysis from European Scleroderma Trial and Research Group. Rheumatology 51 (suppl 2): ii25–ii26.

38. Distler JHW, Jordan S, Airo P, Alegre-Sancho JJ, Allanore Y, et al. (2011) Is there a role for TNF-alpha antagonists in the treatment of SSc? EUSTAR expert consensus development using the Delphi technique. Clin Exp Rheumatol 29: S40–S45.

14

In Vivo Dioxin Favors Interleukin-22 Production by Human CD4+ T Cells in an Aryl Hydrocarbon Receptor (AhR)-Dependent Manner

Nicolò Costantino Brembilla[1]*, Jean-Marie Ramirez[1], Rachel Chicheportiche[1], Olivier Sorg[2], Jean-Hilaire Saurat[2], Carlo Chizzolini[1]

1 Department of Immunology and Allergy, Swiss Centre for Applied Human Toxicology, University Hospital and School of Medicine, Geneva, Switzerland, 2 Department of Dermato-Toxicology, Swiss Centre for Applied Human Toxicology, University Hospital and School of Medicine, Geneva, Switzerland

Abstract

Background: The transcription factor aryl hydrocarbon receptor (AhR) mediates the effects of a group of chemicals known as dioxins, ubiquitously present in our environment. However, it is poorly known how the *in vivo* exposure to these chemicals affects in humans the adaptive immune response. We therefore assessed the functional phenotype of T cells from an individual who developed a severe cutaneous and systemic syndrome after having been exposed to an extremely high dose of 2,3,7,8-tetrachlorodibenzo-*p*-dioxin (TCDD).

Methodology/Principal Findings: T cells of the TCDD-exposed individual were studied for their capacity to produce cytokines in response to polyclonal and superantigenic stimulation, and for the expression of chemokine receptors involved in skin homing. The supernatants from T cells of the exposed individual contained a substantially increased amount of interleukin (IL)-22 but not of IL-17A, interferon (IFN)-γ or IL-10 when compared to nine healthy controls. *In vitro* experiments confirmed a direct, AhR-dependent, enhancing effect of TCDD on IL-22 production by CD4+ T cells. The increased production of IL-22 was not dependent on AhR occupancy by residual TCDD molecules, as demonstrated in competition experiments with the specific AhR antagonist CH-223191. In contrast, it was due to an increased frequency of IL-22 single producing cells accompanied by an increased percentage of cells expressing the skin-homing chemokine receptors CCR6 and CCR4, identified through a multiparameter flow cytometry approach. Of interest, the frequency of CD4+CD25^{hi}FoxP3+ T regulatory cells was similar in the TCDD-exposed and healthy individuals.

Conclusions/Significance: This case strongly supports the contention that human exposure to persistent AhR ligands *in vivo* induce a long-lasting effect on the human adaptive immune system and specifically polarizes CD4+ T cells to produce IL-22 and not other T cell cytokines with no effect on T regulatory cells.

Editor: Bernhard Ryffel, French National Centre for Scientific Research, France

Funding: This work was supported by grant 31003A_124941/1 from the Swiss National Science Foundation to C.C. The funder had no role in study design, data collection and analysis, decision to publish, or preparation of the manuscript. No additional external funding was received for this study.

Competing Interests: The authors have declared that no competing interests exist.

* E-mail: nicolo.brembilla@hcuge.ch

Introduction

2,3,7,8-Tetrachlorodibenzo-*p*-dioxin (TCDD) is the most potent member of a group of halogenated aromatic hydrocarbons, generally known as dioxins [1]. Dioxins are produced when organic material is burned in the presence of chlorine and are therefore widely implicated in many industrial as well as natural processes. Major sources of environmental dioxins include waste incinerators and steel industry as well as the use of herbicide and pesticide containing chlorophenols. Due to their high lipophilicity and poor metabolism, dioxins accumulate in lipid-rich tissues of animals and rapidly climb the food chain up to humans [2]. In addition, dioxins are presents in cigarette smoke. As a consequence, concentrations of dioxins are found in all humans, with higher levels commonly identified in persons living in industrialized countries.

TCDD, considered as the prototypical dioxin, has been shown to have pleiotropic biological effects at low doses in multiple animal species [3,4]. The majority of TCDD effects are mediated via binding and activation of the intracellular aryl hydrocarbon receptor (AhR), as demonstrated by the loss of responsiveness to TCDD in AhR knockout mice [5]. The elevated toxicity of TCDD is caused by its extremely high affinity for AhR and its long half-life (5–10 years in humans [6]). Upon ligand binding AhR undergoes a conformational change and translocates into the nucleus, where it dimerizes with the AhR nuclear translocator (ARNT) and regulates, by binding to xenobiotic response elements (XRE), the expression of a variety of genes, including the xenobiotic metabolizing enzyme *CYP1A1* (cytochrome P450) [7]. In mice, AhR activation is reported to regulate T helper (Th) 17 and T regulatory (Treg) cell differentiation and to modulate immune responses to experimental induced encephalomyelitis in a ligand-dependent manner [8,9,10]. In addition, AhR has been shown to be crucial for interleukin (IL)-22 expression [10] and a regulatory mechanism for IL-22 production via a Notch-AhR axis has been identified [11]. We [12] and others [13] have demonstrated a role for AhR agonists, including TCDD, in promoting the *in vitro* production of IL-22 but not of IL-17 by human CD4 T cells. The possibility that in humans AhR stimulation could participate to the *in vitro* differentiation of IL-10-producing Treg cells has also been suggested [14].

IL-22 is a member of the IL-10 family of cytokines and signals via a receptor consisting of IL-22R and IL-10R2 subunits. IL-22 does not serve the communication between immune cells since cells of hematopoietic origin do not express IL-22R [15]. It mainly acts on epithelial cells of the gastrointestinal tract and the skin, where it promotes antimicrobial defense, protection against damage and regeneration [16]. However, its role in chronic inflammatory disorders may be either protective [17] or highly pathogenetic [18,19]. T cells able to produce IL-22 in the absence of IL-17 and interferon (IFN)-γ, have been named Th22 cells and are enriched in cells expressing the skin-homing chemokine receptors CCR6, CCR4 and CCR10 while lacking CXCR3 [13,20]. Th22 cells have been identified in the skin of individuals suffering of psoriasis and atopic dermatitis [21,22,23] and are thought to be important in skin immunosurveillance and immunopathology [13,20,21].

All the data on the effects of AhR ligands on human T cell subsets have been so far generated *in vitro* and their relevance to *in vivo* situations remains largely unknown. In this report, we extensively characterize the long-term immunological modifications induced by TCDD in one of the two ever reported cases of a human being who survived the *in vivo* exposure to an extremely high dose of the pure compound [24]. Our data indicate for the first time that *in vivo* exposure to TCDD induces a selective increase in the frequency of T cells producing IL-22 but neither IL-17, IL-10, nor IFN-γ, which preferentially express skin-homing chemokine receptors. These data strongly support the *in vivo* existence in humans of Th22 cells that depend on AhR for their expansion.

Materials and Methods

Patient

We obtained written approval from the patient to release peer-reviewed scientific information about his case. Our patient had been intoxicated by pure dioxin (TCDD) presumably in late 2004 at the age of 50. In early January 2005 he arrived under controlled conditions at the Geneva University Hospital, Switzerland, where we identified a TCDD concentration of 108,000 pg/g of lipid weight in his blood serum [24]. Similar levels were identified by an independent laboratory in a sample taken from the same patient in mid-December 2004 [25]. This concentration was more than 50,000 times the averaged TCDD in the general population (normal value: 10–20 pg/g of lipid weight) [26]. The patient was suffering from a severe skin disease, the historically called "chloracne", consisting in what we call now "metabolizing acquired dioxin-induced skin hamartomas" (MADISH) to describe his skin condition [27]. All the experiments shown in this report were performed 4 years after the acute exposure to TCDD, when the patient had a TCDD concentration of 19,000 pg/g of lipid weight in his blood serum and no TCDD-related pathology was anymore clinically apparent. Nine sex and age (52±10 years) matched healthy members of the laboratory served as controls. CD4 and CD8 T cell frequencies in the peripheral blood of the TCDD-exposed individual were within the range of healthy

controls (CD4+CD3+ T cells: 62.4% and 61±7% of living lymphocytes, respectively; CD3+CD8+ T cells: 25.7% and 18±7% of living lymphocytes, respectively). Permission to perform this investigation was granted by Comité departemental de médecine interne et médecine communautère des hôpitaux universitaires de Genève. Written informed consent according to the Helsinki declaration was obtained from each individual involved in this study.

Reagents

Fetal calf serum (FCS), phorbol myristate acetate (PMA), β-mercaptoethanol, staphylococcal enterotoxin B (SEB) and brefeldin A were from Sigma Chemicals (St. Louis, MO); TCDD from Cambridge Isotope Laboratories (Andover, MA); ionomycin from Calbiochem (Merck KGaA, Darmstadt, Germany); RPMI 1640 medium, phosphate buffered saline (PBS), penicillin, streptomycin, L-glutamin, nonessential amino acids, sodium pyruvate from Life Technologies (Carlsbad, CA); human rIL-2 from Biogen (Zug, Switzerland); anti-IL-22-PE from R&D (Minneapolis, MN); anti-CD28 (CD28.2), anti-CD45RA-FITC, anti-CCR6-PercPCy5.5, anti-CCR4-PECy7, anti-CXCR3-APC, anti-CD4-PE-Cy5, anti-CD4-FITC, anti-CD4-APC-Cy7, anti-CD8-APC-Cy7 and anti-CD3-FITC from BD (Franklin Lakes, NJ); anti-IL-17A-FITC, anti-IL10-Alexa 488 and anti-IFN-γ-PE-Cy7 from Biolegend (San Diego, CA); anti-CD25-APC and anti-FoxP3-PE from eBioscience (San Diego, CA); anti-CD3 (OKT3) Ab from ATCC (Manassas, VA); CH-223191 from VWR (Dietikon, Switzerland).

Cell culture

Peripheral blood mononuclear cells (PBMC) were purified by Ficoll-paque Plus (GE Healthcare, Pittsburgh, PA) gradient centrifugation and frozen in liquid nitrogen until use or processed immediately (experiment in Fig. 1A). The cells from the TCDD-exposed individual were treated under the same experimental conditions and in parallel to that of healthy individuals in all experiments shown in this manuscript. PBMC were rested o/n in RPMI 1640 medium supplemented with 10% FCS (complete RPMI, cRPMI) as described [28] and then used in short term (up to 24 h) or long term (7 d) cultures. In short term cultures PBMC were activated for 4.5 h by PMA (50 ng/ml) and ionomycin (1 μM) or for 24 hours in flat-bottom 96-well plates in presence of coated anti-CD3 mAb (1 μg/ml) and soluble anti-CD28 mAb (1 μg/ml). When intracellular cytokine determination was performed, brefeldin A (2.5 μg/ml) was added after 1.5 and 3 hours from the beginning of the activation, respectively. In long-term activation experiments, PBMC were cultured at 1×10^6 cells/ml in 24-well plates in cRPMI in the presence of soluble anti-CD3 Ab (0.1 μg/ml) or SEB (0.2 μg/ml). Culture medium was supplemented with IL-23 (10 ng/ml) and IL-2 (20 U/ml) was added 48 h after culture initiation. When used, TCDD (10 nM, unless otherwise specified) and CH-223191 (3 μM) were added at the beginning of the culture. At day 7 of culture, supernatants were collected and frozen until cytokine determination and the cells were harvested and activated for 4.5 h by PMA and ionomycin for FACS analysis.

Flow cytometry and cytokine assays

Cell surface and intracellular staining were assessed by FACS analysis using FACSCanto (BD) and data were analyzed by FlowJo software 7.5 (Tree Star). For intracellular cytokine determination, cells were stained with anti-CD4-PE-Cy5 or anti-CD4-APC-Cy7 or anti-CD3-FITC mAbs, fixed and stained with anti-IL-17A-FITC or anti-IL-10-Alexa 488, anti-IL-22-PE, anti-IFN-γ-PE-Cy7 and anti-IL-4-APC mAbs using BD Cytofix/

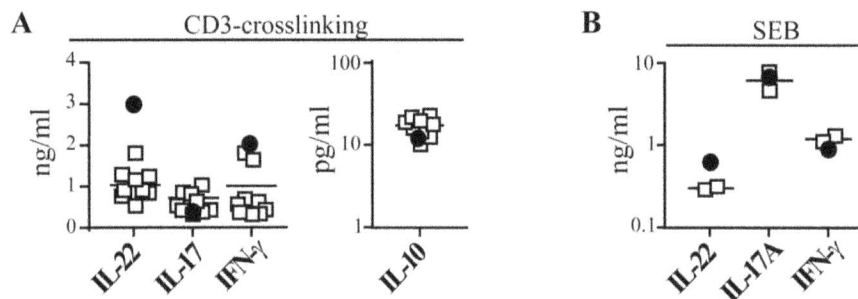

Figure 1. *In vivo* **TCDD-exposure increases IL-22 but does not concomitantly affect IL-17A, IFN-γ and IL-10 production by PBMC.** Cytokine levels were assessed at d 7 in supernatants of PBMC activated by CD3-crosslinking (**A**) or by Staphylococcal Enterotoxin B (SEB) (**B**). IL-2 (20 U/ml) was added 48h after culture initiation. Individual data for a single TCDD-exposed individual (full symbols) and 9 (CD3-crosslinking) or 2 (SEB stimulation) different healthy individuals (empty symbols) are shown.

Cytoperm kit according to manufacturer's instruction. To determine the frequency of Treg cells, PBMC were stained with anti-CD4-APC-Cy7, anti-CD45RA-FITC and anti-CD25-APC, fixed and stained with anti-FoxP3-PE using eBioscience Foxp3 Fixation/Permeabilization buffer according to manufacturer's instruction. In chemokine receptor expression experiments, PBMC were stained with anti-CD4-APC-Cy7, anti-CD45RA-FITC, anti-CCR6-PercPCy5.5, anti-CCR10-PE, anti-CCR4-PECy7 and anti-CXCR3-APC following by FACS analysis.

IFN-γ, IL-22 and IL-10 were quantified in culture supernatants at day 7 of culture by ELISA (R&D Systems or for IL-10 Sanquin, Amsterdam, The Netherlands). IL-17 was quantified by ELISA (R&D) or by Luminex xMAPTM Technology using multiplex beads immunoassay (Fluorokine MAP Multiplex Human Cytokine Panel, R&D).

Real-time quantitative PCR

Total RNA was extracted from resting PBMC using RNAesy micro kit (Quiagen, Hilden, Germany) and cDNA synthesized from 0.25 µg of total RNA using random hexamers and Superscript III reverse transcriptase (Invitrogen, Carlsbad, CA) according to manufacturer's instructions. SYBR Green assays were performed on a SDS 7900 HT instrument (Applied Biosystems). Each reaction was performed in triplicates. Raw Ct values obtained with SDS 2.2.2 software (Applied Biosystems) were analyzed and the more stable housekeeping genes TBP (TATA-box-binding protein) and EEF1A1 (eukaryotic translation elongation factor 1 alpha 1) selected for normalization. All oligonucleotides were obtained from Quiagen: CYP1A1, QT00012341; TBP1, QT00000721; EEF1A1, QT01669934.

Results and Discussion

CD4+ T cells characterized by the preferential production of IL-22 in the absence of IL-17 and IFN-γ have been recently described by us and others in the peripheral blood of healthy individuals [12,13,20]. These cells have been named Th22 cells. Cells with similar characteristics have been detected in the skin of individuals suffering of psoriasis and atopic dermatitis [21,22]. In humans, AhR natural ligands such as the tryptophan photoproduct 6-formylindolo[3,2-b]carbazole (FICZ) and β-naphthoflavone as well as the synthetic ligand TCDD, have been shown to favor the *in vitro* polarization of naïve CD4+ T cells toward IL-22-single producing cells [12,13]. However, whether previous *in vivo* exposure to an AhR-ligand in humans could favor the preferential outgrowth of a particular cell subset, thus affecting the adaptive T cell response, is unknown at present. To test this hypothesis, we

determined the capacity of PBMC of a person surviving the exposure to an extremely high dose of the stable AhR ligand TCDD to produce cell subset discriminating cytokines upon CD3-crosslinking. When compared to those of 9 healthy individuals, the PBMC of the TCDD-exposed individual produced at base-line 3-fold higher levels of IL-22 but similar levels of IL-17A, IFN-γ and IL-10 (**Figure 1A**). Similarly, PBMC of the TCDD-intoxicated individual secreted higher amounts of IL-22 but not of IL-17A and

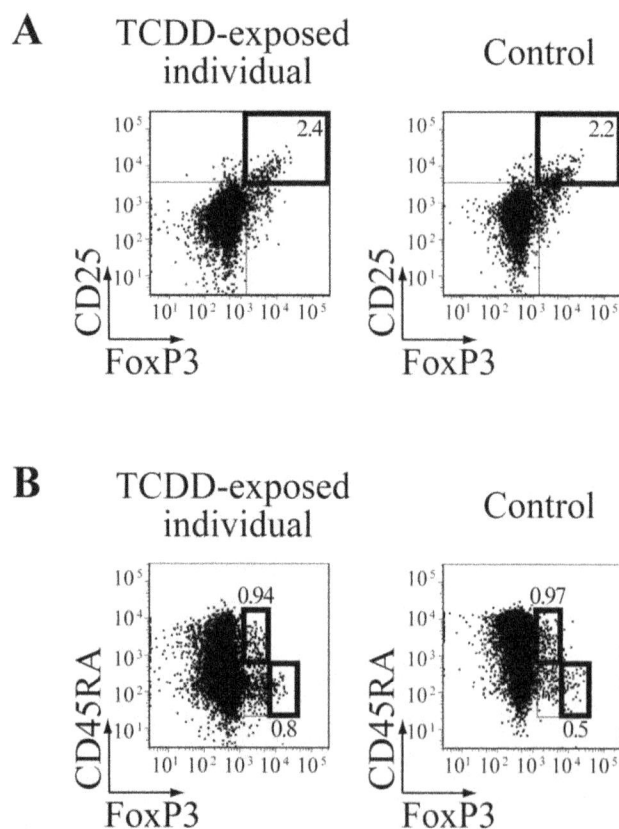

Figure 2. The levels of Treg cells are comparable in the peripheral blood of TCDD-exposed and healthy individuals. Surface staining of *ex-vivo* isolated PBMC from the TCDD-exposed and a representative healthy individual of five tested. Plots are gated on CD4+ T cells, numbers in plots indicate the percentage of CD25^{hi}FoxP3+ Treg cells (**A**) or that of CD45RA+FoxP3^{lo} resting and CD45RA-FoxP3^{hi} activated Treg cells (**B**) in the CD4+ T cell fraction.

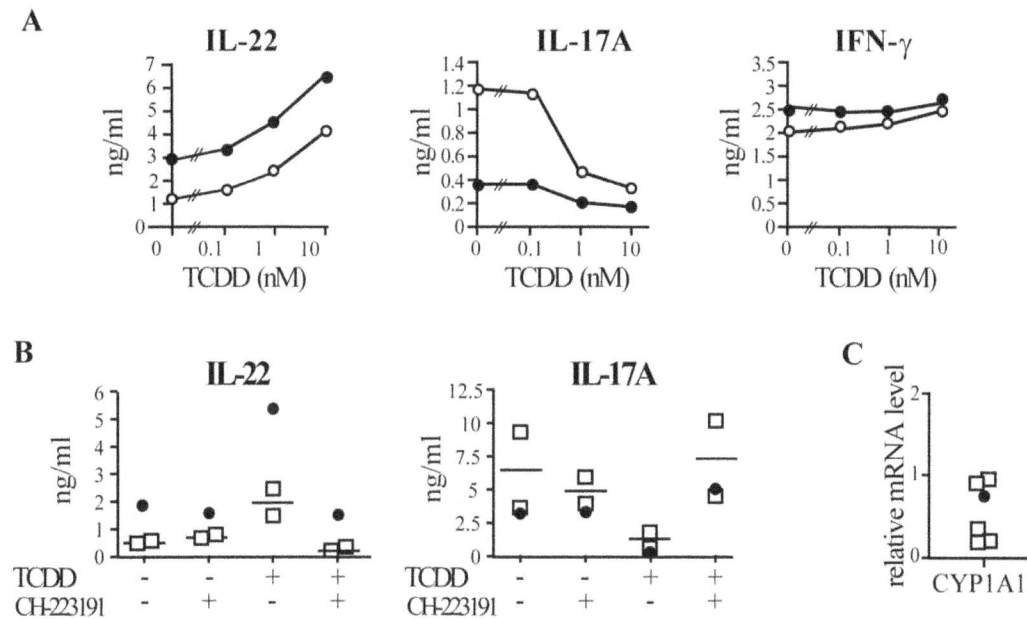

Figure 3. *In vitro* TCDD enhances IL-22 and down-regulates IL-17A production by PBMC in an AhR dependent manner. (A) PBMC were activated by CD3-crosslinking in the presence or absence of TCDD and the specific AhR inhibitor CH-223191. Cytokine levels were assessed in the supernatants harvested at d 7. Dose-dependent responses to TCDD in a single TCDD-exposed individual (full symbols) and one healthy individual (empty symbols). **(B)** Culture conditions as in A. Cytokine determination in a single TCDD-exposed individual (full symbols) and 2 healthy individuals (empty symbols) **(C)** mRNA levels of *CYP1A1* quantified by real-time PCR of resting PBMC from a single TCDD-exposed (full symbols) and five healthy individual (empty symbols). Expression levels have been normalized against the geometric mean of two house-keeping genes (EEF1A1 and TBP).

IFN-γ following superantigen stimulation with Staphylococcal Enterotoxin B (SEB) (**Figure 1B**). SEB is a superantigen able to specifically activate a subset of T cells expressing the T cell receptors Vβ3, Vβ12, Vβ13.2, Vβ14, Vβ15, Vβ17 and Vβ20 chains [29]. Thus, persistent TCDD-exposure *in vivo* does not favor in humans the outgrowth of IL-17 producing Th17 cells, as observed in mice [9,10,30,31], nor of IL-10 producing Tr1 cells, as observed *in vitro* in humans [8,9,14]. In contrast, it selectively favors the production of IL-22, induced in response to both mitogenic and superantigenic stimulation.

To further address the possible expansion of Treg cells upon exposure to TCDD as documented in mice [8,9], we assessed the frequency of CD4+ T cells simultaneously expressing high levels of the IL-2 receptor subunit CD25 and the Treg-specific transcription factor FoxP3 in resting conditions [32]. We observed comparable levels of CD25[hi]FoxP3+ cells in the CD4+ T cell fraction of *ex-vivo* isolated PBMC from the TCDD-exposed and 5 healthy individuals (2.49% and 2.28±1.13% of CD4 T cells, respectively) (**Figure 2A**). Similarly, no difference were identified in the frequency of both resting (CD45RA+FoxP3[lo]: 0.94% and 1.65±0.92% of CD4 T cells, respectively) and activated (CD45RA-FoxP3[hi]: 0.8% and 0.74±0.25% of CD4 T cells, respectively) Treg cells, as defined by the expression of the phosphatase CD45RA and the transcription factor FoxP3 (**Figure 2B**) [32]. Thus, the frequency and subset composition of T cells with regulatory function was unaffected by TCDD exposure, although TCDD levels were still 10,000 times above normal values.

We next tested whether *in vitro* TCDD could modulate the production of IL-22, IL-17A and IFN-γ by PBMC activated upon CD3-crosslinking. We found that TCDD dose-dependently increased further the production of IL-22 in the TCDD-exposed individual and, as expected, boosted IL-22 production in controls.

This increase was specific as far as IFN-γ was not affected while IL-17A production decreased in the presence of TCDD (**Figure 3A**). Thus, exposure to TCDD in our patient did not alter the ability of his lymphocytes to respond to TCDD stimulation and did not result in lymphocyte exhaustion. Together, these data corroborate and expand previous observations demonstrating a direct ability of TCDD to modulate the production of IL-22 cytokine in short-term culture *in vitro* [12].

TCDD is thought to form a long-lived and stable complex with AhR [7]. Thus, the higher amount of IL-22 produced by PBMC of the TCDD-exposed individual in the absence of exogenously added TCDD could result from the persistent action of the ligand on a stable number of cells. Alternatively, it could be explained by an increased frequency of IL-22-producing cells previously primed *in vivo* under the influence of TCDD. To discriminate between these two hypotheses, we cultured the PBMC in the presence of the high-affinity AhR-antagonist CH-223191. If residual TCDD was binding AhR in the TCDD-exposed individual, the AhR antagonist would reduce the amount of IL-22 produced upon T cell activation by displacing at least in part the bound TCDD, otherwise no effects would be observed. The presence of the AhR antagonist CH-223191 in the culture in the absence of TCDD did not decrease the basal level of IL-22 produced by the TCDD-exposed subject to the one observed in healthy individuals (**Figure 3B**). However, the specific AhR antagonist completely reversed the enhanced IL-22 and decreased IL-17A production observed when exogenous TCCD was added to the cultures in both the TCDD-exposed and healthy individuals (**Figure 3B**). To confirm these findings, we assessed the mRNA levels of the AhR-target gene *CYP1A1*, which is readily up-regulated by TCDD ligation [7]. In agreement with the lack of inhibition by CH-223191 in basal conditions, which suggests no occupancy of TCDD binding sequences, no differences were observed in the

A

B

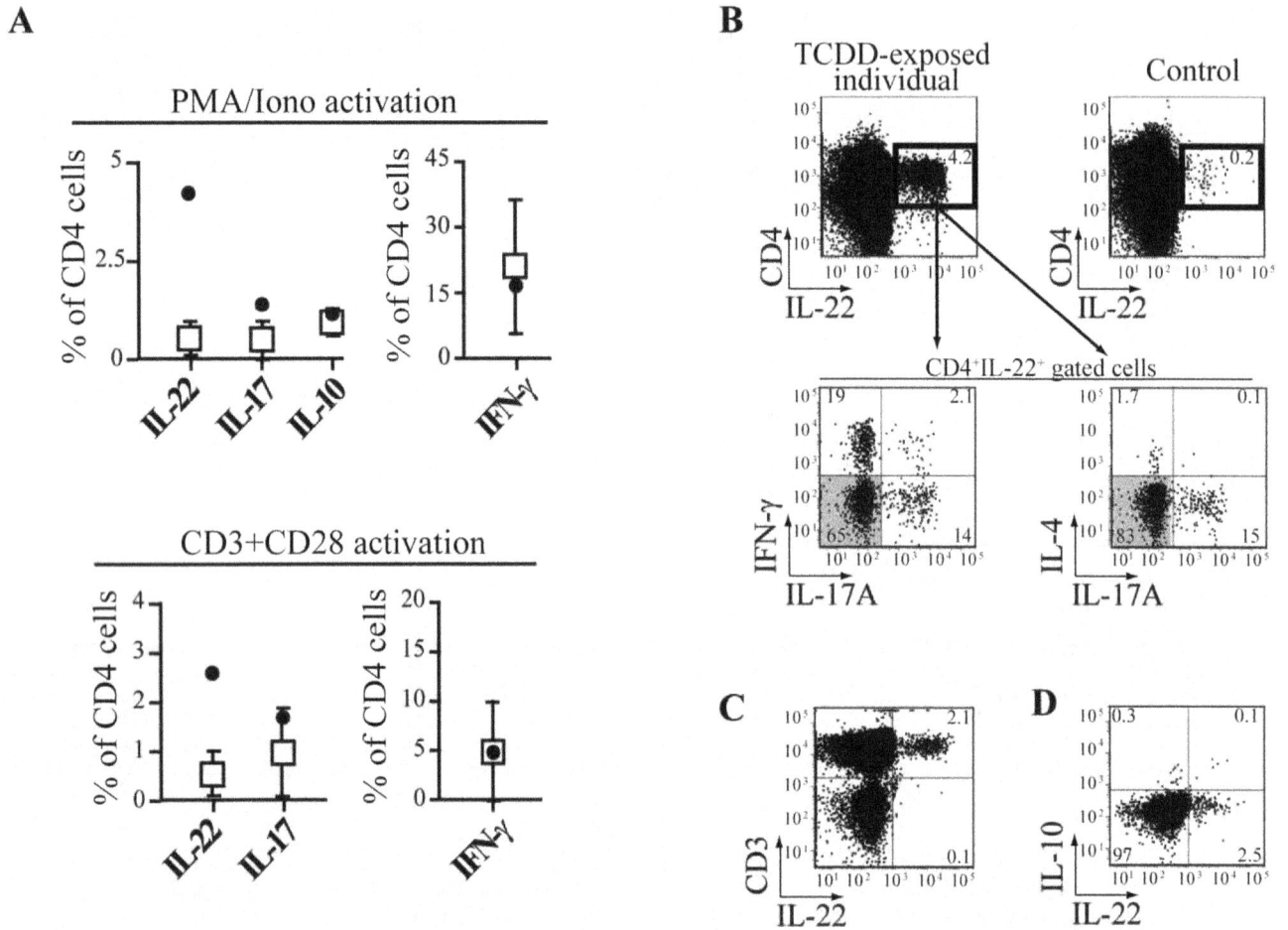

Figure 4. *In vivo* TCDD-exposure favors the expansion of Th22 cells. (A) Intracellular staining of *ex-vivo* isolated PBMC from a TCDD-exposed (full symbols) and healthy individuals (empty symbols) upon activation by PMA/Ionomycin for 4.5 h (n = 5) or CD3/CD28 crosslinking for 24 h (n = 9). **(B, C, D)** Representative FACS plots of cells activated by PMA/Ionomycin from the TCDD-exposed and a control individual (upper right panel in B) after gating on the forward and side scatter of viable PBMC **(B, C)** or on CD4+ cells **(D)**. Numbers in plots indicate the percentage of cells in each quadrant.

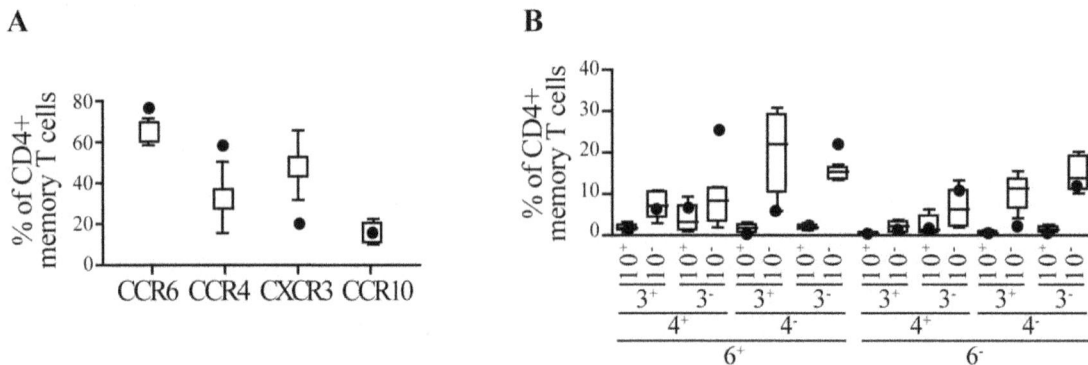

A

B

Figure 5. Increased frequency of CD4+ memory T cells expressing the skin-homing receptors CCR6+ and CCR4+ in an individual exposed *in vivo* to high levels of TCDD. Surface chemokine receptor expression on CD4+CD45RA- memory T cells from *ex-vivo* isolated PBMC in a TCDD-exposed (full symbols) or 5 healthy individuals (empty symbols). **(A)** Mean ± SD of cells expressing CCR6, CCR4, CXCR3 and CCR10. **(B)** Percentage of cells expressing various combinations of CCR6, CCR4, CXCR3 and CCR10. Data from the 5 healthy individuals are expressed as box plots. Box plots were automatically generated using GraphPad Prism version 4.00 for Windows (GraphPad Software). The box represents values between 25th and 75th percentile with a line at the median (50th percentile). The whiskers extend above and below the box to show the highest and the lowest values. 6, 4, 3 and 10 in panel B denote CCR6, CCR4, CXCR3 and CCR10, respectively.

transcription level of CYP1A1 in resting PBMC from the TCDD-exposed and control individuals (**Figure 3C**). These data demonstrate the involvement of AhR in mediating dioxin effects and, most importantly, suggest that the AhR receptor was not anymore occupied in the TCDD-exposed individual at the time of our investigation. Thus, the increased production of IL-22 could be explained by an increased frequency of cells producing IL-22, which accumulated with time while responding to novel antigenic challenges under the polarizing effect exerted by TCDD. To test this hypothesis we assessed the frequency of *ex vivo*-detectable IL-22-secreting CD4+ cells in PBMC from the TCDD-exposed and healthy individuals. We observed that the frequency of CD4+ cells producing IL-22 was at least 3-fold higher in the TCDD-exposed individual compared to controls. By contrast, the frequency of cells producing IL-17A, IL-10 and IFN-γ was similar (**Figure 4A**). The increase in IL-22 producing cells was reproducible in short term cultures across a variety of activation stimuli, which included TCR-dependent (CD3 and CD28 cross-linking) and TCR-independent (PMA and ionomycin) signaling (**Figure 4A and B**). In the CD4+ compartment, IL-22 is mainly produced by CD3+ T cells and to a minor extent by CD3- cells including lymphoid tissue inducer (LTi) cells [33]. In the TCDD exposed individual, all IL-22 producing cells were CD3+, thus indicating that the source of IL-22 was CD4+ T cells (**Figure 4B and C**). Of interest, multiparameter flow cytometry analysis revealed that the majority of the IL-22+ cells in the TCDD-exposed individual did not concomitantly produce IL-17A, IL-4, IFN-γ (**Figure 4B**) and IL-10 (**Figure 4D**). Altogether, these data strongly indicate that *in vivo* exposure to TCDD favors the expansion of CD4+ T cells having the functional properties of Th22 cells.

Since the exposure to dioxin resulted in severe skin manifestations, we tested whether the pattern of chemokine receptors associated with skin homing expressed in CD4+ T cells was skewed in the TCDD-exposed individual [34,35,36,37,38]. We found that the frequency of CCR6+ and CCR4+ cells in the memory CD4 T cell compartment was higher in the TCDD-exposed individual than in controls, while the frequency of CXCR3+ cells was lower (**Figure 5A**). This is remarkable, since Th22 cells were shown to be enriched in CD4+ T cells expressing CCR6, CCR4 and CCR10 in absence of CXCR3 [13,20]. A detailed multiparametric analysis performed at a single cell level, revealed that in the TCDD-exposed individual there was a substantial three-fold increase in the frequency of CD4+ memory T cells with the CCR6+CCR4+CXCR3-CCR10- phenotype and a modest increase in the CCR6+CCR4-CXCR3-CCR10- subset when compared to healthy controls (**Figure 5B**). No differences were identified in the CCR6- compartment, thus stressing the specificity

of our finding. It is noteworthy that we did not observe a concomitant preferential expression of CCR10 in the TCDD-exposed individual as observed by others in Th22 cells [13,20]. This may reflect a specific characteristic of T cell producing IL-22 under the influence of TCDD.

It is tempting to speculate that Th22 may have contributed to some extent to the pathogenesis of the dioxin induced skin lesions [27]. Th22 cells have been shown to be involved in skin disease such as psoriasis and atopic dermatitis [21,22,23] which molecular pathology is very different from the dioxin-induced skin lesions, historically called "chloracne" and now defined as "metabolizing acquired dioxin induced skin hamartomas" which primarily involve sebaceous glands [27]. Further studies are needed to analyze the putative effect, if any, of IL-22 in sebaceous gland pathology. However, It is also possible that the skewed pattern of chemokine receptor expression in the TCDD-exposed individual was only the consequence of the expansion of Th22 cells taking place with time.

In conclusion, we present here strong evidence indicating that prolonged exposure *in vivo* to high dose of TCDD induces a profound, long-lasting, perturbation of the adaptive immune system and specifically polarizes CD4+ T cells to produce IL-22 but not other T cell cytokines in an AhR-dependent manner. The best model explaining our findings suggest that antigenic exposure taking place under the influence of TCDD polarizes T cells to the Th22 subset. While historically relevant environmental disasters [39,40,41] caused people exposure to a mix of toxic agent including TCDD, the case here discussed represents a unique opportunity for investigating the effect of pure dioxin on human T cells. TCDD is one of the major environmental pollutants, present in food and in cigarette smoke. While current doses are largely below those observed in the index case, our observation helps to better understand the effect of dioxin on the human immune system.

Acknowledgments

We are grateful to Montserrat Alvarez and Marie-Elise Truchetet (Immunology and Allergy, Geneva University Hospital, Switzerland) for technical assistance and Lionel Fontao (Dermatology, Geneva University Hospital, Switzerland) for critical discussion.

Author Contributions

Conceived and designed the experiments: JHS OS NCB JMR CC. Performed the experiments: NCB JMR RC. Analyzed the data: NCB JMR OS JHS CC. Contributed reagents/materials/analysis tools: OS JHS. Wrote the paper: NCB CC.

References

1. Poland A, Knutson JC (1982) 2,3,7,8-tetrachlorodibenzo-p-dioxin and related halogenated aromatic hydrocarbons: examination of the mechanism of toxicity. Annu Rev Pharmacol Toxicol 22: 517–554.

2. Schecter A, Cramer P, Boggess K, Stanley J, Papke O, et al. (2001) Intake of dioxins and related compounds from food in the U.S. population. J Toxicol Environ Health A 63: 1–18.

3. Birnbaum LS, Tuomisto J (2000) Non-carcinogenic effects of TCDD in animals. Food Addit Contam 17: 275–288.

4. Schecter A, Birnbaum L, Ryan JJ, Constable JD (2006) Dioxins: an overview. Environ Res 101: 419–428.

5. Fernandez-Salguero PM, Hilbert DM, Rudikoff S, Ward JM, Gonzalez FJ (1996) Aryl-hydrocarbon receptor-deficient mice are resistant to 2,3,7,8-tetrachlorodibenzo-p-dioxin-induced toxicity. Toxicol Appl Pharmacol 140: 173–179.

6. Aylward LL, Brunet RC, Carrier G, Hays SM, Cushing CA, et al. (2005) Concentration-dependent TCDD elimination kinetics in humans: toxicokinetic modeling for moderately to highly exposed adults from Seveso, Italy, and Vienna, Austria, and impact on dose estimates for the NIOSH cohort. J Expo Anal Environ Epidemiol 15: 51–65.

7. Denison MS, Nagy SR (2003) Activation of the aryl hydrocarbon receptor by structurally diverse exogenous and endogenous chemicals. Annu Rev Pharmacol Toxicol 43: 309–334.

8. Funatake CJ, Marshall NB, Steppan LB, Mourich DV, Kerkvliet NI (2005) Cutting edge: activation of the aryl hydrocarbon receptor by 2,3,7,8-tetrachlorodibenzo-p-dioxin generates a population of CD4+ CD25+ cells with characteristics of regulatory T cells. J Immunol 175: 4184–4188.

9. Quintana FJ, Basso AS, Iglesias AH, Korn T, Farez MF, et al. (2008) Control of T(reg) and T(H)17 cell differentiation by the aryl hydrocarbon receptor. Nature 453: 65–71.

10. Veldhoen M, Hirota K, Westendorf AM, Buer J, Dumoutier L, et al. (2008) The aryl hydrocarbon receptor links TH17-cell-mediated autoimmunity to environmental toxins. Nature 453: 106–109.

11. Alam MS, Maekawa Y, Kitamura A, Tanigaki K, Yoshimoto T, et al. (2010) Notch signaling drives IL-22 secretion in CD4+ T cells by stimulating the aryl hydrocarbon receptor. Proc Natl Acad Sci U S A 107: 5943–5948.

12. Ramirez JM, Brembilla NC, Sorg O, Chicheportiche R, Matthes T, et al. (2010) Activation of the aryl hydrocarbon receptor reveals distinct requirements for IL-

22 and IL-17 production by human T helper cells. Eur J Immunol 40: 2450–2459.

13. Trifari S, Kaplan CD, Tran EH, Crellin NK, Spits H (2009) Identification of a human helper T cell population that has abundant production of interleukin 22 and is distinct from T(H)-17, T(H)1 and T(H)2 cells. Nat Immunol 10: 864–871.

14. Gandhi R, Kumar D, Burns EJ, Nadeau M, Dake B, et al. Activation of the aryl hydrocarbon receptor induces human type 1 regulatory T cell-like and Foxp3(+) regulatory T cells. Nat Immunol 11: 846–853.

15. Wolk K, Kunz S, Witte E, Friedrich M, Asadullah K, et al. (2004) IL-22 increases the innate immunity of tissues. Immunity 21: 241–254.

16. Wolk K, Witte E, Witte K, Warszawska K, Sabat R (2010) Biology of interleukin-22. Semin Immunopathol 32: 17–31.

17. Sugimoto K, Ogawa A, Mizoguchi E, Shimomura Y, Andoh A, et al. (2008) IL-22 ameliorates intestinal inflammation in a mouse model of ulcerative colitis. J Clin Invest 118: 534–544.

18. Boniface K, Guignouard E, Pedretti N, Garcia M, Delwail A, et al. (2007) A role for T cell-derived interleukin 22 in psoriatic skin inflammation. Clin Exp Immunol 150: 407–415.

19. Zheng Y, Danilenko DM, Valdez P, Kasman I, Eastham-Anderson J, et al. (2007) Interleukin-22, a T(H)17 cytokine, mediates IL-23-induced dermal inflammation and acanthosis. Nature 445: 648–651.

20. Duhen T, Geiger R, Jarrossay D, Lanzavecchia A, Sallusto F (2009) Production of interleukin 22 but not interleukin 17 by a subset of human skin-homing memory T cells. Nat Immunol 10: 857–863.

21. Eyerich S, Eyerich K, Pennino D, Carbone T, Nasorri F, et al. (2009) Th22 cells represent a distinct human T cell subset involved in epidermal immunity and remodeling. J Clin Invest 119: 3573–3585.

22. Nograles KE, Zaba LC, Shemer A, Fuentes-Duculan J, Cardinale I, et al. (2009) IL-22-producing "T22" T cells account for upregulated IL-22 in atopic dermatitis despite reduced IL-17-producing TH17 T cells. J Allergy Clin Immunol 123: 1244–1252 e1242.

23. Wolk K, Haugen HS, Xu W, Witte E, Waggie K, et al. (2009) IL-22 and IL-20 are key mediators of the epidermal alterations in psoriasis while IL-17 and IFN-gamma are not. J Mol Med 87: 523–536.

24. Sorg O, Zennegg M, Schmid P, Fedosyuk R, Valikhnovskyi R, et al. (2009) 2,3,7,8-tetrachlorodibenzo-p-dioxin (TCDD) poisoning in Victor Yushchenko: identification and measurement of TCDD metabolites. Lancet 374: 1179–1185.

25. Brouwer A, Botschuiver S, Veerhoek D, Besselink HT, Hamm S, et al. (2005) Observation of an extremely high dioxin level in a human serum sample from ukraine by Dr Calux®, which was confirmed to be 2,3,7,8-tetrachlorodibenzo-p-dioxin by GC-HRMS. Organohalogen Compounds 67: 1705–1708.

26. Wittsiepe J, Furst P, Schrey P, Lemm F, Kraft M, et al. (2007) PCDD/F and dioxin-like PCB in human blood and milk from German mothers. Chemosphere 67: S286–294.

27. Saurat JH, Sorg O (2010) Chloracne, a misnomer and its implications. Dermatology 221: 23–26.

28. Chizzolini C, Chicheportiche R, Alvarez M, de Rham C, Roux-Lombard P, et al. (2008) Prostaglandin E2 synergistically with interleukin-23 favors human Th17 expansion. Blood 112: 3696–3703.

29. Deringer JR, Ely RJ, Stauffacher CV, Bohach GA (1996) Subtype-specific interactions of type C staphylococcal enterotoxins with the T-cell receptor. Mol Microbiol 22: 523–534.

30. Kimura A, Naka T, Nohara K, Fujii-Kuriyama Y, Kishimoto T (2008) Aryl hydrocarbon receptor regulates Stat1 activation and participates in the development of Th17 cells. Proc Natl Acad Sci U S A 105: 9721–9726.

31. Veldhoen M, Hirota K, Christensen J, O'Garra A, Stockinger B (2009) Natural agonists for aryl hydrocarbon receptor in culture medium are essential for optimal differentiation of Th17 T cells. J Exp Med 206: 43–49.

32. Miyara M, Yoshioka Y, Kitoh A, Shima T, Wing K, et al. (2009) Functional delineation and differentiation dynamics of human CD4+ T cells expressing the FoxP3 transcription factor. Immunity 30: 899–911.

33. Spits H, Di Santo JP (2009) The expanding family of innate lymphoid cells: regulators and effectors of immunity and tissue remodeling. Nat Immunol 12: 21–27.

34. Fitzhugh DJ, Naik S, Caughman SW, Hwang ST (2000) Cutting edge: C-C chemokine receptor 6 is essential for arrest of a subset of memory T cells on activated dermal microvascular endothelial cells under physiologic flow conditions in vitro. J Immunol 165: 6677–6681.

35. Reiss Y, Proudfoot AE, Power CA, Campbell JJ, Butcher EC (2001) CC chemokine receptor (CCR)4 and the CCR10 ligand cutaneous T cell-attracting chemokine (CTACK) in lymphocyte trafficking to inflamed skin. J Exp Med 194: 1541–1547.

36. Schutyser E, Struyf S, Van Damme J (2003) The CC chemokine CCL20 and its receptor CCR6. Cytokine Growth Factor Rev 14: 409–426.

37. Soler D, Humphreys TL, Spinola SM, Campbell JJ (2003) CCR4 versus CCR10 in human cutaneous TH lymphocyte trafficking. Blood 101: 1677–1682.

38. Homey B, Alenius H, Muller A, Soto H, Bowman EP, et al. (2002) CCL27-CCR10 interactions regulate T cell-mediated skin inflammation. Nat Med 8: 157–165.

39. Michalek JE, Pirkle JL, Needham LL, Patterson DG, Jr., Caudill SP, et al. (2002) Pharmacokinetics of 2,3,7,8-tetrachlorodibenzo-p-dioxin in Seveso adults and veterans of operation Ranch Hand. J Expo Anal Environ Epidemiol 12: 44–53.

40. Steele EJ, Bellett AJ, McCullagh PJ, Selinger B (1990) Reappraisal of the findings on Agent Orange by the Australian Royal Commission. Toxicol Lett 51: 261–268.

41. Yoshimura T (2003) Yusho in Japan. Ind Health 41: 139–148.

15

Distinct Effects of Different Phosphatidylglycerol Species on Mouse Keratinocyte Proliferation

Ding Xie[2¤a], Mutsa Seremwe[2], John G. Edwards[3], Robert Podolsky[4¤b], Wendy B. Bollag[1,2]*

1 Charlie Norwood VA Medical Center, Augusta, Georgia, United States of America, **2** Department of Physiology, Medical College of Georgia at Georgia Regents University, Augusta, Georgia, United States of America, **3** Apeliotus Technologies, Inc., Atlanta, Georgia, United States of America, **4** Center for Biotechnology and Genomic Medicine, Department of Medicine, Medical College of Georgia at Georgia Regents University, Augusta, Georgia, United States of America

Abstract

We have previously shown that liposomes composed of egg-derived phosphatidylglycerol (PG), with a mixed fatty acid composition (comprising mainly palmitate and oleate), inhibit the proliferation and promote the differentiation of rapidly dividing keratinocytes, and stimulate the growth of slowly proliferating epidermal cells. To determine the species of PG most effective at modulating keratinocyte proliferation, primary mouse keratinocytes were treated with different PG species, and proliferation was measured. PG species containing polyunsaturated fatty acids were effective at inhibiting rapidly proliferating keratinocytes, whereas PG species with monounsaturated fatty acids were effective at promoting proliferation in slowly dividing cells. Thus, palmitoyl-arachidonyl-PG (16:0/20:4), palmitoyl-linoleoyl-PG (16:0/18:2), dilinoleoyl-PG (18:2/18:2) and soy PG (a PG mixture with a large percentage of polyunsaturated fatty acids) were particularly effective at inhibiting proliferation in rapidly dividing keratinocytes. Conversely, palmitoyl-oleoyl-PG (16:0/18:1) and dioleoyl-PG (18:1/18:1) were especially effective proproliferative PG species. This result represents the first demonstration of opposite effects of different species of a single class of phospholipid and suggests that these different PG species may signal to diverse effector enzymes to differentially affect keratinocyte proliferation and normalize keratinocyte proliferation. Thus, different PG species may be useful for treating skin diseases characterized by excessive or insufficient proliferation.

Editor: Andrzej T. Slominski, University of Tennessee, United States of America

Funding: This work was supported by NIH grants #AR45212 and AR55022 and an award from the Georgia Research Alliance. WBB is supported by a VA Research Career Scientist Award. The funders had no role in study design, data collection and analysis, decision to publish, or preparation of the manuscript. The contents of this article do not represent the views of the Department of Veterans Affairs or the United States Government.

Competing Interests: Wendy B. Bollag is an inventor on a patent (No. 8,808,715) entitled "Methods and Compositions for Modulating Keratinocyte Function" (USSN 12/164,021) for the use of phosphatidylglycerol species to normalize keratinocyte function submitted by Georgia Regents University. At the time of the collection of the reported data, Apeliotus Technologies, Inc., through its Chief Executive Officer John G. Edwards, licensed this technology and employed Dr. Bollag part-time to oversee this research as part of a National Institutes of Health Small Business Technology Transfer award (#AR55022). However, subsequently, Apeliotus Technologies relinquished its license of the intellectual property, for which patent protection continues to be sought by Georgia Regents University.

* Email: WB@gru.edu

¤a Current address: Department of Family Medicine, Medical College of Georgia at Georgia Regents University, Augusta, Georgia, United States of America
¤b Current address: Department of Family Medicine and Public Health Sciences, Wayne State University, Detroit, Michigan, United States of America

Introduction

Keratinocyte proliferation and differentiation are precisely regulated processes which are essential for proper formation and function of the epidermis of the skin to serve as a physical and water-permeability barrier [1,2]. Because this largest organ of the body serves as the interface between the internal and external environments, the skin senses and responds to a variety of stresses (reviewed in [3]). Defects in the regulation of this growth/ differentiation program, and the epidermis' inability to restore homeostasis when stressed, can result in an abnormal barrier and a variety of skin diseases, such as non-melanoma skin cancer and psoriasis [4].

Previously, our laboratory has shown the existence of a novel cell signaling module composed of the glycerol transporter, aquaporin-3 (AQP3) and phospholipase D2 (PLD2). Phospholipase D (PLD) is a lipid-metabolizing enzyme that can catalyze both phospholipid hydrolysis to produce phosphatidate and a transphosphatidylation reaction using primary alcohols, such as glycerol, to generate phosphatidylalcohols [5]. In addition, we showed that PLD2, one isoform of PLD, colocalizes with AQP3 in, and co-immunoprecipitates from, caveolin-rich membrane microdomains in epidermal keratinocytes [6]. Together these two proteins appear to function to produce phosphatidylglycerol (PG) [7], which is important in the regulation of keratinocyte function [5,6,8,9]. Indeed, manipulating this novel signaling module, the AQP3/PLD2/PG unit, alters keratinocyte proliferation and differentiation [8]. For instance, direct provision of liposomes produced from egg-derived PG (egg PG) results in an inhibition of keratinocyte proliferation in rapidly dividing keratinocytes [8]. Interestingly, however, in slowly dividing cells egg PG liposomes stimulate proliferation, suggesting that egg PG can normalize keratinocyte function [8]. Although there are many questions remaining to be answered about this novel cell signaling module, the ability of egg PG to normalize keratinocyte function is of interest because of the wide range of possible clinical applications to skin diseases characterized by abnormal proliferation and the potential for targeting this PLD2/AQP3/PG signaling modue for their treatment.

Egg PG is comprised of multiple PG species, with different acyl groups identifying the different PG species. Thus, egg PG exhibits the following fatty acid composition (with the first number representing the total number of carbon atoms in the fatty acid and the second number, the number of double bonds): 16:0 (34%) 16:1 (2%), 18:0 (11%), 18:1 (32%), 18:2 (18%) and 20:4 (3%) (Avanti Polar Lipids website). As a first step to define the mechanism underlying the normalization effect of egg PG, we sought to identify the PG species most effective at altering keratinocyte proliferation, with the assumption that the same species of PG would exert both effects on proliferation (inhibition of rapidly proliferating keratinocytes and enhancement of slowly growing cells). Cell proliferation was examined in order to screen a large number of PG species, although as the initial step in differentiation, growth arrest (or reversal of growth arrest) often reflects effects on other differentiation processes, such as involucrin levels as we have shown previously [8]. We found that various PG species affected keratinocyte proliferation differently; these results actually favor the potential clinical applications of different PG species for the treatment of different skin diseases, characterized by hyper- or hypoproliferation.

Materials and Methods

Materials

Dihexanoylphosphatidylglycerol (DHPG), dipalmitoylphosphatidylglycerol (DPPG), distearoylphosphatidylglycerol (DSPG), palmitoyl-oleoylphosphatidylglycerol (POPG), dioleoylphosphatidylglycerol (DOPG), palmitoyl-arachidonoylphosphatidylglycerol (PAPG), palmitoyl-linoleoylphosphatidylglycerol (PLPG), dilinoleoylphosphatidylglycerol (DLPG), soy-derived PG (soy PG), egg-derived PG, and dilinoleoylphosphatidylpropanol (DLPP) were all obtained from Avanti Polar Lipids, Inc. (Alabaster, AL). The composition of egg PG is provided in the Introduction. Soy PG is composed of 16:0 (17%), 18:0 (6%), 18:1 (13%), 18:2 (59%), and 18:3 (5%) (Avanti Polar Lipids website). Calcium-free minimal essential medium and antibiotics were obtained from Biologos, Inc. (Maperville, Illinois). Bovine pituitary extract and epidermal growth factor were purchased from Life Technologies, Inc. (Grand Island, New York). ITS+(6.25 μg insulin per mL, 6.25 μg transferrin per mL, 6.25 ng selenous acid per mL, 5.35 mg linoleic acid per mL, and 0.125% bovine serum albumin) was supplied by Collaborative Biomedical Products (Bedford, Massachusetts).

Keratinocyte Preparation and Cell culture

All animal studies were performed under a protocol approved by the Georgia Regents Institutional Animal Care and Use Committee and adhere to the standards described in the Guide for the Care and Use of Laboratory Animals. Mouse epidermal keratinocyte cell cultures were prepared from ICR strain CD-1 outbred neonatal mice 1–3 days of age as described in detail in [10,11]. Briefly, the skins were harvested and incubated overnight in 0.25% trypsin at 4°C. The epidermis and dermis were separated and the basal keratinocytes scraped from the underside of the epidermis. The cells were collected by centrifugation and incubated overnight in an atmosphere of 95% air/5% CO_2 at 37°C in plating medium [5]. The cells were refed every 1–2 days with serum-free keratinocyte medium (SFKM) also as in [5] until

use. The newborn mice used for preparation of primary keratinocytes were anethetized by hypothermia and euthanized by decapitation. All procedures were conducted in conformity with the Public Health Service Policy on Humane Care and Use of Laboratory Animals and approved by the Institutional Animal Care and Use Committee.

DNA Synthesis Assay

[^{3}H]Thymidine incorporation into DNA was assayed as a measure of keratinocyte proliferation as described in [12]. Briefly, keratinocyte cultures were incubated for 24 hours in SFKM containing various concentrations of different PG species or DLPP, prepared as liposomes by sonication. [^{3}H]Thymidine at a final concentration of 1 μCi/mL, was added to the cells for an additional 1-hour incubation. Reactions were terminated using ice-cold 5% trichloroacetic acid and unincorporated radiolabel removed by washing. Cells were solubilized in 0.3 M NaOH, and the radioactivity incorporated into DNA quantified by liquid scintillation spectroscopy.

Statistical Analysis

Data are expressed as mean ± SEM. Experiments were performed a minimum of three times and analyzed by ANOVA with a Student-Newmann-Keuls or Dunnett's post-hoc test using Instat or Prizm software (Graphpad, La Jolla. CA). $P \leq 0.05$ was considered statistically significant.

To compare the different effects of all of the PGs investigated together, it was necessay to use a mixed model analysis of variance to analyze the effects in different experimental settings. Prior to analysis to improve assumptions of normality and additivity for the models to be used, the data were transformed and grouped. Because one of the treatments had 0 concentration units, we transformed concentration using ln[PG concentration + exp(2.5)], which results in even spacing of the transformed concentrations. Cell proliferation rate (counts per minute; CPM) was transformed using ln(CPM). Because in some experiments cells were quickly proliferating, while in other experiments the cells were not, we grouped experiments that had different responses to egg PG using finite mixture regression models and the flexmix package detailed in [13]. This method clusters each experiment by the regression fit between ln(CPM) and ln(concentration), grouping cultures with similar regression lines in the same cluster. Because the relationship between ln(CPM) and ln(concentration) was not linear, we used quadratic regression for the clustering analysis. The number of clusters was determined using the Bayesian information criterion (BIC). This analysis initially suggested that eight groups of regression lines were present for the egg PG data. Inspection of plots of these groups indicated four patterns were present with some variation within these four patterns, based on the relationship between ln(CPM) and ln(concentration) of egg PG: (1) a linear increasing relationship; (2) a non-linear decreasing relationship; (3) a flat, quadratic relationship; and (4) a decreasing step function relationship. These four general patterns were used as the four groups in subsequent analyses. While the data do support eight clusters, collapsing these clusters together does not affect the subsequent analyses that examined the effects of different PGs on the relationship between ln(CPM) and ln(concentration), since the differences in slopes and intercepts within a cluster can be accommodated within the analyses.

We used a mixed model analysis of variance separately for each of the four grouped clusters identified above to determine how the different PG species affected the relationship between cell proliferation and PG concentration. The model used for this analysis of variance included PG species as a fixed effect that potentially interacted with ln(concentration), and random coefficients for each culture/experiment. This analysis accounts for the different responses for each individual culture/experiment. We focused on three effects from this model: (1) the PG species effect, which reflects the PG species change in intercept; (2) the PG species by ln(concentration) effect, which reflects the PG species change in the linear slope; and (3) the PG species by ln(concentration)^2 effect, which reflects the PG species change in the quadratic regression coefficient. The first effect relates to the overall difference in means between the PG species, although this difference may be dose dependent as reflected by the last two effects. Together, these three effects reveal how PG species change the overall relationship between cell proliferation [ln(CPM)] and PG concentration. The mixed model analysis was conducted using the Proc Mixed procedure in SAS 9.13. $P \leq 0.05$ was deemed as significant.

Results

PG species containing saturated or monounsaturated fatty acids stimulated keratinocyte proliferation

Since previous data indicated an ability of egg PG to inhibit the proliferation of rapidly dividing and stimulate the growth of slowly proliferating keratinocytes [14], we first examined the effect on keratinocyte proliferation of the PG species containing the most abundant acyl groups found in egg PG. Since the major acyl groups associated with egg-derived lipids are palmitic acid (16:0), and oleic acid (18:1), the synthetic PGs, DPPG (16:0/16:0), POPG (16:0/18:1), and DOPG (18:1/18:1) were initially chosen to examine their effects on the proliferation of primary cultures of mouse epidermal keratinocytes. PG prepared in the form of liposomes was provided to the keratinocytes at doses ranging from 0 to 100 μg/mL. In all cases an egg PG comparator dose response was performed for comparison among experiments of the effects of different PG species. POPG and DOPG significantly stimulated DNA synthesis in a dose-dependent manner (Figure 1B and 1C). The initial dose of POPG and DOPG demonstrating a significant stimulatory effect was 100 μg/mL and 50 μg/mL, respectively. Although there was no significant effect of DPPG on DNA synthesis, it followed the same trend (Figure 1A). Contrary to our assumption that a certain PG species would exert both inhibitory and stimulatory effects, these results suggested that some PG species might stimulate keratinocyte proliferation while others might inhibit keratinocyte proliferation. In addition, our data suggested that the monounsaturated fatty acid tails in PG may play a role in this stimulatory effect. We also determined that 100 μg/mL DSPG (18:0/18:0) significantly increased [^{3}H]thymidine incorporation by 36%, suggesting a likely pro-stimulatory effect of saturated fatty acids as well (Figure 1D). Since none of the PG species containing the most abundant fatty acids in egg PG inhibited keratinocyte proliferation, we opted to test additional PG species, containing fatty acids representing a minor fraction of those comprising egg PG.

PG species containing polyunsaturated fatty acids inhibited keratinocyte proliferation

PLPG (16:0/18:2), DLPG (18:2/18:2), and PAPG (16:0/20:4), each possessing at least one polyunsaturated fatty acid, were selected as PG species containing fatty acids comprising a minor fraction of those in egg PG. These PG species, prepared as liposomes, were directly provided to the primary mouse keratinocytes at doses as described above. Synthetic PLPG, DLPG, and PAPG were particularly effective at inhibiting keratinocyte proliferation in a dose-dependent manner (Figure 2A, B, and C).

The initial dose of PLPG, DLPG, and PAPG demonstrating a significant inhibitory effect was 25 μg/mL, 12.5 μg/mL, and 6.25 μg/mL, respectively. Note the apparent trend of increasing inhibitory effects with a greater degree of (poly)unsaturation.

We also tested a synthetic PG with short acyl chains, which should be more soluble in aqueous solution and thus more easily applied, and determined that there was no significant effect of DHPG (6:0/6:0) on keratinocyte proliferation (Figure 2D). This result suggests that the natural, longer chain fatty acid-containing PGs may be more effective in regulating keratinocyte function.

Soy PG inhibited keratinocyte proliferation

Our results with PLPG, DLPG, and PAPG suggested an important role of polyunsaturated fatty acids in PG's antiproliferative effects. However, these synthetic PGs are expensive to produce. Considering the potential medical application of this phospholipid to hyperproliferative skin disorders, we sought to determine the effects on keratinocyte proliferation of soy PG, which is a less expensive PG mixture containing a large percentage of polyunsaturated fatty acids, including linoleic (18:2) and linolenic (18:3) acids (13% and 59%, respectively). Consistent with the effects of synthetic PG species containing polyunsaturated fatty acids, soy PG also significantly inhibited DNA synthesis in a dose-dependent manner (Figure 3). We next sought to determine the most effective of these tested PG species on keratinocyte proliferation in comparison to egg PG for use in further experiments to test potential medical applications.

Comparison of the effects of different PG species on keratinocyte proliferation

It was not technically feasible to conduct all of the tests of PG species reported above in one single set of experiments. Likewise, it was impossible to treat all keratinocytes at exactly the same degree of confluence across the multiple experiments required, as the primary cultures were prepared from neonatal mice of slightly different ages resulting in somewhat different plating efficiencies and thus confluence at treatment. Because epidermal keratinocytes are contact inhibited, these differences in confluence likely resulted in the observed disparate proliferation under control conditions. Consequently, to allow comparison among all the experiments, egg PG was tested as a comparator in each experiment. Note that a total of 38 separate experiments from 38 different keratinocyte preparations/primary cultures were performed, each with its own egg PG control to allow comparison among experiments with different degrees of confluence. Based on the response to egg PG, all of the results could be grouped into four clusters as shown in Figure 4: (1) cluster 1 represented the experiments in which the response to egg PG was stimulatory, and in which the cells were slowly dividing, as indicated by the lower value at the zero concentration on the x-axis compared with those of clusters 2, 3, and 4; (2) cluster 2 represented the experiments in which the response to egg PG was monophasically inhibitory; (3) cluster 3 represented the experiments in which the response to egg PG was relatively flat; and (4) cluster 4 represented the experiments in which the response to egg PG was biphasically inhibitory (Figure 4). We found that in cluster 1, the stimulatory effect of DOPG was significantly more potent than that of egg PG while DPPG was significantly less potent. In cluster 2, POPG, DSPG, and DOPG were significantly less inhibitory than egg PG, whereas DLPG, PAPG, and soy PG were significantly more potent than egg PG at inhibiting proliferation. In cluster 3, in which egg PG had little or no effect on keratinocyte proliferation, soy PG still exhibited a significant inhibitory effect, suggesting greater potency of soy PG. In cluster 4, PAPG's inhibition was significantly more

a

16:0/16:0

b

16:0/18:1

c

18:1/18:1

d

18:0/18:0

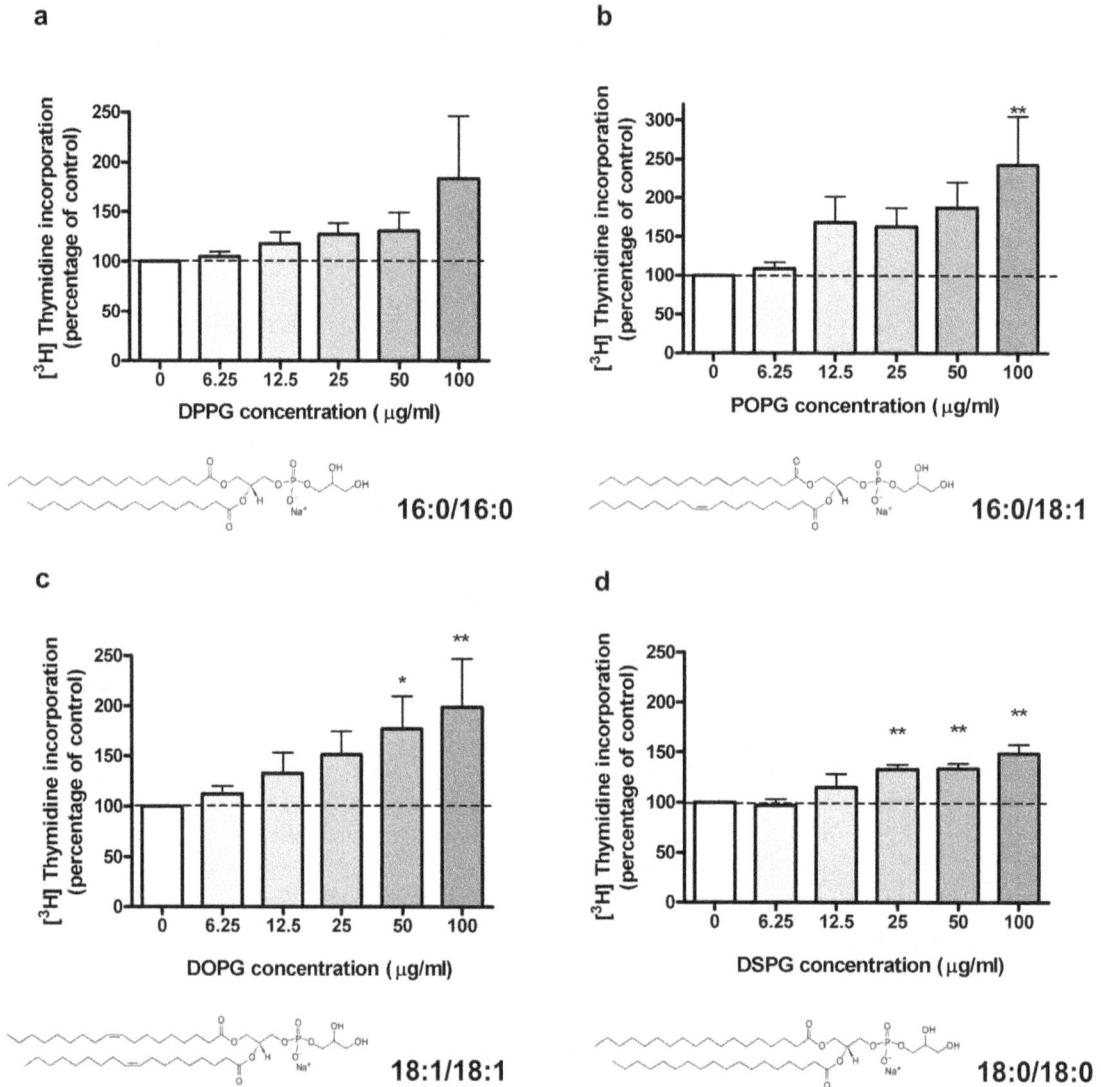

Figure 1. Effects of PG species containing saturated or monounsaturated fatty acids on keratinocyte proliferation. Near-confluent keratinocytes were treated for 24 hrs with the indicated concentrations of liposomes of DPPG (A), POPG (B), DOPG (C) or DSPG (D), prepared via bath sonication of the different PG species in SFKM. [3H]Thymidine incorporation into DNA was then determined as in [10]. Values represent the means ± SEM of 4 to 11 separate experiments performed in duplicate; *$p < 0.05$, **$p < 0.01$ versus the control value (0 µg/mL). [3H]Thymidine incorporation into DNA in the control was 31,300±8,400 cpm/well, 33,600±9,800 cpm/well, 32,200±8,700 cpm/well, and 44,200±1,200 cpm/well for panels A, B, C and D, respectively.

potent than that of egg PG, whereas DPPG, POPG, and DHPG were significantly less inhibitory (or slightly stimulatory) relative to egg PG. These results imply that the acyl groups of PG species play a key role in the effects of this phospholipid signal on keratinocyte proliferation. Because the fatty acid tails can be released from the phospholipids potentially allowing them to exert independent effects on cells, it was important to test whether the glycerol head group, and thus the intact phospholipid, mediates the ability of PG species to modulate keratinocyte proliferation.

Comparison of the effects of DLPG and DLPP on keratinocyte proliferation

In a previous study, we used liposomes composed of dioleoyl- or dipalmitoyl-phosphatidylpropanol (DOPP or DPPP) as a phospholipid control for PG [8]. Note that phosphatidylpropanol has essentially the same structure as PG, lacking only the two hydroxyl

groups at the C2 and C3 positions of the head group. This makes it a good control for determining effects mediated by the glycerol head group. Comparison of the previous study with the present study indicates that the glycerol head group plays a role in the stimulatory effect of PG species containing saturated or monounsaturated fatty acids. Specifically, whereas DPPG tended to increase keratinocyte proliferation and DOPG significantly increased keratinocyte proliferation in the present study (Figure 1), neither DPPP nor DOPP had a significant effect on keratinocyte proliferation in the previous study [8]. To investigate whether the glycerol head group plays a role in the inhibitory effect of PG species containing polyunsaturated fatty acids, we compared the effects of DLPG and DLPP on keratinocyte proliferation. DLPG was selected because it was one of the most effective inhibitory PG species in the present study (Figure 2).

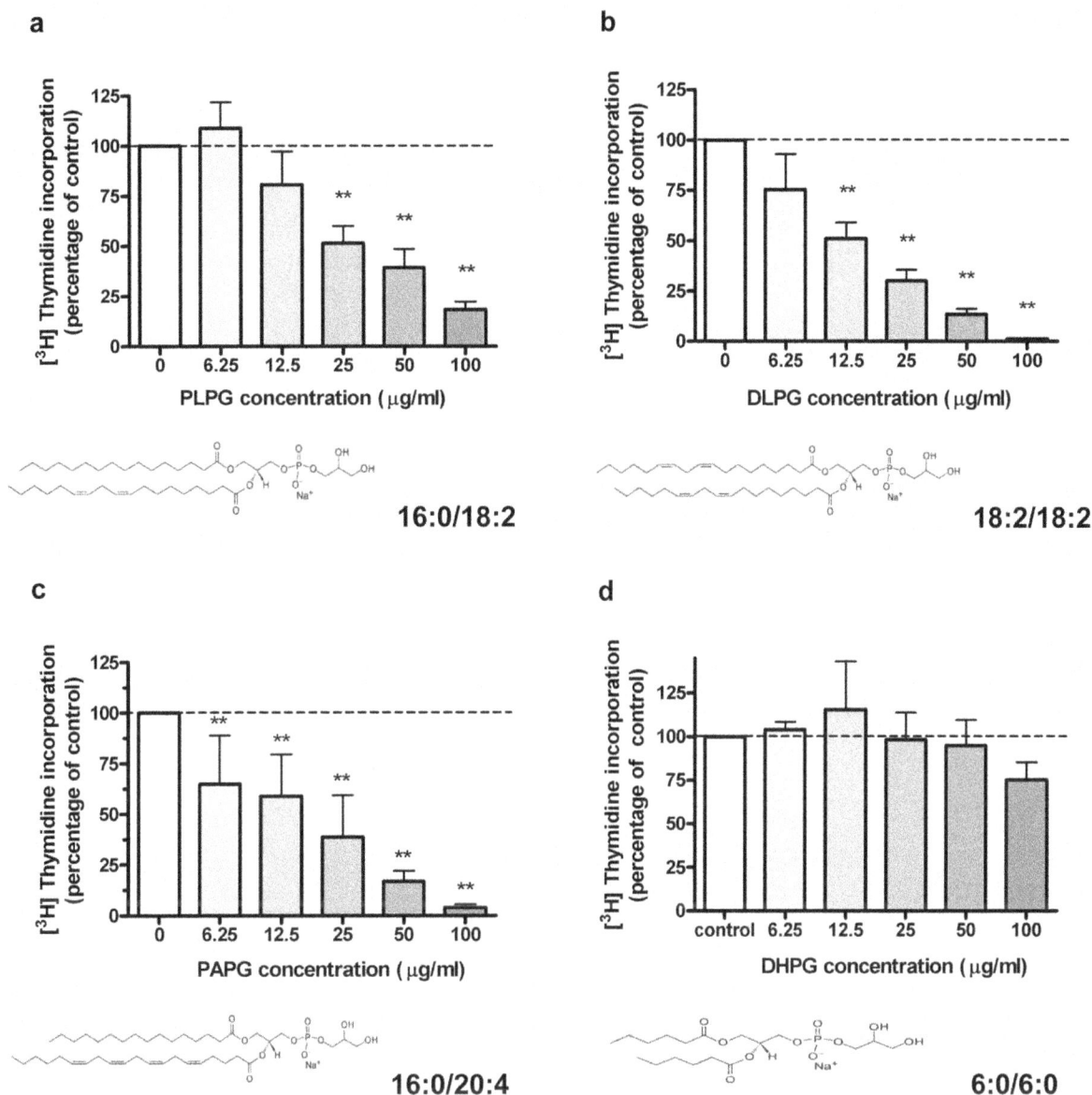

Figure 2. Effects of PG species containing polyunsaturated fatty acids on keratinocyte proliferation. Near-confluent keratinocytes were treated for 24 hrs with the indicated concentrations of liposomes of PLPG (A), DLPG (B), PAPG (C) or DHPG (D), prepared via bath sonication of the different PG species in SFKM. [3H]Thymidine incorporation into DNA was then determined as above. Values represent the means ± SEM of 3 to 5 separate experiments performed in duplicate; *p<0.05, **p<0.01 versus the control value (0 µg/mL level served as control in each panel). [3H]Thymidine incorporation into DNA in the control was 45,300±4,900 cpm/well, 37,700±8,900 cpm/well, 66,000±13,000 cpm/well, and 55,300±8,900 cpm/well for panels A, B, C, and D respectively.

As shown in Figure 5, both DLPG and DLPP, with the same polyunsaturated fatty acid tails, significantly inhibited keratinocyte proliferation compared with control. However, DLPG was more potent, exerting a significantly greater inhibitory effect than DLPP. In particular, DLPP induced a significant inhibition only at 50 µg/mL, and this dose was significantly less inhibitory than that of the corresponding dose of DLPG, whereas DLPG induced significant inhibition at one quarter the dose (12.5 µg/mL). These results suggest that the polar head group of PG does indeed play a role in the effect of PG species on keratinocyte proliferation, whether stimulatory or inhibitory, and argue against the idea that the effect of PG is mediated to any great extent through fatty acids released from the phospholipid.

Discussion

PG is garnering attention as a physiologically active phospholipid with potential involvement in cell signaling. Older studies from the Elias laboratory suggested the existence of a PG-activated protein kinase (PK-P) in human leukemia cells and human spleen [15,16]. A subsequent study indicated that this protein kinase was in fact, protein kinase C (PKC)-θ, which mediates the phosphorylation of the actin-binding sequence of moesin [17]. Similarly, Fields and colleagues published several reports [18–20] detailing the discovery of the role of nuclear PG in activating PKCβII to induce the phosphorylation of lamin B and the subsequent dissolution of the nuclear membrane during cell division in leukemia cell lines. More recent studies have suggested a role for

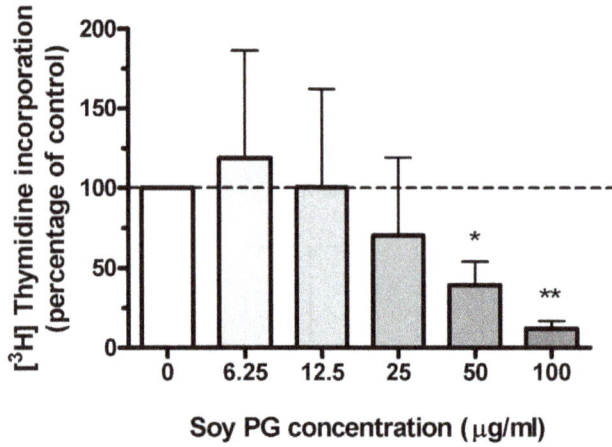

Figure 3. Effects of soy PG on keratinocyte proliferation. Near-confluent keratinocytes were treated for 24 hrs with the indicated concentrations of soy PG liposomes, prepared via bath sonication of the phospholipid in SFKM. [3H]Thymidine incorporation into DNA was then determined as above. Values represent the means ± SEM of 5 separate experiments performed in duplicate; *p<0.05, **p<0.01 versus the control value (0 µg/). [3H]Thymidine incorporation into DNA in the control was 62,600±8,000 cpm/well.

PG in stabilizing membrane proteins [21], activating the ferlin family of proteins that mediate membrane trafficking [22], enhancing protein-protein interaction [23,24] and protecting cells from the harmful effects of mitochondrial cardiolipin deficiency [25].

Our previous study provided evidence for the existence in primary mouse keratinocytes of a novel lipid signaling pathway, for which PG is a key effector in regulating keratinocyte proliferation and differentiation (reviewed in [26]). In particular, we showed that egg PG inhibits keratinocyte proliferation in rapidly dividing keratinocytes and stimulates keratinocyte proliferation in slowly dividing keratinocytes [8]. Since there are many species of PG, with different fatty acid compositions, present in egg PG and in the human body, in this report we sought to identify the most effective PG species able to normalize keratinocyte function, with the idea that this phospholipid could be used to treat skin diseases characterized by excessive or insufficient proliferation.

Unexpectedly, we found that PG with different compositions, that is, monounsaturated versus polyunsaturated fatty acid-containing species, had different effects on keratinocyte proliferation. In detail, PG species containing monounsaturated fatty acids, such as the oleic acid in POPG (16:0/18:1) and DOPG (18:1/18:1), stimulated mouse keratinocyte proliferation, while PG species containing polyunsaturated fatty acids, such as the arachidonic and linoleic acids in PAPG (16:0/20:4), PLPG

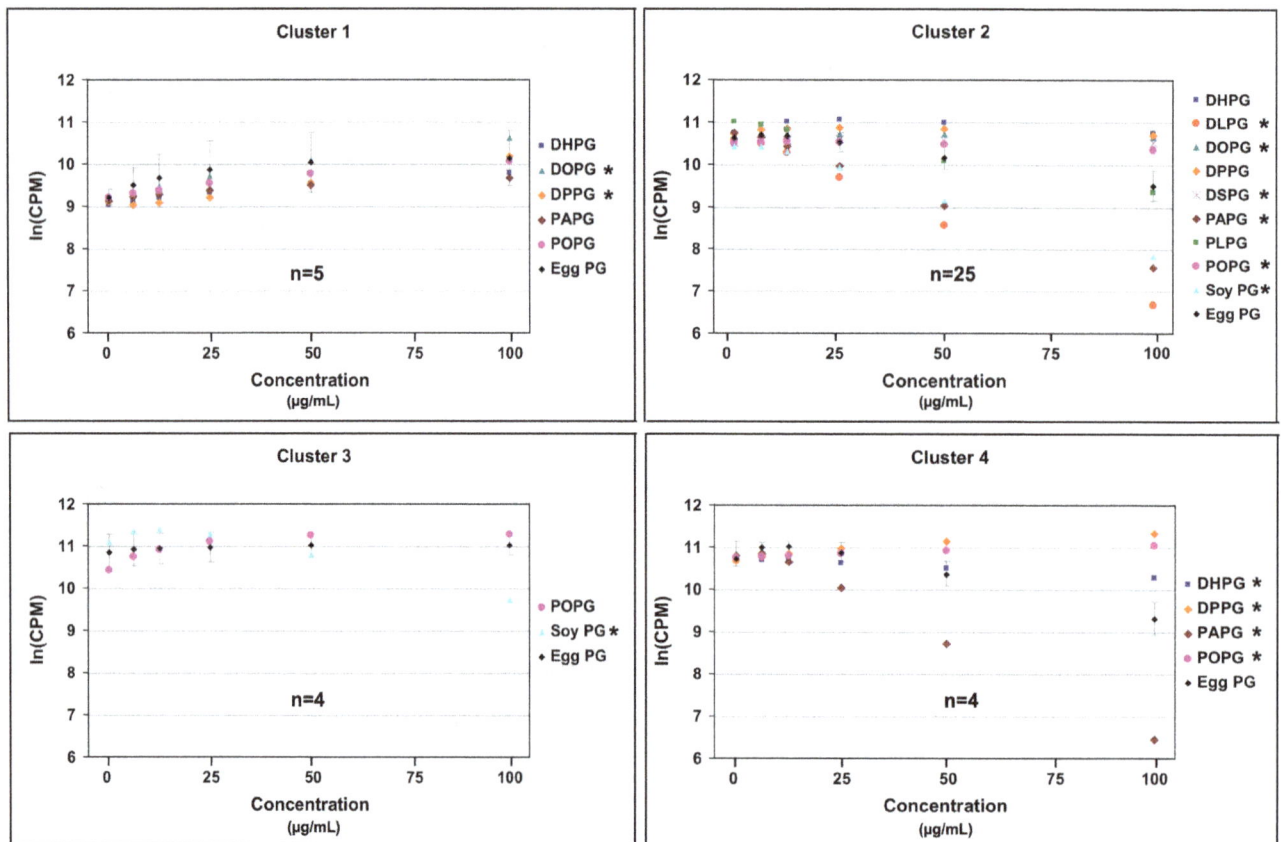

Figure 4. Comparison of Effects of PG Species on Keratinocyte Proliferation. Based on the regression line of the comparative egg PG data, Cluster 1 represents the experiments with a linear increasing relationship between ln(CPM) and ln(concentration) of egg PG, Cluster 2 represents the experiments with a non-linear decreasing relationship between ln(CPM) and ln(concentration), Cluster 3 represents the experiments with a flat, quadratic relationship between ln(CPM) and ln(concentration), and Cluster 4 represents the experiments with a decreasing step function between ln(CPM) and ln(concentration), respectively. Those PG species exhibiting a statistically significant difference from egg PG (either a greater or lesser effect) are marked by asterisks. The number of different experiments for which the egg PG comparator was performed is indicated.

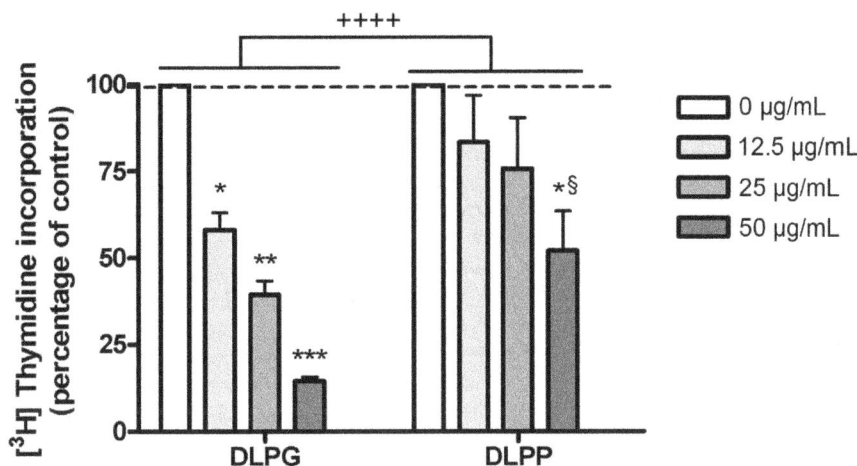

Figure 5. Comparison of the Effects of DLPG and DLPP on Keratinocyte Proliferation. Near-confluent to confluent keratinocytes were treated for 24 hrs with the indicated concentrations of liposomes composed of DLPG or DLPP, prepared via bath sonication of the phopholipid in SFKM. [^{3}H]Thymidine incorporation into DNA was then determined. Values represent the means ± SEM of more than 3 separate experiments performed in duplicate; **p<0.01, ***p<0.001 versus the control value (0 µg/mL); §p<0.05 versus the corresponding concentration of DLPG; ++++ p<0.0001 as indicated. [^{3}H]Thymidine incorporation into DNA in the control was 50,400±7,500 cpm/well, and 53,300±6,400 cpm/well for DLPG and DLPP, respectively.

(16:0/18:2) and DLPG (18:2/18:2), inhibited mouse keratinocyte proliferation. It is perhaps not surprising that PG species with different acyl groups have different signaling functions since in the lung saturated PG cannot block the anti-inflammatory effects of surfactant protein A on lipopolysaccharide (LPS)-treated macrophages while unsaturated PG can [27]. Nevertheless, to our knowledge, ours represents the first report of opposite effects of two species within the same phospholipid class on a particular cellular response. Our previous studies suggested that PG liposomes might be an ideal treatment to normalize skin function under both pathological and physiological conditions [8]. The discovery reported here suggests that specific PG species might be used under different conditions.

The efficacy of linoleic acid-containing PGs is intriguing considering the fact that this fatty acid is the predominant species in the epidermis. Thus, Marcello and colleagues found that linoleic acid represents over 20% of the fatty acid species in the epidermis [28]. Interestingly, linoleic acid percentage was higher in the suprabasal layers of the epidermis (27.4%) in comparison with the basal layer (20.7%). In addition, polyunsaturated fatty acids compose 37% of the fatty acids of suprabasal epidermis [28]. This result suggests the possibility that PGs containing polyunsaturated fatty acids are physiologically relevant in terms of regulating keratinocyte proliferation. Furthermore, it would suggest that PG formed from the action of PLD2 on phosphatidylcholine in the presence of glycerol (provided by AQP3) may contain a high proportion of polyunsaturated fatty acids.

For each PG species we tested, we also tested at the same time within the same cell preparation the effects of egg PG as a comparator. By performing an egg PG dose response in all experiments, a later assessment among experiments could be accomplished. As demonstrated previously [8], we observed both inhibitory and stimulatory effects of this phospholipid on keratinocyte proliferation (Figure 4). Egg PG exhibited an inhibitory effect on proliferation in rapidly proliferating cells (clusters 2–4 of Figure 4), while in slowly proliferating keratinocytes, egg PG showed stimulatory effects on cell proliferation (cluster 1 of Figure 4). This result suggested that under different physiologic or pathologic conditions, specific PG species can exert

opposite effects to "normalize" keratinocyte proliferation, although the current report suggests that this normalization reflects, at least in part the presence in egg PG of more than one PG species with different signaling functions.

Although synthetic polyunsaturated fatty acid-containing PGs, and in particular DLPG, seemed most effective at inhibiting keratinocyte proliferation in vitro, the expense of these PGs could potentially preclude their use as a treatment for psoriasis. Therefore, we also investigated the ability of soy PG, a mixture of PG species containing a high proportion of polyunsaturated fatty acids, to inhibit keratinocyte proliferation. This lipid also has the advantage of being a natural product, and our results in vitro indicated its efficacy (Figure 3).

Previously, we had also shown that neither DOPP nor DPPP altered keratinocyte proliferation [8]; however, the corresponding PG species either tended to stimulate keratinocyte proliferation (DPPG) or significantly stimulated keratinocyte proliferation (DOPG). Likewise, although both DLPG and DLPP (18:2/18:2) inhibited keratinocyte proliferation, the effect of DLPG was significantly greater than that of DLPP. Together these results indicate the importance of the head group in determining the effects of PG and argue against the idea that the fatty acids are being released from the PG phospholipid to induce the disparate effects observed.

Several questions remain. For example, what downstream targets of the specific PG species exert the inhibitory or stimulatory effects on keratinocyte proliferation? We speculate that PG exerts different effects through different effector pathways. One potential mechanism stems from the observation by Murray and Fields [18] that in human leukemia cells PG binds to and stimulates protein kinase CβII (PKCβII), an important protein kinase mediating proliferation in these cells. Furthermore, these authors demonstrated that specific PG species exhibit different activities but that other phospholipids (phosphatidylserine and phosphatidylcholine) do not mimic the effect of PG, suggesting that the ability of PG to activate PKCβII resides in the head group [18]. A role for the fatty acid side chain constituents is also provided by the finding that DOPG was significantly more potent at stimulating PKCβII activity than the other PG species tested [18]. Likewise, DOPG produced a potent stimulatory effect on DNA synthesis, suggesting the possibility that PKCβII might underlie the growth effects of PG [18]. On the other hand, many PKC isoforms trigger differentiation rather than proliferation in keratinocytes [29,30]. Moreover, Murray and Fields [18] did not determine the efficacy of PG species containing polyunsaturated fatty acids (the only species tested were DOPG, DPPG, POPG, and DSPG). Therefore, it is possible that PKCβII stimulated by polyunsaturated fatty acid-containing PG may instead be prodifferentiative in keratinocytes. Indeed, in other experiments we have determined that overexpression of PKCβII appears to sensitize keratinocytes to the differentiating effects of PG as well as of an elevated extracellular calcium concentration (manuscript in preparation), which stimulates the production of PG [5].

PG might also function by an ability to modify pattern recognition receptor signaling, such as occurs upon activation of toll-like receptors (TLR). Pattern recognition receptors can be activated not only in reponse to pathogen-associated molecular patterns but also damage-associated molecular patterns arising from cell injury (reviewed in [31,32]). For example, PG, produced by alveolar cells as a significant component of pulmonary surfactant, inhibits TLR signaling in macrophages exposed to LPS *in vitro*, acting at multiple sites to disrupt TLR4 signaling [33], as well as TLR2 pathway activation in response to bacterial and mycoplasma byproducts *in vitro* [34]. PG also protects the lungs from inflammation initiated by LPS exposure *in vivo* [33]. In addition, PG inhibits infection of airway epithelial cells by respiratory syncytial virus and influenza A *in vitro* and protects the lungs from the deleterious effects of these viruses *in vivo* [35,36]. Finally, in eukaryotes PG is a precursor of cardiolipin [37], a key mitochondrial lipid that plays a role in mitochondrial function and energy production as well as apoptosis (reviewed in [38]). Indeed, PG can partially substitute for cardiolipin in several

cellular functions [25]. Moreover, PG can inhibit cell death in response to apoptosis-inducing agents and/or cardiolipin deficiency [25,39], suggesting another possible mechanism by which this lipid signal might regulate keratinocyte growth and differentiation.

In summary, we showed that PG species containing polyunsaturated fatty acids were effective at inhibiting rapidly proliferating keratinocytes, whereas PG species with monounsaturated and saturated fatty acids were effective at promoting proliferation in slowly dividing keratinocytes. Our results support the idea that these effects require both the glycerol headgroup and the fatty acid tails because (1) different fatty acids had disparate actions and (2) phospholipids similar to PG but lacking the glycerol headgroup (phosphatidypropanol) were less efficacious than the corresponding PG in promoting proliferation or differentiation. To our knowledge these findings also represent the first (and so far only) demonstration of the ability of different species within a given phospholipid class to induce opposite effects in intact cells. Future investigation is ongoing to determine the downstream targets of the AQP3-PLD2-PG signaling pathway and the mechanism by which the different PGs exert these disparate effects. Since abnormal keratinocyte proliferation and differentiation characterize a wide range of skin diseases, the findings of this study may open new avenues for treatment of these diseases. Furthermore, our results suggest that different PG species may be useful for treating various skin diseases characterized by excessive or insufficient proliferation.

Author Contributions

Conceived and designed the experiments: DX JGE WBB. Performed the experiments: DX MS. Analyzed the data: DX RP WBB. Contributed to the writing of the manuscript: DX RP WBB.

References

1. Goldsmith LA (1991) Physiology, Biochemistry, and Molecular Biology of the Skin. New York: Oxford University Press.
2. Yuspa SH, Hennings H, Tucker RW, Kilkenny A, Lee E, et al. (1990) The Regulation of Differentiation in Normal and Neoplastic Keratinocytes. New York: Wiley-Liss, Inc. 211–222 p.
3. Slominski AT, Zmijewski MA, Skobowiat C, Zbytek B, Slominski RM, et al. (2012) Sensing the environment: regulation of local and global homeostasis by the skin's neuroendocrine system. Adv Anat Embryol Cell Biol 212: v, vii, 1–115.
4. Langley R (2005) Psoriasis: everything you need to know. New York: Firefly Books, Inc.
5. Zheng X, Ray S, Bollag WB (2003) Modulation of phospholipase D-mediated phosphatidylglycerol formation by differentiating agents in primary mouse epidermal keratinocytes. Biochim Biophys Acta 1643: 25–36.
6. Zheng X, Bollag WB (2003) Aquaporin 3 colocates with phospholipase D2 in caveolin-rich membrane microdomains and is downregulated upon keratinocyte differentiation. J Invest Dermatol 121: 1487–1495.
7. Zheng X, Ray S, Bollag WB (2003) Modulation of phospholipase D-mediated phosphatidylglycerol formation by differentiating agents in primary mouse epidermal keratinocytes. Biochim Biophys Acta 1643: 25–36.
8. Bollag WB, Xie D, Zheng X, Zhong X (2007) A potential role for the phospholipase D2-aquaporin-3 signaling module in early keratinocyte differentiation: production of a phosphatidylglycerol signaling lipid. J Invest Dermatol 127: 2823–2831.
9. Bollag WB, Zhong X, Dodd ME, Hardy DM, Zheng X, et al. (2005) Phospholipase d signaling and extracellular signal-regulated kinase-1 and -2 phosphorylation (activation) are required for maximal phorbol ester-induced transglutaminase activity, a marker of keratinocyte differentiation. J Pharmacol Exp Ther 312: 1223–1231.
10. Griner RD, Qin F, Jung EM, Sue-Ling CK, Crawford KB, et al. (1999) 1,25-Dihydroxyvitamin D3 induces phospholipase D-1 expression in primary mouse epidermal keratinocytes. J Biol Chem 274: 4663–4670.
11. Bollag WB, Ducote J, Harmon CS (1993) Effects of the selective protein kinase C inhibitor, Ro 31-7549, on the proliferation of cultured mouse epidermal keratinocytes. J Invest Derm 100: 240–246.
12. Griner RD, Qin F, Jung EM, Sue-Ling CK, Crawford KB, et al. (1999) 1,25-Dihydroxyvitamin D3 induces phospholipase D-1 expression in primary mouse epidermal keratinocytes. J Biol Chem 274: 4663–4670.

13. Grün B, Leisch F (2007). Fitting finite mixtures of generalized linear regressions in R Computational Statistics & Data Analysis 51: 5247–5252.
14. Bollag WB, Xie D, Zhong X, Zheng X (2007) A potential role for the phospholipase D2-aquaporin-3 signaling module in early keratinocyte differentiation: Production of a novel phosphatidylglycerol lipid signal. J Invest Dermatol 127: 2823–2831.
15. Klemm DJ, Elias L (1988) Phosphatidylglycerol-modulated protein kinase activity from human spleen. II. Interaction with phospholipid vesicles. Arch Biochem Biophys 265: 506–513.
16. Klemm DJ, Elias L (1988) Purification and assay of a phosphatidylglycerol-stimulated protein kinase from murine leukemic cells and its perturbation in response to IL-3 and PMA treatment. Exp Hematol 16: 855–860.
17. Pietromonaco SF, Simons PC, Altman A, Elias L (1998) Protein kinase C-q phosphorylation of moesin in the actin-binding sequence. J Biol Chem 273: 7594–7603.
18. Murray NR, Fields AP (1998) Phosphatidylglycerol is a physiologic activator of nuclear protein kinase C. J Biol Chem 273: 11514–11520.
19. Gökmen-Polar Y, Fields AP (1998) Mapping of a molecular determinant for protein kinase C bII isozyme function. J Biol Chem 273: 20261–20266.
20. Murray NR, Burns DJ, Fields AP (1994) Presence of a beta II protein kinase C-selective nuclear membrane activation factor in human leukemia cells. J Biol Chem 269: 21385–21390.
21. Laganowsky A, Reading E, Allison TM, Ulmschneider MB, Degiacomi MT, et al. (2014) Membrane proteins bind lipids selectively to modulate their structure and function. Nature 510: 172–175.
22. Marty NJ, Holman CL, Abdullah N, Johnson CP (2013) The C2 domains of otoferlin, dysferlin, and myoferlin alter the packing of lipid bilayers. Biochemistry 52: 5585–5592.
23. Bao H, Duong F (2013) Phosphatidylglycerol directs binding and inhibitory action of EIIAGlc protein on the maltose transporter. J Biol Chem 288: 23666–23674.
24. Kruse O, Hankamer B, Konczak C, Gerle C, Morris E, et al. (2000) Phosphatidylglycerol is involved in the dimerization of photosystem II. J Biol Chem 275: 6509–6514.
25. Potting C, Tatsuta T, Konig T, Haag M, Wai T, et al. (2013) TRIAP1/PRELI complexes prevent apoptosis by mediating intramitochondrial transport of phosphatidic acid. Cell Metab 18: 287–295.

26. Qin H, Zheng X, Zhong X, Shetty AK, Elias PM, et al. (2011) Aquaporin-3 in keratinocytes and skin: Its role and interaction with phospholipase D2. Arch Biochem Biophys 508: 138–143.

27. Chiba H, Piboonpocanun S, Mitsuzawa H, Kuronuma K, Murphy RC, et al. (2006) Pulmonary surfactant proteins and lipids as modulators of inflammation and innate immunity. Respirology 11: S2–S6.

28. Terashi H, Izumi K, Rhodes LM, Marcelo CL (2000) Human stratified squamous epithelia differ in cellular fatty acid composition. J Dermatol Sci 24: 14–24.

29. Yuspa SH, Ben T, Hennings H, Lichti U (1982) Divergent responses in epidermal basal cells exposed to the tumor promoter 12-O-tetradecanoylphorbol-13-acetate. Cancer Res 42: 2344–2349.

30. Stanwell C, Denning MF, Rutberg SE, Cheng C, Yuspa SH, et al. (1996) Staurosporine induces a sequential program of mouse keratinocyte terminal differentiation through activation of PKC isozymes. J Invest Dermatol 106: 482–489.

31. McCarthy CG, Goulopoulou S, Wenceslau CF, Spitler K, Matsumoto T, et al. (2014) Toll-like receptors and damage-associated molecular patterns: novel links between inflammation and hypertension. Am J Physiol Heart Circ Physiol 306: H184–196.

32. Modlin RL (2012) Innate immunity: ignored for decades, but not forgotten. J Invest Dermatol 132: 882–886.

33. Kuronuma K, Mitsuzawa H, Takeda K, Nishitani C, Chan ED, et al. (2009) Anionic pulmonary surfactant phospholipids inhibit inflammatory responses from alveolar macrophages and U937 cells by binding the lipopolysaccharide-interacting proteins CD14 and MD-2. J Biol Chem 284: 25488–25500.

34. Kandasamy P, Zarini S, Chan ED, Leslie CC, Murphy RC, et al. (2011) Pulmonary surfactant phosphatidylglycerol inhibits Mycoplasma pneumoniae-stimulated eicosanoid production from human and mouse macrophages. J Biol Chem 286: 7841–7853.

35. Numata M, Chu HW, Dakhama A, Voelker DR (2010) Pulmonary surfactant phosphatidylglycerol inhibits respiratory syncytial virus-induced inflammation and infection. Proc Natl Acad Sci U S A 107: 320–325.

36. Numata M, Kandasamy P, Nagashima Y, Posey J, Hartshorn K, et al. (2012) Phosphatidylglycerol suppresses influenza A virus infection. Am J Respir Cell Mol Biol 46: 479–487.

37. Tan BK, Bogdanov M, Zhao J, Dowhan W, Raetz CR, et al. (2012) Discovery of a cardiolipin synthase utilizing phosphatidylethanolamine and phosphatidylglycerol as substrates. Proc Natl Acad Sci U S A 109: 16504–16509.

38. Osman C, Voelker DR, Langer T (2011) Making heads or tails of phospholipids in mitochondria. J Cell Biol 192: 7–16.

39. Shaban H, Borras C, Vina J, Richter C (2002) Phosphatidylglycerol potently protects human retinal pigment epithelial cells against apoptosis induced by A2E, a compound suspected to cause age-related macula degeneration. Exp Eye Res 75: 99–108.

16

Increased Levels of Eotaxin and MCP-1 in Juvenile Dermatomyositis Median 16.8 Years after Disease Onset; Associations with Disease Activity, Duration and Organ Damage

Helga Sanner[1,2,9], Thomas Schwartz[3,4,5*,9], Berit Flatø[1,5], Maria Vistnes[3,4], Geir Christensen[3,4], Ivar Sjaastad[3,4,6]

1 Section of Rheumatology, Oslo University Hospital-Rikshospitalet, Oslo, Norway, 2 Norwegian Competence Centre of Pediatric and Adolescent Rheumatology, Oslo University Hospital-Rikshospitalet, Oslo, Norway, 3 Institute for Experimental Medical Research, Oslo University Hospital-Ullevål, Oslo, Norway, 4 KG Jebsen Cardiac Research Center and Center for Heart Failure Research, University of Oslo, Oslo, Norway, 5 Institute for Clinical Medicine, University of Oslo, Oslo, Norway, 6 Department of Cardiology, Oslo University Hospital-Ullevål, Oslo, Norway

Abstract

Objective: To compare cytokine profiles in patients with juvenile dermatomyositis (JDM) after medium to long-term follow-up with matched controls, and to examine associations between cytokine levels and disease activity, disease duration and organ damage.

Methods: Fifty-four JDM patients were examined median 16.8 years (2–38) after disease onset (follow-up) and compared with 54 sex- and age-matched controls. Cytokine concentrations in serum were quantified by Luminex technology. In patients, disease activity score (DAS), myositis damage index (MDI) and other disease parameters were collected by chart review (early parameters) and clinical examination (follow-up).

Results: Serum levels of eotaxin, monocyte chemoattractant protein-1 (MCP-1) and interferon-inducible protein 10 (IP-10) were elevated in JDM patients compared to controls (31.5%, 37.2% and 43.2% respectively, all $p < 0.05$). Patients with active ($n = 28$), but not inactive disease ($n = 26$) had a higher level of MCP-1 than their respective controls. Levels of eotaxin and MCP-1 correlated with disease duration ($r = 0.47$ and $r = 0.64$, both $p < 0.001$) and age in patients, but not with age in controls. At follow-up, MDI was associated with MCP-1 (standardized $\beta = 0.43$, $p = 0.002$) after adjusting for disease duration and gender. High MDI 1 year post-diagnosis predicted high levels of eotaxin and MCP-1 at follow-up (standardized $\beta = 0.24$ and 0.29, both $p < 0.05$) after adjusting for disease duration and gender.

Conclusion: Patients with JDM had higher eotaxin, MCP-1 and IP-10 than controls. High eotaxin and MCP-1 at follow-up was predicted by early disease parameters, and MCP-1 was associated with organ damage at follow-up, highlighting a role of these chemokines in JDM.

Editor: Paul Proost, University of Leuven, Rega Institute, Belgium

Funding: The authors have no support or funding to report.

Competing Interests: The authors have declared that no competing interests exist.

* E-mail: thomas.schwartz@medisin.uio.no

⑨ These authors contributed equally to this work.

Introduction

Juvenile dermatomyositis (JDM) is a systemic autoimmune vasculopathy of childhood, involving proximal muscle weakness and characteristic skin lesions. While the mortality rate has decreased (now ∼3%) [1], still 30–61% of patients have signs of sustained disease activity and 60–90% develop organ damage 7.2–16.8 years after disease onset [1–3]. Thus new therapeutic targets could improve patient care; however, the pathogenesis of JDM is not fully understood.

Cytokines are small signal molecules, produced by endothelial-immune- and muscle cells. They mediate and regulate innate and adaptive immune responses and inflammatory reactions through a number of mechanisms including recruitment and activation of leukocytes [4]. During the last decade, the role of cytokines and chemokines (chemotactic cytokines) in the pathogenesis in myositis has been an area of interest [5,6]. However, most studies performed on cytokines consist of mixed patients groups with polymyositis (PM), adult dermatomyositis (DM) and juvenile DM and if controlled, the studies are small. Increased plasma levels of interleukine 18 (IL-18) [7] and IL-15 [8] are reported in patients with DM/PM early in the disease course (first year and median 1 year, respectively). IL-15 was also shown to correlate with disease activity [8]. In a controlled study on 37 DM and 19 JDM patients (median disease duration 2 years), several chemokines including monocyte attractant protein-1 (MCP-1) and interferon-inducible protein 10 (IP-10) were increased [9]. Recently, criteria for clinically inactive disease state in JDM were proposed by the Paediatric Rheumatology International Trials Organization (PRINTO) [10]; however it is not clear whether disease state is associated with a specific signature of cytokines or inflammatory parameters.

Knowledge about cytokine abundance in myositis, in particular JDM, is limited. Specifically there is lack of studies with long-term follow up. Our sex- and age-matched patient-control pairs [11,12] provide a unique opportunity to compare the cytokine profile in JDM patients after medium to long-term follow-up and to explore how cytokine levels correlate with measures of disease activity and damage at follow-up and at 1 year post-diagnosis.

Materials and Methods

Patients and controls

Inclusion criteria were a probable or definitive diagnosis of DM according to the Bohan and Peter criteria [13], disease onset before 18 years, minimum 24 months disease duration and age ≥6 years at inclusion. We identified a retrospective inception cohort of 66 JDM patients diagnosed between January 1970 and June 2006 in Norway, previously described in detail [2,14,15]. Four of the patients were deceased; the remaining 62 could all be tracked through the Norwegian population register, and 59 (95%) participated in the study.

Sex- and age-matched controls were randomly drawn from the National Population Register. Exclusion criteria in the controls were: mobility problems, inflammatory rheumatic disease, other autoimmune conditions treated with immunosuppressive agents, and heart or lung disease (except for mild asthma). After cytokine analyses, statistical calculations to detect outliers were performed and 5 pairs were excluded (see statistical analysis). The data presented are based on the remaining 54 patients and 54 controls.

Ethics statement

Written informed consent was obtained from all patients and controls (and their parents if aged below 16 years), according to the Declaration of Helsinki. The study was approved by the South-Eastern Regional Ethics Committee for Medical Research.

Data collection and clinical measures

At Oslo University Hospital from September 2005 to May 2009, a single physician (HS) performed clinical examination of all patients, median 16.8 years (range 2–38 years) after disease onset (follow-up), and matched controls. In patients, disease activity was assessed by Disease Activity Score (DAS) for JDM [16] (range 0–20, 0 = no activity), which consists of DAS skin (0–9) and DAS muscle (0–11). Cumulative organ damage was measured by Myositis Damage Index (MDI, range 0–35/40) [17]. In addition, retrospective scoring of DAS and MDI from the first year post-diagnosis were performed, based on chart review [2]. From the criteria proposed by PRINTO (2012), inactive disease was defined as at least 3 of the following 4: manual muscle test (MMT-8) ≥78 (0–80), physician global assessment of muscle activity (phyGlo-VAS) ≤0.2, Childhood Myositis Assessment Scale (CMAS) ≥48 and creatine kinase (CK) ≤150 [10,18]. JDM patients with inactive disease are referred to as JDM-inactive and the remaining patients are called JDM-active. Physical health was measured by the Short Form-36 (SF-36) physical component summary score (PCS) [19]. The Health Assessment Questionnaire (HAQ) [20] and the Childhood HAQ [21] were used to measure physical

function in patients aged ≥18 years (n = 35) and <18 years (n = 19), respectively. At time of follow-up, none of the study participants had clinical signs of infection. Disease onset was defined as the time of the first muscle or skin symptom clearly related to JDM (by chart review) and disease duration as the time from disease onset to follow-up examination. History of medication was obtained from study cases and by chart review.

Laboratory analyses

At follow-up examination, venous blood samples were collected and serum concentrations of 29 cytokines analysed. IL-1β, IL-1 receptor antagonist (Ra), IL-2, IL-4, IL-5, IL-6, IL-7, IL-8 (CXCL8), IL-9, IL-10, IL-12, IL-13, IL-15, IL-17, basic fibroblast growth factor (bFGF), granulocyte-colony-stimulating factor (G-CSF), granulocyte-macrophage colony-stimulating factor (GM-CSF), interferon γ (IFN-γ), IP-10 (CXCL10), MCP-1 (CCL2), macrophage inflammatory protein 1α (MIP-1α) (CCL3), MIP-1β (CCL4), eotaxin (CCL11), platelet-derived growth factor bb (PDGF), TNF-α, and vascular endothelial growth factor (VEGF) were quantified using Bio-Plex protein array systems (Bio-Rad, Hercules, CA), based on xMAP technology (Luminex, Austin, TX). The Luminex analyses were performed according to manufacturer's protocol, with minor modifications [22], including selection of high-sensitivity standard curve to optimize measurements of non-septic concentrations of cytokines. However, the high-sensitivity standard curve yielded physiological concentrations of Regulated upon Activation, Normal T-cell Expressed, and Secreted (RANTES/CCL5) above detection limit. RANTES was therefore excluded for further analyses. An intra-assay variation with a coefficient of variation (CV) of 7.49±0.81 was calculated based on measurements of standards. To diminish the effect of the inter-assay variation, all samples were analyzed in a randomized fashion. Three of the 29 cytokines, IFN-α, IL-18 and transforming growth factor β1 (TGF-β1), were analysed with enzyme-linked immunosorbent assay (ELISA) technique.

Along with cytokine analyses, Th1/Th2 cell balance (ratio between CD4+ Th1 helper cells that produce IFN-γ and IL-2 and CD4+ Th2 helper cells that produce IL-4, IL-5, IL-6, IL-10 and IL-13) was evaluated by calculating the ratio of IFN-γ/IL-4 [23]. Erythrocyte sedimentation rates (ESR) were assessed and high-sensitive serum concentration of C-reactive protein (CRP) analysed.

Statistical analysis

Differences between patients and matched controls were tested by the paired sample t-test for normally distributed continuous variables. Two tailed tests were used for all calculations except for comparisons where a priori patients, based on the literature were likely not to have lower values than controls (e.g. ESR and CRP). Bonferroni correction was performed when appropriate. Correlations were determined by Spearman correlation coefficient (r). Association between eotaxin and MCP-1 (dependent variables) and MDI, DAS skin and DAS muscle measured 1 year post-diagnosis and at follow-up (independent variables) were tested in multivariate linear regression models with forward deletion of the variables after controlling for age and gender. Age was not included in the linear regression model due to high intercorrelation (r = 0.9) with disease duration. p value <0.05 was considered significant. SPSS version 20.0 (SPSS, Chicago, Il) was used for statistical analyses.

To detect outlying individuals, we calculated the mean cytokine levels for all groups and found the Mahalanobis distance from the cytokine level of each individual to its respective group mean. Bonferroni corrected p values were obtained based on an approximation of the Mahalanobis distance to a chi square distribution with the number of cytokines as degrees of freedom. One patient and four controls had samples with a p value <0.001 and were therefore considered to be outliers. These five and their matched control or patient were removed from the data set before the remaining statistical analyses, hence data from 54 pairs were analyzed and presented.

Results

Characteristics and serum cytokine levels in JDM patients and controls

Characteristics of the 54 JDM patients and 54 sex- and age-matched controls are shown in Table 1. Eotaxin-, MCP-1- and IP-10-levels were higher in patients than in controls (31.5%, 37.2% and 43.2% respectively, all p<0.05, Table 2). No differences between patients and controls in levels of the other 26 cytokines, Th1/Th2 ratio (Table 2), CRP or ESR were found (Table 1).

Cytokines and inflammatory parameters in JDM-active vs JDM-inactive and in JDM-active and JDM-inactive vs controls

According to PRINTO criteria, 26 (48%) of the patients had inactive disease. No differences were found between JDM-active and JDM-inactive in ESR (8.5 (6.1) vs 5.9 (4.7) mm, p = 0.09),

CRP (2.7 (2.8) vs 1.8 (3.7) mg/L, p = 0.36) or in the 29 cytokines studied (Table 2).

However, the 28 JDM-active had 47.9% higher level of MCP-1 (35.5 (19.9) vs 24.0 (10.7) pg/ml, p = 0.012) than their matched controls; between JDM-inactive and their controls, no such difference in MCP-1 levels were seen (33.8 (24.2) vs 26.8 (12.2) pg/ml, p = 0.18.

Associations between cytokines, age and disease parameters at follow-up

Eotaxin and MCP-1 both correlated with disease duration (r = 0.64 and r = 0.47, p's<0.001, Table 3 and Figure 1) and age in patients. However, when exploring the association between age and serum cytokine levels in controls, no associations were found. IP-10 correlated neither with disease duration nor with age in patients or controls.

Both Eotaxin and MCP-1, but not IP-10, correlated with MDI at follow-up (Table 3). High MCP-1 was associated with high CRP, low SF-36 PCS, high CHAQ/HAQ and high cumulative prednisolone dose. Eotaxin and MCP-1 intercorrelated stronger in patients than in controls. No intercorrelation between IP-10 and IFN-α was seen neither in patients nor in controls (r = −0.12 and r = 0.11). No correlations were seen neither between eotaxin, MCP-1 nor IP-10 and disease activity (DAS) at follow-up. In a multivariate linear regression analysis, MDI at follow-up was associated with MCP-1 (standardized β = 0.43, p = 0.002, R² final

Table 1. Characteristics and disease parameters in 54 patients with juvenile dermatomyositis and in 54 controls.

Characteristics	JDM patients	Controls
Females	32 (59)	32 (59)
Age at symptom onset (years)	7.7 (1.4–17.3)	NA
Age at diagnosis (years)	8.5 (2.1–19.3)	NA
Variables assessed median 16.8 years after disease onset (follow-up)		
Age (years) at follow-up	22.0 (6.7–55.4)	22.1 (6.2–55.4)
Duration from disease onset (years)	16.8 (2.0–38.1)	NA
CRP (<4 mg/L)	2.3 (3.3)	1.4 (3.1)
ESR (<17 mm)[†]	7.0 (5.7)	5.7 (4.8)
SF 36 PCS[‡] (0–100)	54.3 (26.9–60.9)	56.9 (32.1–63.7)*
CHAQ/HAQ (0–3)	0 (0–1.38)	NA
MDI total (0–40)	3 (0–13)	NA
DAS skin (0–9)	4 (0–7)	NA
DAS muscle (0–11)	1 (0–8)	NA
DAS total (0–20)	5 (0–13)	NA
Prednisolone dosis, cumulative (g)	10.6 (12.3)	NA
Prednisolone or DMARDs	16 (30)	NA
Variables assessed 1 year post- diagnosis		
MDI total (0–40)	1 (0–7)	NA
DAS skin (0–9)	4 (0–8)	NA
DAS muscle (0–11)	1 (0–7)	NA
DAS total (0–20)	5 (0–15)	NA

Values are number (%), median (range) or mean (SD). JDM: juvenile dermatomyositis; NA: not applicable; CRP: C-reactive protein; ESR: erythrocyte sedimentation rate; SF-36 PCS: Short Form 36 physical component Summary; CHAQ: Childhood Health Assessment Questionnaire; DMARDs: disease modifying anti-rheumatic drugs; MDI: Myositis Damage Index; DAS: Disease Activity Score.
*p<0.05.
[‡]n = 46 pairs, only assessed in those >13 years;
[†]n = 50 pairs.

Table 2. Cytokine levels in patients with juvenile dermatomyositis assessed median 16.8 years after disease onset, and in controls.

	JDM active	JDM inactive	All JDM	Controls	p value
MCP-1	35.5 (19.9)	33.8 (24.2)	34.7 (21.9)	25.3 (11.4)	0.006
IP-10	1598 (1631)	1361 (877)	1484 (1316)	1036 (475)	0.026
Eotaxin	150 (118)	133 (90)	142 (105)	108 (63.6)	0.039
IL-6	8.4 (14.1)	4.9 (4.0)	6.7 (10.6)	4.0 (2.0)	0.060
TNF-α	23.3 (25.7)	21.4 (18.0)	22.4 (22.2)	16.3 (7.2)	0.065
IL-13	2.7 (4.7)	2.8 (4.6)	2.8 (4.6)	1.6 (0.9)	0.078
IL-8	11.3 (3.3)	10.6 (2.0)	10.9 (2.7)	10.2 (2.2)	0.080
IL-1Ra	204 (396)	134 (140)	170 (301)	98.7 (61.5)	0.084
IFN-γ	62.0 (86.8)	49.1 (43.5)	54.7 (70.5)	40.2 (20.9)	0.134
IL-10	6.1 (23.2)	3.5 (6.8)	4.8 (17.3)	1.7 (1.6)	0.183
IL-15	2.3 (3.1)	2.4 (3.0)	2.4 (3.0)	1.7 (1.7)	0.210
IL-18	422 (152)	415 (213)	419 (182)	391 (154)	0.336
TGF-β1	28000 (6770)	29900 (10700)	28900 (8860)	29500 (7360)	0.703
IL-4	2.1 (0.57)	2.1 (0.55)	2.1 (0.55)	2.0 (0.57)	0.794
IL-1β	0.96 (0.90)	1.1 (1.1)	1.0 (1.0)	1.0 (0.9)	0.946
Th1/Th2	27.6 (35.3)	23.8 (22.6)	25.8 (29.6)	19.7 (9.4)	0.780
IFN-α	11.9 (1.8)	11.1 (0.8)	11.5 (1.5)	12.0 (1.4)	0.07

Values for cytokine levels are mean (SD) pg/ml; n: all JDM = 54, controls = 54, JDM active = 28, JDM inactive = 26. p value when comparing cytokine levels in all JDM and controls; for the comparison active vs inactive JDM, no differences were detected. The cytokines shown were selected based on associations seen in the present and/or previous studies on dermatomyositis or other rheumatic diseases. JDM: juvenile dermatomyositis; MCP: monocyte chemoattractant protein; IP: interferon-inducible protein; IL: interleukine; TNF: tumor necrosis factor; Ra: receptor antagonist; TGF: transforming growth factor; Th1/Th2, IFN-γ/IL-4.

model = 40%), none of the control measures (age and gender) were significant. A borderline significant association was seen between MDI and eotaxin (standardized $\beta = 0.25$, $p = 0.054$) in a similar linear regression analysis.

Early predictors of elevated eotaxin and MCP-1 levels

MDI and DAS total assessed 1 year post-diagnosis, correlated both with eotaxin and MCP-1 (Table 4). DAS skin, but not DAS muscle correlated with eotaxin and borderline with MCP-1.

In a linear regression analysis, MDI 1 year post-diagnosis predicted high MCP-1 (standardized $\beta = 0.29$, $p = 0.025$). Of the control measures, disease duration contributed significantly (standardized $\beta = 0.32$, $p = 0.014$), but not gender (R^2 final model = 34%).

Accordingly, MDI 1 year post-diagnosis also predicted high eotaxin (standardized $\beta = 0.24$, $p = 0.049$), both of the control measures were significant (gender, standardized $\beta = 0.23$, $p = 0.045$; disease duration, standardized $\beta = 0.41$, $p = 0.001$; R^2 final model = 41%).

Discussion

In our study we have investigated cytokine abundance in JDM patients and found, median 16.8 years after disease onset, increased serum levels of eotaxin, MCP-1 and IP-10, compared to matched controls. When stratified in JDM-active and JDM-inactive, MCP-1 was elevated in JDM-active in comparison to their respective controls; not in JDM-inactive compared to controls. Eotaxin and MCP-1 both correlated with disease duration, and increased levels were predicted by high score of organ damage early in the disease course. MCP-1 was associated with cumulative organ damage at follow-up. To our knowledge,

no other controlled study has investigated circulating cytokine profile in an unselected JDM cohort after long-term follow up.

We have previously described the representativeness of our cohort [2], which we believe contains the vast majority of Norwegian JDM patients diagnosed between 1970 and 2006. Our cohort is comparable with other hospital or registry based cohorts with regards to female predominance, age at diagnosis, medication and muscle weakness at disease onset [24,25]. The representativeness of the patients and the sex- and age matching with controls drawn randomly from the National Population Register, represent strengths of our study.

We aimed at detecting differences in circulating levels of cytokines in JDM patients compared to controls, and found a significant increase in 3 and a numeric increase with p values of 0.06–0.08 for 5 of 28 cytokines. Eotaxin and MCP-1 correlated with disease duration and therefore, necessarily with age. For patients, age was substantially stronger correlated with eotaxin and MCP-1 than for controls, indicating that the correlation between disease duration and CC chemokines is not driven by aging per se. In previous studies on cytokines, DM and JDM patients have been investigated at time of diagnosis or early in disease course [8,9]. Increased serum levels of eotaxin, MCP-1 and IP-10, were found in a study of 9 JDM patients with clinically active disease [26]. The association between MCP-1 and active disease is supported by our findings: when stratified according to the recently (2012) proposed PRINTO criteria [10], differences in MCP-1 levels compared to controls were seen in JDM-active but not in JDM-inactive. Although we should be careful with our conclusions; we may have been underpowered to detect differences between JDM-active and JDM-inactive. However, the association with disease duration in all patients suggests that eotaxin and MCP-1 may contribute to a sustained inflammation and continue to play a role in JDM throughout the disease course as well.

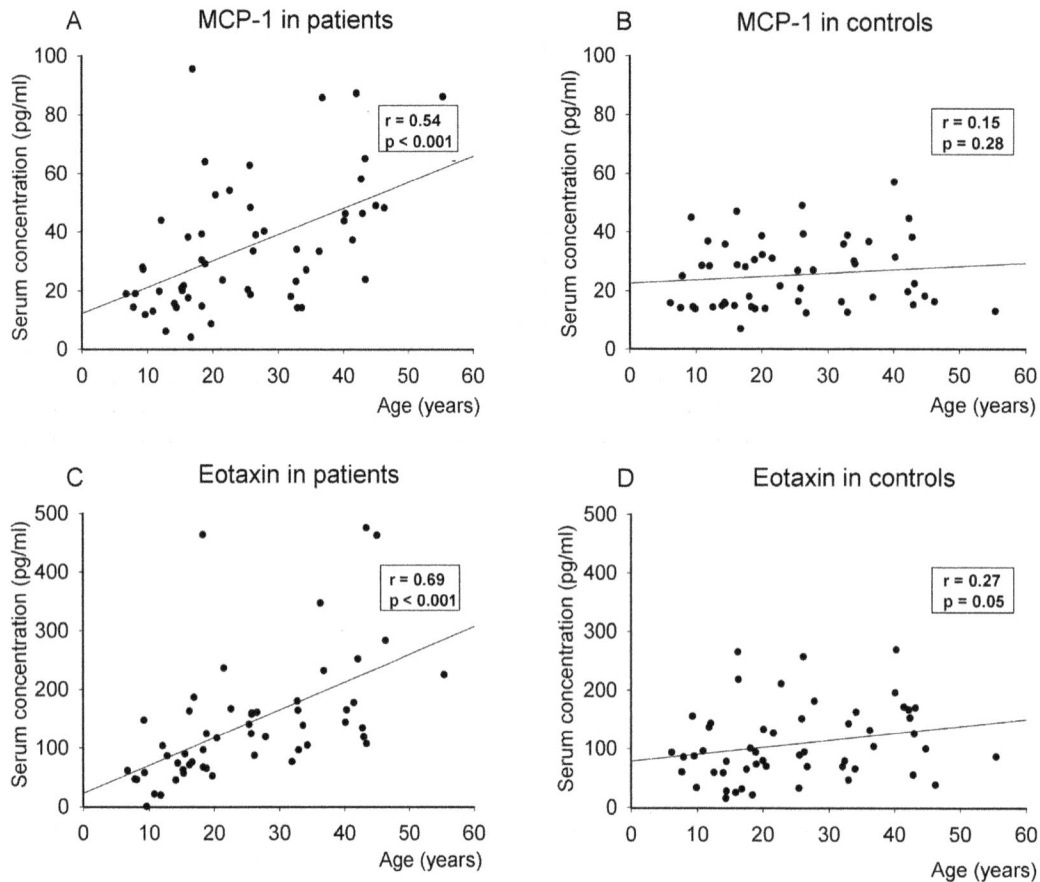

Figure 1. Correlations between monocyte chemoattractant protein-1 (MCP-1) (A and B) and eotaxin (C and D) and age, in 54 patients with juvenile dermatomyositis and sex- and age-matched controls. r, Spearman correlation coefficient.

Table 3. Correlations between MCP-1, eotaxin and clinical and disease variables in patients with juvenile dermatomyositis assessed median 16.8 years after disease onset, and in controls.

	MCP-1		Eotaxin	
Clinical variables	**Patients**	**Controls**	**Patients**	**Controls**
Male gender	0.37*	0.21	0.33*	0.39*
Age	0.54**	0.15	0.69**	0.27*
Disease duration	0.47**	NA	0.64**	NA
ESR	−0.05	−0.08	−0.10	−0.20
CRP	0.27*	0.15	0.09	0.01
Eotaxin	0.70**	0.56**	NA	NA
MDI	0.52**	NA	0.52**	NA
DAS total	0.25	NA	0.18	NA
DAS skin	0.17	NA	0.20	NA
DAS muscle	0.20	NA	0.09	NA
Prednisolone	0.28*	NA	0.22	NA
SF 36 PCS	−0.36*	0.09	−0.24	0.11
CHAQ/HAQ	0.32*	NA	0.21	NA

Values are r = Spearman correlation coefficient. MCP: monocyte chemoattractant protein; ESR: erythrocyte sedimentation rate; CRP: C-reactive protein; MDI: Myositis Damage Index; DAS: Disease Activity Score; Prednisolone: cumulative prednisolone dose during disease course; CHAQ: Childhood Health Assessment Questionnaire; SF-36 PCS: Short Form 36 physical component Summary. *p<0.05; **p<0.001.

Table 4. Correlations between MCP-1, eotaxin and disease variables in patients with juvenile dermatomyositis 1 year post - diagnosis.

	MCP-1		Eotaxin	
	r	p value	r	p value
MDI	0.35	0.01	0.40	0.003
DAS total	0.28	0.039	0.36	0.007
DAS skin	0.27	0.053	0.36	0.008
DAS muscle	0.18	0.20	0.18	0.21

MCP: monocyte chemoattractant protein; r: Spearman correlation coefficient; MDI: Myositis Damage Index; DAS: Disease Activity Score.

Several studies suggest a role of IFN-α activity in adult and juvenile dermatomyositis [27,28]. Since IFN-α was comparable in patients and controls, we did not analyze correlations with disease parameters.

Our observation that eotaxin correlated with early DAS skin, indicates a link between eotaxin and skin affection, in JDM. Some studies associate eotaxin to fibrosis in different tissues as heart, liver and lungs [29–31]. In JDM, eotaxin might induce similar tissue fibrosis, either by recruiting granulocytes that release pro-fibrotic substances, or by itself. Furthermore, we found a correlation between eotaxin and organ damage (MDI) at follow-up, and in this context a pro-fibrotic effect could be relevant. The increased eotaxin and MCP-1 levels in patients could support a hypothesis of low-grade sustained inflammation in JDM, contributing to accumulate organ damage as suggested in juvenile idiopathic arthritis [32]. Furthermore, correlation between eotaxin at follow-up, and disease activity and organ damage at 1 year post-diagnosis could indicate that this is a process initiated early in the course of the disease.

It is reasonable to believe that JDM patients have a more widespread and pronounced inflammation at the time of diagnosis than at long-term follow-up. A large study from Sweden in 2010 showed that in rheumatoid arthritis (RA), many cytokines, including eotaxin and MCP-1, were increased even before disease onset, with further increase at the time of diagnosis [33]. In JDM, a small study showed initial inflammation by measuring increased serum level of IL-18 at time of diagnosis; the level then decreased through the first year of the disease [23]. In our study, extensive information about disease course was obtained through data from patients with disease duration ranging from 2 to 38 years. It is noteworthy that none of the cytokines showed a negative correlation with disease duration as one perhaps might expect. Whether there is a continuous increase in eotaxin abundance after the initial active disease, remains unknown. Given the cross-sectional nature of the study, we did not have data on the cytokine levels from the initial years of the disease. One could speculate in a biphasic response: a high initial level of eotaxin, then a decline until, again, a steady climb after 2 years and onwards based on the data in our study. This could be pursued by comparing our long-term results with a prospective study with serial cytokine samples, during the early phase of the disease.

MCP-1 is an attractor and activator of monocytes and T-lymphocytes and is more studied than eotaxin. Besides being an important actor in the immune response, MCP-1 is involved in inflammation, angiogenesis and formation of atherosclerosis [34]. The angiogenetic effect is especially interesting since JDM is a vasculopathy, this could be evaluated by capillaroscopy.

Homology between eotaxin and MCP-1 is 49% and they share 64% of the protein structure [35]; our data also show intercor-

relation between the two. Eotaxin is the natural agonist of CC chemokine receptor 3 (CCR3), thus elevated circulating levels of this chemokine may potentially increase the recruitment of CCR3-expressing cells, thereby maintaining chronic inflammation. However, eotaxin has also been shown to be a partial agonist of the receptor CCR2 for which MCP-1 is a full agonist [36]. Thus, eotaxin can partially block MCP-1 effects and could for instance modulate monocyte recruitment in inflammatory condition which is a main effect of MCP-1. Such interactions may well be present in JDM, although this has not yet been studied.

MCP-1 correlated consistently with organ damage and early disease activity and, as well as with other inflammatory parameters such as CRP. Also, the association with cumulative prednisolone dosis is interesting, possibly reflecting longstanding active disease. In the DM/JDM patients studied by Bilgic et al [9], correlation between MCP-1, IP-10, IL-6 and global disease activity was also found the first two years of the disease. In our study, high early organ damage predicted elevated levels of both eotaxin and MCP-1. This suggests that eotaxin and MCP-1 measured at follow-up could be useful biomarkers of disease outcome in JDM; particularly since they are both associated with long-term cumulative organ damage. Also since eotaxin and MCP-1 are up regulated in the acute phase of JDM [26] one could speculate that these cytokines could be early biomarkers of organ damage late in disease course.

Eotaxin and MCP-1 may represent targets for biological treatment in JDM. Anti-CCL2/MCP-1 [37], anti-CCL11/eotaxin (bertilimumab) and CCR3 antagonist [38] are available and potential treatment options. However, effects of cytokines are diverse and complex. For example: in the literature, IP-10 is considered as a type1 interferon (IFN-α) regulated cytokine [27], despite this, we saw no correlations between IP-10 and IFN-α in our study. Furthermore, one study showed no clinical improvement in RA by blocking CCR2 [37], whereas another study on a mouse model of RA surprisingly showed exacerbation of arthritis when CCR2 was knocked out [39]. Thus, it is not obvious whether modulation MCP-1 or eotaxin targets will have beneficial effects in JDM, and interactions at receptor level between eotaxin and MCP-1 can obscure interpretation of the results.

In conclusion; in 54 JDM patients seen median 16.8 years after symptom onset, we have shown higher levels of eotaxin, MCP-1 and IP-10, compared to controls. On a subgroup level, increased MCP-1 compared to controls was seen only in JDM-active, not in JDM-inactive. Both eotaxin and MCP-1 correlated with disease duration and organ damage; for IP-10, such correlations were not seen. It is not clear whether eotaxin and MCP-1 per se cause sustained inflammation and represent possible therapeutic targets. They might also be markers for disease damage as a result of disease activity caused by other unknown mechanisms. Either way, the novel knowledge on these substances can improve insight and treatment modalities of JDM.

Acknowledgments

We thank Ståle Nygård for helpful statistical advices and Hilde Dishington for laboratory assistance.

Author Contributions

Conceived and designed the experiments: HS TS BF IS. Performed the experiments: HS MV. Analyzed the data: HS TS BF MV GC IS. Contributed reagents/materials/analysis tools: HS MV. Wrote the paper: HS TS IS. Made critical review and approved the final version of the manuscript: HS TS BF MV GC IS. Had full access to all of the data in the study and take responsibility for the integrity of the data and the accuracy of the data analysis: HS TS BF MV GC IS.

References

1. Ravelli A, Trail L, Ferrari C, Ruperto N, Pistorio A, et al. (2010) Long-term outcome and prognostic factors of juvenile dermatomyositis: a multinational, multicenter study of 490 patients. Arthritis Care Res (Hoboken) 62: 63–72.
2. Sanner H, Gran JT, Sjaastad I, Flato B. (2009) Cumulative organ damage and prognostic factors in juvenile dermatomyositis: a cross-sectional study median 16.8 years after symptom onset. Rheumatology 48: 1541–7.
3. Mathiesen PR, Zak M, Herlin T, Nielsen SM. (2010) Clinical features and outcome in a Danish cohort of juvenile dermatomyositis patients. Clin Exp Rheumatol 28: 782–9.
4. Oppenheim JJ, Feldman M. (2001) Introduction to the role of cytokines in innate and defense and adaptive immunity. In: Oppenheim JJ FM, ed. Cytokine Reference.New York: Academic Press 3–20.
5. De PB, Creus KK, De Bleecker JL. (2009) Role of cytokines and chemokines in idiopathic inflammatory myopathies. Curr Opin Rheumatol 21: 610–6.
6. Zong M, Lundberg IE. (2011) Pathogenesis, classification and treatment of inflammatory myopathies. Nat Rev Rheumatol 7: 297–306.
7. Gono T, Kawaguchi Y, Sugiura T, Ichida H, Takagi K, et al. (2010) Interleukin-18 is a key mediator in dermatomyositis: potential contribution to development of interstitial lung disease. Rheumatology (Oxford) 49: 1878–81.
8. Mielnik P, Chwalinska-Sadowska H, Wiesik-Szewczyk E, Maslinski W, Olesinska M. (2012) Serum concentration of interleukin 15, interleukin 2 receptor and TNF receptor in patients with polymyositis and dermatomyositis: correlation to disease activity. Rheumatol Int 32: 639–43.
9. Bilgic H, Ytterberg SR, Amin S, McNallan KT, Wilson JC, et al. (2009) Interleukin-6 and type I interferon-regulated genes and chemokines mark disease activity in dermatomyositis. Arthritis Rheum 60: 3436–46.
10. Lazarevic D, Pistorio A, Palmisani E, Miettunen P, Ravelli A, et al. (2013) The PRINTO criteria for clinically inactive disease in juvenile dermatomyositis. Ann Rheum Dis 72: 686–93.
11. Schwartz T, Sanner H, Husebye T, Flato B, Sjaastad I. (2011) Cardiac dysfunction in juvenile dermatomyositis: a case-control study. Ann Rheum Dis 70: 766–71.
12. Sanner H, Aalokken TM, Gran JT, Sjaastad I, Johansen B, et al. (2011) Pulmonary outcome in juvenile dermatomyositis: a case-control study. Ann Rheum Dis 70: 86–91.
13. Bohan A, Peter JB. (1975) Polymyositis and dermatomyositis (first of two parts). N Engl J Med 292: 344–7.
14. Sanner H, Kirkhus E, Merckoll E, Tollisen A, Roisland M, et al. (2010) Long term muscular outcome, predisposing and prognostic factors in Juvenile Dermatomyositis: - A case control study. Arthritis Care Res 62: 1103–11.
15. Schwartz T, Sanner H, Gjesdal O, Flato B, Sjaastad I. (2013) In juvenile dermatomyositis, cardiac systolic dysfunction is present after long-term follow-up and is predicted by sustained early skin activity. Ann Rheum Dis; doi:10.1136/annrheumdis-2013-.
16. Bode RK, Klein-Gitelman MS, Miller ML, Lechman TS, Pachman LM. (2003) Disease activity score for children with juvenile dermatomyositis: reliability and validity evidence. Arthritis Rheum 49: 7–15.
17. Isenberg DA, Allen E, Farewell V, Ehrenstein MR, Hanna MG, et al. (2004) International consensus outcome measures for patients with idiopathic inflammatory myopathies. Development and initial validation of myositis activity and damage indices in patients with adult onset disease. Rheumatology (Oxford) 43: 49–54.
18. Sanner H, Sjaastad I, Flato B. (2014) The myositis disease activity assessment tool and the PRINTO criteria for clinically inactive disease applied after long-term follow-up in juvenile onset dermatomyositis. Rheumatology (Oxford): In Press.
19. Sultan SM, Ioannou Y, Moss K, Isenberg DA. (2002) Outcome in patients with idiopathic inflammatory myositis: morbidity and mortality. Rheumatology (Oxford) 41: 22–6.
20. Fries JF, Spitz P, Kraines RG, Holman HR. (1980) Measurement of patient outcome in arthritis. Arthritis Rheum 23: 137–45.

21. Feldman BM, Ayling-Campos A, Luy L, Stevens D, Silverman ED, et al. (1995) Measuring disability in juvenile dermatomyositis: validity of the childhood health assessment questionnaire. J Rheumatol 22: 326–31.
22. Vistnes M, Waehre A, Nygard S, Sjaastad I, Andersson KB, et al. (2010) Circulating cytokine levels in mice with heart failure are etiology dependent. J Appl Physiol 108: 1357–64.
23. Tucci M, Quatraro C, Dammacco F, Silvestris F. (2006) Interleukin-18 overexpression as a hallmark of the activity of autoimmune inflammatory myopathies. Clin Exp Immunol 146: 21–31.
24. McCann LJ, Juggins AD, Maillard SM, Wedderburn LR, Davidson JE, et al. (2006) The Juvenile Dermatomyositis National Registry and Repository (UK and Ireland)—clinical characteristics of children recruited within the first 5 yr. Rheumatology (Oxford) 45: 1255–60.
25. Pachman LM, Abbott K, Sinacore JM, Amoruso L, Dyer A, et al. (2006) Duration of illness is an important variable for untreated children with juvenile dermatomyositis. J Pediatr 148: 247–53.
26. Szodoray P, Alex P, Knowlton N, Centola M, Dozmorov I, et al. (2010) Idiopathic inflammatory myopathies, signified by distinctive peripheral cytokines, chemokines and the TNF family members B-cell activating factor and a proliferation inducing ligand. Rheumatology (Oxford) 49: 1867–77.
27. Baechler EC, Bilgic H, Reed AM. (2011) Type I interferon pathway in adult and juvenile dermatomyositis. Arthritis Res Ther 13: 249.
28. Niewold TB, Kariuki SN, Morgan GA, Shrestha S, Pachman LM. (2009) Elevated serum interferon-alpha activity in juvenile dermatomyositis: associations with disease activity at diagnosis and after thirty-six months of therapy. Arthritis Rheum 60: 1815–24.
29. Zweifel M, Matozan K, Dahinden C, Schaffner T, Mohacsi P. (2010) Eotaxin/CCL11 levels correlate with myocardial fibrosis and mast cell density in native and transplanted rat hearts. Transplant Proc 42: 2763–6.
30. Tacke F, Trautwein C, Yagmur E, Hellerbrand C, Wiest R, et al. (2007) Up-regulated eotaxin plasma levels in chronic liver disease patients indicate hepatic inflammation, advanced fibrosis and adverse clinical course. J Gastroenterol Hepatol 22: 1256–64.
31. Huaux F, Gharaee-Kermani M, Liu T, Morel V, McGarry B, et al. (2005) Role of Eotaxin-1 (CCL11) and CC chemokine receptor 3 (CCR3) in bleomycin-induced lung injury and fibrosis. Am J Pathol 167: 1485–96.
32. de Jager W, Hoppenreijs EP, Wulffraat NM, Wedderburn LR, Kuis W, et al. (2007) Blood and synovial fluid cytokine signatures in patients with juvenile idiopathic arthritis: a cross-sectional study. Ann Rheum Dis 66: 589–98.
33. Kokkonen H, Soderstrom I, Rocklov J, Hallmans G, Lejon K, et al. (2010) Up-regulation of cytokines and chemokines predates the onset of rheumatoid arthritis. Arthritis Rheum 62: 383–91.
34. Yadav A, Saini V, Arora S. (2010) MCP-1: chemoattractant with a role beyond immunity: a review. Clin Chim Acta 411: 1570-9.
35. Garcia-Zepeda EA, Rothenberg ME, Ownbey RT, Celestin J, Leder P, et al. (1996) Human eotaxin is a specific chemoattractant for eosinophil cells and provides a new mechanism to explain tissue eosinophilia. Nat Med 2: 449–56.
36. Martinelli R, Sabroe I, LaRosa G, Williams TJ, Pease JE. (2001) The CC chemokine eotaxin (CCL11) is a partial agonist of CC chemokine receptor 2b. J Biol Chem 276: 42957–64.
37. Vergunst CE, Gerlag DM, Lopatinskaya L, Klareskog L, Smith MD, et al. (2008) Modulation of CCR2 in rheumatoid arthritis: a double-blind, randomized, placebo-controlled clinical trial. Arthritis Rheum 58: 1931–9.
38. Morokata T, Suzuki K, Masunaga Y, Taguchi K, Morihira K, et al. (2006) A novel, selective, and orally available antagonist for CC chemokine receptor 3. J Pharmacol Exp Ther 317: 244–50.
39. Fujii H, Baba T, Ishida Y, Kondo T, Yamagishi M, et al. (2011) Ablation of the Ccr2 gene exacerbates polyarthritis in interleukin-1 receptor antagonist-deficient mice. Arthritis Rheum 63: 96–106.

17

In Vitro Differential Diagnosis of Clavus and Verruca by a Predictive Model Generated from Electrical Impedance

Chien-Ya Hung[1], Pei-Lun Sun[2], Shu-Jen Chiang[3], Fu-Shan Jaw[1]*

1 Institute of Biomedical Engineering, National Taiwan University, Taipei, Taiwan, **2** Department of Dermatology, Mackay Memorial Hospital, Taipei, Taiwan, **3** Institute of Zoology, National Taiwan University, Taipei, Taiwan

Abstract

Background: Similar clinical appearances prevent accurate diagnosis of two common skin diseases, clavus and verruca. In this study, electrical impedance is employed as a novel tool to generate a predictive model for differentiating these two diseases.

Materials and Methods: We used 29 clavus and 28 verruca lesions. To obtain impedance parameters, a LCR-meter system was applied to measure capacitance (C), resistance (R_e), impedance magnitude (Z), and phase angle (θ). These values were combined with lesion thickness (d) to characterize the tissue specimens. The results from clavus and verruca were then fitted to a univariate logistic regression model with the generalized estimating equations (GEE) method. In model generation, log Z_{SD} and θ_{SD} were formulated as predictors by fitting a multiple logistic regression model with the same GEE method. The potential nonlinear effects of covariates were detected by fitting generalized additive models (GAM). Moreover, the model was validated by the goodness-of-fit (GOF) assessments.

Results: Significant mean differences of the index d, R_e, Z, and θ are found between clavus and verruca ($p<0.001$). A final predictive model is established with Z and θ indices. The model fits the observed data quite well. In GOF evaluation, the area under the receiver operating characteristics (ROC) curve is 0.875 (>0.7), the adjusted generalized R^2 is 0.512 (>0.3), and the p value of the Hosmer-Lemeshow GOF test is 0.350 (>0.05).

Conclusions: This technique promises to provide an approved model for differential diagnosis of clavus and verruca. It could provide a rapid, relatively low-cost, safe and non-invasive screening tool in clinic use.

Editor: Johanna M. Brandner, University Hospital Hamburg-Eppendorf, Germany

Funding: This study was supported by grants from the National Science Council (NSC 100-2923-E-002-007-MY3, and NSC 101-2221-E-002-016), Taiwan. The funders had no role in study design, data collection and analysis, decision to publish, or preparation of the manuscript.

Competing Interests: The authors have declared that no competing interests exist.

* E-mail: jaw@ntu.edu.tw

Introduction

Verruca and clavus are two skin disorders commonly encountered in dermatological clinics. Verruca, also referred to as wart, is an infection by human papillomaviruses. Based on the involved site and morphology, verruca can be categorized into several clinical forms, such as verruca vulgaris, plantar and palmar warts, verruca plana, anogenital warts, condyloma, etc. [1]. The former two forms are far more common than the others. These two forms are single or multiple keratotic spiny papules or nodules on hands and/or feet. They are symptomless but can cause pain when grow endophytically on soles. Punctate black dots in verruca, which result from thrombosed capillaries, can be observed by dermoscopy. Verruca lesions may increase in size and number with time and can be contagious.

Although verruca and clavus resemble each other in clinical symptoms, appearances and predilection sites, the latter unlike the former is not contagious. Clavus results from prolonged pressure and friction on the skin [2]. Clavus lesions are painful hard keratotic papules and nodules on soles and palms. Under a dermoscope, a clavus has a compact, homogeneous translucent central core. There may be some hemorrhages resulting from ruptured capillaries due to shearing forces on skin. No punctate black dots are observed in clavus (Figure S1).

Differential diagnosis between verruca and clavus is mainly based on etiology, pathogenesis, treatment, and means of prevention. The standard treatment for verruca is liquid nitrogen cryotherapy. Other therapeutic modalities include curettage, surgical excision, chemical caustics, and immunotherapies. On the other hand, paring of central radix of corn and topical keratolytics are used in treating clavus [1,2]. Histopathology is of great diagnostic value for these two diseases. In typical verruca, there are hyperkeratosis, parakeratosis and acanthosis of epidermis with koilocytes at the upper epidermis and dilated, thrombosed dermal capillaries. As to clavus, there is a prominent parakeratotic plug in the stratum corneum with an underlying atrophied stratum Malpighian layer. Although dermoscopy is a useful non-invasive tool to make the differential diagnosis, its clinical application is operator-dependent, especially in those cases where typical features are lacking. Therefore, finding an effective alternative approach for differentiating between clavus and verruca is highly desirable for clinical diagnosis.

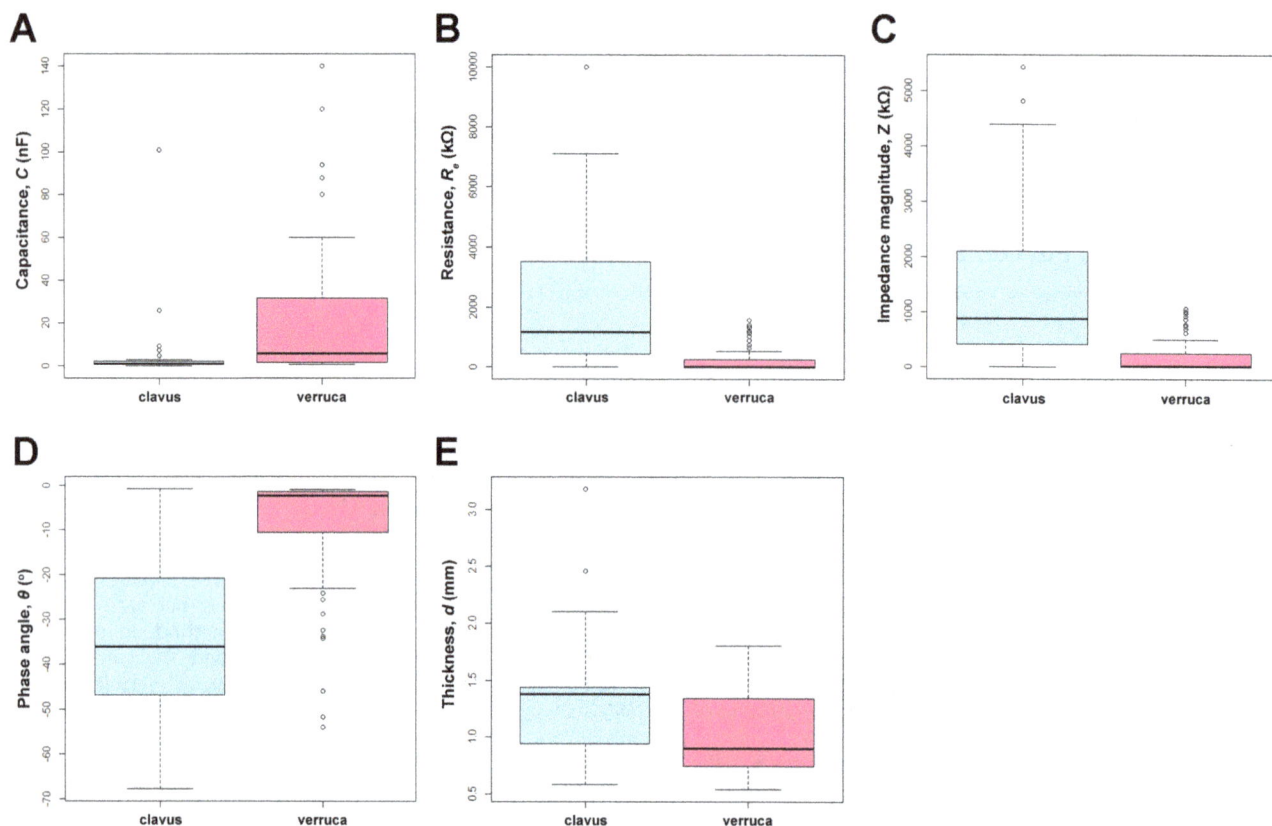

Figure 1. Conditional box plots of the all five measured indices, stratified by clavus and verruca. The lower edge, middle line, and upper edge of the box represent the 25th, 50th, and 75th percentiles of the distribution of the measured index, at 80 Hz. The box plots, A, B, C, D, and E, are for capacitance (C), resistance (R_e), impedance magnitude (Z), phase angle (θ) and thickness (d), respectively.

Electrical impedance, known as a rapid, safe tool with a relatively low cost, has recently been used in measuring skin or stratum corneum hydration [3–12]. It has also been applied to distinguish allergic and irritant contact dermatitis by evaluating the degree of irritation in human skin [13–15]. In addition, the electrical impedance values have been assessed to discriminate skin tumors, such as melanoma, dysplastic nevi, nodular basal cell carcinoma, superficial basal cell carcinoma, as well as benign and malignant skin lesions [16–22]. Clavus has a much thicker stratum corneum and a thinner epidermis than verruca. It is thus expected that their differential thickness and capacitance of stratum corneum will cause differences in their electrical impedance, which can be used as a predictive tool for diagnosing the two types of skin disorders.

In this study, we employed electrical impedance to differentiate between clavus and verruca. The electrical properties of target tissues were measured after a small current or voltage had been applied to them. The resulting impedance values reflected well the different histological constituents of clavus and verruca. It appears quite promising that our study will help build an electrical impedance system for clinical use in the future to quickly and unequivocally discern between clavus and verruca.

Materials and Methods

On the basis of dermoscopic features, specimens were diagnosed and collected by dermatologists from clavus and verruca patients at out-patient clinic. A total of 57 lesions obtained from hands or feet of 29 patients consisted of 29 clavus and 28 verruca lesions.

The criteria for a valid specimen were as follows: Each specimen was (1) diagnosed unequivocally under a dermoscope, (2) greater than 3 mm in diameter, (3) collected from a patient whose lesion has not been treated before, and, (4) regarded as independent if more than one lesion was removed from the same patient. All the samples were processed in accordance with standard treatment protocols for clavus and verruca at our hospital, *i.e.* paring the outer part of the lesions, and applying triacetic acid solution and liquid nitrogen cryotherapy on clavus and verruca, respectively. All the samples were subjected to impedance measuring without any patient information, except the diagnosis. After measuring, all the samples were discarded and disinfected. No patient medical profiles were recorded, thus no linkage between the patients and the samples could be retrieved thereafter.

Impedance measurement

To assemble an electrical impedance system, both sides of each specimen were sealed by two pieces of insulation tape, each with a 3 mm hole in the center. Two holes on each side of the insulation tape were allocated on opposing sides. Therefore, a controlled area of the specimen was used for measurement. This was followed by attaching a pair of pre-gelled electrodes (MEDI-TRACE Mini, Kendall/Tyco, USA) to the two tape holes. Next, the sample was placed in a shielding chamber to reduce noises. Its electrical properties were then measured by a commercial LCR-meter (LCR-821, Instek, Taiwan) under 1 V, at the frequencies of 50 Hz, 80 Hz, 100 Hz, 200 Hz, 1 kHz, 2 kHz, 5 kHz, 10 kHz, 100 kHz, and 1 MHz. The data acquisitions were immediately performed after setup, at 30 min and 60 min. The impedance

Table 1. Comparison of impedance data between clavus and verruca at 80 Hz.

	Clavus	Verruca	Total	p value
Number of subjects	15	14	29	
Number of lesions	29	28	57	
Number of observations	87	84	171	
Measured variable:				
C (nF)	4.21±15.31	19.85±28.66	11.84±24.07	0.099
	1.24 (0.17, 101)	5.85 (0.80, 140)	2.10 (0.17, 140.00)	
R_e (kΩ)	1874.58±2095.43	209.02±397.98	1061.63±1734.63	<0.001
	1153.50 (1.90, 10000)	10.20 (0.74, 1559)	307.50 (0.74, 10000)	
Z (kΩ)	1280.19±1279.58	181.15±311.53	753.70±1094.39	<0.001
	873.90 (2.56, 5436)	16.24 (0.73, 1063)	357.30 (0.73, 5436)	
θ (°)	−33.71±18.36	−8.84±12.69	−21.80±20.16	<0.001
	−36.00 (−67.70, −0.81)	−2.36 (−53.90, −0.99)	−18.30 (−67.70, −0.81)	
d (mm)	1.34±0.55	1.02±0.36	1.19±0.49	<0.001
	1.38 (0.58, 3.18)	0.90 (0.54, 1.80)	1.10 (0.54, 3.18)	
Transformed variable:				
C_{SD}	−0.06±0.85	0.80±1.59	0.36±1.33	0.100
	−0.23 (−0.29, 5.30)	0.03 (−0.25, 7.46)	−0.18 (−0.29, 7.46)	
R_{eSD}	1.11±1.74	−0.27±0.33	0.43±1.44	<0.001
	0.51 (−0.45, 7.85)	−0.44 (−0.45, 0.85)	−0.19 (−0.45, 7.85)	
Z_{SD}	1.13±1.61	−0.26±0.39	0.46±1.38	<0.001
	0.61 (−0.48, 6.35)	−0.46 (−0.48, 0.85)	−0.04 (−0.48, 6.35)	
θ_{SD}	−0.33±0.88	0.87±0.61	0.24±0.97	<0.001
	−0.44 (−1.96, 1.25)	1.18 (−1.30, 1.24)	0.41 (−1.96, 1.25)	
log Z_{SD}	1.02±0.75	−0.43±1.02	0.32±1.15	<0.001
	1.19 (−1.41, 2.01)	−0.58 (−1.96, 1.28)	0.79 (−1.96, 2.01)	
log d	0.22±0.39	−0.04±0.34	0.09±0.39	<0.001
	0.32 (−0.54, 1.16)	−0.11 (−0.62, 0.59)	0.10 (−0.62, 1.16)	

Notes: The measured variables, d, C, R_e, Z, and θ, indicate thickness, capacitance, resistance, impedance magnitude, and phase angle, respectively. The transformed variables, C_{SD}, R_{eSD}, Z_{SD}, and θ_{SD}, signify standardized C, R_e, Z, and θ values, respectively. The transformed variables, log d and log Z_{SD} denote logarithmized d value and standardized logarithmized Z value. The listed values were mean ± standard deviation (SD) on the upper row and median (range) on the lower one. All p-values of group comparisons are obtained by fitting univariate logistic regression models with the generalized estimating equations (GEE) method to account for the correlations between repeated measurements.

indices include capacitance (C), resistance (R_e), impedance magnitude (Z), and phase angle (θ). Additionally, the thickness (d) of the sample was measured by vernier caliper. Temperature and relative humility were recorded.

Statistics analysis

Statistical analysis of the electrical impedance system was performed using the R 3.0.2 software (R Foundation for Statistical Computing, Vienna, Austria) [23]. In statistical testing, two-sided p value ≤0.05 was considered statistically significant. To compare the differentiating powers across frequencies, all observations from 10 frequencies were standardized and examined by conditional plots. After scrutinizing the differences in the conditional plots at 10 frequencies, and also referring to previous studies about keratinized tissues [4], we chose 80 Hz as the optimal frequency due to its differentiating capability (Text S1). For univariate analysis, the measured indices, d, C, R_e, Z, and θ, at 80 Hz were standardized and/or logarithmized to be log d, C_{SD}, R_{eSD}, Z_{SD}, log Z_{SD} and θ_{SD}, respectively. The distributional properties of these continuous variables were expressed by mean ± standard

deviation (SD). These indices were then analyzed by fitting univariate logistic regression model with the generalized estimating equations (GEE) method for examination on the discrimination abilities between clavus and verruca data. Note that the use of the GEE method was to account for the correlations between the repeated measurements within subjects on the lesions.

To generate a best model with predictive factors, multivariate analysis was further performed by fitting multivariate logistic regression model with the same GEE method. The two indices, log Z_{SD} and θ_{SD}, were identified as predictive factors by a stepwise variable selection procedure. To validate the model, the basic model-fitting techniques were applied for (1) variable selection, (2) goodness-of-fit (GOF) assessment, and (3) regression diagnostics and remedies. The GOF assessments the estimated area under the receiver operating characteristic (ROC) curve, adjusted generalized R^2, and the Hosmer-Lemeshow GOF test. In practice, the value of the c statistic ($0 \leq c \leq 1$) ≥0.7 suggests an acceptable level of discrimination power. Adjusted generalized R^2 ≥0.30 indicates an acceptable fit of a logistic regression model. And, larger p values of the Hosmer-Lemeshow GOF test indicate better fits. As regards to

A

B

C

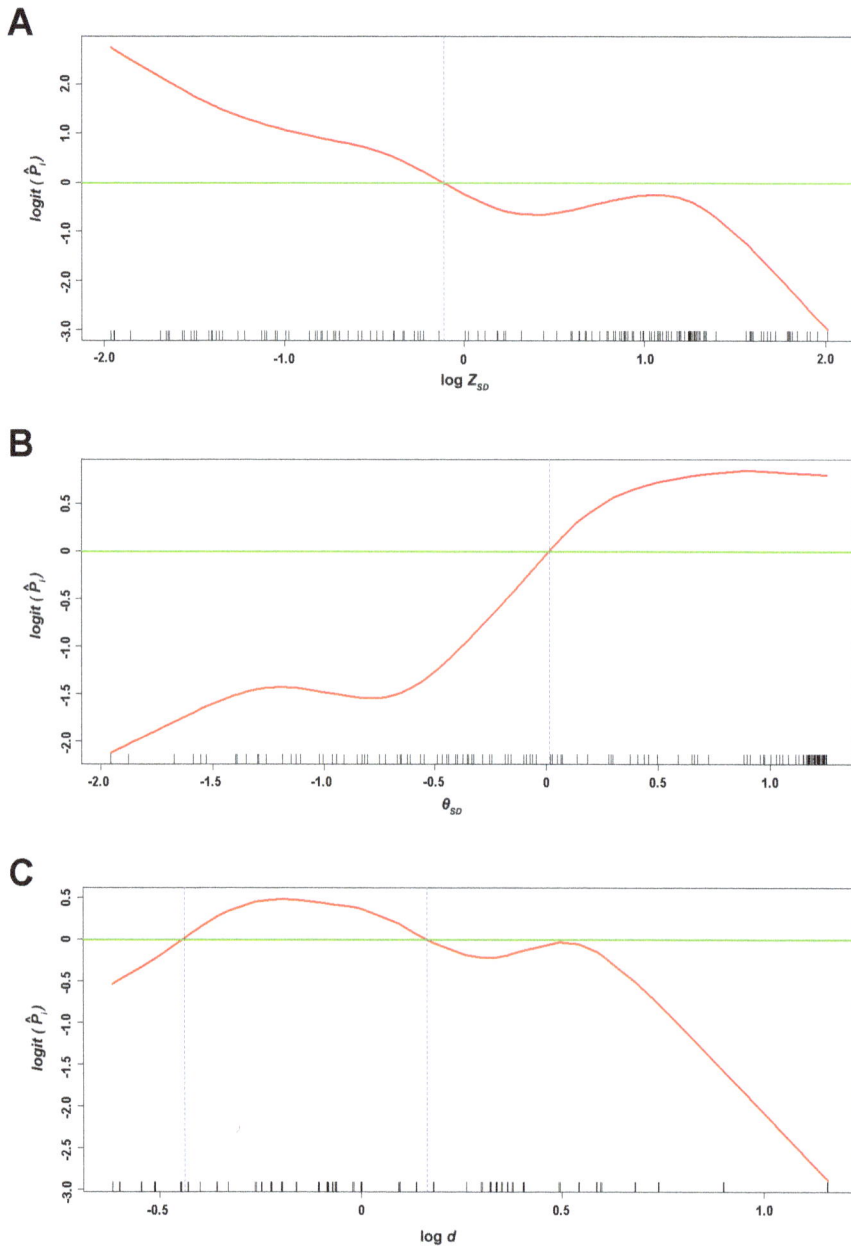

Figure 2. The GAM plots of the predictors, log Z_{SD} (A), θ_{SD} (B), and log d (C) respectively. The generalized additive models plots reveal the smoothed partial effects of the predictors in modeling the probability of being verruca. The distribution of the observed values of log Z_{SD}, θ_{SD}, and log d are shown by the rugs on the X-axes. The Y-axes are the *logit* of the estimated probability of being verruca ($\hat{P}_i$), i.e., $\log\left(\frac{\hat{P}_i}{1-\hat{P}_i}\right)$. The horizontal green line indicates the place where $\hat{P}_i = 0.5$.

regression diagnostics, the non-linear effects of continuous covariates were detected by the generalized additive models (GAM), such that faults in the model can be exposed.

Results

To discriminate the electrical properties between clavus and verruca, the measured and transformed indices of clavus at 80 Hz are compared with those of verruca in Table 1. For statistical analysis, 87 clavus and 84 verruca observations were used. By fitting univariate logistic regression analysis with the GEE method, all impedance indices are significantly different between clavus and verruca ($p<0.001$), except C and C_{SD}. In Figure 1, the

conditional box plots of the measured indices further demonstrate that the absolute value of θ index of clavus is higher than that of verruca. Moreover, R_e and Z values of clavus are approximately ten times higher than those of verruca. These results indicate that high impedance is associated with clavus, whereas low impedance in verruca. Moreover, R_e and Z indices can be used to best distinguish clavus and verruca.

To generate a model for estimating the probability of being verruca versus clavus, all the indices, are analyzed using multivariate logistic regression with the GEE method. Moreover, the GAM plots of Figures 2A and 2B depict the approximately linear partial effects of predictors, log Z_{SD} and θ_{SD}, for the

Table 2. Multivariate analysis of the predictors of verruca at 80 Hz by fitting multiple logistic regression model with the generalized estimating equations (GEE) method.

Covariate	Estimate regression coefficient	Robust Standard Error	Chi-Square test	p Value	Estimated Odds Ratio	95% Confidence Interval of Odds Ratio
Intercept	−0.0198	0.5613	0.0012	0.9719	-	-
log Z_{SD}	−0.9008	0.5670	2.5245	0.1121	0.406	0.134-1.234
θ_{SD}	0.8347	0.7112	1.3773	0.2406	2.304	0.572-9.288

Goodness-of-fit assessment: Number of clusters = 57, number of observations = 166, the estimated area under the Receiver Operating Characteristic (ROC) curve = 0.875>0.7, adjusted generalized R^2 = 0.512>0.3, and Hosmer-Lemeshow goodness-of-fit F test $p = 0.350>0.05$ (df = 9, 156).

Prediction: To calculate the estimated probability of being verruca (i.e., the *predicted value*, $\hat{P}_i$) given the observed covariate values, one can use the following formula. According to the above fitted multiple logistic regression model

$$\text{logit}(\hat{P}_i) = \log\left(\frac{\hat{P}_i}{1-\hat{P}_i}\right) = -0.0198 - 0.9008 \times \log Z_{SD} + 0.8347 \times \theta_{SD} \text{ the } \textit{predicted value} \text{ of observation } i \text{ is}$$

$$\hat{P}_i = \frac{1}{1+\exp[-(-0.0198-0.9008 \times \log Z_{SD}+0.8347 \times \theta_{SD})]} \text{ where } \log Z_{SD} = \text{ logarithmized standardized } Z \text{ value, and } \theta_{SD} = \text{ standardized } \theta \text{ value.}$$

probability of being verruca respectively, but Figure 2C reveals an apparently nonlinear partial effect of log d and identified two appropriate cut-off points in discretizing. Therefore, one of the best models is selected (Text S2). In the final model, the estimated odds ratios (ORs) of predictors, log Z_{SD} and θ_{SD}, are 0.406 ($p = 0.1121$) and 2.304 ($p = 0.2406$), respectively (Table 2). The probability of being verruca (i.e., the predicted value) can be estimated by

$$\hat{P}_i = \frac{1}{1+\exp(0.0198+0.9008 \times \log Z_{SD}-0.8347 \times \theta_{SD})}$$

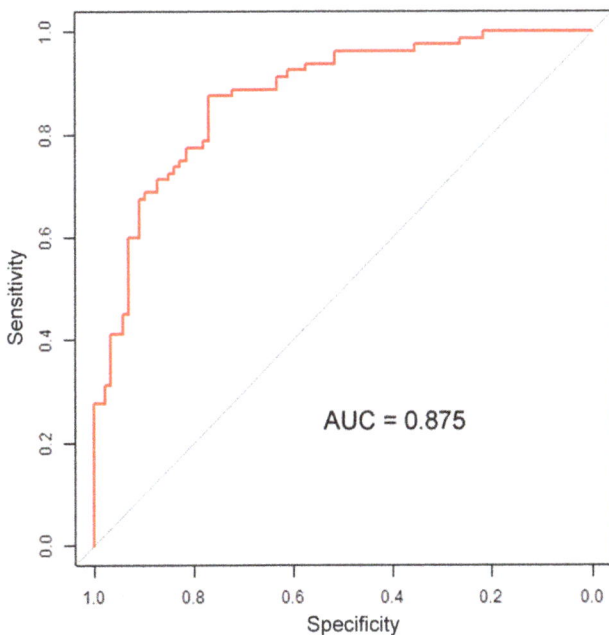

Figure 3. The Receiver Operating Characteristic (ROC) curve for the prediction of verruca. The estimated area under the ROC curve (AUC) is 0.875.

As $\hat{P}_i$ value approaches 1, the more probable the sample is associated with verruca. If $\hat{P}_i$ value approaches 0, the more likely the sample is clavus. Furthermore, based on the above model, GOF assessment is used to validate the performance of the model. The area under the ROC is 0.875 (>0.7) (Figure 3), the adjusted generalized R^2 is 0.512 (>0.3), and the p value of the Hosmer-Lemeshow GOF test is 0.350 (>0.05). These results all pass the tests for best model-fitting techniques. Overall, a model with log Z_{SD} and θ_{SD} as predictive factors is generated for differentiating verruca from clavus, and the validity of the model is determined by GOF method.

Discussion

Impedance is proposed in this study to reflect the different histological constituents of clavus and verruca, so as to assemble a new electrical impedance system for differentiating these two lesion types. Research have disclosed that the impedance/resistivity of stratum corneum is greater than those of other tissues in the human body [24,25], whereas hydration of intact skin decreases the impedance [10,11]. In other words, impedance is high in stratum corneum and correlates reversely with the degree of hydration and admittance. Therefore, the relative high impedance values of clavus lesion found in the study may be resulted from its massive hyperkeratosis and relative thin, atrophic epidermis, which in turn point to the translucent central core under a dermoscope and biopsies. On the contrary, the components of verruca-relative thin stratum corneum, acanthosis proliferated by keratinocytes, and capillary proliferation-may explain why low impedance values are measured. Such differences in impedance values elucidate electrical impedance to be a competitive modality for discriminating the heterogeneous components of clavus from those of verruca.

To identify predictive factor from electrical impedance for model generation, this study discerns statistic differences between clavus and verruca, regarding resistance, impedance magnitude, phase angle, and thickness, but not capacitance. More importantly, resistance and impedance magnitude between clavus and verruca can differ by a factor of ten. However, only the model generated from the two parameters-impedance magnitude and phase angle-fits the data most. This can be explained by the following two equations [18]:

$$Z = \sqrt{R^2 + X^2}$$

$$\theta = \tan^{-1}\left(\frac{X}{R}\right)$$

Here, impedance is defined as total resistance of a biological conductor on alternating current. Simultaneously, it is comprised of two parts: one is resistance, and the other is reactance, defined as X. The reason why impedance magnitude and phase angle are the two parameters for model generation is clear. Furthermore, the advantage of using these two parameters is that they are transformed and calibrated values and as a result of that the predictive procedure becomes far less complicated. It is worthy to note that the use of these two indices in model design has been revealed in previous research, though relating neither to clavus nor to verruca. Impedance magnitude is found to be one of the important indices in analyzing electrical impedance spectra [6,10,12,18–20,26,27]. While, phase angle is in association with the studies concerning cancers, chronic obstructive pulmonary disease, HIV, hospital mortality of geriatric patients, and skin condition test [10,12,26,28,29].

After discussion on the three indices in question, attention is driven to the parameters, thickness and capacitance. Thickness parameter, although showing capabilities in distinguishing between clavus and verruca, is observed to pose problems in impedance analysis, due partly to the difficulties in specifying measured locations, and due partly to its variations caused by biological factors and environmental conditions [10,27]. In addition to this, the thickness of the sample, unlike all the other indices acquired by LCR-meter, is measured manually. Therefore, a model generated without thickness as predictor not only eliminates uncertainties embedded within, but also simplifies its procedure. As for capacitance, it is the only index derived from electrical impedance delivers otherwise result.

Last but not the least, the limitations of the model are detected by the GAM plots. Theoretically, the plots should be linear, but a partial linear is plotted. The non-linear effects of continuous covariates expose the inadequacies of the model. That is to say, misdiagnosis may occur, when lesions are not typical. Non-typical lesions include verruca with very thick corneal layer and few capillary proliferation, and clavus with exceeding hydration.

Conclusions

In conclusion, we employed electrical impedance as a novel tool to postulate a predictive model for differential diagnosis of clavus and verruca. From electrical impedance, log Z_{SD} and θ_{SD}, were two predictive factors derived for estimating the probability of being verruca versus clavus. Moreover, the validity of the model was approved by GOF and GAM methods. In spite of certain limitations, this study provides a rapid, low cost, safe and non-invasive alternative modality for physicians' clinic practice. Further application on *in vivo* diagnosis and investigation on circuit design for size reduction are expected.

Supporting Information

Figure S1 The stereoscopic features of (A) clavus and (B) verruca.

Text S1 Frequency selection.

Text S2 Final model selection.

Author Contributions

Conceived and designed the experiments: PLS FSJ. Performed the experiments: CYH PLS. Analyzed the data: CYH PLS SJC FSJ. Wrote the paper: CYH PLS SJC.

References

1. Androphy EJ, Kirnbauer R (2012). Human papilloma virus infections. In: Goldsmith LA, Katz SI, Gilchrest BA, Paller AS, Leffell DJ, Wolff K, editors. Fitzpatrick's Dermatology in General Medicine, 8th edition. McGraw-Hill Professional. pp. 2421–2433.
2. DeLauro TM, DeLauro NM (2012). Corns and calluses. In: Goldsmith LA, Katz SI, Gilchrest BA, Paller AS, Leffell DJ, Wolff K, editors. Fitzpatrick's Dermatology in General Medicine, 8th edition. McGraw-Hill Professional. pp. 1111–1114.
3. Johnsen GK, Martinsen OG, Grimnes S (2009). Estimation of *in vivo* water content of the stratum corneum from electrical measurements. Open Biomed Eng J 3: 8–12.
4. Martinsen OG, Grimnes S, Sveen O (1997). Dielectric properties of some keratinised tissues. Part 1: Stratum corneum and nail in situ. Med Biol Eng Comput 35: 172–176.
5. Yamamoto T, Yamamoto Y (1976). Electrical properties of the epidermal stratum corneum. Med Biol Eng 14: 151–158.
6. Nicander I, Norlen L, Brockstedt U, Rozell BL, Forslind B, et al. (1998). Electrical impedance and other physical parameters as related to lipid content of human stratum corneum. Skin Res Technol 4: 213–221.
7. Grimnes S (1983). Skin impedance and electro-osmosis in the human epidermis. Med Biol Eng Comput 21: 739–749.
8. Martinsen OG, Grimnes S (2001). Facts and myths about electrical measurement of stratum corneum hydration state. Dermatology 202: 87–89.
9. Lindholm-Sethson B, Han S, Ollmar S, Nicander I, Jonsson G, et al. (1998). Multivariate analysis of skin impedance data in long-term type 1 diabetic patients. Chemometr Intell Lab Syst 44: 381–394.
10. Birgersson U, Birgersson E, Aberg P, Nicander I, Ollmar S (2011). Non-invasive bioimpedance of intact skin: mathematical modeling and experiments. Physiol Meas 32: 1–18.
11. Curdy C, Naik A, Kalia YN, Alberti I, Guy RH (2004). Non-invasive assessment of the effect of formulation excipients on stratum corneum barrier function *in vivo*. Int J Pharm 271: 251–256.
12. Nicander I, Nyren M, Emtestam L, Ollmar S (1997). Baseline electrical impedance measurements at various skin sites _ related to age and sex. Skin Res Technol 3: 252–258.
13. Ollmar S, Nyren M, Nicander I, Emtestam L (1994). Electrical impedance compared with other non-invasive bioengineering techniques and visual scoring for detection of irritation in human skin. Br J Dermatol 130: 29–36.
14. Nicander I, Ollmar S, Eek A, Lundh Rozell B, Emtestam L (1996). Correlation of impedance response patterns to histological findings in irritant skin reactions induced by various surfactants. Br J Dermatol 134: 221–228.
15. Nyren M, Kuzmina N, Emtestam L (2003). Electrical impedance as a potential tool to distinguish between allergic and irritant contact dermatitis. J Am Acad Dermatol 48: 394–400.
16. Glickman YA, Filo O, David M, Yayon A, Topaz M, et al. (2003). Electrical impedance scanning: a new approach to skin cancer diagnosis. Skin Res Technol 9: 262–268.
17. Kuzmina N, Talme T, Lapins J, Emtestam L (2005). Non-invasive preoperative assessment of basal cell carcinoma of nodular and superficial types. Skin Res Technol 11: 196–200.
18. Åberg P, Nicander I, Holmgren U, Geladi P, Ollmar S (2003). Assessment of skin lesions and skin cancer using simple electrical impedance indices. Skin Res Technol 9: 257–261.
19. Beetner DG, Kapoor S, Manjunath S, Zhou X, Stoecker WV (2003). Differentiation among basal cell carcinoma, benign lesions, and normal skin using electric impedance. IEEE Trans Biomed Eng 50: 1020–1025.
20. Aberg P, Nicander I, Hansson J, Geladi P, Holmgren U, et al. (2004). Skin cancer identification using multifrequency electrical impedance-a potential screening tool. IEEE Trans Biomed Eng 51: 2097–2102.

21. Emtestam L, Nicander I, Stenstrom M, Ollmar S (1998). Electrical impedance of nodular basal cell carcinoma: a pilot study. Dermatology 197: 313–316.

22. Dua R, Beetner DG, Stoecker WV, Wunsch DC (2004). Detection of basal cell carcinoma using electrical impedance and neural networks. IEEE Trans Biomed Eng 51: 66–71.

23. R Core Team (2010). R: A Language and Environment for Statistical Computing. Vienna, Austria: R Foundation for Statistical Computing.

24. Faes TJ, van der Meij HA, de Munck JC, Heethaar RM (1999). The electric resistivity of human tissues (100 Hz–10 MHz): a meta-analysis of review studies. Physiol Meas 20: R1–10.

25. Miklavčič D, Pavšelj N, Hart FX (2006). Electric properties of tissues. In: Wiley Encyclopedia of Biomedical Engineering, John Wiley & Sons, Inc., pp. 1–12.

26. M, Fischer H, Polat H, Helm EB, Frenz M, et al. (1995). Bioelectrical impedance analysis as a predictor of survival in patients with human immunodeficiency virus infection. J Acquir Immune Defic Syndr Hum Retrovirol 9: 20–25.

27. Mize MM, Aguirre Vila-Coro A, Prager TC (1989). The relationship between postnatal skin maturation and electrical skin impedance. Arch Dermatol 125: 647–650.

28. Gupta D, Lammersfeld CA, Burrows JL, Dahlk SL, Vashi PG, et al. (2004). Bioelectrical impedance phase angle in clinical practice: implications for prognosis in advanced colorectal cancer. Am J Clin Nutr 80: 1634–1638.

29. Wirth R, Volkert D, Rosler A, Sieber CC, Bauer JM (2010). Bioelectric impedance phase angle is associated with hospital mortality of geriatric patients. Arch Gerontol Geriatr 51: 290–294.

18

Persistent Release of IL-1s from Skin Is Associated with Systemic Cardio-Vascular Disease, Emaciation and Systemic Amyloidosis: The Potential of Anti-IL-1 Therapy for Systemic Inflammatory Diseases

Keiichi Yamanaka[1]*, **Takehisa Nakanishi**[1], **Hiromitsu Saito**[2], **Junko Maruyama**[3], **Kenichi Isoda**[1], **Ayumu Yokochi**[4], **Kyoko Imanaka-Yoshida**[5,6], **Kenshiro Tsuda**[1], **Masato Kakeda**[1], **Ryuji Okamoto**[7], **Satoshi Fujita**[7], **Yoichiro Iwakura**[8], **Noboru Suzuki**[2], **Masaaki Ito**[7], **Kazuo Maruyama**[4], **Esteban C. Gabazza**[9], **Toshimichi Yoshida**[5,6], **Motomu Shimaoka**[10], **Hitoshi Mizutani**[1]

1 Department of Dermatology, Mie University, Graduate School of Medicine, Tsu, Mie, Japan, 2 Department of Animal Genomics, Functional Genomics Institute, Mie University Life Science Research Center, Tsu, Mie, Japan, 3 Department of Clinical Engineering, Suzuka University of Medical Science, Suzuka, Mie, Japan, 4 Anesthesiology and Critical Care Medicine, Mie University, Graduate School of Medicine, Tsu, Mie, Japan, 5 Pathology and Matrix Biology, Mie University, Graduate School of Medicine, Tsu, Mie, Japan, 6 Mie University Research Center for Matrix Biology, Tsu, Mie, Japan, 7 Cardiology, Mie University, Graduate School of Medicine, Tsu, Mie, Japan, 8 Division of Experimental Animal Immunology, Tokyo University of Science, Noda, Chiba, Japan, 9 Immunology, Mie University, Graduate School of Medicine, Tsu, Mie, Japan, 10 Molecular Pathology and Cell Adhesion Biology, Mie University, Graduate School of Medicine, Tsu, Mie, Japan

Abstract

The skin is an immune organ that contains innate and acquired immune systems and thus is able to respond to exogenous stimuli producing large amount of proinflammatory cytokines including IL-1 and IL-1 family members. The role of the epidermal IL-1 is not limited to initiation of local inflammatory responses, but also to induction of systemic inflammation. However, association of persistent release of IL-1 family members from severe skin inflammatory diseases such as psoriasis, epidermolysis bullosa, atopic dermatitis, blistering diseases and desmoglein-1 deficiency syndrome with diseases in systemic organs have not been so far assessed. Here, we showed the occurrence of severe systemic cardiovascular diseases and metabolic abnormalities including aberrant vascular wall remodeling with aortic stenosis, cardiomegaly, impaired limb and tail circulation, fatty tissue loss and systemic amyloid deposition in multiple organs with liver and kidney dysfunction in mouse models with severe dermatitis caused by persistent release of IL-1s from the skin. These morbid conditions were ameliorated by simultaneous administration of anti-IL-1α and IL-1β antibodies. These findings may explain the morbid association of arteriosclerosis, heart involvement, amyloidosis and cachexia in severe systemic skin diseases and systemic autoinflammatory diseases, and support the value of anti-IL-1 therapy for systemic inflammatory diseases.

Editor: Masataka Kuwana, Keio University School of Medicine, Japan

Funding: K. Yamanaka (26461690) and H. Mizutani (24591647) received grants for scientific research from the Ministry of Education, Culture, Sports, Science and Technology, Japan. The funders had no role in study design, data collection and analysis, decision to publish, or preparation of the manuscript.

Competing Interests: Hitoshi Mizutani is an adviser of Oriental Yeast Co., which has commercial interest in the results of this research and technology (KCASP1Tg). The other authors declare no competing financial interests.

* Email: yamake@clin.medic.mie-u.ac.jp

Introduction

Cardiovascular diseases, obesity, liver and renal diseases are going to be the major pathologies of the 21th century. A significant interaction between systemic inflammatory changes and systemic organ disease during the metabolic syndromes has been reported. Skin is a prototype of immune system that can respond to exogenous stimuli triggering systemic inflammation by promoting the migration of bone-derived hematopoietic cells. Cardiovascular and other systemic disorders have been reported in severe systemic skin diseases including psoriasis, epidermolysis bullosa (EB),

hidradenitis suppurativa, atopic dermatitis (AD) and desmoglein-1 deficiency [1–4]. However, the mechanistic pathways of systemic organ involvement during inflammatory skin diseases are unclear.

The role of epidermal keratinocytes is to trigger local and systemic inflammation by releasing stored IL-1s leading to activation of the immune system and the cytokine cascade. Skin scratching, cracking by xerosis and dermatitis promote the release of active IL-1α through a calcium-activated protease calpain [5] and/or CTL/NK protease granzyme B mechanism [6]. IL-1β is stored as an inactive precursor and can be activated by specific enzymes (e.g. caspase-1/IL-1β converting enzyme) before being secreted. IL-1 plays a key role in allergic dermatitis [7].

Chronic inflammation can cause aberrant remodeling of vascular and fatty tissues, potentially resulting in atherosclerosis and obesity/lipodystrophy [8]. Anti-inflammatory agents have been used as a novel therapeutic approach to reverse these pathological conditions [9]; for example, clinical trials using inhibitors of IL-1 have been carried out to treat atherosclerosis [10]. IL-1 is believed to affect primarily surrounding cells at sites of tissue injury. Bone marrow-derived hematologic cells (e.g., monocytes/macrophages) migrate into vascular walls where they secrete IL-1 that can stimulate resident cells (e.g. vascular smooth muscle cells, endothelial cells), and thereby contribute to the pathogenesis of atherosclerosis [11]. In addition to its primary role as a local mediator, excessive expression of IL-1 can spill over into the systemic circulation and affect remote organs. Sustained skin inflammation in severe epidermal inflammation patients including psoriasis, EB, AD can lead to aberrant secretion of IL-1, which can potentially cause vascular and visceral pathologies. The pathological effects of hypercytokinemia have been well documented in some cases of acute and usually self-limiting inflammation, typically caused by infections (e.g., cytokine storm in severe influenza virus infection-associated acute respiratory distress syndrome) [12] as well as in cases of cancer-associated chronic inflammation leading to cachexia [13]. However, the exact morbid conditions induced by high systemic levels of IL-1 during severe diseases with persistent and intensive epidermis injury remains largely unknown.

We addressed this problem by using keratin-14 driven caspase-1 transgenic mice (KCASP1Tg) [14] and a keratinocyte-specific mature IL-18-transgenic mice line (KIL-18Tg) that we have previously developed [7]. Here, we show that KCASP1Tg and KIL-18Tg mice with dermatitis have severe pathology in systemic organs other than the skin including aberrant remodeling of fatty and connective tissues, and extensive amyloid deposition with organ dysfunction, and that these abnormalities improved with the use of anti IL-1α/β antibodies.

Materials and Methods

Transgenic mice

Transgenic mice in which keratinocytes specifically overexpress the human caspase-1 gene with the K14 promoter, designated as KCASP1Tg, were used in this study [14]. A keratinocyte-specific mature IL-18-transgenic mice line (KIL-18Tg) that has been previously characterized was also used [7]. C57BL/6 littermate mice were used as controls. We closely monitored these mice until they were 6-months old. KIL-18Tg mice of less than 1-year old showed no findings of dermatitis; these mice are referred as KIL-18Tg(−). After 1-year old, the KIL-18Tg mice develop chronic dermatitis; these mice are referred as KIL-18Tg(+). Animal care was performed according to current ethical guidelines, and the experimental protocol was approved by the Mie University Board Committee for Animal Care and Use (#22-39).

Percentage of skin alteration and measurement of body weight

Skin alterations and body weight were observed at two-week intervals. Skin lesions and total body surface area were evaluated by marking on lucent plastic film, and then expressed as the percentage of area versus the total-body surface (n = 10, each group). Long-term observation was also performed in KIL-18Tg mice (n = 7, each group).

Computed tomography and 3-dimensional analysis

Under total anesthesia using isoflurane inhalation (Abbott, Abbott Park, IL), mice underwent micro X-ray CT angiography (Rigaku, Tokyo, Japan), and the data was analyzed using i-VIEW-R software (Rigaku). Body fat percentage was calculated and 3-dimensional graphics were obtained (n = 6, each group).

Plasma cytokine and cholesterol concentration

Plasma samples were collected from 6-months old mice (n = 10, each group) and eighteen-months old KIL-18Tg(+) mice (n = 7). Plasma cytokine levels were measured by specific ELISA kits (IL-1α, β: R&D systems, Minneapolis, MN, USA, IL-18: MBL, Nagoya, Japan) according to the manufacturer's instructions. TG, HDL, LDL cholesterol levels, liver and renal functions were measured with commercially available systems. Serum leptin (R&D systems), adiponectin (Otsuka, Tokyo, Japan) and amyloid A protein levels (Life Technologies, Carlsbad, CA) were measured by specific ELISA following the manufacturer's instructions.

IL-1 neutralization in KCASP1Tg mice

Ten μg of anti-IL-1α, β and α plus β neutralizing antibodies (BioLegend, CA, USA) were injected intraperitoneally into KCASP1Tg mice once-a-week from 1-month to 6-months old. PBS-treated KCASP1Tg littermates were used as controls (n = 7, each group).

Intra-peritoneal injection of recombinant protein

Intra-peritoneal injection of 1 μg of recombinant protein (IL-1α or IL-1 β (BioLegend)) into normal mice was performed 3 times/week during the period the mice were 6 to 16 weeks old, and physical changes were compared with normal PBS-treated mice (n = 6, each group).

Histological analysis

Abdominal adipose tissue and aorta specimens were fixed in 10% buffered neutral formaldehyde and embedded in paraffin. Histological sections were 6-μm thick and stained with hematoxylin and eosin (H&E). The aorta sections were also stained with Elastica van Gieson stain (EVG). The sections for liver, kidney, and spleen were stained with H&E and with Congo-red (n = 7, each group).

Culture of adipocytes with conditioned medium from skin culture

Skin culture was prepared by taking 1 cm² skin sections from 6-months-old normal or KCASP1Tg mice, minced with scissors, and harvested in 2 mL of RPMI 1640 containing 10% FCS, 2 mM L-glutamine, 100 U/ml penicillin, and 100 μg/ml streptomycin plated in a 24-well culture plate (Coster, NY, USA). In some experiments the skin post culture medium was treated with 1 μg of anti-IL-1α, anti-IL-1β, or a mixture of anti IL-1α and β neutralizing antibodies (BioLegend), and then incubated for 2 hours. The mouse embryonic fibroblast adipose-like cell line 3T3-L1 (ATCC, Manassas, VA) was cultured as previously reported for 10 days [15], and then differentiated into mature adipocytes. The medium was changed using the following supplementation: skin culture supernatant derived from normal mice, KCASP1Tg, anti-IL-1α and/or anti-IL-1β neutralizing antibodies-treated KCASP1Tg skin supernatant. On day 14, cultured cells were rinsed with PBS, stained with oil red O (Sigma-Aldrich, St. Louis, MO) and haematoxylin, and then observed under microscope (n = 7, each group).

A

B

Normal   KCASP1Tg   KIL-18Tg (-)   KIL-18Tg (+)

C

D

(TG mg/dl)   (HDL mg/dl)   (LDL mg/dl)   (leptin ng/ml)   (adiponectin ng/ml)

E

IL-1α (pg/mL)   IL-1β (pg/mL)   IL-18 (ng/mL)

Figure 1. KCASP1Tg and KIL-18Tg(+) mice showed emaciation and altered lipid metabolism in addition to dermatitis. A) KCASP1Tg mice had erosive dermatitis at week 8, which spread across the entire face and trunk when mice were 5-months old. KIL-18Tg mice showed no dermatitis at 6 months of age, KIL-18Tg(−). Weight loss began at 10 weeks in KCASP1Tg mice, but not in age matched KIL-18Tg mice (n = 10, each group). The left Y-axis shows body weight and the right Y-axis shows the percentage of dermatitis. KIL-18Tg mice developed dermatitis at 1-year old, followed by weight loss, KIL-18Tg(+) (n = 7, each group) (*p<0.05, **p<0.001, ***p<0.0001). **B)** CT scan of KCASP1Tg mice at 6 months of age revealed a dramatic decrease in visceral fat as shown in yellow compared to normal control or KIL-18Tg(−) mice. Eighteen-year old KIL-18Tg(+) showed decreased visceral fat. Subcutaneous fat (in orange color) was also decreased in KCASP1Tg and KIL-18Tg(+). **C)** A comparison of the somatic fat ratio across the three groups determined by CT scan at 2, 4 and 6 months of age, and a decrease was observed in KCASP1Tg mice compared to the other two groups (n = 6, each group). **D)** Six-month-old KCASP1Tg mice showed decreased plasma HDL cholesterol and leptin levels, as well as increased triglyceride levels. LDL cholesterol and adiponectin levels remained normal. Eighteen-months old KIL-18Tg(+) mice showed decreased leptin levels. No significant change was identified in the triglyceride, HDL and LDL cholesterol, and adiponectin levels in KIL-18Tg(+) mice. **E)** Plasma IL-1α and β levels were elevated in 6-months old KCASP1Tg mice. IL-1 levels were under the detection limit in KIL-18Tg(−) mice, but were elevated in 18-months old KIL-18Tg(+) mice. Plasma IL-18 levels were increased in both KCASP1Tg and KIL-18Tg mice (n = 10).

Cytokine measurement in skin culture supernatant

IL-1α and IL-β levels were measured in skin culture supernatant with FlowCytomix (eBioscience) following the manufacturer's instructions (n = 7, each group).

Snapping tension of abdominal aorta

Mice were anesthetized with sodium pentobarbital (50 mg/kg, i.p.), and the abdominal arteries were isolated, gently cleaned of fat and connective tissue, and cut into rings (1 mm in length) as previously reported [16]. Rings were suspended vertically between stainless steel hooks in organ baths (20 ml) with modified Krebs–Henseleit solution (room temperature) containing (in mM): NaCl 115, KCl 4.7, CaCl2 2.5, MgCl2 1.2, NaHCO3 25, KH2PO4 1.2, and dextrose 10 in order to record the tension. The changes in isometric tension were measured with a force–displacement transducer (TB-651T; Nihon Kohden, Tokyo, Japan) connected to a carrier amplifier (EF601G; Nihon Kohden) and recorded with a pen recorder (WT-645G; Nihon Kohden). The bath medium was maintained at 37°C and bubbled continuously with 95% air and 5% CO2. Arterial rings were washed and allowed to equilibrate for 30 min. To measure the tension when the aortic ring snapped, the isometric tension was gradually increased (n = 12, each group).

Peripheral blood pressure and thermography

Blood pressure was measured when mice were 6 months old using the BP-98A tail cuff system (Softron, Tokyo, Japan). This was done while the animals were still conscious as previously described [17][18], and the peripheral blood circulation was measured by thermography (FLIR systems, Boston, MA) (n = 10, each group). These measurements were also performed in eighteen-months old KIL-18Tg(+) mice (n = 7).

Statistical analysis

Statistical analysis was performed using the Friedman test. Student t test was used for the analysis of snapping tension results. P<0.05 was considered as significant.

Results

KCASP1Tg and KIL-18Tg mice with dermatitis show emaciation and altered lipid metabolism

The dermatitis in KCASP1Tg mice gradually spreads across the entire face and trunk, covering approximately 15% of the body surface when the mouse was 5-months old. Notably, KCASP1Tg mice gradually became emaciated as the dermatitis spreads. In these mice, weight loss began at week 10 (Fig. 1A). CT scans revealed a dramatic decrease in somatic and subcutaneous fat tissues (Fig. 1B,C). Caspase-1 is the converting enzyme for

immature IL-1β and IL-18, therefore to rule out the possibility that this emaciation was primarily induced by high circulating level of IL-18, further studies were performed using the IL-18 transgenic mice (KIL-18Tg)[7]. KIL-18Tg of less than one-year of age did not show any phenotype; these mice are referred as KIL-18Tg(-) (Fig. 1A). After becoming 1-year old, the KIL-18Tg mice develop dermatitis followed by weight loss; these mice are referred as KIL-18Tg(+) (Fig. 1A,B). Six-months old KCASP1Tg mice showed decreased plasma levels of HDL cholesterol and leptin but elevated plasma level of triglycerides (Fig. 1D). Eighteen-months old KIL-18Tg(+) mice showed decreased plasma level of leptin but no significant changes were observed in the levels of triglyceride, HDL and LDL cholesterol, and adiponectin.

In addition, KCASP1Tg mice have increased levels of IL-1α, IL-1β, and IL-18 (Fig. 1E); this increase in plasma levels was due to leakage of IL-1α from injured keratinocytes and to conversion of the precursors of IL-1β and IL-18 by the transgene encoded caspase-1. The plasma concentration of IL-18 was already elevated in KIL-18Tg(−), but the IL-1 level was under the detection limit. Both IL-1α and IL-1β were dramatically increased in KIL-18Tg(+) mice after onset of dermatitis. We postulate that IL-1α in KIL-18Tg(+) mice is released from injured keratinocytes, and that pro-IL-1β is converted by endogenous caspase-1 before its release. These data suggest that skin derived IL-1α and IL-1β rather than IL-18 are the primary cause of emaciation.

IL-1α and IL-1β are the primary cause of fat tissue remodeling

We treated KCASP1Tg mice with anti-IL-1α and/or IL-1β neutralizing antibodies when they were between 4 to 24 weeks old. Antibody treatment ameliorated body weight loss. Simultaneous injections of IL-1α and IL-1β antibodies produced additive effects (Fig. 2A). CT scans revealed that IL-1 antibody treatment prevented a decrease in the amount of somatic fat (Fig. S1B). The IL-1 antibodies also delayed the onset and progression of dermatitis, thereby supporting the idea that the skin pathology is accelerated by IL-1 [7]. Furthermore, to substantiate the pathogenic role of IL-1 in dermatitis and wasting syndrome, we treated normal healthy mice with recombinant IL-1α or IL-1β. Administration of either recombinant protein into wild-type mice caused a similar decrease in body weight within 10 weeks (Fig. 2B).

To study the underlying mechanisms by which sustained exposure of adipocytes to IL-1 induced emaciation, histopathological analysis of adipocytes was performed. While adipocytes from normal healthy mice appear as "plump nourished cells", those from KCASP1Tg and KIL-18Tg(+) mice were small and round (Fig. 2C). Using a mouse embryonic fibroblast adipose cell line, we studied whether this atrophy of adipocyte was a direct

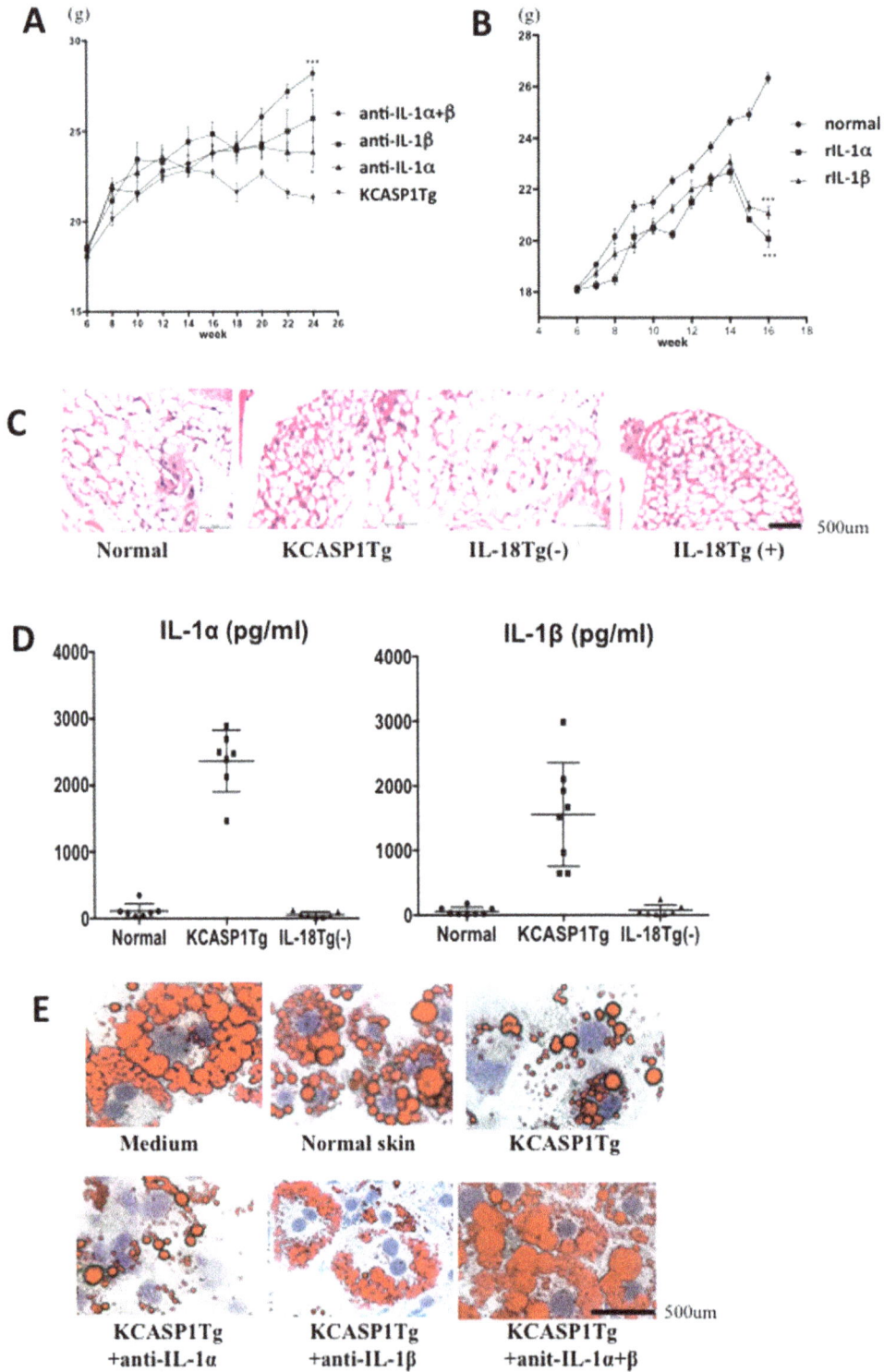

Figure 2. IL-1α and IL-1β trigger fat tissue remodeling. A) KCASP1Tg mice were treated once-a-week with an intra-peritoneal injection of 10 μg anti-IL-1α and/or IL-1β neutralizing antibodies between 4 to 24 weeks of age. PBS-treated KCASP1Tg littermates were used as controls. The body weight loss was ameliorated by either anti-IL-1α, anti-IL-1β or anti-IL-1α/β administration, (n = 7, each group). **B)** Emaciation was reproduced by administering 1 μg of recombinant IL-1α or IL-1β protein 3 times per week from 6 to 16 weeks of age to wild type mice compared to PBS-injected mouse controls from 6 to 16 weeks (n = 6, each group). **C)** H&E staining of abdominal adipose tissue revealed that the adipocytes were large and plump in shape in normal control and 6-months old KIL-18Tg(−) mice; they were small and round, however, in 6-month-old KCASP1Tg and 18-months old KIL-18Tg(+) mice. The number of infiltrating mononuclear cells was similar among these groups (n = 7, each group). **D)** Cytokine levels in the skin culture supernatant were measured by flow cytometry. IL-1α and IL-1β were detected in conditioned medium from the skin culture of normal control mice and KIL-18Tg(−) mice, but was significantly higher in medium from skin culture of KCASP1Tg mice (n = 7, each group). **E)** Mouse adipose cells cultured in regular medium contained abundant lipid drops on day 14. The addition of supernatant from normal skin culture revealed a decrease

in the number of plump adipocytes containing lipids as stained with oil red O, which was reversed by supplementing with supernatant from KCASP1Tg mice skin culture. The pretreatment of KCASP1Tg mice skin culture medium with anti-IL-1α or anti-IL-1β neutralizing antibodies partially ameliorated the inhibitory effects on adipose cells, which were almost abrogated by simultaneous treatment with both antibodies (n = 7, each group).

effect of skin-derived cytokines. The skin culture supernatant from normal control mice and KIL-18Tg(−) mice contained low levels of IL-1α and IL-1β, whereas the skin culture supernatant from KCASP1Tg mice contained increased levels of those cytokines

(Fig. 2D). The adipocytes cultured in normal media exhibited a plump shape containing abundant lipid particles (as stained with oil red O) (Fig. 2E). The addition of culture supernatant from normal skin resulted in a mild reduction of cytoplasmic lipid

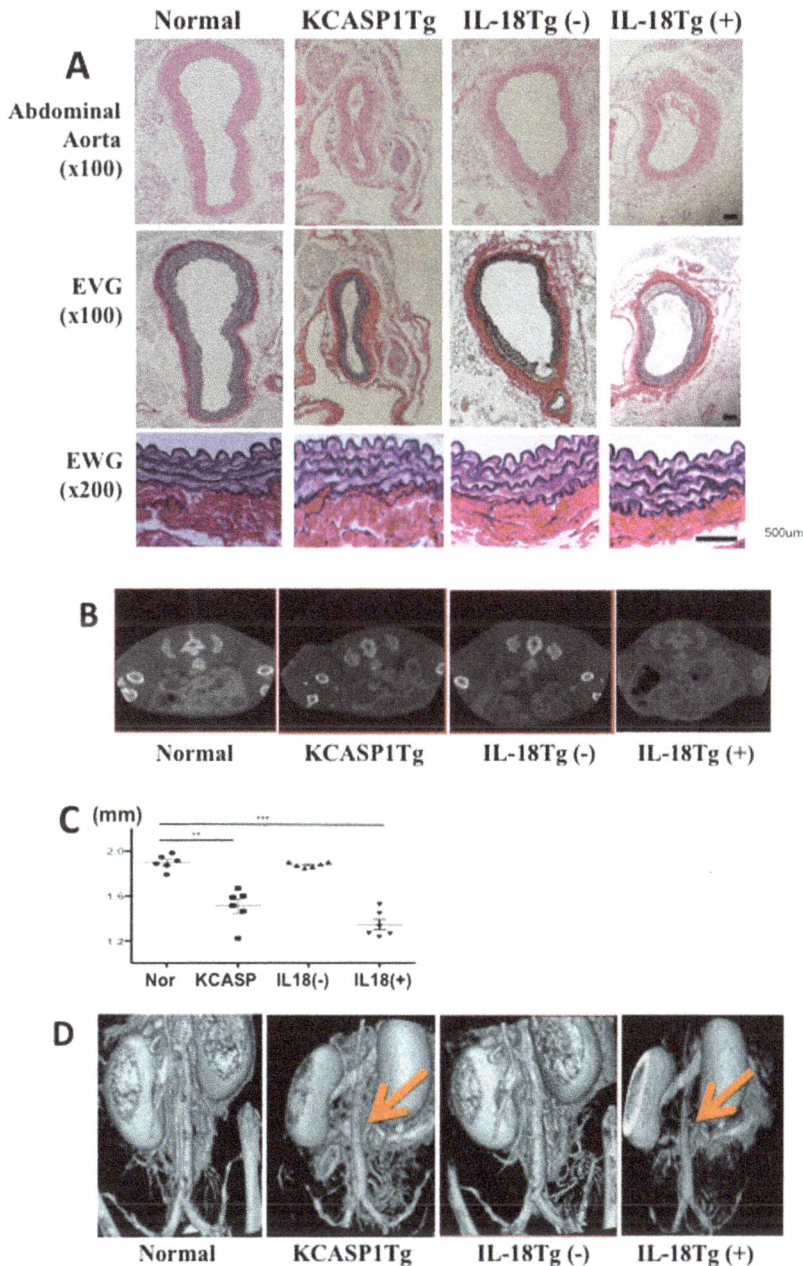

Figure 3. KCASP1Tg and KIL-18Tg(+) mice developed arteriosclerosis with impaired peripheral blood circulation. A) H and E staining of aorta sections revealed stenosis in 6-months old KCASP1Tg and 18-months old KIL-18Tg(+) mice. EVG staining revealed no significant changes in terms of periaortic lesions or elastic fibers. **B**) Enhanced CT scans revealed the presence of aortic stricture in KCASP1Tg and KIL-18Tg(+) mice. **C**) The aorta diameter in KCASP1Tg and KIL-18Tg(+) mice was decreased compared to normal control and KIL-18Tg(−) mice (n = 6, each group). **D**) Three-dimensional CT images showed the presence of aortic stenosis in KCASP1Tg and KIL-18Tg(+) mice.

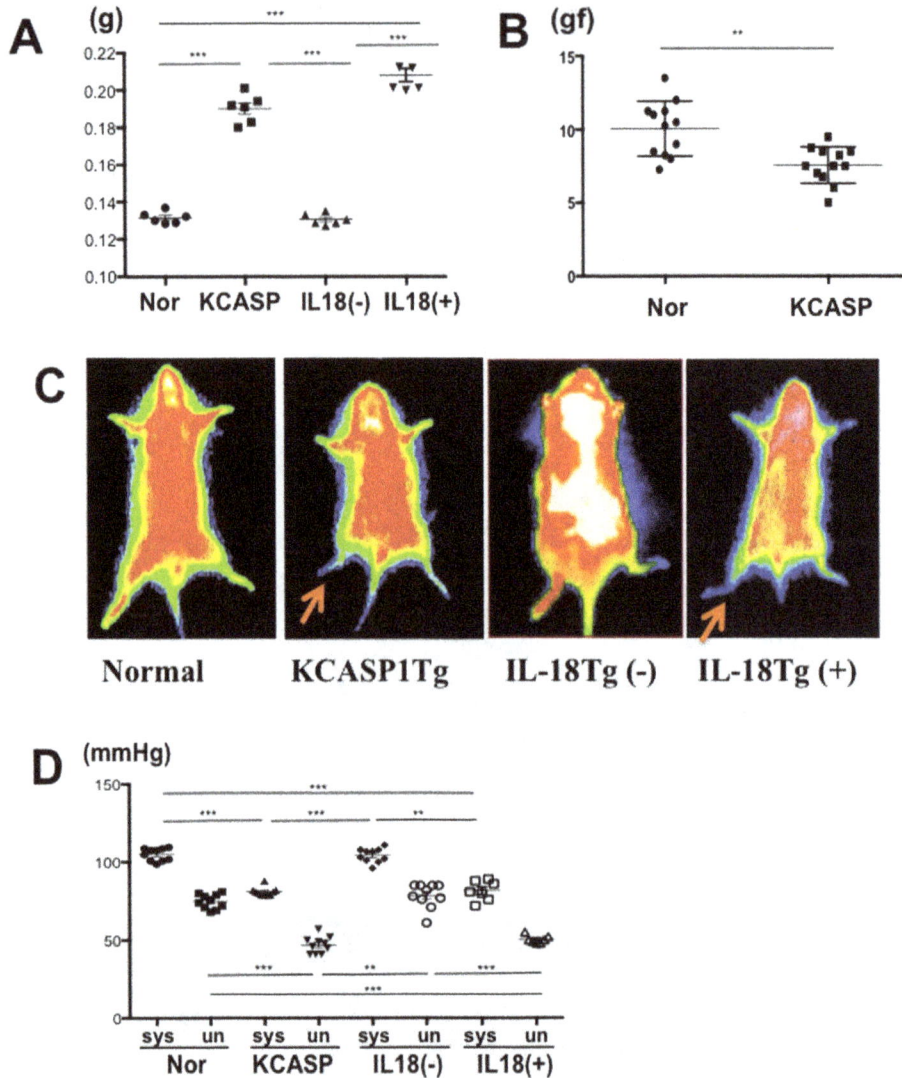

Figure 4. Cardiovascular findings in KCASP1Tg and KIL-18Tg(+). A) Six-months old KCASP1Tg mice had significantly heavier hearts compared to normal control and KIL-18Tg(−) mice. The heart weight of 18-months old KIL-18Tg(+) mice was also increased (n = 6, each group). **B)** The maximal tension produced in an 1 mm ring segment obtained from normal and KCASP1Tg mice is shown. The strength of the snapping point of the aorta ring from KCASP1Tg mice was significantly lower than in those from control mice (n = 12, each group). **C)** Thermography showed deterioration of peripheral blood circulation in the lower limbs and tail in 6-months old KCASP1Tg and 18-months old KIL-18Tg(+) mice. **D)** Both systolic and diastolic pressures were significantly lower in KCASP1Tg and KIL-18Tg(+) mice, (n = 10, each group) compared to control or KIL-18Tg(−) mice.

particles, thereby rendering the adipocytes less plump as a result of the cytokines released from the cultured normal skin. Furthermore, the addition of the KCASP1Tg mice skin culture supernatant induced severe reductions of lipid particles in adipocytes. The ability of KCASP1Tg mice skin supernatant to inhibit lipid particle growth was partially neutralized by either anti-IL-1α or IL-1β antibody. Indeed, this effect was abolished completely by simultaneous treatment with both antibodies (Fig. 2E).

KCASP1Tg and KIL-18Tg(+) mice developed arteriosclerosis with impaired peripheral blood circulation and cardiomegaly

We next examined vessel structures. Aortic stenosis was observed in 6-months old KCASP1Tg mice and in 18-months old KIL-18Tg(+) mice (Fig. 3A). The smooth muscle (data not shown) and elastic fibers appeared normal in the vascular wall of stenotic aorta. We did not see any significant changes in the mRNA expression of the pro-fibrotic cytokine TGF-β1 and the anti-fibrotic cytokines IFN-γ and TNF-α in the aortas of controls or KCASP1Tg mice (data not shown). Atherosclerotic plaques were not detected. Enhanced CT scans revealed that the aorta diameter in KCASP1Tg and KIL-18Tg(+) mice was significantly reduced (Fig. 3B,C). Three-dimensional CT images of the

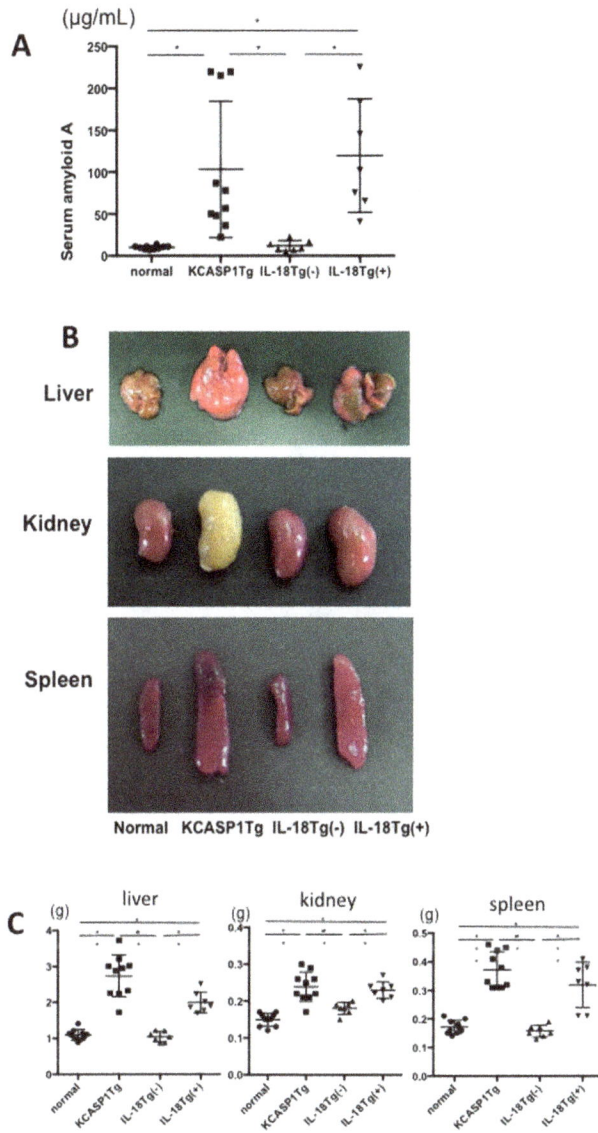

Figure 5. High serum amyloid A protein and organomegaly in KCASP1Tg and KIL-18Tg(+) mice. A) Serum amyloid A protein (SAA) levels were significantly higher in KCASP1Tg mice than in normal control and 6-months old KIL-18Tg(−) mice. Eighteen-months old KIL-18Tg(+) mice also showed elevated SAA concentration (n = at least 7). **B) C)** The liver, kidney, and spleen of both KCASP1Tg and KIL-18Tg(+) mice were significantly enlarged compared to control and KIL-18Tg(−) mice.

abdominal aorta in KCASP1Tg and KIL-18Tg(+) mice clearly showed the presence of vascular stricture (Fig. 3D). In addition, these mice exhibited cardiomegaly with left ventricular hypertrophy (Fig. 4A). Ultrasonic echocardiography revealed no obvious left ventricular dysfunction in 6-months old KCASP1Tg mice (data not shown). Cardiomegaly was probably a secondary sign; it likely represents a compensatory response to aortic stenosis, and a consequence of reduced firmness and pliability of the aorta wall (Fig. 4B). Thermographic analysis revealed hampered circulation in lower limbs and tail of KCASP1Tg and KIL-18Tg (+) mice (Fig. 4C). Peripheral blood circulation further deteriorated after cold stimulation (data not shown), which is similar to that observed

in patients with severe arteriosclerosis. The aortic stenosis was associated with impaired peripheral perfusion. The blood pressure measured at the tail was low during the systolic and diastolic phases in KCASP1Tg and KIL-18Tg(+) mice (Fig. 4D), thereby confirming impairment of peripheral circulation observed in the thermographic analysis.

KCASP1Tg and KIL-18Tg(+) developed amyloidosis in the liver, kidney and spleen

Chronic inflammation is often associated with amyloidosis. We investigated this by measuring the levels of serum amyloid A protein (SAA) and found significantly higher levels in KCASP1Tg and KIL-18Tg(+) mice than in control mice (Fig. 5A). The liver, kidney and spleen were hypertrophic in KCASP1Tg and KIL-18Tg(+) mice compared to normal controls (Fig. 5B,C). Histological examinations showed a dense amyloid deposition (Congo-red staining) and loss of normal architecture. Hepatocytes were replaced by dense deposits in the liver, and the damage of glomeruli and renal tubules were apparent in the kidneys, and lymph follicles were absent in the spleen (Fig. 6A). Liver damage as assessed by the serum level of transaminases was worse in KCASP1Tg mice than in control mice. Kidney function was mildly impaired in KCASP1Tg mice, and it was significantly deteriorated in KIL-18Tg(+) mice (Fig. 6B).

Discussion

Several studies have shown the occurrence of systemic complications such as arteriosclerosis, cardiomyopathy, abnormal fat metabolism, renal sclerosis and systemic amyloidosis in severe inflammatory skin disorders. Here we demonstrated that sustained circulating level of IL-1 derived from severe skin inflammation causes weight loss, vascular sclerotic changes, cardiomegaly and severe systemic amyloidosis in multiple organs. Surprisingly, these pathologies were ameliorated by simultaneous treatment with anti-IL-1α and anti-IL-1β antibodies (Fig. 2A, Fig. S1 and S2). We hypothesized that mice generated by crossing KCASP1Tg with IL-1α/β double knock-out mice [18] (KCASP1Tg/IL-1α/β double knock-out mice) would have milder symptoms than KCASP1Tg mice due to overexpression of caspase-1 in a background lacking both IL-1α and IL-1β. Similar to the beneficial effects obtained with the antibody treatment, KCASP1Tg/IL-1α/β double knock-out mice also showed an improvement in the pathological phenotypes described here (Fig. S1 and S2). Although the number of KCASP1Tg/IL-1α/β double knockout mice is few due to the difficulty of mating, the significance between KCASP1Tg and KCASP1Tg/IL-1α/β double knockout mice reached the significance. Amelioration of emaciation was not complete in the crossed mice, however, suggesting the involvement of other inflammatory cytokines in the mechanism of emaciation; this is currently under investigation in our laboratory.

Leakage of IL-1α and IL-1β from injured keratinocytes induces atrophy of fat tissue/adipocytes, resulting in decreased somatic and subcutaneous fat. IL-1 is involved in the pathogenesis of arteriosclerosis obliterans (ASO) and atherosclerosis [19], monocytes being the source of IL-1 in ASO. Atheroma and sclerosis are characteristic findings of ASO. In many animal models of ASO, hyperlipidemia occurs prior to atheroma formation. Interestingly, KCASP1Tg and KIL-18Tg(+) mice showed no atheroma plaque formation, suggesting that, *in vivo*, IL-1 can induce arteriosclerosis without atheroma formation. Vascular atherosclerotic changes have also been reported in auto-inflammatory diseases including familial Mediterranean fever (FMF); in this disease, intermittent

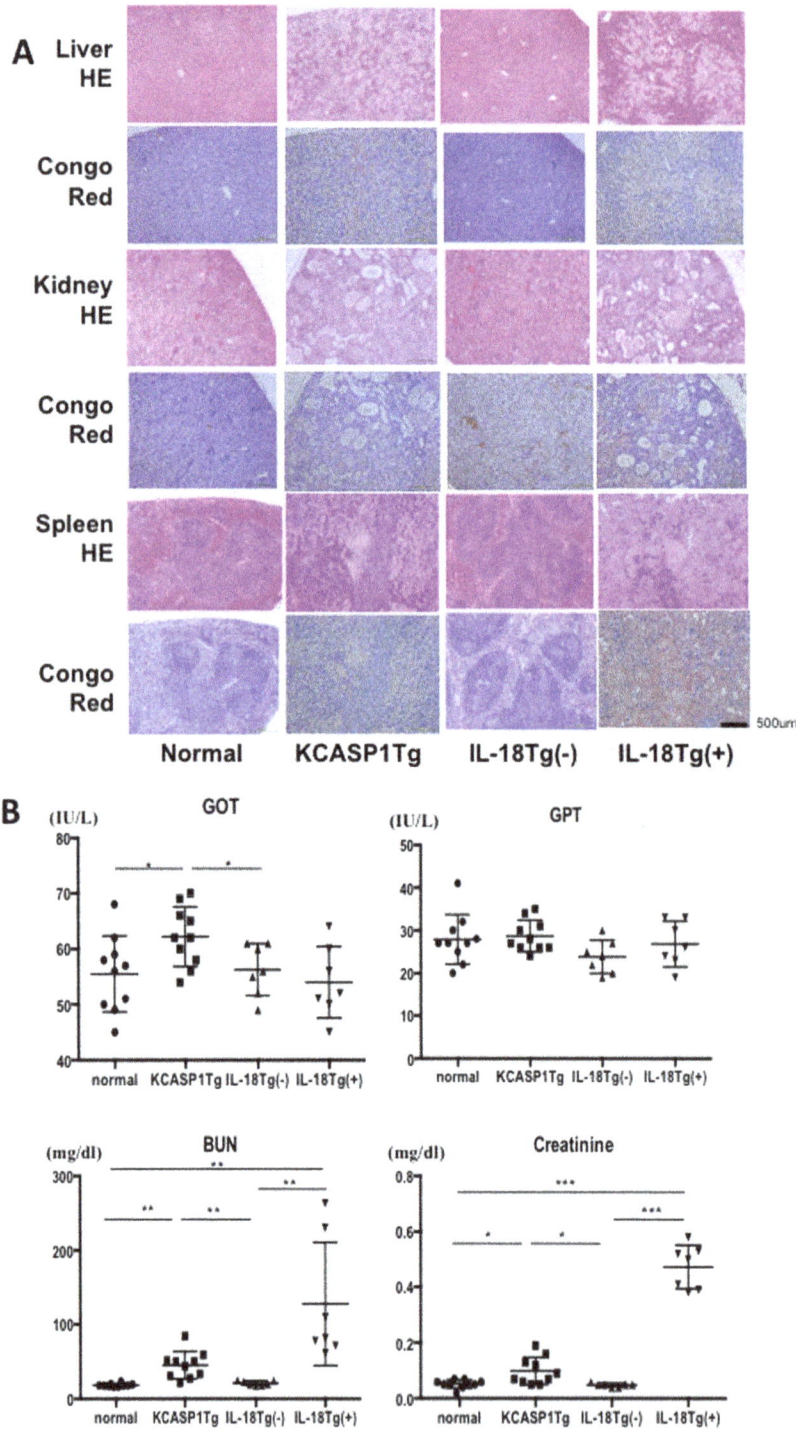

Figure 6. KCASP1Tg and KIL-18Tg(+) mice developed amyloidosis in the liver, kidney and spleen. A) Histological analyses showed loss of normal architecture: hepatocytes were replaced by dense deposits in the liver, the glomeruli and renal tubules were damaged in the kidney, and lymph-follicles were absent in the spleen. Dense amyloid deposition was detected in KCASP1Tg and KIL-18Tg(+) mice by Congo-red staining. **B)** KCASP1Tg mice showed mild liver and kidney dysfunction while renal function had significantly deteriorated in KIL-18Tg(+) mice (n = at least 7).

exposure to IL-1 [20] only leads to scant atheroma formation. The total and HDL cholesterol levels in FMF patients are usually low compared to levels observed in KCASP1Tg mice. The plasma IL-18 levels in KIL-18Tg mice began to rise at a young age (i.e., 4-weeks old) but within one-year of age these mice develop no

vascular complications and have no elevation in the serum level of IL-1 suggesting a secondary role of IL-18 in the mechanism of sclerosis [7].

The results of the present study not only provide a valuable *in vivo* example for systemic pathologies caused by chronic and sustained high circulating level of IL-1, but also have important clinical connotations; for example, a massive release of IL-1 from the skin can occur if severe AD patients intensely and repeatedly scratch their itchy skin, further worsening skin damage. The results of the present study suggest the need to avoid scratching to improve the clinical control of inflammatory skin diseases including AD. Psoriasis is another chronic inflammatory disease of the skin characterized by an elevated circulating level of IL-1 induced by local overexpression of TNF-α or IL-12/23 p40; the increased circulating level of IL-1 has been shown to be a risk factor for cardiovascular disorders [21]. Biologics therapy targeting TNF-α or IL-12/23 p40 suppress skin lesions and by this mechanism reduces the risk of vascular complications [22]. In EB, The skin pathological phenotype of EB is caused by inflammation and by minor trauma as previous demonstrated [23,24]. The IL-1β signaling is constitutively activated in EB keratinocytes [25], and the serum IL-1α and IL-1β levels are several-fold increased even in the mild type of EB [26]. Sustained skin disruption in EB patients can lead to aberrant skin secretion with high circulating level of IL-1 that may potentially cause emaciation, vascular disorder, systemic amyloidosis and other visceral pathologies. Recently, a hereditary disease with a new syndrome featuring severe dermatitis, multiple allergies and metabolic wasting syndrome (SAM syndrome) caused by homozygous mutations in DSG1 has been described [4]. DSG1 encodes desmoglein 1, a major constituent of desmosomes, which have a crucial role in maintaining epidermal integrity and barrier function. Mutations that cause SAM syndrome may lead to loss of cell-to-cell adhesion, induce calcium flux in keratinocytes with IL-1α release.

The results of the present study provide evidence supporting the morbid association of chronic and severe inflammation of the skin with cardiovascular complications. These novel observations may also explain the involvement of systemic organs in the hereditary inflammatory skin diseases such as EB, severe AD and SAM syndrome. Successful inhibition of complications in other systemic organs by the treatment with anti-IL-1 antibodies provides a tool for preventing the disease and to improve prognosis in this kind of patients. This is not limited to skin diseases but also to other disorders such as autoinflammatory disorders.

Supporting Information

Figure S1 Amelioration of clinical and pathological findings by neutralization and knockout of IL-1 in KCASP1Tg mice. A) IL-1s neutralization with antibodies ameliorated the impaired peripheral circulation as demonstrated by thermography and aorta histopathological changes. IL-1α and IL-1β double knockout KCASP1Tg developed neither peripheral circulatory changes nor histopathological changes in aorta. **B**) Body fat ratio improved by IL-1 neutralization (n = 7) and by its deficiency (n = 4) in. KCASP1Tg mice. The data of normal and KCASP1Tg are taken from Figure 1C.

Figure S2 Organ amyloidosis was ameliorated by neutralization and knockout of IL-1 in KCASP1Tg mice. A) The H&E and Congo-red staining revealed that IL-1 neutralization or deficiency ameliorate amyloid deposition in the liver, kidney and spleen.

Author Contributions

Conceived and designed the experiments: KY ECG TY MS HM. Performed the experiments: KY TN HS JM AY KI KT MK RO SF. Analyzed the data: KY TN HS JM KI AY KI-Y YI NS MI KM. Contributed reagents/materials/analysis tools: KY TN HS JM AY KI-Y KT MK RO SF. Contributed to the writing of the manuscript: KY ECG TY MS HM.

References

1. Davidovici BB, Sattar N, Prinz J, Puig L, Emery P, et al. (2010) Psoriasis and systemic inflammatory diseases: potential mechanistic links between skin disease and co-morbid conditions. The Journal of investigative dermatology 130: 1785–1796.

2. Fine JD, Hall M, Weiner M, Li KP, Suchindran C (2008) The risk of cardiomyopathy in inherited epidermolysis bullosa. Br J Dermatol 159: 677–682.

3. Fine JD, Johnson LB, Weiner M, Stein A, Cash S, et al. (2004) Inherited epidermolysis bullosa and the risk of death from renal disease: experience of the National Epidermolysis Bullosa Registry. American journal of kidney diseases: the official journal of the National Kidney Foundation 44: 651–660.

4. Samuelov L, Sarig O, Harmon RM, Rapaport D, Ishida-Yamamoto A, et al. (2013) Desmoglein 1 deficiency results in severe dermatitis, multiple allergies and metabolic wasting. Nature genetics 45: 1244–1248.

5. Watanabe N and Kobayashi Y (1994) Selective release of a processed form of interleukin 1 alpha. Cytokine 6: 597–601.

6. Afonina IS, Tynan GA, Logue SE, Cullen SP, Bots M, et al. (2011) Granzyme B-dependent proteolysis acts as a switch to enhance the proinflammatory activity of IL-1alpha. Molecular cell 44: 265–278.

7. Konishi H, Tsutsui H, Murakami T, Yumikura-Futatsugi S, Yamanaka K, et al. (2002) IL-18 contributes to the spontaneous development of atopic dermatitis-like inflammatory skin lesion independently of IgE/stat6 under specific pathogen-free conditions. Proceedings of the National Academy of Sciences of the United States of America 99: 11340–11345.

8. Herrero L, Shapiro H, Nayer A, Lee J, Shoelson SE (2010) Inflammation and adipose tissue macrophages in lipodystrophic mice. Proceedings of the National Academy of Sciences of the United States of America 107: 240–245.

9. Dinarello CA, Simon A, van der Meer JW (2012) Treating inflammation by blocking interleukin-1 in a broad spectrum of diseases. Nature reviews Drug discovery 11: 633–652.

10. Ridker PM, Thuren T, Zalewski A, Libby P (2011) Interleukin-1beta inhibition and the prevention of recurrent cardiovascular events: rationale and design of the Canakinumab Anti-inflammatory Thrombosis Outcomes Study (CANTOS). American heart journal 162: 597–605.

11. Tabas I (2010) Macrophage death and defective inflammation resolution in atherosclerosis. Nature reviews Immunology 10: 36–46.

12. Peiris JS, Cheung CY, Leung CY, Nicholls JM (2009) Innate immune responses to influenza A H5N1: friend or foe? Trends in immunology 30: 574–584.

13. Tsoli M, Robertson G (2012) Cancer cachexia: malignant inflammation, tumorkines, and metabolic mayhem. Trends in endocrinology and metabolism: TEM.

14. Yamanaka K, Tanaka M, Tsutsui H, Kupper TS, Asahi K, et al. (2000) Skin specific caspase-1 transgenic mouse expresses cutaneous apoptosis and pre-endotoxin shock condition with a high serum level of IL-18. Journal of Immunology 165: 997–1003.

15. Green H, Meuth M (1974) An established pre-adipose cell line and its differentiation in culture. Cell 3: 127–133.

16. Maruyama J, Yokochi A, Maruyama M, Nosaka S (1999) Acetylcholine-induced endothelium-derived contracting factor in hypoxic pulmonary hypertensive rats. J Appl Physiol 86: 1687–1695.

17. Nishioka T, Suzuki M, Onishi K, Takakura N, Inada H, et al. (2007) Eplerenone attenuates myocardial fibrosis in the angiotensin II-induced hypertensive mouse: involvement of tenascin-C induced by aldosterone-mediated inflammation. Journal of cardiovascular pharmacology 49: 261–268.

18. Horai R, Asano M, Sudo K, Kanuka H, Suzuki M, et al. (1998) Production of mice deficient in genes for interleukin (IL)-1alpha, IL-1beta, IL-1alpha/beta, and IL-1 receptor antagonist shows that IL-1beta is crucial in turpentine-induced fever development and glucocorticoid secretion. The Journal of experimental medicine 187: 1463–1475.

19. Merhi-Soussi F, Kwak BR, Magne D, Chadjichristos C, Berti M, et al. (2005) Interleukin-1 plays a major role in vascular inflammation and atherosclerosis in male apolipoprotein E-knockout mice. Cardiovascular research 66: 583–593.

20. Akdogan A, Calguneri M, Yavuz B, Arslan EB, Kalyoncu U, et al. (2006) Are familial Mediterranean fever (FMF) patients at increased risk for atherosclerosis? Impaired endothelial function and increased intima media thickness are found in FMF. Journal of the American College of Cardiology 48: 2351–2353.

21. Yu AP, Tang J, Xie J, Wu EQ, Gupta SR, et al. (2009) Economic burden of psoriasis compared with the general population and stratified by disease severity. Current medical research and opinion 25: 2429–2438.

22. Ahlehoff O, Skov L, Gislason G, Lindhardsen J, Kristensen SL, et al. (2013) Cardiovascular disease event rates in patients with severe psoriasis treated with

systemic anti-inflammatory drugs: a Danish real-world cohort study. Journal of internal medicine 273: 197–204.

23. Retief CR, Malkinson FD, Pearson RW (1999) Two familial cases of epidermolysis bullosa simplex successfully treated with tetracycline. Archives of dermatology 135: 997–998.

24. Veien NK, Buus SK (2000) Treatment of epidermolysis bullosa simplex (EBS) with tetracycline. Archives of dermatology 136: 424–425.

25. Wally V, Lettner T, Peking P, Peckl-Schmid D, Murauer EM, et al. (2013) The pathogenetic role of IL-1beta in severe epidermolysis bullosa simplex. The Journal of investigative dermatology 133: 1901–1903.

26. Samavedam UK, Kalies K, Scheller J, Sadeghi H, Gupta Y, et al. (2013) Recombinant IL-6 treatment protects mice from organ specific autoimmune disease by IL-6 classical signalling-dependent IL-1ra induction. Journal of autoimmunity 40: 74–85.

Chronic Stress Suppresses the Expression of Cutaneous Hypothalamic–Pituitary–Adrenocortical Axis Elements and Melanogenesis

Silin Pang[1,2], Huali Wu[1,2], Qian Wang[1,2], Minxuan Cai[1,2], Weimin Shi[3], Jing Shang[1,2]*

1 New Drug Screening Center, China Pharmaceutical University, Nanjing, China, **2** State Key Laboratory of Natural Medicines, China Pharmaceutical University, Nanjing, China, **3** Shanghai First People Hospital, Shanghai, China

Abstract

Chronic stress can affect skin function, and some skin diseases might be triggered or aggravated by stress. Stress can activate the central hypothalamic–pituitary–adrenocortical (HPA) axis, which causes glucocorticoid levels to increase. The skin has HPA axis elements that react to environmental stressors to regulate skin functions, such as melanogenesis. This study explores the mechanism whereby chronic stress affects skin pigmentation, focusing on the HPA axis, and investigates the role of glucocorticoids in this pathway. We exposed C57BL/6 male mice to two types of chronic stress, chronic restraint stress (CRS) and chronic unpredictable mild stress (CUMS). Mice subjected to either stress condition showed reduced melanogenesis. Interestingly, CRS and CUMS triggered reductions in the mRNA expression levels of key factors involved in the HPA axis in the skin. In mice administered corticosterone, decreased melanin synthesis and reduced expression of HPA axis elements were observed. The reduced expression of HPA axis elements and melanogenesis in the skin of stressed mice were reversed by RU486 (a glucocorticoid receptor antagonist) treatment. Glucocorticoids had no significant inhibitory effect on melanogenesis in vitro. These results suggest that, high levels of serum corticosterone induced by chronic stress can reduce the expression of elements of the skin HPA axis by glucocorticoid-dependent negative feedback. These activities can eventually result in decreased skin pigmentation. Our findings raise the possibility that chronic stress could be a risk factor for depigmentation by disrupting the cutaneous HPA axis and should prompt dermatologists to exercise more caution when using glucocorticoids for treatment.

Editor: Andrzej T Slominski, University of Tennessee, United States of America

Funding: This work was supported by 2012–2014 National Science and Technology Infrastructure Program (2012BAI30B001), PI 2011–2013 Mega-projects of Science Research for the 12th Five-Year Plan of China (2011ZX09401-007), PI. The funders had no role in study design, data collection and analysis, decision to publish, or preparation of the manuscript.

Competing Interests: The authors have declared that no competing interests exist.

* E-mail: shangjing21cn@163.com

Introduction

Substantial evidence suggests that chronic stress can affect the function of multiple physiological systems, including skin function [1–4]. Stress has been associated with the onset and aggravation of many skin disorders, such as psoriasis, alopecia, atopic dermatitis, and vitiligo [5–10]. The "brain–skin connection" may underlie skin diseases triggered or aggravated by stress [3,4,7,11].

During exposure to stressful events, the central hypothalamic–pituitary–adrenocortical (HPA) axis is activated. In brief, during stress, corticotropin-releasing hormone (CRH) is synthesized and released, which increases pro-opiomelanocortin (POMC) expression. POMC is converted into adrenocorticotropic hormone (ACTH) and other melanocortin peptides, such as α-MSH. ACTH then binds to the melanocortin type 2 receptor (MC2R) of the adrenal cortex and stimulates glucocorticoid synthesis and secretion into systemic circulation to exert various physiological effects. In the adrenal cortex, P450scc (Gene symbol: CYP11A1) acts as a key enzyme in glucocorticoid synthesis. Glucocorticoid binding to glucocorticoid receptors (GRs) in hypophysiotropic neurons and the anterior pituitary gland can inhibit the release of

CRH and ACTH to allow for negative feedback regulation of the HPA axis [12–15].

The skin is the largest organ in the human body and can be regulated by the immune and neuroendocrine systems [3,16–18]. Skin reacts to environmental stressors, such as ultraviolet radiation (UVR), in a strikingly similar manner to the activities of the central HPA axis [3,19,20]. The skin and its major appendages express key molecules, including CRH or urocortin (UCN1), POMC, and P450scc, along the classical HPA axis. CRH or UCN1 can interact with CRH receptor type 1 (CRHR1) to produce POMC-derived peptides, with the latter stimulating the local production of glucocorticoids [21–28]. After exposure to UVR, the gene expression levels of CRH or UCN1, POMC, and CYP11A1 in the skin increase [19,29]. Simultaneously, the skin is also the target organ of CRH and the related urocortin peptide, POMC-derived peptides, and glucocorticoids [3,4,22,23,26,27,30]. Treating melanocytes with CRH has been shown to induce melanogenesis [22,26,31]. POMC, ACTH, and α-MSH also increase melanogenesis in melanocytes [31–33]. Thus, skin pigmentation has a close relationship with cutaneous HPA axis activation.

Because of the evolutionary conservation of HPA-like networks at the central and cutaneous levels, interactions may exist between these systems, and such interactions could affect the functions of each system [4,34]. For example, UVR of the skin results in excitation of the central nervous system [3,35], and skin disorder is associated with higher central HPA axis activity [36]. The possibility of communication between the cutaneous and systemic HPA axes poses an interesting question for research [3]. However, to our knowledge, very few studies have investigated the influence of the higher central HPA axis on the skin. Thus, this study aimed to explore the effects of chronic stress on skin function and to test whether the cutaneous HPA axis is involved. Here, C57BL/6 male mice were subjected to two types of chronic stress, and the effects of these stresses on skin were observed. Because high levels of serum corticosterone were observed in stressed mice, normal mice were administered corticosterone and stressed mice were administered a glucocorticoid receptor antagonist to explore the role of glucocorticoids in the effects of stress on the skin.

Materials and Methods

Animals

Male C57BL/6 mice (5 weeks old, 20.6 ± 2.1 g) were obtained from the Laboratory Animal Services Center of the Yangzhou University. Animals were maintained on a 12-h light/dark cycle at a regulated temperature ($22 \pm 2°C$), humidity ($50 \pm 10\%$) and fed a standard diet and water ad libitum. Animals were acclimatized for 7 days. This study was carried out in strict accordance with the guidelines of the "Principles of Laboratory Animal Care" (NIH Publication No. 80–23, revised in 1996). This study was specifically approved by the Animal Experimentation Ethics Committee of the Chinese Pharmaceutical University (Approval ID: SCXK - (Su) 2011–0003). All efforts were made to minimize suffering.

Chronic stress application

Mice were randomly divided into the following three groups: (1) control group, (2) chronic restraint stress (CRS) group, and (3) chronic unpredictable mild stress (CUMS) group. The CRS procedure was performed as described before [37]. The CUMS procedure was performed as described before with adjustments [38]. In brief, CUMS consisted of a variety of unpredictable stressors, namely, 14-h food deprivation, 14-h water deprivation, 3-min swimming, 1-min tail pinch, 0.5 h cage shock, 24-h soiled cage, and overnight illumination. One of these stressors was given every day for 21 days.

Drugs

Corticosterone was purchased from Sigma-Aldrich (MO, USA). Mice were randomly divided into control and corticosterone (CORT) groups. Mice received corticosterone injections (20 mg/kg, subcutaneously), once per day for 21 days.

RU486 (a glucocorticoid receptor antagonist) was purchased from Sigma-Aldrich. Mice were randomly divided into the following three groups: (1) control group, (2) CUMS group with no drug injection and the application of CUMS, and (3) CUMS+ RU486 group with the application of CUMS concomitant with 100 mg/kg/day of RU486 injected subcutaneously for 21 days.

Depilation and tissue sample collection

On day 9, all mice received epilation with rosin and paraffin (1:1, w:w) to induce anagen of the hair cycle (Fig. 1) [39]. Mice were maintained under intraperitoneal anesthesia with chloral hydrate (300 mg/kg) during epilation. On day 22, mice were sacrificed after taking blood samples from eyes under anesthesia between 09:00 am and 10:00 am. Blood was incubated at room temperature for 1 h to allow clotting to occur, and serum was then

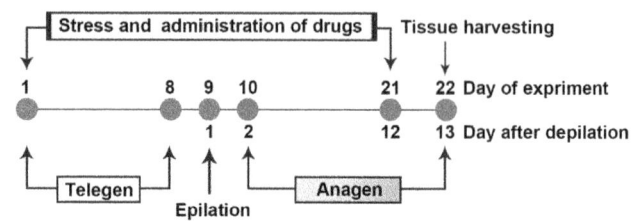

Figure 1. Time table of the experiments. CRS or CUMS was administered beginning on day 1 and continued for 21 days. Drugs were also administered from day 1 for 21 days. All mice received epilation to induce anagen of the hair cycle at day 9. Mice were photographed on days 10 and 22, which were 2 and 13 days post-depilation. Tissue samples were collected on day 22.

separated by centrifugation and stored at $-70°C$ until use. The back skin of mice was collected and stored in liquid nitrogen until use.

Cell culture

The B16F10 murine melanoma cells were purchased from the Cell Bank of the Chinese Academy of Sciences. Cell culture was performed as described before [40]. α-MSH and dexamethasone (DEX) were purchased from Sigma-Aldrich (MO, USA). To detect the effects of DEX and α-MSH on melanogenesis, cells were incubated with 1 μM DEX or 50 nM α-MSH. B16F10 cells at passage numbers between 5 and 7 were used for the experiments.

Normal human epidermal melanocytes were derived from young male adult foreskins (ethnic Han/aged 18–22 years) obtained at circumcision following standard protocols [41]. Melanocytes were incubated with MCDB153 medium (Sigma-Aldrich, USA) containing 1 nM choleratoxin (Sigma-Aldrich, USA), 0.1 mM 3-isobutyl-1-methylxanthine (Sigma-Aldrich, USA), 1.6 nM phorbolesters (Sigma-Aldrich, USA), 5 μg/mL insulin (Sigma-Aldrich, USA) and incubated at $37°C$ in a humidified atmosphere containing 5% CO_2. To detect the effects of DEX and α-MSH on melanogenesis, cells were incubated with 1 μM DEX or 50 nM α-MSH. Melanocytes at passage numbers between 3 and 6 were used for the experiments. The studies on human material were approved by Nanjing Drum Tower Hospital, Medical Ethics Committee. All participants provided their written informed consent to participate in this study. This consent procedure was approved by the Nanjing Drum Tower Hospital, Medical Ethics Committee.

Measurement of body weight and corticosterone analysis

The body weight of all mice were recorded on days 3, 6, 9, 12, 15, 18, and 21. Serum corticosterone concentrations were measured using the IBL-AMERICA Corticosterone rat/mouse ELISA kit (IBL, USA) according to the manufacturer's instructions. Serum samples were incubated at room temperature and then directly used for detection. The lowest detectable concentration of corticosterone that could be distinguished from the "zero calibrator" was 4.1 ng/mL.

Assessment of skin pigmentary response

All mice were photographed with a digital camera (Canon, Japan) once every day after depilation. The grayscale (0–255) of specific area in the photographs (the region from neck to tail) were analyzed by Image J software and presented as ratios (grayscale/255).

Table 1. Primer sequences.

Genes	Species	Forward (F) and Reverse (R) primer sequences		Product size (bp)
MITF	mouse	F	TGCTCGCCTGATCTGGTGAAT	152
		R	GTGCCGAGGTTGTTGGTAAAGG	
TYR	mouse	F	GATGGAACACCTGAGGGACCACTAT	150
		R	GCTGAAATTGGCAGTTCTATCCATT	
Hsd11b1	mouse	F	CTCCTCCCGATCCTGGTGCTCT	132
		R	TGCCATTTCTCTTCCAATCCCTTT	
Hsd11b2	mouse	F	GTTAACAACGCTGGCCTCAATA	160
		R	CAACGGTCACAATACGTCCCT	
Nr3c1	mouse	F	GGATGACCAAATGACCCTTCTACAG	112
		R	ATCAGGAGCAAAGCATAGCAGGTT	
CRHR1	mouse	F	CTCACGTACTCCACCGACCG	130
		R	TGCCAAACCAGCACTTTTCA	
CRHR2	mouse	F	CCCTGTGGACACTTTTGGAGC	183
		R	GGGTCGTGTTGTACTTGATGCC	
MC1R	mouse	F	GGCTGTCGTGGGCATCTGGA	204
		R	ATGGACCGCCGCCTTTTGTG	
MC2R	mouse	F	ACCATCATCACCCTAACAAT	136
		R	GACACAGGATAAAAACCAGC	
UCN1	mouse	F	CACTGTCCATCGACCTCACCTTC	117
		R	ACTTGCCCACCGAATCGAATA	
POMC	mouse	F	TTGCTGAGAACGAGTCGGC	86
		R	GACCTGCTCCAAGCCTAATGG	
CYP11A1	mouse	F	AGATGCCTGGAAGAAAGACCGAA	199
		R	GATGGACTCAAAGGAAAAGCGGA	
Actb	Mouse	F	CAGGTCATCACTATTGGCAACGAG	87
		R	GATGCCACAGGATTCCATACCC	
MITF	Human	F	ACGAGAACAGCAACGCGCAAA	145
		R	GCAGAGACCCGTGGATGGAATA	
TYR	Human	F	GTTGCGGTGGGAACAAGAAATC	164
		R	AGAAGAATGATGCTGGGCTGAGTAA	
GAPDH	Human	F	CGCTGAGTACGTCGTGGAGTC	172
		R	GCTGATGATCTTGAGGCTGTTGTC	

Measurement of melanin contents

Cells were incubated with compounds for 72 hours. After they were washed twice with ice-cold phosphate-buffered saline (PBS), cells were lysed by incubation in cell lysis buffer [20 mM Tris PH 7.5, 150 mMNaCl, 1% TritonX-100, 2.5 mM sodium pyrophosphate, 1 mM EDTA, 1%Na3VO4, 0.5 μg/ml leupeptin, 1 mM phenylmethanesulfonyl fluoride (PMSF)] (Biyuntian, China) at 4°C for 10 min, then the lysates were centrifuged at 14,000 rpm for 15 min. The supernatant containing protein was removed and conserved. Protein concentrations were determined by BCA Protein Assay kit (Biyuntian, China) with bovine serum albumin (BSA) (Sigma-Aldrich, USA) as a standard. The precipitate containing total melanin was dissolved in 100 μL of 1N NaOH/10%DMSO for 2 h at 80°C. Total melanin content was estimated by absorbance at 405 nm and comparison made with total protein concentration, then calculated as a percent of the control.

Western blotting

The protein suspension of skin tissues was obtained using a Total Protein Extraction Kit (APPLYGEN, China) and the protein concentrations were detected by BCA Protein Assay kit with BSA as a standard. The same amount of total protein was assayed for each Western blot. Proteins were separated by SDS-PAGE and transferred to nitrocellulose membranes. The membranes were incubated with primary antibodies: POMC (1:200, Santa Cruz Biotechnology Inc, USA) and β-Actin (1:4000, Sigma-Aldrich, USA) for 1.5 h at room temperature then washed with Tris-buffered saline, including 0.1% Tween-20, exposed to peroxidase-conjugated secondary antibodies (1:4000, Sigma-Aldrich, USA) for 1 h at room temperature, washed. Proteins were visualized using an enhanced chemiluminescence detection system. Densitometric analysis was performed by using Quantity One (Bio-Rad, USA). Three animals were used for each data point. Western blot assay results reported here are representative

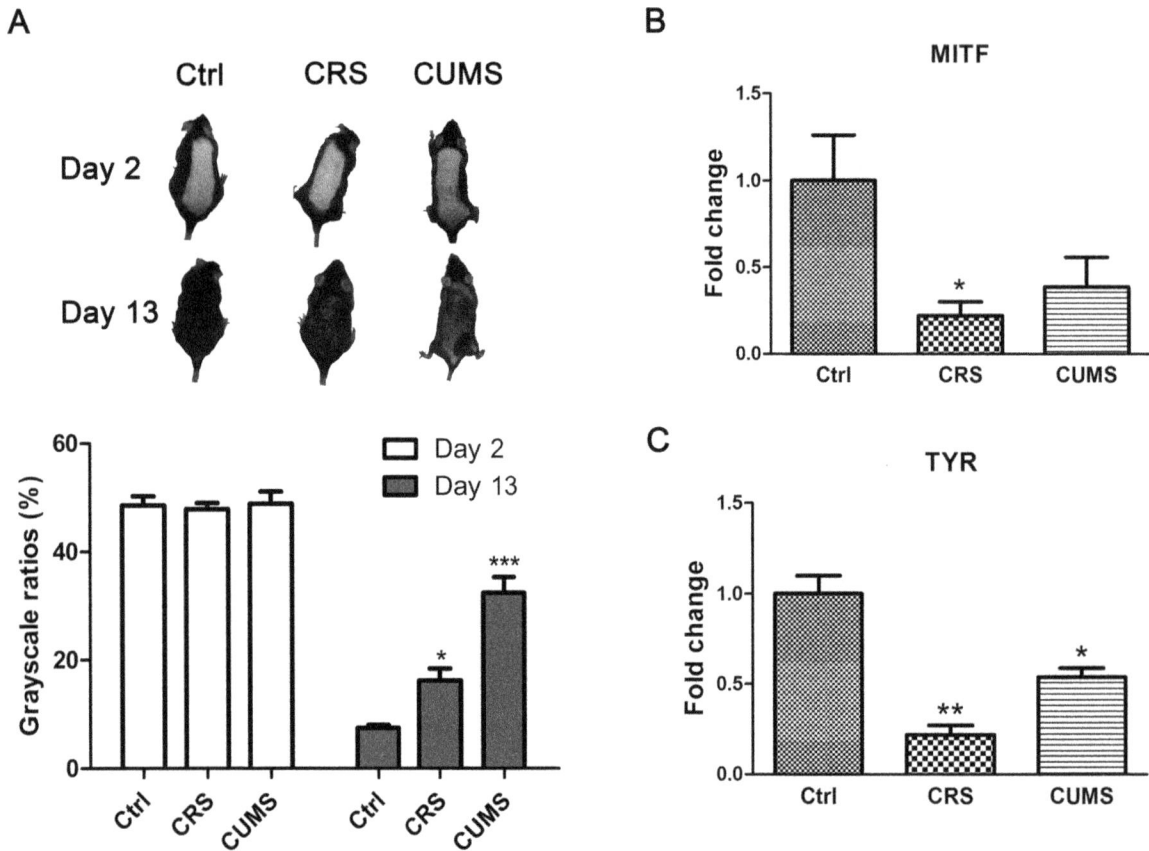

Figure 2. Chronic stress causing reduction of melanogenesis in mice dorsal skin. A: Photographs of mice back skin on day 2 and day 13 after epilation showing the reduction of melanin in the skin of CRS and CUMS group mice on day 13. **B**: The mRNA expression levels of microphthalmia-associated transcription factor (MITF) in mouse skin. **C**: The mRNA expression levels of tyrosinase (TYR) in mouse skin. The expression levels of each gene were normalized against β-Actin then calculated as fold change using the comparative $2^{-\Delta\Delta CT}$ method. Data are showed in mean ± SEM, n = 8, and the data were analyzed by one-way ANOVA with Tukey's post hoc test. * $P<0.05$, ** $P<0.01$, *** $P<0.001$, compared with control.

of three independent experiments. The related protein bands, cut and displayed in the same figure, are from the same membrane.

Quantitative real-time PCR

Total RNA was extracted from cells or mouse dorsal skin using TRIZOL reagent (Gibco-BRL, USA) and total RNA concentration was quantified spectrophotometrically. First strand cDNA was synthesized with PrimeScript RT Master Mix (Takara, Japan) according to the manufacturer's instructions. The quantitative real-time PCR was performed on an iQ5 multicolor real-time PCR detection system (Bio-Rad, USA) by using SYBR Premix Ex TaqTM2 (Takara, Japan) according to the manufacturer's instructions. Primer sequences are shown in Table 1. Real-time PCR conditions were: 1 cycle of 2 min at 50°C, 95°C for 10 min, followed by 40 cycles of 95°C cDNA denaturation for 20 s, 60°C primer annealing for 30 s and 72°C extension for 30 s. Melting curve analyses were performed to confirm absence of nonspecific bands. The expression levels of each gene were normalized against β-Actin (Gene symbol: Actb) or GAPDH, then calculated as fold change using the comparative $2^{-\Delta\Delta CT}$ method and the results were from at least three independent experiments according to the manufacturer's protocols [42].

Statistical analysis

Statistical analysis was performed using GraphPadPrismVersion 5.0c (GraphPad Software). Data were analyzed by unpaired, two-tailed Student's t test or by one-way ANOVA with Tukey's post hoc test, as appropriate. P<0.05 was regarded as significant. Results are presented as mean ± SEM.

Results

Effects of chronic stress on the mouse dorsal skin melanogenesis

Mice were photographed after epilation. Upon visual examination, all groups of mice had a similar skin color on the second day after epilation. However, on the thirteenth day, the skin color showed visible differences, and stressed mice showed lighter skin color than control mice (Fig. 2A).

Experiments were performed to detect any changes in microphthalmia-associated transcription factor (MITF) or tyrosinase (TYR) mRNA expression levels in the dorsal skin. MITF is a key transcription factor for melanogenesis that effectively transactivates the TYR genes by binding to an M-box motif in the TYR promoter [43]. Tyrosinase is the rate-limiting enzyme in two critical steps in melanogenesis [44]. The CRS mice showed reduced mRNA expression levels of MITF (P<0.05) and TYR (P<0.01) (Fig. 2B, C). The CUMS mice showed reduced mRNA expression levels of TYR (P<0.05) (Fig. 2C).

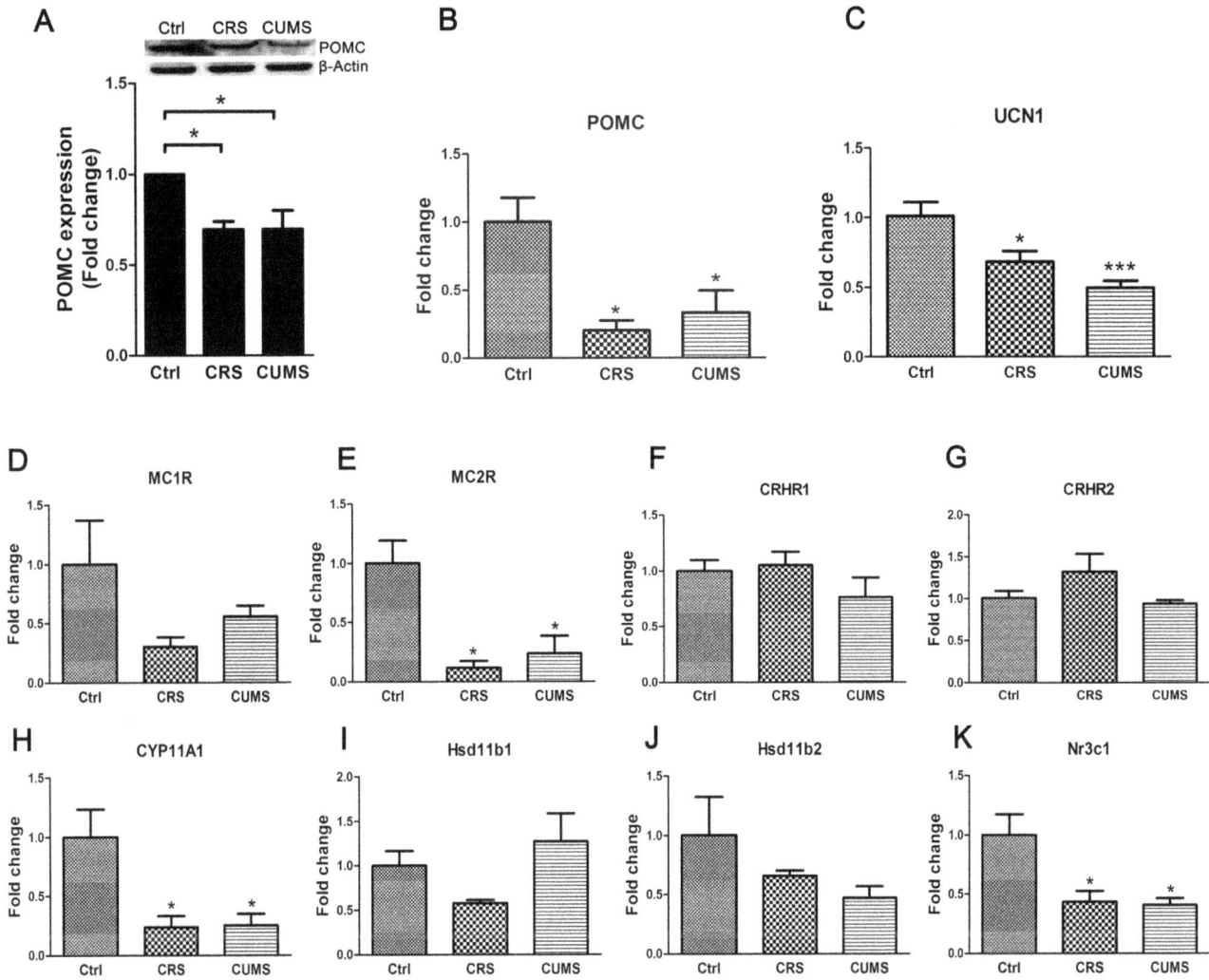

Figure 3. Chronic stress causing disrupted expressions of cutaneous HPA axis elements. A: POMC expression was analyzed by immunoblotting. β-Actin expression was indicated as a loading control. Western blot assay are representative of three experiments. Densitometric scanning of band intensities obtained from three separate experiments was used to quantify change of proteins expression. Three animals were used for each data point. Data are showed in mean ± SEM. **B–K:** The mRNA expression levels of POMC, UCN1, MC1R, MC2R, CRHR1, CRHR2, CYP11A1, Hsd11b1, Hsd11b2, and Nr3c1 in mouse skin. The expression levels of each gene were normalized against β-Actin then calculated as fold change using the comparative $2^{-\Delta\Delta CT}$ method. Data are showed in mean ± SEM, n = 8. Data were analyzed by one-way ANOVA with Tukey's post hoc test. * $P<0.05$, ** $P<0.01$, compared with control.

Effects of chronic stress on the cutaneous HPA axis

The expression of POMC was examined in mouse skin. POMC expression levels were reduced by both CRS ($P<0.05$) and CUMS ($P<0.05$) (Fig. 3A). Similarly, the mRNA expression levels of POMC in mouse skin were also reduced by CRS ($P<0.05$) and CUMS ($P<0.05$) (Fig. 3B). The mRNA expression levels of POMC cleavage product receptors were also measured, and chronic stress reduced MC2R mRNA expression levels (Fig. 3E). Although there were decreased mRNA expression levels of MC1R in the skin of stressed mice, the changes were not significantly different from the levels in control mice (Fig. 3D).

Alterations of POMC expression in the skin of stressed mice may be caused by changes in UCN1 expression, thereby affecting the cutaneous HPA axis, and may lead to changes in the expression of CYP11A1. To test this possibility, experiments were performed to measure mRNA expression of UCN1 and CYP11A1, and both genes were found to be reduced in the skin of stressed mice (Fig. 3C, H). UCN1 exerts biological effects by

binding to its receptors [28,45,46]. The mRNA expression levels of CRHR1 and CRHR2 did not significantly change in the skin of stressed mice (Fig. 3F, G). 11β-hydroxysteroid dehydrogenase type 1 (11β-HSD1, Gene symbol: HSD11b1), 11β-hydroxysteroid dehydrogenase type 2 (11β-HSD2, Gene symbol: HSD11b2), and glucocorticoid receptor (GR) play key roles in the regulation of glucocorticoid activities [47–50]. The expression of the genes that encode 11β-HSD1 (Hsd11b1) and 11β-HSD2 (Hsd11b2) showed no significant changes in the skin of stressed mice, whereas the expression of the gene that encodes GR (Gene symbol: Nc3r1) was reduced (Fig. 3I–K).

Effects of chronic stress on body weight and serum corticosterone levels

Our data indicated that CRS and CUMS did not significantly inhibit mouse body weight gain compared to the control group (Fig. 4A).

A

B

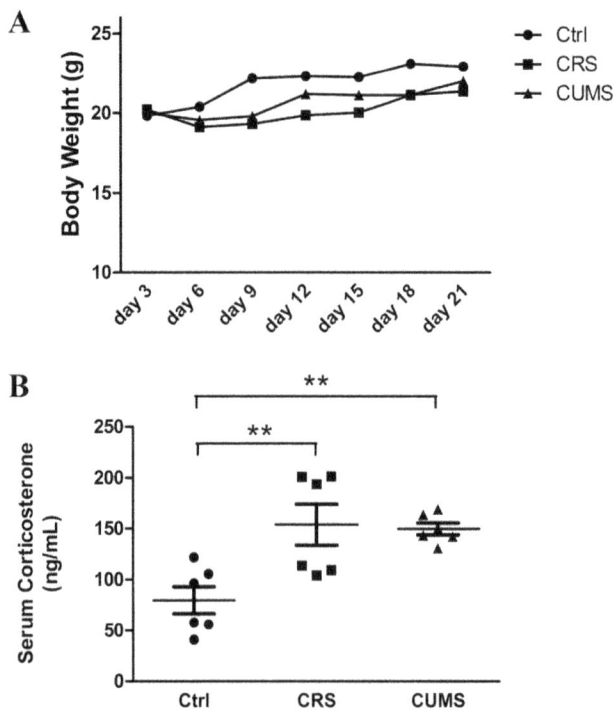

Figure 4. Effects of chronic stress on mice body weight gain and serum corticosterone levels. A: On days 3, 6, 9, 12, 15, 18, and 21, CRS and CUMS did not inhibit mice body weight gain significantly compared with control. **B**: The serum corticosterone levels in mice of different group. Serum for corticosterone measurement was collected on day 22, one day after the final stressor. Data are showed in mean ± SEM, n = 6, and the data were analyzed by one-way ANOVA with Tukey's post hoc test. ** $P<0.01$, compared with control.

Sustained activation of the central HPA axis by chronic stress can lead to elevated glucocorticoid levels [51]. Compared to controls (Ctrl, 79.72±12.08 ng/mL), chronic stress caused a significant elevation of serum corticosterone levels (CRS, 153.83±18.36 ng/mL; CUMS, 149.75±5.31 ng/mL) (Fig. 4B).

Effects of corticosterone on the dorsal skin of mice

Considering that chronic stress caused a marked elevation of serum corticosterone levels, further studies were conducted to investigate whether corticosterone affects the dorsal skin of mice in vivo. On the thirteenth day after epilation, mice that received corticosterone injections had a significantly lighter observable skin color than controls (Fig. 5A). In the CORT group, mice had significantly lower MITF expression (Fig. 5B). These results suggest that corticosterone reduces skin melanogenesis.

The expression levels of key factors along the HPA axis were evaluated in the dorsal skin of mice that received chronic corticosterone injections. POMC expression was reduced after corticosterone injections (Fig. 5C). Corticosterone also significantly suppressed mRNA expression levels of UCN1, POMC, CYP11A1, MC2R, CRHR1, CRHR2 and Nr3c1 (Fig. 5D).

Effects of RU486 on the dorsal skin of stressed mice

Because chronic stress caused a marked elevation of serum corticosterone levels, further studies were conducted to test whether RU486 (a glucocorticoid receptor antagonist) could reverse the effects of CUMS on the dorsal skin of mice in vivo. On the thirteenth day after epilation, mice that received RU486

injections had a significantly darker observable skin color than CUMS mice (Fig. 6A). The CUMS mice showed reduced expression of MITF and TYR, but RU486 reversed this effect (Fig. 6B, C). Additionally, administration of RU486 significantly ameliorated the CUMS-induced reduction of POMC expression (Fig. 6D). Furthermore, RU486 also normalized the CUMS-induced reduction of mRNA expression levels of UCN1, POMC, and CYP11A1 (Fig. 6E). These results suggested that stress-induced alterations of these mediators might be mediated by glucocorticoids.

Effects of HPA axis-related hormones on melanin synthesis in vitro

To determine whether corticosterone could directly inhibit melanogenesis, NHEMs or B16F10 cells were incubated with α-MSH or DEX, a synthetic corticosteroid. In NHEMs, both α-MSH and DEX significantly increased melanin content, and α-MSH showed a stronger effect than DEX (Fig. 7A). Next, we used RT-PCR to examine the effects of these hormones on the expression of genes associated with melanogenesis. Both α-MSH and DEX increased mRNA expression levels of MITF and TYR, and again α-MSH showed a stronger effect than DEX (Fig. 7B, C). In B16F10 cells, α-MSH significantly increased the melanin content, whereas DEX showed no significant effect (Fig. 7D). We found that α-MSH increased the mRNA expression levels of MITF and TYR, whereas DEX showed no significant effect (Fig. 7E, F). These results suggested that glucocorticoids showed no inhibitory effects on melanogenesis in B16F10 cells and that glucocorticoids promoted melanogenesis in NHEMs.

Discussion

Our data demonstrate that chronic stress can suppress cutaneous melanogenesis and the expression levels of cutaneous HPA axis elements. Moreover, chronic stress can cause the elevation of serum corticosterone levels, suggesting that increased corticosterone levels may contribute to the suppression of chronic stress. Consistent with this possibility, mice that received subcutaneous injections of corticosterone showed reduced expression of cutaneous HPA axis elements and decreased pigmentation. Additionally, the glucocorticoid receptor antagonist increased the CUMS-induced reductions of melanogenesis and cutaneous HPA axis element expression levels. These findings suggest that stress can suppress the activation of the cutaneous HPA axis through glucocorticoids and thereby cause reduced melanogenesis.

In a study of human hair follicles in vitro, the glucocorticoid receptor agonist hydrocortisone could reduce follicular CRH expression [22]. The skin of DEX-treated mice shows attenuated production of POMC mRNA [52]. These data, along with our observations that subcutaneous injections of corticosterone can reduce the expression of HPA axis hormones in the skin of mice, suggest that the skin has HPA axis-like regulatory feedback systems that are mediated by glucocorticoids. Stress is the main factor that drives increased central HPA axis activation [1]. Both CRS and CUMS cause sustained responsiveness of the central HPA axis [53,54] and caused high levels of serum glucocorticoids in our study. These results imply that stress may attenuate the activation of the cutaneous HPA axis. Some researchers have reported that 2 h restraint stress treatment could suppress cutaneous POMC mRNA expression levels [55]. Together with the inhibitory effect of chronic stress on the cutaneous HPA axis, it is possible that this phenomenon is caused by glucocorticoid-dependent negative feedback.

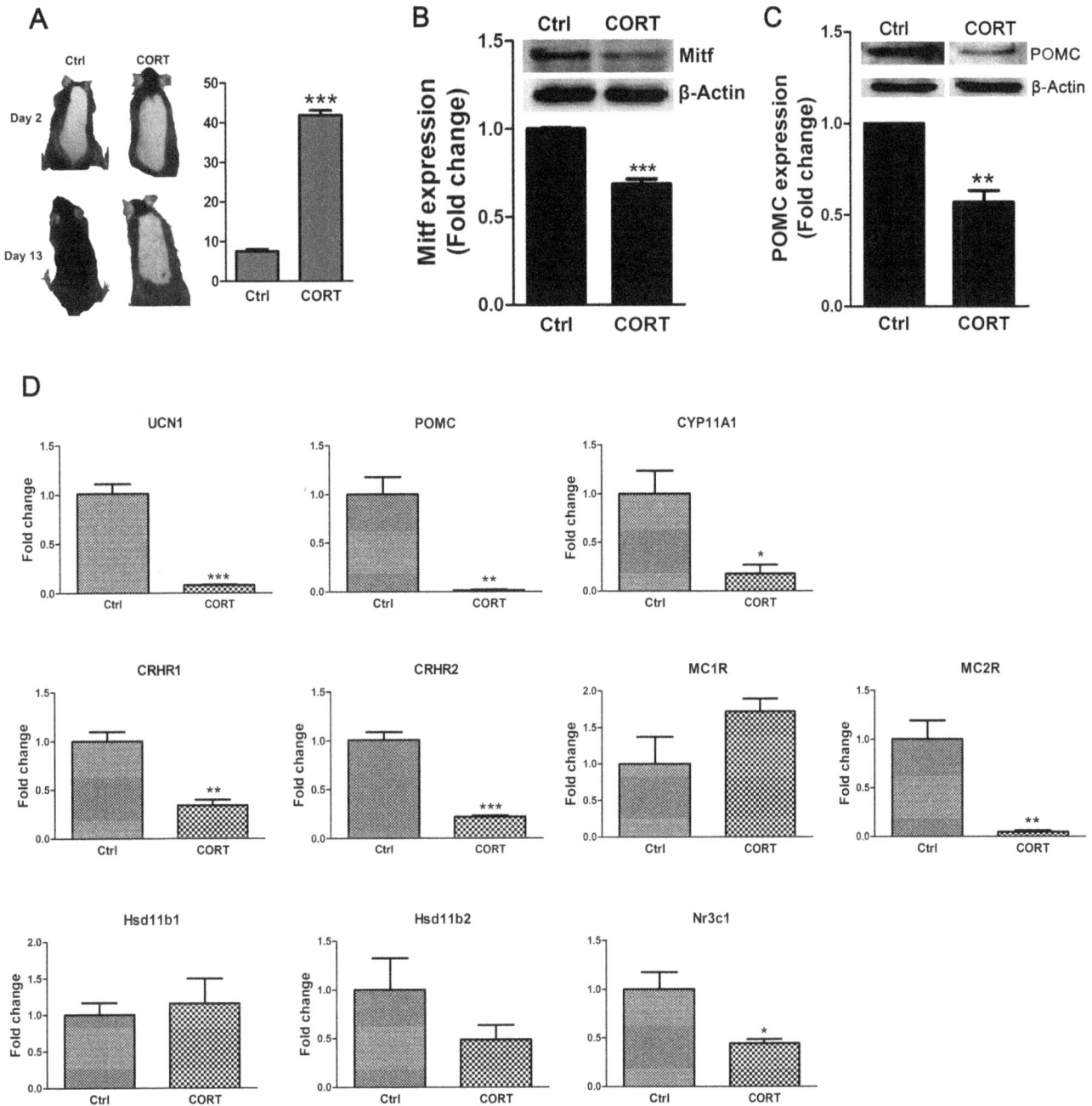

Figure 5. Corticosterone causing reduction of melanogenesis and disrupted expressions of cutaneous HPA axis elements. A: Photographs of mice back skin on day 2 and day 13 after epilation showing the reduction of melanin in corticosterone treated mice on day 13. **B**: MITF expression was analyzed by immunoblotting. **C**: POMC expression was analyzed by immunoblotting. β-Actin expression was indicated as a loading control. Western blot assay are representative of three experiments. Densitometric scanning of band intensities obtained from three separate experiments was used to quantify change of proteins expression. Three animals were used for each data point. Data are showed in mean ± SEM. **D**: The mRNA expression levels of UCN1, POMC, CYP11A1, CRHR1, CRHR2, MC1R, MC2R, Hsd11b1, Hsd11b2, and Nr3c1 in mouse skin. The expression levels of each gene were normalized against β-Actin then calculated as fold change using the comparative $2^{-\Delta\Delta CT}$ method. Data are showed in mean ± SEM, n = 8. Data were analyzed by Student's t test. * $P<0.05$, ** $P<0.01$, *** $P<0.001$, compared with control.

In addition to the decreased expression of hormones along the cutaneous HPA axis in situ, chronic stress also leads to changes in the expression of cognate receptors for these hormones. Mice that experienced chronic stress or long-term corticosterone injections exhibited reduced MC2R mRNA expression levels in skin. ACTH binds to MC2R to promote glucocorticoid synthesis [56]. Reduced expression of MC2R and POMC may cause a reduction in

glucocorticoid synthesis, which is consistent with the reduced expression of CYP11A1 observed in our experiments. CRHR1 and CRHR2 are important receptors of the HPA axis. Hypothalamic CRHR1 gene transcription in mice has been shown to be inhibited by glucocorticoid administration [56]. Corticosterone-treated mice had decreased cutaneous expression levels of CRHR1 and CRHR2, whereas stressed mice showed no

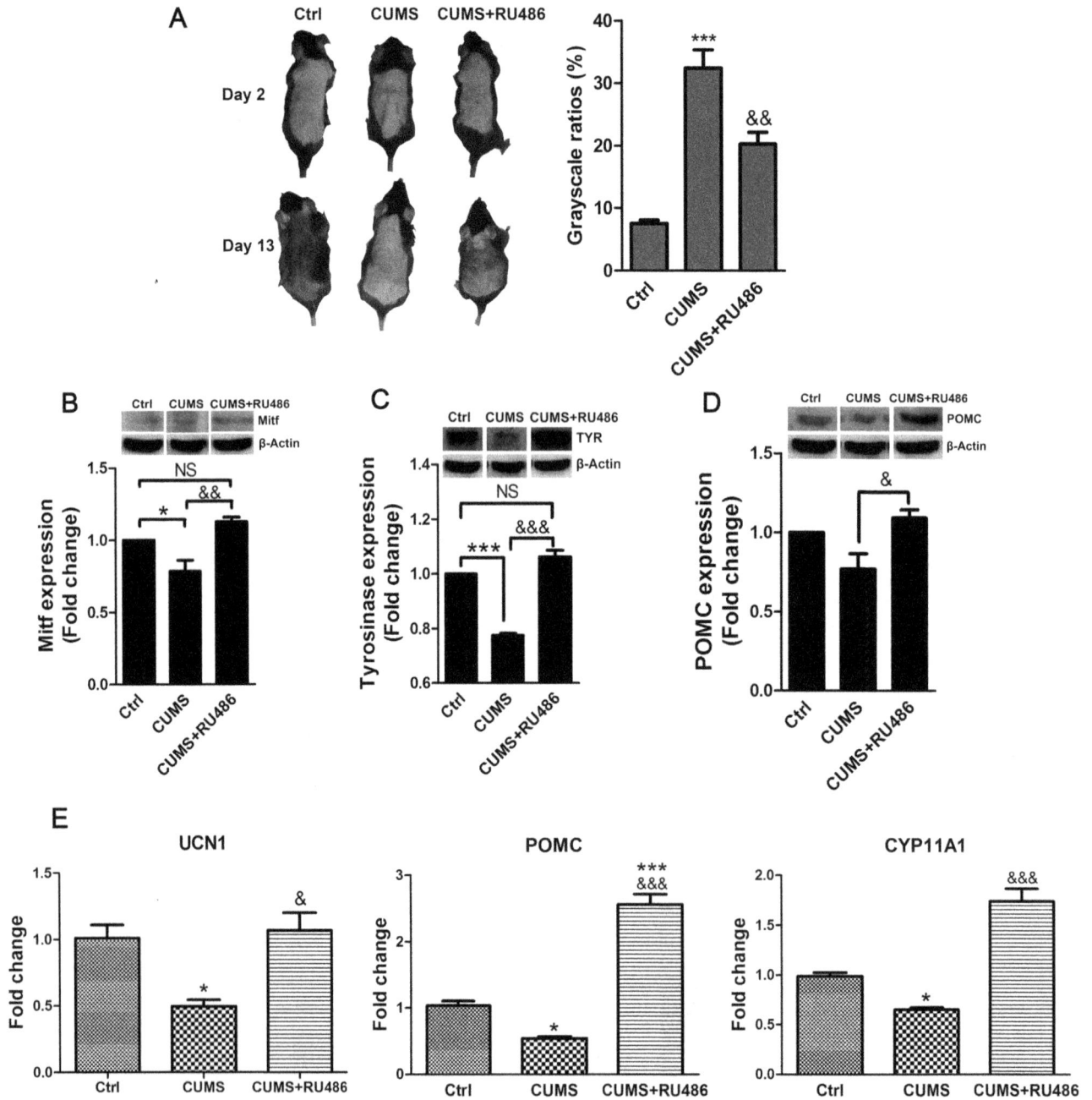

Figure 6. Effects of RU486 on the dorsal skin of stressed mice. A: Photographs of mice back skin on day 2 and day 13 after epilation showing that the mice received RU486 injection had a significantly darker observable skin color than CUMS mice. **B**: MITF expression was analyzed by immunoblotting. **C**: TYR expression was analyzed by immunoblotting. **D**: POMC expression was analyzed by immunoblotting. β-Actin expression was indicated as a loading control. Western blot assay are representative of three experiments. Densitometric scanning of band intensities obtained from three separate experiments was used to quantify change of proteins expression. Three animals were used for each data point. Data are showed in mean ± SEM. **E**: The mRNA expression levels of UCN1, POMC, and CYP11A1 in mouse skin. The expression levels of each gene were normalized against β-Actin then calculated as fold change using the comparative $2^{-\Delta\Delta CT}$ method. Data are showed in mean ± SEM, n = 8. The data were analyzed by one-way ANOVA with Tukey's post hoc test. * $P<0.05$, *** $P<0.001$, compared with control; $^{\&}P<0.05$, $^{\&\&}P<0.01$, $^{\&\&\&}P<0.001$, compared with CUMS.

significant differences. Substance P can increase the expression of CRHR1 in mast cells in human skin [57]. There is increased Substance P protein expression in cutaneous peripheral nerve fibers in chronically stressed mice [58]. The involvement of other factors that increase in response to stress in skin might underlie the differential expression of CRHR1 and CRHR2 in chronically stressed and corticosterone-treated mice.

Based on our findings, glucocorticoids play an important role in the regulation of chronic stress. In humans, two key enzymes that regulate local cortisol availability are 11β-HSD1 and 11β-HSD2, which induce intracellular conversion of cortisol, and, together with GR, play a key role in regulating glucocorticoid activities [47–50]. Expression of 11β-HSD1, 11β-HSD2, and GR has been detected in human skin [59,60]. We found that the mRNA

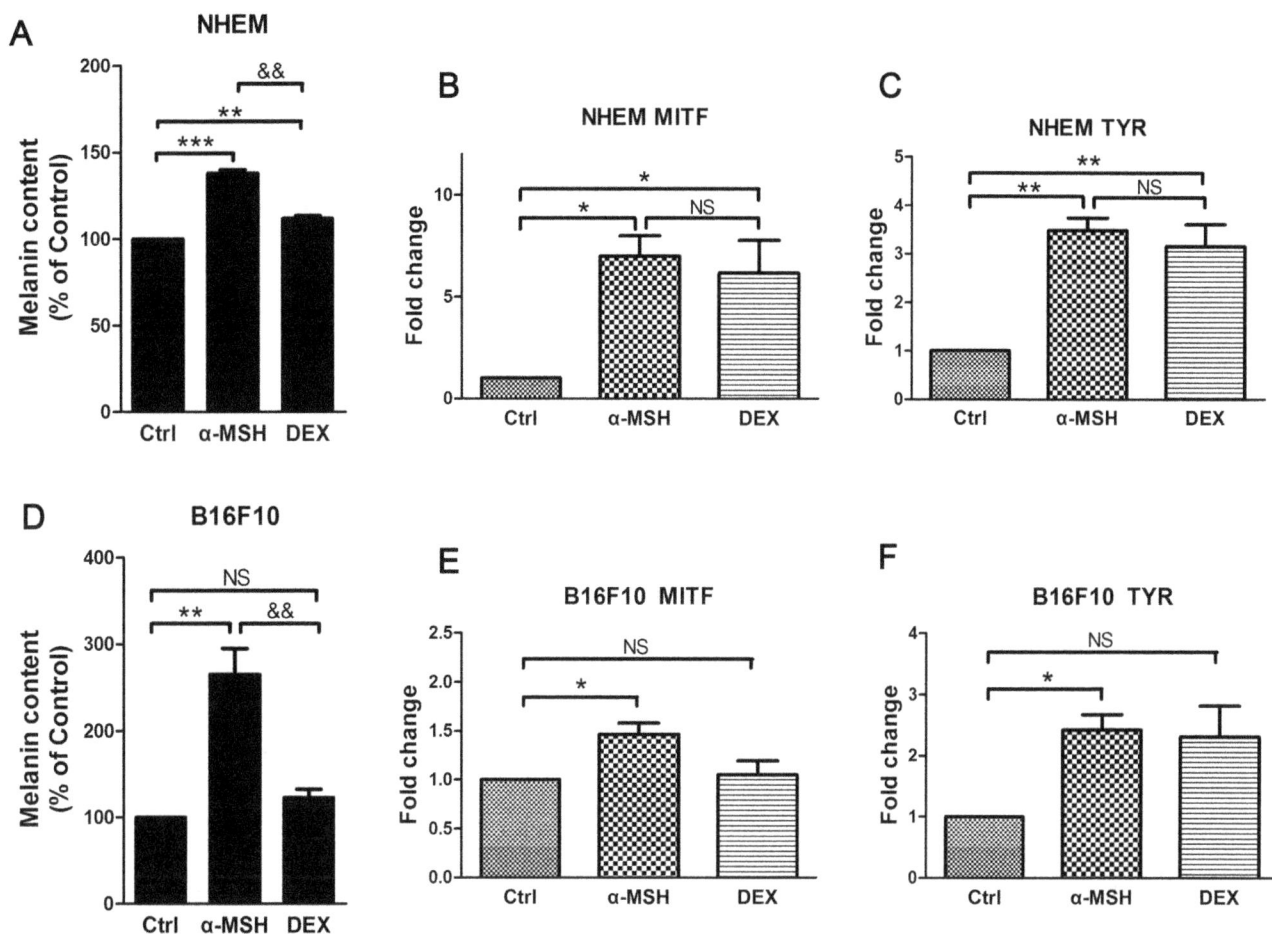

Figure 7. Effects of HPA axis-related hormones on melanin synthesis in vitro. A: Measurement of melanin contents in normal human epidermal melanocytes (NHEMs) after treatment with 50 nM α-MSH or 1 μM DEX for 72 h. **D**: Measurement of melanin contents in B16F10 cells after treatment with 50 nM α-MSH or 1 μM DEX for 72 h. **B–C**: The mRNA expression levels of MITF and TYR in NHEMs after treatment with 50 nM α-MSH or 1 μM DEX for 24 h. **E–F**: The mRNA expression levels of MITF and TYR in B16F10 cells after treatment with 50 nM α-MSH or 1 μM DEX for 24 h. The expression levels of each gene were normalized against β-Actin or GAPDH then calculated as fold change using the comparative $2^{-\Delta\Delta CT}$ method. Data are combined from three separate experiments and showed in mean ± SEM, and the data were analyzed by one-way ANOVA with Tukey's post hoc test. * $P<0.05$, ** $P<0.01$, *** $P<0.001$, compared with control; $^{\&\&}P<0.01$, compared with α-MSH.

expression levels of HSD11b1 and HSD11b2 could be detected in the skin of mice and that the expression level of these genes was not affected by chronic stress or corticosterone injections. Recent studies have shown that chronic stress can reduce GR expression in the brain, and this effect may be mediated by elevated glucocorticoid levels [61,62]. We found that both chronically stressed and corticosterone-treated mice showed reduced mRNA expression of Nr3c1. This phenomenon may be caused by desensitization of skin exposed to high glucocorticoid concentrations.

human skin expresses mRNAs for three obligatory enzymes of steroid synthesis including cytochromes P450scc, P450c17 and P450c21 [63]. P450scc also shows pleiotropic effects in cutaneous secosteroidal system [3,64,65]. Since chronic stress and corticosterone treatment suppressed mRNA expression levels of CYP11A1, we propose that chronic stress and glucocorticoids treatment may affect steroidogenesis and secosteroidogenesis in the skin.

Clinically, glucocorticoids are used to treat many skin diseases [66–68]. Although the precise role of the cutaneous HPA axis in skin function remains to be determined, the multiple functions of

HPA axis-derived hormones on the skin adds further evidence to the role of the cutaneous HPA axis in maintaining homeostasis in the skin microenvironment [11,20,69]. In addition to some direct effects of glucocorticoids on skin [68,70,71], local glucocorticoid treatment may affect skin function by restraining the activation of the cutaneous HPA axis. Moreover, skin disorder is accompanied by psychological pressure, which can lead to elevated cortisol levels [2]. Based on our data, we speculate that these patients could have attenuated expression of cutaneous HPA axis elements. Our findings should prompt dermatologists to be more cautious when using glucocorticoids for treatment.

Melanogenesis is an important function of the skin that protects the body against radiation and helps maintain homeostasis of the skin microenvironment [33,72,73]. Melanogenesis is closely related to activation of the skin HPA axis. In patients with depigmentation, decreased epidermal POMC processing and α-MSH levels have been previously reported [74]. In this study, we found no significant inhibitory effect of glucocorticoids on melanogenesis in B16F10 cells. In NHEMs, glucocorticoids could promote melanogenesis, however this effect was weaker than α-MSH treatment. However, administering corticosterone to mice resulted in reduced melanin synthesis, which is consistent with a previous report that the application of DEX to the skin of mice decreased tyrosinase protein concentration [52]. The inhibitory effect of corticosterone and chronic stress on melanogenesis in vivo appears to be indirect. The reduced pigmentation may be caused by the repressed expression of skin HPA axis elements, which are caused by glucocorticoids. Taking into account that glucocorticoids promotes melanin synthesis and that glucocorticoids exert their biological effects by binding to their receptor, the reduced expression of glucocorticoid receptor in chronically stressed and corticosterone-treated mice may have also caused the reduced pigmentation.

In summary, our data demonstrate that chronic stress can suppress the expression of skin HPA axis-related genes and proteins. This restriction of the cutaneous HPA axis may be caused by negative feedback control via high glucocorticoid concentrations induced by stress. Additionally, the suppressed expression of elements of the cutaneous HPA axis is accompanied by reduced pigmentation, emphasizing that chronic stress may be a risk factor for the development of skin problems.

Acknowledgments

We thank Feng Wang, Liangliang Zhou and Jinpeng Lv for expert technical assistance.

Author Contributions

Conceived and designed the experiments: SP JS. Performed the experiments: SP HW QW MC. Analyzed the data: SP HW. Contributed reagents/materials/analysis tools: JS WS. Wrote the paper: SP.

References

1. McEwen BS (2008) Central effects of stress hormones in health and disease: Understanding the protective and damaging effects of stress and stress mediators. Eur J Pharmacol 583: 174–185.
2. Schut C, Weik U, Tews N, Gieler U, Deinzer R, et al. (2013) Psychophysiological effects of stress management in patients with atopic dermatitis: a randomized controlled trial. Acta Derm Venereol 93: 57–61.
3. Slominski AT, Zmijewski MA, Skobowiat C, Zbytek B, Slominski RM, et al. (2012) Sensing the environment: regulation of local and global homeostasis by the skin's neuroendocrine system. Adv Anat Embryol Cell Biol. 212: v, vii, 1–115.
4. Slominski AT, Zmijewski MA, Zbytek B, Tobin DJ, Theoharides TC, et al. (2013) Key Role of CRF in the Skin Stress Response System. Endocr Rev 34: 827–884
5. Evers AW, Verhoeven EW, Kraaimaat FW, de Jong EM, de Brouwer SJ, et al. (2010) How stress gets under the skin: cortisol and stress reactivity in psoriasis. Br J Dermatol 163: 986–991.
6. Hadshiew IM, Foitzik K, Arck PC, Paus R (2004) Burden of hair loss: stress and the underestimated psychosocial impact of telogen effluvium and androgenetic alopecia. J Invest Dermatol 123: 455–457.
7. Hall JM, Cruser D, Podawiltz A, Mummert DI, Jones H, et al. (2012) Psychological Stress and the Cutaneous Immune Response: Roles of the HPA Axis and the Sympathetic Nervous System in Atopic Dermatitis and Psoriasis. Dermatol Res Pract 2012: 403908.
8. Hunter HJ, Griffiths CE, Kleyn CE (2013) Does psychosocial stress play a role in the exacerbation of psoriasis? Br J Dermatol 169: 965–974.
9. Lonne-Rahm SB, Rickberg H, El-Nour H, Marin P, Azmitia EC, et al. (2008) Neuroimmune mechanisms in patients with atopic dermatitis during chronic stress. J Eur Acad Dermatol Venereol 22: 11–18.
10. Manolache L, Benea V (2007) Stress in patients with alopecia areata and vitiligo. J Eur Acad Dermatol Venereol 21: 921–928.
11. Arck PC, Slominski A, Theoharides TC, Peters EM, Paus R (2006) Neuroimmunology of stress: skin takes center stage. J Invest Dermatol 126: 1697–1704.
12. Vale W, Spiess J, Rivier C, Rivier J (1981) Characterization of a 41-residue ovine hypothalamic peptide that stimulates secretion of corticotropin and beta-endorphin. Science 213: 1394–1397.
13. Rivier C, Vale W (1983) Modulation of stress-induced ACTH release by corticotropin-releasing factor, catecholamines and vasopressin. Nature 305: 325–327.
14. Munck A, Guyre PM, Holbrook NJ (1984) Physiological functions of glucocorticoids in stress and their relation to pharmacological actions. Endocr Rev 5: 25–44.
15. Bamberger CM, Schulte HM, Chrousos GP (1996) Molecular determinants of glucocorticoid receptor function and tissue sensitivity to glucocorticoids. Endocr Rev 17: 245–261.
16. Tanida M, Katsuyama M, Sakatani K (2007) Relation between mental stress-induced prefrontal cortex activity and skin conditions: a near-infrared spectroscopy study. Brain Res 1184: 210–216.
17. Dhabhar FS (2013) Psychological stress and immunoprotection versus immunopathology in the skin. Clin Dermatol 31: 18–30.
18. Slominski A, Wortsman J (2000) Neuroendocrinology of the skin. Endocr Rev 21: 457–487.
19. Skobowiat C, Dowdy JC, Sayre RM, Tuckey RC, Slominski A (2011) Cutaneous hypothalamic-pituitary-adrenal axis homolog: regulation by ultraviolet radiation. Am J Physiol Endocrinol Metab 301: E484–493.
20. Slominski A, Mihm MC (1996) Potential mechanism of skin response to stress. Int J Dermatol 35: 849–851.
21. Slominski A, Zbytek B, Nikolakis G, Manna PR, Skobowiat C, et al. (2013) Steroidogenesis in the skin: Implications for local immune functions. J Steroid Biochem Mol Biol 137: 107–123

22. Ito N, Ito T, Kromminga A, Bettermann A, Takigawa M, et al. (2005) Human hair follicles display a functional equivalent of the hypothalamic-pituitary-adrenal axis and synthesize cortisol. FASEB J 19: 1332–1334.
23. Slominski A, Zbytek B, Szczesniewski A, Semak I, Kaminski J, et al. (2005) CRH stimulation of corticosteroids production in melanocytes is mediated by ACTH. Am J Physiol Endocrinol Metab 288: E701–706.
24. Slominski A, Zjawiony J, Wortsman J, Semak I, Stewart J, et al. (2004) A novel pathway for sequential transformation of 7-dehydrocholesterol and expression of the P450scc system in mammalian skin. Eur J Biochem 271: 4178–4188.
25. Slominski A, Pisarchik A, Tobin DJ, Mazurkiewicz JE, Wortsman J (2004) Differential expression of a cutaneous corticotropin-releasing hormone system. Endocrinology 145: 941–950.
26. Slominski A, Wortsman J, Luger T, Paus R, Solomon S (2000) Corticotropin releasing hormone and proopiomelanocortin involvement in the cutaneous response to stress. Physiol Rev 80: 979–1020.
27. Slominski A, Wortsman J, Pisarchik A, Zbytek B, Linton EA, et al. (2001) Cutaneous expression of corticotropin-releasing hormone (CRH), urocortin, and CRH receptors. FASEB J 15: 1678–1693.
28. Slominski A, Zbytek B, Zmijewski M, Slominski RM, Kauser S, et al. (2006) Corticotropin releasing hormone and the skin. Front Biosci 11: 2230–2248.
29. Skobowiat C, Nejati R, Lu L, Williams RW, Slominski AT (2013) Genetic variation of the cutaneous HPA axis: An analysis of UVB-induced differential responses. Gene 530: 1–7
30. Talaber G, Jondal M, Okret S (2013) Extra-adrenal glucocorticoid synthesis: Immune regulation and aspects on local organ homeostasis. Mol Cell Endocrinol 380: 89–98
31. Kauser S, Slominski A, Wei ET, Tobin DJ (2006) Modulation of the human hair follicle pigmentary unit by corticotropin-releasing hormone and urocortin peptides. FASEB J 20: 882–895.
32. Rousseau K, Kauser S, Pritchard LE, Warhurst A, Oliver RL, et al. (2007) Proopiomelanocortin (POMC), the ACTH/melanocortin precursor, is secreted by human epidermal keratinocytes and melanocytes and stimulates melanogenesis. FASEB J 21: 1844–1856.
33. Slominski A, Tobin DJ, Shibahara S, Wortsman J (2004) Melanin pigmentation in mammalian skin and its hormonal regulation. Physiol Rev 84: 1155–1228.
34. Slominski A (2007) A nervous breakdown in the skin: stress and the epidermal barrier. J Clin Invest 117: 3166–3169.
35. Kourosh AS, Harrington CR, Adinoff B (2010) Tanning as a behavioral addiction. Am J Drug Alcohol Abuse 36: 284–290.
36. Zhang X, Yu M, Yu W, Weinberg J, Shapiro J, et al. (2009) Development of alopecia areata is associated with higher central and peripheral hypothalamic-pituitary-adrenal tone in the skin graft induced C3H/HeJ mouse model. J Invest Dermatol 129: 1527–1538.
37. Zhao X, Seese RR, Yun K, Peng T, Wang Z (2013) The role of galanin system in modulating depression, anxiety, and addiction-like behaviors after chronic restraint stress. Neuroscience 246: 82–93.
38. Willner P, Towell A, Sampson D, Sophokleous S, Muscat R (1987) Reduction of sucrose preference by chronic unpredictable mild stress, and its restoration by a tricyclic antidepressant. Psychopharmacology (Berl) 93: 358–364.
39. Muller-Rover S, Handjiski B, van der Veen C, Eichmuller S, Foitzik K, et al. (2001) A comprehensive guide for the accurate classification of murine hair follicles in distinct hair cycle stages. J Invest Dermatol 117: 3–15.
40. Ping F, Shang J, Zhou J, Song J, Zhang L (2012) Activation of neurokinin-1 receptor by substance P inhibits melanogenesis in B16-F10 melanoma cells. Int J Biochem Cell Biol 44: 2342–2348.
41. Kim NS, Cho JH, Kang WH (2000) Behavioral differences between donor site-matched adult and neonatal melanocytes in culture. Arch Dermatol Res 292: 233–239.
42. Bustin SA, Benes V, Garson JA, Hellemans J, Huggett J, et al. (2009) The MIQE guidelines: minimum information for publication of quantitative real-time PCR experiments. Clin Chem 55: 611–622.

43. Yasumoto K, Yokoyama K, Shibata K, Tomita Y, Shibahara S (1995) Microphthalmia-associated transcription factor as a regulator for melanocyte-specific transcription of the human tyrosinase gene. Mol Cell Biol 15: 1833.

44. Sulaimon SS, Kitchell BE (2003) The biology of melanocytes. Vet Dermatol 14: 57–65.

45. Perrin MH, Vale WW (1999) Corticotropin releasing factor receptors and their ligand family. Ann N Y Acad Sci 885: 312–328.

46. Krause K, Schnitger A, Fimmel S, Glass E, Zouboulis CC (2007) Corticotropin-releasing hormone skin signaling is receptor-mediated and is predominant in the sebaceous glands. Horm Metab Res 39: 166–170.

47. Bujalska I, Shimojo M, Howie A, Stewart PM (1997) Human 11 beta-hydroxysteroid dehydrogenase: studies on the stably transfected isoforms and localization of the type 2 isozyme within renal tissue. Steroids 62: 77–82.

48. Bujalska IJ, Walker EA, Hewison M, Stewart PM (2002) A switch in dehydrogenase to reductase activity of 11β-hydroxysteroid dehydrogenase type 1 upon differentiation of human omental adipose stromal cells. Journal of Clinical Endocrinology & Metabolism 87: 1205–1210.

49. Draper N, Stewart PM (2005) 11beta-hydroxysteroid dehydrogenase and the pre-receptor regulation of corticosteroid hormone action. J Endocrinol 186: 251–271.

50. Tomlinson JW, Walker EA, Bujalska IJ, Draper N, Lavery GG, et al. (2004) 11beta-hydroxysteroid dehydrogenase type 1: a tissue-specific regulator of glucocorticoid response. Endocr Rev 25: 831–866.

51. Raone A, Cassanelli A, Scheggi S, Rauggi R, Danielli B, et al. (2007) Hypothalamic-pituitary-adrenal modifications consequent to chronic stress exposure in an experimental model of depression in rats. Neuroscience 146: 1734–1742.

52. Ermak G, Slominski A (1997) Production of POMC, CRH-R1, MC1, and MC2 receptor mRNA and expression of tyrosinase gene during the hair cycle and dexamethasone treatment in the C57BL/6 mouse skin. J Invest Dermatol 108: 160–165.

53. Aguilera G, Kiss A, Lu A, Camacho C (1996) Regulation of adrenal steroidogenesis during chronic stress. Endocr Res 22: 433–443.

54. Joels M, Karst H, Alfarez D, Heine VM, Qin Y, et al. (2004) Effects of chronic stress on structure and cell function in rat hippocampus and hypothalamus. Stress 7: 221–231.

55. Flint MS, Morgan JB, Shreve SN, Tinkle SS (2003) Restraint stress and corticotropin releasing hormone modulation of murine cutaneous POMC mRNA. Stress 6: 59–62.

56. Chen A, Perrin M, Brar B, Li C, Jamieson P, et al. (2005) Mouse corticotropin-releasing factor receptor type 2alpha gene: isolation, distribution, pharmacological characterization and regulation by stress and glucocorticoids. Mol Endocrinol 19: 441–458.

57. Asadi S, Alysandratos KD, Angelidou A, Miniati A, Sismanopoulos N, et al. (2012) Substance P (SP) induces expression of functional corticotropin-releasing hormone receptor-1 (CRHR-1) in human mast cells. J Invest Dermatol 132: 324–329.

58. Liu N, Wang LH, Guo LL, Wang GQ, Zhou XP, et al. (2013) Chronic restraint stress inhibits hair growth via substance P mediated by reactive oxygen species in mice. PLoS One 8: e61574.

59. Tiganescu A, Walker EA, Hardy RS, Mayes AE, Stewart PM (2011) Localization, age- and site-dependent expression, and regulation of 11beta-hydroxysteroid dehydrogenase type 1 in skin. J Invest Dermatol 131: 30–36.

60. Skobowiat C, Sayre RM, Dowdy JC, Slominski AT (2013) Ultraviolet radiation regulates cortisol activity in a waveband-dependent manner in human skin ex vivo. Br J Dermatol 168: 595–601.

61. Chiba S, Numakawa T, Ninomiya M, Richards MC, Wakabayashi C, et al. (2012) Chronic restraint stress causes anxiety- and depression-like behaviors, downregulates glucocorticoid receptor expression, and attenuates glutamate release induced by brain-derived neurotrophic factor in the prefrontal cortex. Prog Neuropsychopharmacol Biol Psychiatry 39: 112–119.

62. Meyer U, van Kampen M, Isovich E, Flugge G, Fuchs E (2001) Chronic psychosocial stress regulates the expression of both GR and MR mRNA in the hippocampal formation of tree shrews. Hippocampus 11: 329–336.

63. Slominski A, Ermak G, Mihm M (1996) ACTH receptor, CYP11A1, CYP17 and CYP21A2 genes are expressed in skin. J Clin Endocrinol Metab 81: 2746–2749.

64. Slominski AT, Kim TK, Chen J, Nguyen MN, Li W, et al. (2012) Cytochrome P450scc-dependent metabolism of 7-dehydrocholesterol in placenta and epidermal keratinocytes. Int J Biochem Cell Biol 44: 2003–2018.

65. Slominski AT, Kim T-K, Shehabi HZ, Semak I, Tang EK, et al. (2012) In vivo evidence for a novel pathway of vitamin D3 metabolism initiated by P450scc and modified by CYP27B1. The FASEB Journal 26: 3901–3915.

66. Luger T, Loske KD, Elsner P, Kapp A, Kerscher M, et al. (2004) [Topical skin therapy with glucocorticoids—therapeutic index]. J Dtsch Dermatol Ges 2: 629–634.

67. Schafer-Korting M, Kleuser B, Ahmed M, Holtje HD, Korting HC (2005) Glucocorticoids for human skin: new aspects of the mechanism of action. Skin Pharmacol Physiol 18: 103–114.

68. Werth VP (2013) The safe and appropriate use of systemic glucocorticoids in treating dermatologic disease. J Am Acad Dermatol 68: 177–178.

69. Slominski A, Wortsman J (2007) Differential expression of HPA axis homolog in the skin. Mol Cell Endocrinol 265–266: 143–149.

70. Kao JS, Fluhr JW, Man MQ, Fowler AJ, Hachem JP, et al. (2003) Short-term glucocorticoid treatment compromises both permeability barrier homeostasis and stratum corneum integrity: inhibition of epidermal lipid synthesis accounts for functional abnormalities. J Invest Dermatol 120: 456–464.

71. Zoller NN, Kippenberger S, Thaci D, Mewes K, Spiegel M, et al. (2008) Evaluation of beneficial and adverse effects of glucocorticoids on a newly developed full-thickness skin model. Toxicol In Vitro 22: 747–759.

72. Agar N, Young AR (2005) Melanogenesis: a photoprotective response to DNA damage? Mutat Res 571: 121–132.

73. Slominski A, Wortsman J, Plonka PM, Schallreuter KU, Paus R, et al. (2005) Hair follicle pigmentation. J Invest Dermatol 124: 13–21.

74. Spencer JD, Gibbons NC, Rokos H, Peters EM, Wood JM, et al. (2007) Oxidative stress via hydrogen peroxide affects proopiomelanocortin peptides directly in the epidermis of patients with vitiligo. J Invest Dermatol 127: 411–420.

The Flavonoid Luteolin Inhibits Fcγ-Dependent Respiratory Burst in Granulocytes, but Not Skin Blistering in a New Model of Pemphigoid in Adult Mice

Eva Oswald[1,2,4], **Alina Sesarman**[2], **Claus-Werner Franzke**[2], **Ute Wölfle**[3], **Leena Bruckner-Tuderman**[2,5,6], **Thilo Jakob**[1], **Stefan F. Martin**[1], **Cassian Sitaru**[2,5]*

1 Allergy Research Group, Department of Dermatology, University Freiburg Medical Center, Freiburg, Germany, 2 Molecular Dermatology, Department of Dermatology, University Freiburg Medical Center, Freiburg, Germany, 3 Competence Centre Skintegral, Department of Dermatology, University Freiburg Medical Center, Freiburg, Germany, 4 Faculty of Biology, University of Freiburg, Freiburg, Germany, 5 BIOSS Centre for Biological Signalling Studies, Freiburg, Germany, 6 Freiburg Institute for Advanced Studies, Freiburg, Germany

Abstract

Bullous pemphigoid is an autoimmune blistering skin disease associated with autoantibodies against the dermal-epidermal junction. Passive transfer of antibodies against BP180/collagen (C) XVII, a major hemidesmosomal pemphigoid antigen, into neonatal mice results in dermal-epidermal separation upon applying gentle pressure to their skin, but not in spontaneous skin blistering. In addition, this neonatal mouse model precludes treatment and observation of diseased animals beyond 2–3 days. Therefore, in the present study we have developed a new disease model in mice reproducing the spontaneous blistering and the chronic course characteristic of the human condition. Adult mice were pre-immunized with rabbit IgG followed by injection of BP180/CXVII rabbit IgG. Mice pre-immunized against rabbit IgG and injected 6 times every second day with the BP180/CXVII-specific antibodies (n = 35) developed spontaneous sustained blistering of the skin, while mice pre-immunized and then treated with normal rabbit IgG (n = 5) did not. Blistering was associated with IgG and complement C3 deposits at the epidermal basement membrane and recruitment of inflammatory cells, and was partly dependent on Ly-6G-positive cells. We further used this new experimental model to investigate the therapeutic potential of luteolin, a plant flavonoid with potent anti-inflammatory and anti-oxidative properties and good safety profile, in experimental BP. Luteolin inhibited the Fcγ-dependent respiratory burst in immune complex-stimulated granulocytes and the autoantibody-induced dermal-epidermal separation in skin cryosections, but was not effective in suppressing the skin blistering *in vivo*. These studies establish a robust animal model that will be a useful tool for dissecting the mechanisms of blister formation and will facilitate the development of more effective therapeutic strategies for managing pemphigoid diseases.

Editor: Dominik Hartl, University of Tübingen, Germany

Funding: The authors acknowledge support by grants from the Deutsche Forschungsgemeinschaft SI-1281/4-1 (CS), MA-1567/9-1 (SM), SFB850-B6 (LB-T, C-WF), and BIOSS (LB-T,CS), from the Medical Faculty of the Freiburg University (CS) and by the Freiburg Institute for Advanced Studies (LB-T). The funders had no role in study design, data collection and analysis, decision to publish, or preparation of the manuscript.

Competing Interests: The authors have declared that no competing interests exist.

* E-mail: cassian.sitaru@uniklinik-freiburg.de

Introduction

Pemphigoids are autoimmune blistering disorders associated with autoimmunity against hemidesmosomal proteins [1]. Collagen XVII (CXVII) is a major autoantigen in different pemphigoid diseases, including bullous pemphigoid (BP), pemphigoid gestationis, linear IgA disease, mucous membrane pemphigoid and lichen planus pemphigoides [1]. BP is a prototypical organ-specific autoimmune diseases of the skin associated with subepidermal blisters and autoimmunity against the hemidesmosomal proteins CXVII and BP230 at the dermal-epidermal junction (DEJ) [1,2]. While the plakin protein BP230 is an intracellular hemidesmosomal component [3,4], CXVII also known as the bullous pemphigoid antigen of 180 kDa (BP180) is a transmembrane collagen with its N-terminus intracellularly located, its ectodomain spanning the lamina lucida, and its C-terminus reaching the lamina densa of the basement membrane [5,6]. The ectodomain of BP180/CXVII consists of 15 interrupted collagenous regions

and contains major epitopes of pemphigoid autoantibodies and autoreactive T cells within its 16th non-collagenous (NC16A) region [7–9]. Further antigenic determinants in pemphigoid diseases were shown on both intra- and extracellular domains of BP180/CXVII [10,11].

The pathogenic significance of autoantibodies against BP180/CXVII is supported by several lines of evidence: (1) serum levels of circulating autoantibodies against BP180/CXVII correlate with disease activity in patients with BP [12–15]; (2) pemphigoid autoantibodies and rabbit antibodies generated against BP180/CXVII recruit leukocytes to the DEJ and induce dermal-epidermal separation of human skin [16,17]; (3) rabbit antibodies generated against BP180/CXVII induce subepidermal blistering when injected into mice and hamsters [18,19]; (4) the passive transfer of autoantibodies from BP patients into CXVII-humanized mice induces dermal-epidermal separation [20,21]; (5) the transfer of maternal antibodies against human BP180/CXVII induces spontaneous skin blistering in pups humanized for the autoantigen [22]; (6) the transfer of splenocytes from mice immunized against human BP180/CXVII into Rag2$^{-/-}$/CXVII-humanized mice results in a sustained production of blister-inducing autoantibodies, partially mimicking the features of the disease in humans [23]. While the pathogenic role of autoantibodies to BP230 was suggested by several observations in patients and experimental animals, the contribution of anti-BP230 reactivity to disease pathogenesis still needs further investigation [15,24–26].

Previous attempts to induce blistering by injecting BP patient IgG into wildtype mice have failed [27,28]. To circumvent this problem, elegant alternative models have been developed using the passive transfer of antibodies generated against the murine autoantigens or, more recently, by the use of patients' autoantibodies in transgenic mice expressing human BP180/CXVII [18–21]. These ingenious models reproduce most of the major disease features and offer unique opportunities to elucidate the pathomechanisms underlying autoantibody-induced tissue damage in pemphigoid diseases. However, major shortcomings of these models are: 1) the fact that neonatal mice injected with BP180/CXVII-specific antibodies do not develop spontaneous skin blistering and 2) by their experimental design, the models in neonatal mice have a short observation period and do not allow for adequately reproducing the course of the chronic pemphigoid disease for pathogenic and therapeutic studies.

Therefore, in the present study we set out to develop a pemphigoid disease model in adult mice reproducing the spontaneous blistering and the chronic course characteristic of human condition. In a model of progressive antibody-induced glomerulonephritis it has been shown that pre-immunization with rabbit IgG in complete Freund's adjuvant several days prior to injection of rabbit anti-mouse glomerular basement membrane (GBM) antiserum results in strong inflammation with deposition of IgG and complement C3 and glomerular lesions [29]. Using this information, we pre-immunized mice with rabbit IgG before passively transferring rabbit IgG generated against BP180/CXVII. Mice pre-immunized against rabbit IgG and repeatedly injected with the BP180/CXVII-specific IgG developed spontaneous sustained blistering of the skin. In addition, blistering was associated with complement activation and recruitment of inflammatory cells and partly dependent on Ly-6G-positive cells. In further ex vivo and animal experiments, we investigated the therapeutic potential of luteolin, a plant flavonoid with potent anti-inflammatory and anti-oxidative properties [30]. Luteolin inhibited the Fcγ-dependent respiratory burst in immune complex (IC)-stimulated granulocytes and the autoantibody-induced dermal-epidermal separation in skin cryosections, but was not effective in suppressing the skin blistering in the new animal model of BP.

Results

Generation and characterization of rabbit antibodies against murine BP180/CXVII

Rabbit antibodies were generated against different fragments of murine BP180/CXVII by immunizing the animals with a mixture of the respective recombinant proteins. These antibodies were shown to bind to the basement membrane zone of murine skin by indirect immunofluorescence (IF) microscopy (**Figure S1A and B**). By immunoblotting, we showed that the generated antibodies recognized a 180 kDa protein band in extracts of BP180/CXVII-expressing COS-7 cells (**Figure S1C**).

Complement-activating capacity of rabbit IgG specific for murine BP180/CXVII

The complement-activating capacity of BP180/CXVII-specific IgG was evaluated by an in vitro complement-binding test (**Figure 1**). BP180/CXVII-specific IgG (**Figure 1A**), in contrast to normal rabbit IgG (**Figure 1B**), fixed complement at the epidermal basement membrane.

Granulocyte-activating capacity of rabbit IgG specific for murine BP180/CXVII

To analyze the ability of ICs composed of rabbit IgG and murine BP180/CXVII to activate granulocytes, we performed luminol chemiluminescence assays with granulocytes from healthy donors (**Figure 2A**). Incubation of granulocytes with BP180/CXVII-specific IgG complexed with the antigen, but not with the antigen alone, resulted in the production of reactive oxygen species (ROS) (**Figure 2A**). To assess the capacity of BP180/CXVII-specific rabbit antibodies to induce granulocyte-dependent dermal-epidermal separation in human skin, IgG from pre-immune rabbits and animals immunized with murine BP180/CXVII was incubated with skin cryosections, and subsequently with leukocytes. After the addition of leukocytes, BP180/CXVII-specific IgG induced subepidermal splits in skin cryosections (**Figure 2B**), in contrast normal rabbit IgG failed to induce dermal-epidermal separation in cryosections (**Figure 2C**).

Pre-immunization of mice against rabbit IgG

To accelerate and increase the inflammatory reaction triggered by binding of IgG autoantibodies at the DEJ of murine skin, we pre-immunized mice with purified rabbit IgG mixed with complete Freund's adjuvant. Subsequently, mice were injected with BP180/CXVII-specific or control rabbit IgG. The immunization induced the production of high levels of mouse IgG against rabbit IgG as shown by ELISA (**Figure S2A**). None of the mice pre-immunized with rabbit IgG showed skin disease clinically and histologically nor deposition of mouse IgG or complement C3 at the DEJ. However, injection of mice with BP180/CXVII-specific IgG, but not with normal rabbit IgG, resulted in deposition of mouse IgG at the murine epidermal basement membrane as detailed below.

Adult mice injected with BP180/CXVII-specific IgG develop spontaneous skin blistering

Adult SJL (n = 2), BALB/c (n = 31), C57BL/6 (n = 3) and C57BL/10 (n = 2) mice pre-immunized with rabbit IgG were

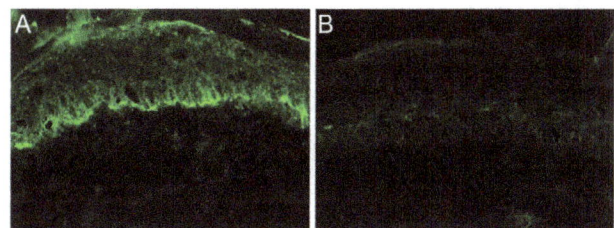

Figure 1. Complement-binding capacity of BP180/CXVII-specific rabbit antibodies. Frozen murine skin sections were incubated with rabbit antibodies and subsequently with fresh human serum as a source of complement. Bound C3 was visualized at the dermal-epidermal junction by fluorochrome-labeled antibody. (**A**) Deposits of C3 in sections incubated with BP180/CXVII-specific rabbit antibody. (**B**) No C3 deposition in sections incubated with normal rabbit IgG (magnification, ×400).

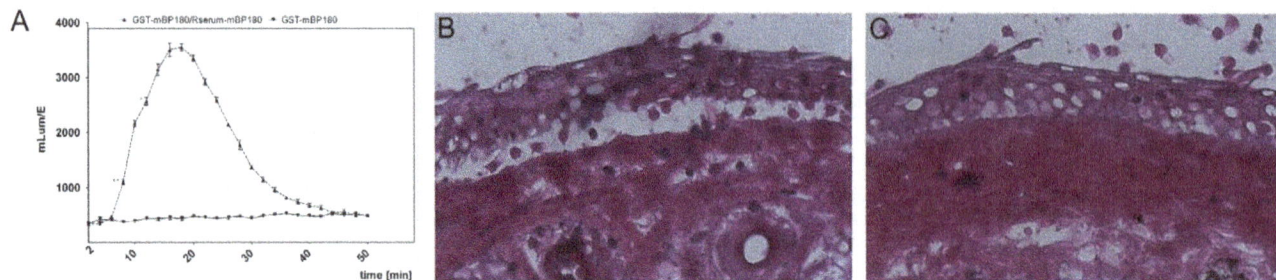

Figure 2. *Ex vivo* **granulocyte-activation capacity of BP180/CXVII-specific rabbit IgG antibodies. (A)** Leukocytes (3×10^7/ml) were stimulated with rabbit ICs consisting of 5 µg recombinant BP180/CXVII/well and 100 µl of 50-fold diluted BP180/CXVII-specific rabbit serum. ROS production was measured over a period of 60 min. Data are represented as mean ± SD; p<0.001. **(B, C)** Frozen skin sections were incubated with IgG and with 3×10^7 leukocytes/ml. Dermal-epidermal separation was observed in sections treated with **(B)** BP180/CXVII-specific IgG, but not with **(C)** normal rabbit IgG (magnification, ×400).

injected intraperitoneally (i.p.) or subcutaneously (s.c.) every second day with 15 mg of IgG purified from rabbit serum for 12 days. Mice (n = 35) injected i.p. (**Figure 3**) or s.c. (**Figure 4**) with IgG from rabbits immunized against murine BP180/CXVII developed skin lesions, including erythema, blisters and erosions. In contrast, mice injected with normal rabbit IgG (n = 5) did not show signs of skin disease (**Figure 3D–F and 4D**). Interestingly, the blistering phenotype induced by the i.p. injection was different when compared with the one triggered by the s.c. injection. While administration of BP180/CXVII-specific IgG by the i.p. route induced blisters at distant sites, including the ears, paws, eyes and snouts (**Figure 3A–C**), the s.c. injections of the BP180/CXVII-specific IgG resulted in lesions mainly restricted to skin areas in the proximity of the injection site (**Figure 4A–C**). Histologically dermal-epidermal separation of the skin with infiltration of inflammatory cells is found (**Figure 5A–C**). Infiltrates were dominated by neutrophils, with few eosinophils (**Figure 5A–B**).

The blistering phenotype in mice is associated with tissue-bound immunoreactants

Direct IF microscopy of perilesional skin revealed linear deposits of rabbit IgG (**Figure 6A**) and murine complement C3

(**Figure 6B**) at the epidermal basement membrane in adult mice that received IgG specific for BP180/CXVII. In addition, deposition of murine IgG was found at the basement membrane in mice injected with BP180/CXVII-specific IgG (**Figure 6C**), but not in animals treated with normal rabbit IgG (**Figure 6F**). In mice injected with normal rabbit IgG no deposition of IgG (**Figure 6D**) and complement C3 (**Figure 6E**) was detected by IF microscopy.

Repeated injection of antibodies induces stable extensive blistering skin disease in mice

In mice injected with rabbit IgG against murine BP180/CXVII, blistering of the skin started at 3–5 days after the first injection and developed during the observation period of 19 days to a full-blown skin blistering disease (**Figure 7**). The extent of the skin disease was scored and serum samples were obtained before the first injection of rabbit IgG (day 0) at day 3 as well as every second day thereafter. Circulating BP180/CXVII-specific rabbit IgG was detected in serum samples by ELISA (**Figure S2B**). During the observation time, disease activity was increasing until it reached a plateau around day 10. Subsequently, while new lesions continued to appear, some areas re-epithelized showing alopecia without scarring.

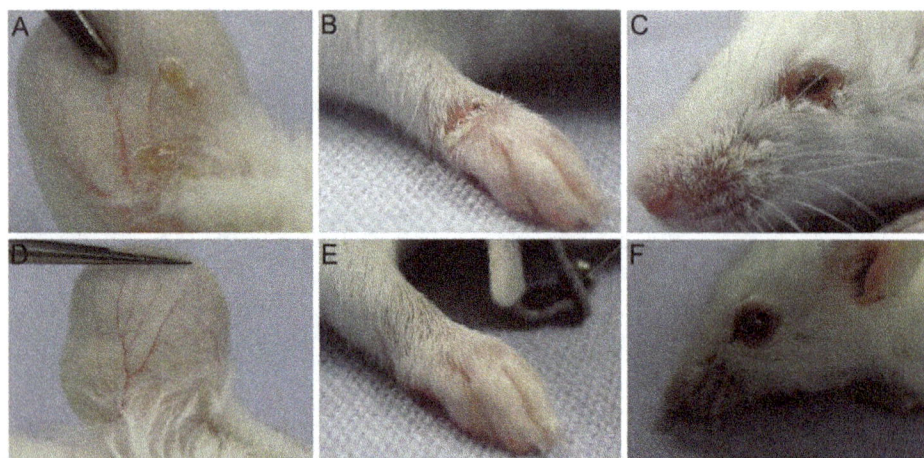

Figure 3. Intraperitoneal injection of BP180/CXVII-specific IgG induces blister formation in adult mice. Skin lesions, including blisters, erosions, and crusts developed on the **(A)** ear, **(B)** front leg and **(C)** periocular area in a BALB/c mouse pre-sensitized with rabbit IgG and subsequently receiving, over a period of 10 days, 6 i.p. injections of IgG, each containing 15 mg of IgG, from a rabbit immunized against murine BP180/CXVII. **(D, E, F)** A control mouse pre-sensitized with rabbit IgG and challenged with the same dose of normal rabbit IgG showed no skin alterations.

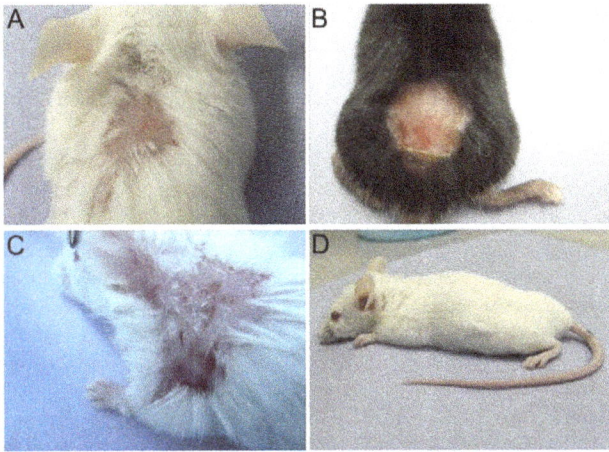

Figure 4. Subcutaneous injection of BP180/CXVII-specific IgG induces blister formation in adult mice. Skin lesions, including blisters, erosions crusts, and alopecia developed in (**A**) BALB/c, (**B**) C57BL6, and (**C**) SJL-1 mice pre-sensitized with rabbit IgG and subsequently receiving, over a period of 10 days, 6 s.c. injections of IgG, each containing 15 mg of IgG, from a rabbit immunized against murine BP180/CXVII. (**D**) A control mouse pre-sensitized with rabbit IgG and challenged with the same dose of normal rabbit IgG showed no skin alterations.

Neutrophil depletion partly inhibits blister formation *in vivo*

Since inflammatory infiltrates in our model were mostly composed of neutrophils, we supposed that these cells mediate tissue damage. Therefore, to deplete neutrophils we have used a Ly-6G-specific monoclonal antibody, which induced a severe reduction of neutrophils from around 30% prior to depletion to less than 6% of leukocytes in the peripheral blood. The depletion was maintained for 4 days with a subsequent increase of

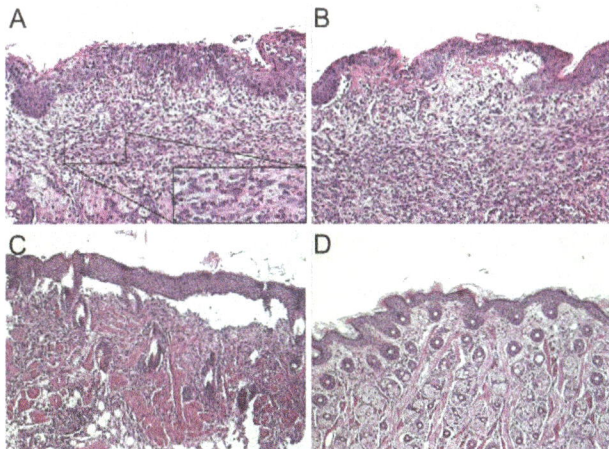

Figure 6. IgG and complement C3 deposition at the basement membrane in experimental bullous pemphigoid. IF microscopy, performed on frozen sections of a perilesional mouse skin biopsy reveals linear deposition of (**A**) rabbit IgG, (**B**) murine C3, and (**C**) murine IgG at the epidermal basement membrane in a diseased mouse. No deposits of (**D**) rabbit IgG, (**E**) murine C3, and (**F**) murine IgG of a control mouse showing no skin lesions (magnification, ×400).

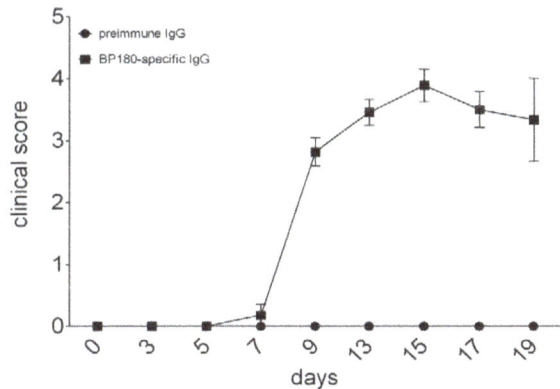

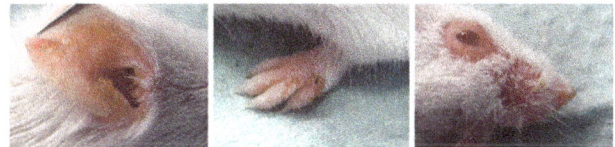

Figure 5. Dermal-epidermal separation in mice injected with BP180/CXVII-specific antibodies. Skin biopsies from mice pre-sensitized with rabbit IgG and subsequently injected with rabbit IgG were stained with hematoxylin and eosin. (**A**) Dense inflammatory infiltrates dominated by granulocytes in a BALB/c mouse receiving BP180/CXVII-specific IgG; (**B**) Subepidermal split and dense inflammatory infiltrates dominated by granulocytes; (**C**) Extensive dermal-epidermal separation; (**D**) Normal histological appearance in a control mouse receiving normal rabbit IgG (magnification, ×400).

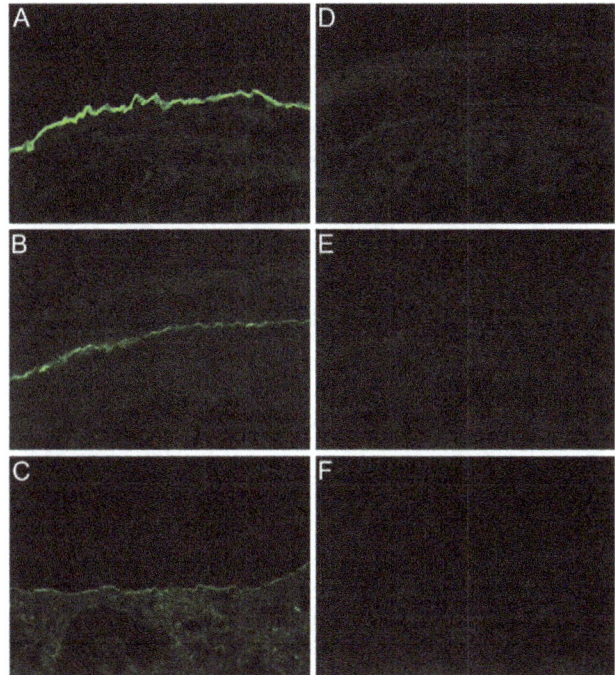

Figure 7. Repeated injections of antibodies against murine BP180/CXVII induce extensive skin blistering. The extent of disease was scored as described in Methods. Means of individual clinical scores of mice injected with BP180/CXVII-specific antibodies (n = 9) and mice injected with normal rabbit IgG (n = 5) are shown before the first injection as well as every subsequent second day for 19 days. The lower panel shows BALB/c mice at day 12 after the first i.p. injection.

neutrophils to normal frequency in the peripheral blood within 1 day. Mice pre-immunized with rabbit IgG and injected with rabbit IgG specific for BP180/CXVII developed skin blisters (**Figure 8A and B**). The transient depletion of neutrophils significantly reduced the skin blistering disease in the group of mice treated with the LyG6-specific compared with group treated with the mock antibody (n = 5/group; **Figure 8C**).

Luteolin inhibits IC-induced ROS production by leukocytes

Luteolin, a plant-derived flavonoid with potent anti-oxidative and anti-inflammatory properties, is a promising, small molecule for the treatment in several inflammatory diseases both by systemic and local application [30]. Therefore, we have addressed the effects of luteolin on the autoantibody-induced granulocyte activation and tissue damage in our model. Human leukocytes were stimulated with ICs consisting of BP180/CXVII-specific antibodies and antigen and treated with different concentrations of luteolin (50–200 µg/ml). Under these conditions, we have observed an inhibition of ROS production in a dose-dependent manner (**Figure 9A**). ROS production may play an important role in the secretion of gelatinase B (MMP-9) from activated neutrophils and is believed to be involved in tissue damage in BP. Therefore, we have asked whether luteolin also inhibits the release of MMP-9 from leukocytes stimulated with ICs. We show that the

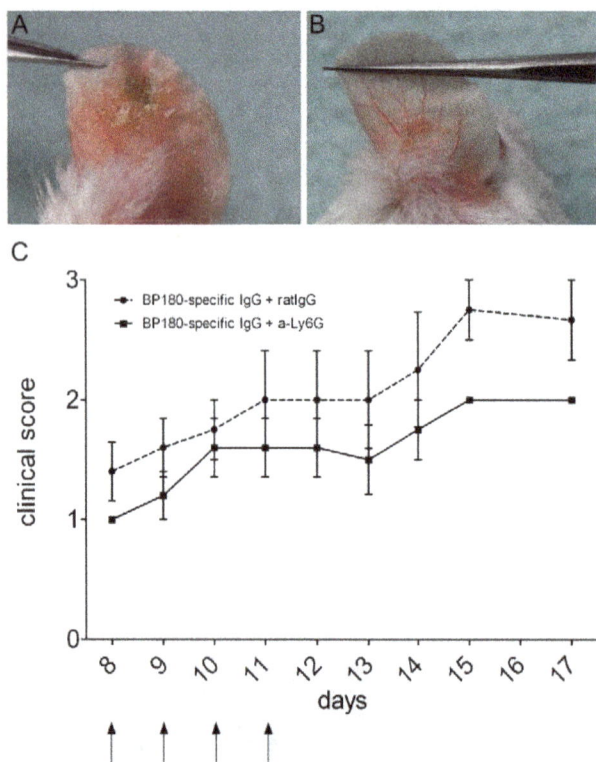

Figure 8. Neutrophil depletion partly inhibits skin blistering induced by BP180/CXVII-specific IgG in mice. Mice pre-immunized with rabbit IgG and injected i.p. with BP180/CXVII-specific rabbit IgG were treated with (**A**) a Ly-6G-specific monoclonal or (**B**) a mock antibody as described in Materials and Methods (arrows). (**C**) Disease activity during the depletion of Ly-6G-positive cells is significantly reduced in the group of mice treated with Ly-6G-specific antibody (n = 5) compared with the group treated with mock antibody (n = 5; p<0.05). Data are shown as mean ± SD.

in vitro stimulation of human leukocytes for 3 h with ICs and different concentrations of luteolin does not inhibit the production and activation of MMP-9 in the supernatant of these cultures as detected and quantified by gelatine zymography (**Figure 9B**).

Luteolin inhibits partly autoantibody-induced granulocyte-dependent dermal-epidermal separation *ex vivo*

We have investigated the effects of luteolin on tissue damage using an *ex vivo* cryosection model of autoantibody-induced granulocyte-dependent dermal-epidermal separation. Cryosections were treated either with sera from BP patients and BP180/CXVII-specific rabbit serum or with control sera from healthy donors and pre-immune rabbits followed by incubation with granulocytes from healthy donors. Addition of luteolin, but not vehicle alone, resulted in a significant reduction of the autoantibody-induced dermal-epidermal separation (**Figure 9C**).

Systemic and local application of luteolin does not significantly impact antibody-induced blistering *in vivo*

Based on the promising *ex vivo* results, we have extended the investigation of the luteolin effects on the autoimmune injury in our mouse model of BP. We pre-sensitized BALB/c mice with rabbit IgG and injected them every second day s.c. with BP180/CXVII-specific IgG or with pre-immune IgG. These mice were treated every day i.p. either with vehicle alone (n = 8) or with 1 mg of luteolin (n = 8). Luteolin administration did not significantly influence the antibody-induced skin blistering. Mice in both groups showed similar disease scores and antibodies to rabbit IgG throughout the experiment (**Figure 10C and Figure S3**). In a subsequent experiment, we have also evaluated the effects of a luteolin-rich topical preparation on the blistering induced in the ears of mice. For this purpose, we have injected s.c. 1.5 mg BP180/CXVII-specific (n = 14) or control IgG (n = 3) into the mouse ears and applied the luteolin-containing RF-40 (n = 10) preparation or vehicle alone (n = 7) every day for 4 days (**Figure 10A and B**). No significant changes were observed in mice topically treated with luteolin compared to those receiving vehicle alone.

Discussion

Pemphigoid diseases are associated with autoantibodies against BP180/CXVII and BP230. Data from experimental pemphigoid models suggest that BP180/CXVII-specific autoantibodies induce subepidermal skin blistering. Current pemphigoid disease models use neonatal mice injected with antibodies to BP180/CXVII. However, in these models, skin blistering does not occur spontaneously and is only induced when mechanical stress is applied to the skin. In addition, the experimental design using the neonatal mouse model of BP allows for observation periods of only up to 3 days. To address these shortcomings, in the present study we generated a pemphigoid disease model in adult mice pre-immunized against rabbit IgG, which developed a spontaneous extensive blistering skin disease upon injection of murine BP180/CXVII-specific rabbit antibodies and allowed for longer observation times.

The passive transfer of pemphigoid patients' autoantibodies into mice does not result in skin blistering. This is likely due to both a limited cross-reactivity of human autoantibodies with the murine autoantigens and to their lower capacity to activate mouse complement and leukocytes [28,31]. Therefore, alternative models using the passive transfer of murine BP180/CXVII-specific antibodies generated in rabbits into neonatal mice or neonatal

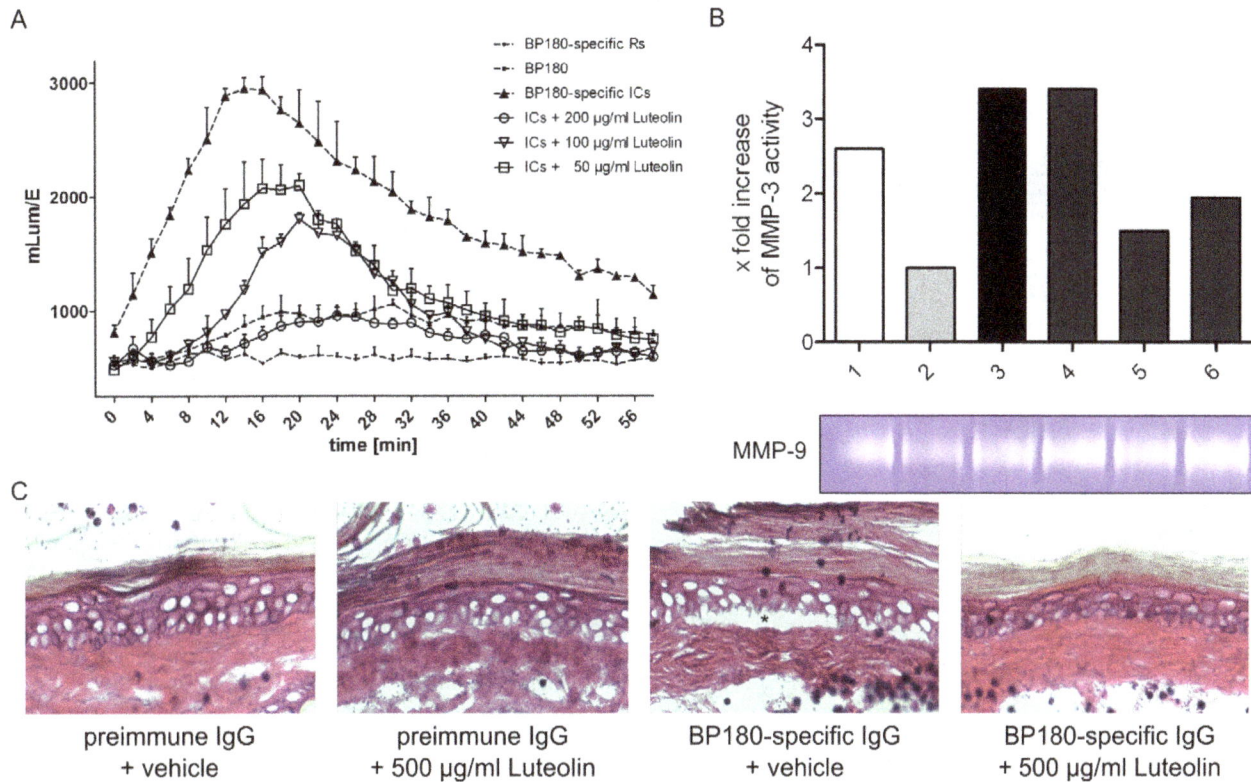

Figure 9. Luteolin inhibits ROS production, but not the release of MMP-9 from IC-stimulated leukocytes. (A) Leukocytes (3×10^7/ml) were pre-incubated with luteolin in different concentrations or vehicle alone and stimulated with rabbit ICs consisting of 5 µg recombinant BP180/CXVII/well and 100 µl of 50-fold diluted rabbit serum. ROS production was measured over a period of 60 min. Data are represented as mean ± SD; $p < 0.05$. (B) 3×10^7/ml leukocytes were stimulated with rabbit ICs consisting of 5 µg recombinant BP180/CXVII/well and 100 µl of 50-fold diluted rabbit serum for 3 h at 37°C. MMP-9 activation was evaluated by zymography in 50-fold diluted supernatants of these cultures of cells stimulated with BP180/CXVII (lane 1), BP180/CXVII-specific rabbit IgG (lane 2), ICs (lane 3), ICs with 1000, 500 and 200 µg/ml Luteolin (lanes 4, 5, and 6 respectively). (C) Luteolin inhibits dermal-epidermal separation in cryosection assays *ex vivo*. Frozen murine skin sections were incubated with pre-immune rabbit serum or BP180/CXVII-specific rabbit serum. Significantly less dermal-epidermal separation was observed in sections treated with 500 µg/ml luteolin compared with those treated with vehicle alone (magnification, ×400).

human CXVII-transgenic mice injected with patient IgG have been devised [18,20,21]. In a separate study, we could show that purified rabbit IgG antibodies generated against murine BP180/CXVII transferred into adult mice results indeed in spontaneous blistering [32]. However, the disease onset was slower and the overall disease activity lower compared with other models for autoimmune subepidermal blistering disease [33] and typical patients with full-blown disease. To further improve the model, in the present study, we have applied an approach initially devised for the autoantibody-induced glomerulonephritis [29,34]. This progressive nephrotoxic serum nephritis in mice is a prototypic type II hypersensitivity response in the kidney induced by antibodies directed against the GBM. Pre-sensitization of mice with rabbit IgG prior to challenge with rabbit nephrotoxic serum results in IC formation leading to accelerated glomerular injury and renal dysfunction that resembles aspects of Goodpasture syndrome in humans [29]. In our pemphigoid model in adult mice, pre-sensitization with rabbit IgG resulted in accelerated onset and enhanced activity of the induced pemphigoid disease most likely due to IC formation of mouse anti-rabbit IgG and the tissue-bound rabbit anti-BP180/CXVII.

Our results show the induction of spontaneous skin blisters by the passive transfer of BP180/CXVII-specific IgG. For the induction of subepidermal skin blistering, we used purified rabbit IgG antibodies with high reactivity against the epidermal

basement membrane. Similar to autoantibodies from BP patients [35] or to rabbit antibodies against collagen VII [33], our rabbit antibodies fixed complement *ex vivo* as assessed by an *in vitro* complement-binding assay, which measures complement activation by the classical pathway [36]. We also observed complement C3 deposits *in vivo* in our model reproducing the immunopathological finding of C3 deposits in BP patients.

The infiltration of leukocytes, dominated by granulocytes, into the upper dermis of the lesional skin is a further major pathological feature of human BP. We have seen constantly inflammatory infiltrates consisting predominantly of granulocytes in the skin of our mice. We could also show that *in situ*-bound and soluble ICs of rabbit IgG and BP180/CXVII activated granulocytes resulting in respiratory burst and dermal-epidermal separation *ex vivo*. However, while in approximately 50% of BP patients' eosinophils represent the major fraction of recruited cells, in our present model neutrophils were the main cell type observed. Thus similar to previous *in vivo* studies [18–21], eosinophil infiltration, an important histopathological feature of human BP, is not fully reproduced in our present model and should be addressed in further studies.

An interesting observation relates to the different clinical phenotypes induced in mice injected with BP180/CXVII-specific IgG depending on the administration route. The i.p. injection of antibodies resulted in generalized skin blistering with predilection

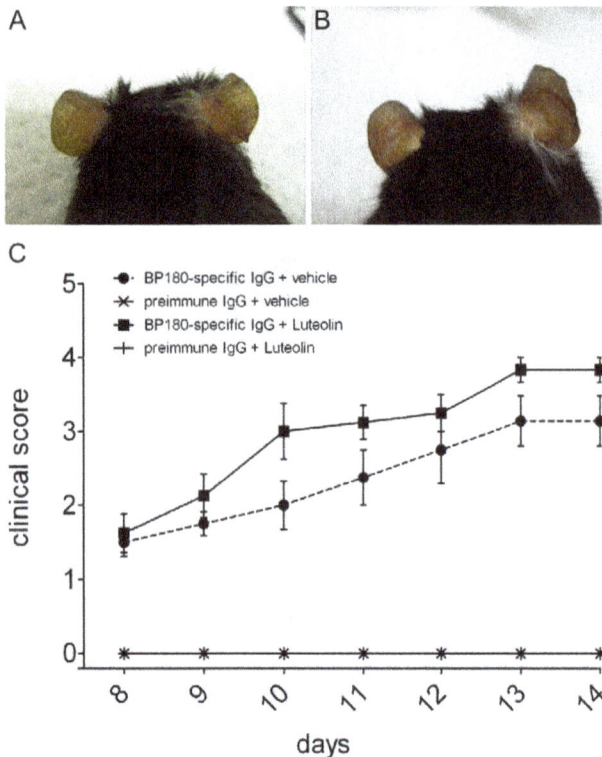

Figure 10. *In vivo* **luteolin treatment does not significantly inhibit blistering in adult mice.** BALB/c mice were pre-immunized with rabbit IgG and injected s.c. with BP180/CXVII-specific IgG. Control mice were pre-sensitized with rabbit IgG and challenged with the same dose of normal rabbit IgG showed no skin alterations. Topical treatment of mice with (**A**) luteolin at concentrations of 5.24 µM/ear did not result in different outcome compared with (**B**) animals treated topically with vehicle alone. (**C**) Treatment of mice with 1 mg luteolin i.p. daily (n = 8) did not significantly influence disease activity when compared to mice treated with vehicle alone (n = 8, p>0.5). Data are shown as mean ± SEM.

on the ears, legs, snout and periocular areas. The s.c. injection of the same IgG preparation triggered extensive skin disease mainly limited to the proximity of the injection area, although a few lesions at distant sites were also observed. The cause of this phenomenon is not known, but is not likely related to a lower systemic availability of pathogenic antibodies, since the levels of circulating BP180/CXVII-specific IgG in the two groups were similar. A further unresolved issue is why lesions develop at predilection sites when the pathogenic IgG is injected intraperitoneally. This site-specificity of the autoimmune attack, which resembles findings in the passive transfer model of epidermolysis bullosa acquisita [33], may be explained by the obvious exposure to increased mechanical trauma and/or by particularities of the vasculature at these sites that were shown to be relevant in antibody-dependent models of rheumatoid arthritis [37].

Results from a neonatal model of BP and our previous data from the *ex vivo* cryosection model of BP showed that granulocyte activation is a prerequisite for autoantibody-induced dermal-epidermal separation [16,38]. In our present study, depletion of neutrophils using a Ly-6G-specific antibody only partly inhibited skin blistering induced by BP180/CXVII-specific IgG. While a straightforward explanation for the relatively modest effect of neutrophil depletion on skin blistering in the adult model of BP is difficult to give at this time, a combination of factors is likely to

have contributed to this outcome. First, the *ex vivo* cryosection model has an obvious limitation due to the fact that the skin sections are dead tissue containing damaged cells precluding more active, keratinocyte-dependent mechanisms to be reproduced in this model. Second, in the neonatal model granulocytes are needed for inducing the "epidermal wrinkling" sign by rubbing the mouse skin. It is however, not known how these cells impact the development of spontaneous blistering reproduced in the new animal model presented here. Importantly, as recently suggested, different mechanisms of autoantibody-induced blister formation may be in place in BP [39,40], which due to the longer observation time in the new BP model may have become apparent in our present study.

Luteolin (3′,4′,5,7-tetrahydroxyflavone), a plant flavonoid with potent anti-inflammatory and anti-oxidative properties and a good safety profile is being investigated as new therapy in inflammatory autoimmune disease and allergy [30]. Therefore, the aim of a further set of experiments was to investigate the therapeutic potential of luteolin in exprimental BP. Initial *ex vivo* experiments demonstrated that luteolin inhibited the FcγR-dependent production of ROS by leukocytes and partly the pemphigoid autoantibody-induced granulocyte-dependent dermal-epidermal separation of skin sections. However, mice treated with luteolin i.p. or by topical application did not show a lower pemphigoid disease activity upon challenge with blister-inducing rabbit IgG. Taken together these results suggest that luteolin is not acting on key pathogenic mechanisms in experimental BP *in vivo* and therefore do not qualify this compound for further exploring its therapeutic potential for the human pemphigoid disease.

In conclusion, this study demonstrates that the passive transfer of BP180/CXVII-specific IgG antibodies induces spontaneous blistering in adult mice and recapitulates the main clinical, histological, and immunopathological features of human pemphigoid disease. A further salient feature of this model is the fact that it allows longer observation times of the diseased mice. Using this model we could show that granulocytes significantly contribute to the autoantibody-triggered tissue damage. Promising *ex vivo* results using the anti-inflammatory flavonoid luteolin were not validated as effective systemic or topical therapy in the experimental pemphigoid model *in vivo*. These studies establish an animal model that will be a useful tool for dissecting the cellular and molecular mechanisms of blister formation in BP. In addition, this experimental system will facilitate the development of more effective therapeutic strategies for managing this chronic autoimmune disorder.

Materials and Methods

Mice

The animal's welfare is checked regularly, and the University Freiburg Medical Center animal facility complies with the national and international laws and regulations. The experiments were approved by the Animal Care and Use Committee (Regierungspräsidium Freiburg, Germany; no. G-10/14 and G-10/84) and performed by certified personnel. 6 to 8-week-old BALB/c, C57BL/6J, C57BL/10 and SJL female mice with a body weight of approximately 20 g were obtained from Charles River, Germany. All injections and bleedings were performed on mice narcotized by inhalation of isoflurane or intraperitoneal administration of a mixture of ketamine (100 µg/g) and xylazine (15 µg/g).

Generation of antibodies against murine BP180/CXVII

Polyclonal antibodies were produced by immunizing rabbits with 200 µg of a mixture containing purified glutathione S-transferase (GST)-mCXVII-EC1, GST-mCXVII-EC3, GST-mCXVII-EC7 and GST-mCXVII-IC2 in a 2:1:1:1 molar ratio in complete Freund's adjuvant. The recombinant fragments designated GST-mCXVII-EC1, GST-mCXVII-EC3, GST-mCXVII-EC7 and GST-mCXVII-IC2 contain murine collagen XVII sequences stretching from amino acid positions 498–580, 856–901, 1030–1134, and 186–475, respectively [31]. These GST-fusion proteins containing sequences of murine BP180/CXVII were cloned and purified as previously described [31,41]. Briefly, recombinant GST fusion and His-tagged proteins were expressed in *E. coli* TOP10 and XL1-Blue and purified by gluthatione agarose and metallochelate affinity chromatography, respectively as described [16,42]. The animals were boosted twice (at 15-day interval) with the same protein preparation in incomplete Freund's adjuvant. Immune sera were obtained at regular intervals and characterized by IF microscopy on cryosections of murine skin.

Affinity purification of rabbit IgG

IgG from rabbit serum or Amicon Ultra-15 filter-concentrated supernatants from hybridoma cells (clone NIMP-R14) was purified using Protein G Sepharose Fast Flow affinity column chromatography (Amersham Biosciences) as described [43]. Briefly, antibodies were eluted with 0.1 M glycine buffer (pH 2.5), neutralized with 1.5 M Tris-HCl (pH 10), and concentrated under extensive washing with PBS (pH 7.2) using Amicon Ultra-15 filters (Millipore). Purified IgG was filter-sterilized (pore size, 0.22 μm; Millipore) and the protein concentration was measured spectrophotometrically at 280 nm. Reactivity of IgG fractions was analyzed by IF microscopy on murine skin.

Passive transfer experiments and clinical scoring of disease activity

Adult mice were pre-immunized on day 0 with 200 μg of rabbit IgG and injected starting with day 3 every second day subcutaneously (s.c.) or intraperitoneally (i.p.) six times with 15 mg of rabbit IgG against murine BP180/CXVII with end-titer on adult mouse skin of 1:16,000–32,000. Control mice received 15 mg of pre-immune IgG purified from rabbits. For neutrophil depletion *in vivo* BALB/c mice were injected i.p. with 0.125 mg of the depleting rat anti-Ly-6G antibody or control rat IgG starting 3 days after injection of BP180/CXVII-specific rabbit IgG on days 5, 7, 8, 9, 10, and 11. Luteolin 98 MM was obtained from International Development and Manufacturing (MMD), dissolved in 1 M NaOH and diluted 1:10 in PBS to produce a stock solution of 10 mg/ml (pH 8.5). For the luteolin treatment *in vivo*, BALB/c mice were injected i.p. with 1 mg of luteolin dissolved in PBS (pH 8.5) or vehicle alone every day. In mice the LD50 values are of >180 mg/kg by i.p. injection [44]. For topical therapy, mice were injected twice s.c. in the ears with 1.5 mg IgG and the luteolin-rich *Reseda luteola l.* extract (RF-40) was topically used at luteolin concentrations of 5.24 μM/site [45]. All skin samples were examined by IF microscopy for IgG and complement C3 deposition and by light microscopy (H&E staining) for signs of dermal-epidermal separation and/or inflammatory infiltrates, as previously described [46,47]. Mice were weighed daily and examined for their general condition and for evidence of cutaneous lesions (i.e., erythema, blisters, erosions, and crusts). Intact blisters or erosions were counted and the extent of skin disease was scored as follows: 0, no lesions; 1, fewer than 20 lesions or less than 10% of the skin surface; 2, more than 20 lesions or 10–20% of the skin surface; 3, 20–40% of the skin surface; 4, 40–60% of the skin surface; and 5, more than 60% of the skin surface.

To evaluate the correlation of antibody titers with the extent of disease, sera were obtained from adult mice at different time points, including before starting the treatment and 2 days after the last injection. Sera were assayed for antibody titers by ELISA. Biopsies of lesional and perilesional skin and esophagus were obtained 2–3 days after the last injection and prepared for examination by histopathology and IF microscopy.

IF microscopy

Indirect and direct IF microscopy using rabbit or mouse sera was performed as described previously [33]. Briefly, indirect IF was carried out on frozen murine skin sections from untreated mice, which were incubated 1 h with 100-fold diluted rabbit serum. Direct IF microscopy was performed using frozen skin sections from treated mice. Bound immunoreactants were visualized using a 100-fold diluted AlexaFluor 488-conjugated antibodies specific for rabbit IgG, mouse C3 and mouse IgG (all Invitrogen). Complement-fixing activity of antibodies to the DEJ was determined as described [43]. Briefly, sections of normal mouse skin were incubated 1 h with 1-fold diluted rabbit sera against BP180/CXVII or control IgG, followed by washing with PBS (pH 7.2), twice for 10 min. Subsequently, sections were treated for 1 h with fresh human serum as a source of complement, diluted 1:5 with Gelatin Veronal Buffer (Sigma). *In situ* complement deposition was visualized using a 100-fold diluted AlexaFluor-488-conjugated antibody specific for human C3 (Invitrogen).

ROS measurement by luminol chemiluminescence

Human leukocytes were isolated from the peripheral blood of healthy donors. For the experiments conducted with human leukocytes, we obtained approval from the Ethics Committee of the Medical Faculty of the University of Freiburg, Germany (Institutional Board Project no. 407/08). We obtained written informed consent from the donors whose material was used in the study, in adherence to the Helsinki Principles. After 3% dextran sedimentation erythrocytes were lysed using a hypotonic solution of 0.2% NaCl. Leukocytes were washed in DMEM medium without supplements and resuspended at a final density of 3×10^7 cells/ml. Cell viability was tested with trypan blue; only preparations with a viability greater than 95% were used. Plate bound murine ICs were formed using the recombinant fragments of murine collagen XVII (GST-mCXVII-EC1, -EC3, -EC7 and IC2) and rabbit sera from rabbits immunized against BP180/CXVII. Briefly, 96-well microtiter plates were coated with 5 μg of equimolar amounts of GST-mCXVII-fragments in 0.1 M bicarbonate buffer (pH 9.6). The wells were washed five times with PBS (pH 7.2) containing 0.05% Tween 20, after each step. After blocking for 1 h with PBS-Tween containing 1% bovine serum albumin (fraction V; Sigma-Aldrich, Germany), wells were incubated for 2 h with a 50-fold diluted rabbit sera against mouse BP180/CXVII. ROS production was measured using luminol-chemiluminescence. Leukocytes were pre-incubated for 5 min at 37°C with 150 μM luminol (Sigma) and, subsequently, 100 μl of cell suspension was added to each well. To study the effects of luteolin, leukocytes were pre-incubated with luteolin to a final concentration of 50, 100, 200 μg/ml or with vehicle alone for 10 min. All procedures were performed in the dark. Unless otherwise specified the chemiluminescence intensity was recorded continuously for 1 h. Kinetic measurement of ROS production in leukocytes stimulated with PMA (500 nM; Sigma) was conducted as control.

MMP-9 activity measurement by gelatine zymography

Human leukocytes were isolated from the peripheral blood of healthy donors and treated as described for ROS production. For the analysis of the effects of luteolin on MMP-9 release and activation by IC-stimulated leukocytes, the cells were pre-incubated with luteolin to a final concentration of 1000, 500 and 200 µg/ml or with vehicle alone in DMEM for 3 h at 37°C. The supernatant was collected, diluted 1:50 in PBS and sample buffer without reducing agents was added. All samples were loaded and separated for 1–2 h on a 8% SDS-PAGE gel containing 1% gelatine under non-reducing conditions. Subsequently, the gel was stained with Coomassie Brillant Blue staining solution for 1 h, followed by destaining the gel for 2 h as described [48].

Flow Cytometry

Blood samples were lysed with ACK lysis buffer, Fc-blocked with anti-mouse CD16/CD32 and then stained for FACS analysis with anti-mouse Ly-6G-FITC and anti-mouse Gr-1-PE or isotype controls as described previously [49,50]. Neutrophils were defined as $Gr-1^+ Ly-6G^+$ cells. All antibodies were from BD Pharmingen. FACS analysis was performed with FACS Canto II (Becton Dickinson).

Cryosection assay

IgG from rabbits or patients was diluted 1:5 in PBS and the protein concentration was measured using absorbance at 280 nm. Six-micrometer cryosections of murine or human skin were washed in PBS to remove embedding medium and incubated with 100 µl of diluted antibody preparations for 2–3 h at 37°C. Sections were washed twice with PBS and chambers were prepared as previously described [41]. Human leukocytes were isolated from the peripheral blood of healthy donors. For the experiments conducted with human leukocytes, we obtained approval from the Ethics Committee of the Medical Faculty of the University of Freiburg, Germany (Institutional Board Project no. 407/08). We obtained written informed consent from the donors whose material was used in the study, in adherence to the Helsinki Principles. After 3% dextran sedimentation erythrocytes were lysed using a hypotonic solution of 0.2% NaCl. Leukocytes were washed in DMEM medium without supplements and resuspended at a final density of 3×10^7 cells/ml. Cell viability was tested with trypan blue; only preparations with a viability greater than 95% were used. In some experiments, leukocytes were pre-incubated with luteolin to a final concentration of 1000, 500 or 200 µg/ml or with vehicle alone for 10 min. Leukocyte suspensions were injected into the chambers and incubated for 3 h at 37°C. Chambers were then disassembled and sections washed in PBS, air dried, and stained with hematoxylin and eosin.

Histology

Biopsies of lesional and perilesional skin and esophagus were fixed in 3.7% buffered formalin. Sections from paraffin-embedded tissues were stained with H&E.

Immunoblot analysis

For immunoblotting, subconfluent COS-7 cells transformed with murine full length BP180/CXVII cDNA or NIMP-R14 hybridoma cells were lysed for 30 min on ice in a buffer containing 1% Triton X-100, 0.137 M NaCl, 20 mM Tris/HCl pH 8.0 (pH 8.0), 2 mM EDTA, and 1 mM Na_3VO_4, 10% glycerol and 1 mM PMSF [33]. The samples were separated by SDS-PAGE on 6% polyacrylamide gels, followed by transfer onto nitrocellulose membrane. 200-fold diluted polyclonal rabbit antibodies directed against murine BP180/CXVII as described above were used.

After incubation with a chicken anti-rabbit IgG HRP-conjugated secondary antibody (Novus biologicals), signals were visualized by 3,3′-diaminobenzidine (Merck) [41].

ELISA

ELISA was used to measure circulating mouse IgG against rabbit IgG following established protocols with minor modification [51]. Briefly, 500 ng purified normal rabbit IgG were immobilized on 96-well microtiter plates using 0.1 M bicarbonate buffer (pH 9.6). After each step, the wells were washed four times with PBS (pH 7.2) containing 0.05% Tween 20, unless otherwise specified. After blocking for 1–2 h with PBS-Tween containing 1% bovine serum albumin (fraction V; Sigma-Aldrich), wells were incubated for 2 h with a 250-fold dilution of mouse sera. Bound antibodies were detected using a 3,000-fold dilution of an HRP-labeled goat anti-mouse IgG antibodies (BioRad) and orthophenylene diamine (Dako) as a chromophore (490 nm).

ELISA was used to measure circulating rabbit IgG against BP180/CXVII following established protocols with minor modification [51]. Briefly, 300 ng of the purified His-tagged murine BP180/CXVII (EC1 fragment) was immobilized on 96-well microtiter plates using 0.1 M bicarbonate buffer (pH 9.6). After each step, the wells were washed four times with PBS (pH 7.2) containing 0.05% Tween 20, unless otherwise specified. After blocking for 2 h with PBS-Tween containing 1% bovine serum albumin (Sigma-Aldrich), wells were incubated for 2 h with a 100-fold dilution of mouse sera. Bound antibodies were detected using a 3,000-fold dilution of a chicken anti-rabbit IgG HRP (NOVUS biologicals) and orthophenylene diamine (Dako) as a chromophore (492 nm).

Statistical analysis

All analyzes were performed using GraphPad Prism Version 5.03. Continuous variables were compared using the Man-Whitney U or Students' t test. P<0.05 was considered statistically significant.

Supporting Information

Figure S1 Reactivity and specificity of IgG antibodies from rabbits immunized with murine BP180/CXVII. Frozen skin sections were incubated with 100-fold diluted serum from a rabbit (**A**) immunized against BP180/CXVII or (**B**) pre-immune rabbit serum. (**C**) Extracts of the NIMP-R14 hybridoma cell line (*lanes 1 and 3*) and of BP180/CXVII-expressing COS-7 cells (*lanes 2 and 4*) were separated by 6% SDS-PAGE and immunoblottted with 200-fold diluted pre-immune rabbit serum (*lanes 1 and 2*) or serum from a rabbit immunized against BP180/CXVII (*lanes 3 and 4*).

Figure S2 (A) Serum levels of mouse IgG antibodies against rabbit IgG. Levels of murine IgG in serum samples of pre-immunized mice, which were subsequently injected with BP180/CXVII-specific (n = 5) or control (n = 3) rabbit IgG were measured by an ELISA using rabbit IgG as antigen as described in Materials and Methods. Data are shown as mean ± SD. (**B**) **Serum levels of rabbit IgG against BP180/CXVII in mice.** Levels of rabbit IgG autoantibodies in serum samples of mice injected with BP180/CXVII-specific (n = 9) or control (n = 5) rabbit IgG were measured by an ELISA using recombinant BP180/CXVII, as described in Materials and Methods. Data are shown as mean ± SD.

Figure S3 Luteolin therapy does not influence levels of the injected pathogenic BP180/CXVII-specific IgG and of rabbit IgG-specific mouse IgG antibodies. (A) Serum levels of mouse IgG antibodies against rabbit IgG. Levels of murine IgG in serum samples of pre-immunized mice, which were subsequently injected with BP180/CXVII-specific (n = 16) or control (n = 11) rabbit IgG and treated with luteolin (n = 14) or vehicle (n = 13) were measured by an ELISA using rabbit IgG as antigen as described in Materials and Methods. Data are shown as mean ± SD. **(B) Serum levels of rabbit IgG against BP180/CXVII in mice.** Levels of rabbit IgG autoantibodies in serum samples of mice injected with BP180/CXVII-specific (n = 16) or control (n = 11) rabbit IgG and subsequently treated with luteolin (n = 14) or vehicle (n = 13) were measured by an ELISA using recombinant BP180/CXVII, as described in Materials and Methods. Data are shown as mean ± SD.

Acknowledgments

We thank Jessika Batt, Freiburg, Germany, for excellent technical assistance.

Author Contributions

Conceived and designed the experiments: EO CS. Performed the experiments: AS C-WF EO. Analyzed the data: LB-T SM TJ UW AS EO. Contributed reagents/materials/analysis tools: C-WF LB-T UW AS SM. Wrote the paper: EO CS LB-T SM TJ. Read and approved the final manuscript: CS EO AS C-WF LB-T TJ SM UW.

References

1. Mihai S, Sitaru C (2007) Immunopathology and molecular diagnosis of autoimmune bullous diseases. J Cell Mol Med 11: 462–81.
2. Sitaru C (2009) Bullous pemphigoid: a prototypical antibody-mediated organ-specific autoimmune disease. J Invest Dermatol 129: 822–4.
3. Stanley JR, Hawley-Nelson P, Yuspa SH, Shevach EM, Katz SI (1981) Characterization of bullous pemphigoid antigen: a unique basement membrane protein of stratified squamous epithelia. Cell 24: 897–903.
4. Stanley JR, Tanaka T, Mueller S, Klaus-Kovtun V, Roop D (1988) Isolation of complementary DNA for bullous pemphigoid antigen by use of patients' autoantibodies. J Clin Invest 82: 1864–70.
5. Diaz LA, Ratrie H, Saunders WS, Futamura S, Squiquera HL, et al. (1990) Isolation of a human epidermal cDNA corresponding to the 180-kD autoantigen recognized by bullous pemphigoid and herpes gestationis sera. J Clin Invest 86: 1088–94.
6. Giudice GJ, Emery DJ, Diaz LA (1992) Cloning and primary structural analysis of the bullous pemphigoid autoantigen BP180. J Invest Dermatol 99: 243–50.
7. Giudice GJ, Emery DJ, Zelickson BD, Anhalt GJ, Liu Z, et al. (1993) Bullous pemphigoid and herpes gestationis autoantibodies recognize a common non-collagenous site on the BP180 ectodomain. J Immunol 151: 5742–50.
8. Büdinger L, Borradori L, Yee C, Eming R, Ferencik S, et al. (1998) Identification and characterization of autoreactive T cell responses to bullous pemphigoid antigen 2 in patients and healthy controls. J Clin Invest 102: 2082–9.
9. Lin MS, Gharia MA, Swartz SJ, Diaz LA, Giudice GJ (1999) Identification and characterization of epitopes recognized by T lymphocytes and autoantibodies from patients with herpes gestationis. J Immunol 162: 4991–7.
10. Egan CA, Taylor TB, Meyer LJ, Petersen MJ, Zone JJ (1999) Bullous pemphigoid sera that contain antibodies to BPAg2 also contain antibodies to LABD97 that recognize epitopes distal to the NC16A domain. J Invest Dermatol 112: 148–52.
11. Perriard J, Jaunin F, Favre B, Büdinger L, Hertl M, et al. (1999) IgG autoantibodies from bullous pemphigoid (BP) patients bind antigenic sites on both the extracellular and the intracellular domains of the BP antigen 180. J Invest Dermatol 112: 141–7.
12. Haase C, Büdinger L, Borradori L, Yee C, Merk HF, et al. (1998) Detection of IgG autoantibodies in the sera of patients with bullous and gestational pemphigoid: ELISA studies utilizing a baculovirus-encoded form of bullous pemphigoid antigen 2. J Invest Dermatol 110: 282–6.
13. Schmidt E, Obe K, Bröcker EB, Zillikens D (2000) Serum levels of autoantibodies to BP180 correlate with disease activity in patients with bullous pemphigoid. Arch Dermatol 136: 174–8.
14. Iwata Y, Komura K, Kodera M, Usuda T, Yokoyama Y, et al. (2008) Correlation of IgE autoantibody to BP180 with a severe form of bullous pemphigoid. Arch Dermatol 144: 41–8.
15. Di Zenzo G, Thoma-Uszynski S, Fontao L, Calabresi V, Hofmann SC, et al. (2008) Multicenter prospective study of the humoral autoimmune response in bullous pemphigoid. Clin Immunol 128: 415–26.
16. Sitaru C, Schmidt E, Petermann S, Munteanu LS, Bröcker E, et al. (2002) Autoantibodies to bullous pemphigoid antigen 180 induce dermal-epidermal separation in cryosections of human skin. J Invest Dermatol 118: 664–71.
17. Herrero-Gonzalez JE, Brauns O, Egner R, Rönspeck W, Mascaro JM, et al. (2006) Immunoadsorption against two distinct epitopes on human type XVII collagen abolishes dermal-epidermal separation induced in vitro by autoantibodies from pemphigoid gestationis patients. Eur J Immunol 36: 1039–48.
18. Liu Z, Diaz LA, Troy JL, Taylor AF, Emery DJ, et al. (1993) A passive transfer model of the organ-specific autoimmune disease, bullous pemphigoid, using antibodies generated against the hemidesmosomal antigen, BP180. J Clin Invest 92: 2480–8.
19. Yamamoto K, Inoue N, Masuda R, Fujimori A, Saito T, et al. (2002) Cloning of hamster type XVII collagen cDNA, and pathogenesis of anti-type XVII collagen antibody and complement in hamster bullous pemphigoid. J Invest Dermatol 118: 485–92.
20. Nishie W, Sawamura D, Goto M, Ito K, Shibaki A, et al. (2007) Humanization of autoantigen. Nat Med 13: 378–83.
21. Liu Z, Sui W, Zhao M, Li Z, Li N, et al. (2009) Subepidermal blistering induced by human autoantibodies to BP180 requires innate immune players in a humanized bullous pemphigoid mouse model. J Autoimmun 31: 331–8.
22. Nishie W, Sawamura D, Natsuga K, Shinkuma S, Goto M, et al. (2009) A novel humanized neonatal autoimmune blistering skin disease model induced by maternally transferred antibodies. J Immunol 183: 4088–93.
23. Ujiie H, Shibaki A, Nishie W, Sawamura D, Wang G, et al. (2010) A novel active mouse model for bullous pemphigoid targeting humanized pathogenic antigen. J Immunol 184: 2166–74.
24. Hall RP3, Murray JC, McCord MM, Rico MJ, Streilein RD (1993) Rabbits immunized with a peptide encoded for by the 230-kD bullous pemphigoid antigen cDNA develop an enhanced inflammatory response to UVB irradiation: a potential animal model for bullous pemphigoid. J Invest Dermatol 101: 9–14.
25. Kiss M, Husz S, Jánossy T, Marczinovits I, Molnár J, et al. (2005) Experimental bullous pemphigoid generated in mice with an antigenic epitope of the human hemidesmosomal protein BP230. J Autoimmun 24: 1–10.
26. Feliciani C, Caldarola G, Kneisel A, Podstawa E, Pfütze M, et al. (2009) IgG autoantibody reactivity against bullous pemphigoid (BP) 180 and BP230 in elderly patients with pruritic dermatoses. Br J Dermatol 161: 306–12.
27. Naito K, Morioka S, Ikeda S, Ogawa H (1984) Experimental bullous pemphigoid in guinea pigs: the role of pemphigoid antibodies, complement, and migrating cells. J Invest Dermatol 82: 227–30.
28. Anhalt GJ, Diaz LA (1987) Animal models for bullous pemphigoid. Clin Dermatol 5: 117–25.
29. Neale TJ, Wilson CB (1982) Glomerular antigens in glomerulonephritis. Springer Semin Immunopathol 5: 221–49.
30. Seelinger G, Merfort I, Schempp CM (2008) Anti-oxidant, anti-inflammatory and anti-allergic activities of luteolin. Planta Med 74: 1667–1677.
31. Sesarman A, Oswald E, Chiriac MT, Csorba K, Vuta V, et al. (2012) Interaction of human IgG autoantibodies with murine innate immunity factors: implications for disease models using the passive transfer of IgG in mice. submitted.
32. Chiriac MT, Licarete E, Rados AM, Sas AG, Lupan I, et al. (2012) A novel model of adult bullous pemphigoid in wild-type mice. submitted.
33. Sitaru C, Mihai S, Otto C, Chiriac MT, Hausser I, et al. (2005) Induction of dermal-epidermal separation in mice by passive transfer of antibodies specific to type VII collagen. J Clin Invest 115: 870–8.
34. Nagai H, Takizawa T, Nishiyori T, Koda A (1982) Experimental glomerulonephritis in mice as a model for immunopharmacological studies. Jpn J Pharmacol 32: 1117–24.
35. Mihai S, Chiriac M, Herrero-Gonzales J, Goodall M, Jefferis R, et al. (2007) IgG4 autoantibodies induce dermal-epidermal separation. J Cell Mol Med 11: 1117–28.
36. Katz SI, Hertz KC, Yaoita H (1976) Herpes gestationis. Immunopathology and characterization of the HG factor. J Clin Invest 57: 1434–41.
37. Binstadt BA, Patel PR, Alencar H, Nigrovic PA, Lee DM, et al. (2006) Particularities of the vasculature can promote the organ specificity of autoimmune attack. Nat Immunol 7: 284–92.
38. Liu Z, Giudice GJ, Zhou X, Swartz SJ, Troy JL, Fairley JA, Till GO, Diaz LA (1997) A major role for neutrophils in experimental bullous pemphigoid. J Clin Invest 100: 1256–1263.
39. Iwata Y, Komura K, Kodera M, Usuda T, Yokoyama Y, Hara T, Muroi E, Ogawa F, Takenaka M, Sato S (2008) Correlation of ige autoantibody to bp180 with a severe form of bullous pemphigoid. Arch Dermatol 144: 41–48.
40. Sitaru C (2009) Bullous pemphigoid: a prototypical antibody-mediated organ-specific autoimmune disease. J Invest Dermatol 129: 822–824.
41. Csorba K, Sesarman A, Oswald E, Feldrihan V, Fritsch A, et al. (2010) Cross-reactivity of autoantibodies from patients with epidermolysis bullosa acquisita with murine collagen VII. Cell Mol Life Sci 67: 1343–51.

42. Sesarman A, Sitaru AG, Olaru F, Zillikens D, Sitaru C (2008) Neonatal Fc receptor deficiency protects from tissue injury in experimental epidermolysis bullosa acquisita. J Mol Med 86: 951–9.

43. Sesarman A, Mihai S, Chiriac MT, Olaru F, Sitaru AG, et al. (2008) Binding of avian IgY to type VII collagen does not activate complement and leucocytes and fails to induce subepidermal blistering in mice. Br J Dermatol 158: 463–71.

44. Chen C, Peng W, Tsai K, Hsu S (2007) Luteolin suppresses inflammation-associated gene expression by blocking NF-kappaB and AP-1 activation pathway in mouse alveolar macrophages. Life Sci 81: 1602–14.

45. Woelfle U, Simon-Haarhaus B, Merfort I, Schempp CM (2010) Reseda luteola l. extract displays antiproliferative and pro-apoptotic activities that are related to its major flavonoids. Phytother Res 24: 1033–1036.

46. Sitaru C, Kromminga A, Hashimoto T, Bröcker EB, Zillikens D (2002) Autoantibodies to type VII collagen mediate Fcgamma-dependent neutrophil activation and induce dermal-epidermal separation in cryosections of human skin. Am J Pathol 161: 301–11.

47. Shimanovich I, Mihai S, Oostingh GJ, Ilenchuk TT, Bröcker E, et al. (2004) Granulocyte-derived elastase and gelatinase B are required for dermal-epidermal separation induced by autoantibodies from patients with epidermolysis bullosa acquisita and bullous pemphigoid. J Pathol 204: 519–27.

48. Liu Z, Zhou X, Shapiro SD, Shipley JM, Twining SS, et al. (2000) The serpin alpha1-proteinase inhibitor is a critical substrate for gelatinase B/MMP-9 in vivo. Cell 102: 647–55.

49. Shimanovich I, Mihai S, Oostingh GJ, Ilenchuk TT, Bröcker E, et al. (2004) Granulocyte-derived elastase and gelatinase b are required for dermal-epidermal separation induced by autoantibodies from patients with epidermolysis bullosa acquisita and bullous pemphigoid. J Pathol 204: 519–527.

50. Sitaru AG, Sesarman A, Mihai S, Chiriac MT, Zillikens D, et al. (2010) T cells are required for the production of blister-inducing autoantibodies in experimental epidermolysis bullosa acquisita. J Immunol 184: 1596–1603.

51. Sitaru C, Chiriac MT, Mihai S, Büning J, Gebert A, et al. (2006) Induction of complement-fixing autoantibodies against type VII collagen results in subepidermal blistering in mice. J Immunol 177: 3461–8.

Activation of PPARβ/δ Causes a Psoriasis-Like Skin Disease In Vivo

Malgorzata Romanowska[1,9]**, Louise Reilly**[1,9]**, Colin N. A. Palmer**[2]**, Mattias C. U. Gustafsson**[3]**, John Foerster**[1]*****

1 Division of Experimental Medicine, University of Dundee, Dundee, United Kingdom, **2** Biomedical Research Institute, University of Dundee, Dundee, United Kingdom, **3** Department of Laboratory Medicine, Division of Medical Microbiology, Lund University, Lund, Sweden

Abstract

Background: Psoriasis is one of the most frequent skin diseases world-wide. The disease impacts enormously on affected patients and poses a huge financial burden on health care providers. Several lines of evidence suggest that the nuclear hormone receptor peroxisome proliferator activator (PPAR) β/δ, known to regulate epithelial differentiation and wound healing, contributes to psoriasis pathogenesis. It is unclear, however, whether activation of PPARβ/δ is sufficient to trigger psoriasis-like changes in vivo.

Methodology/Principal Findings: Using immunohistochemistry, we define the distribution of PPARβ/δ in the skin lesions of psoriasis. By expression profiling, we confirm that PPARβ/δ is overexpressed in the vast majority of psoriasis patients. We further establish a transgenic model allowing inducible activation of PPARβ/δ in murine epidermis mimicking its distribution in psoriasis lesions. Upon activation of PPARβ/δ, transgenic mice sustain an inflammatory skin disease strikingly similar to psoriasis, featuring hyperproliferation of keratinocytes, dendritic cell accumulation, and endothelial activation. Development of this phenotype requires the activation of the Th17 subset of T cells, shown previously to be central to psoriasis. Moreover, gene dysregulation in the transgenic mice is highly similar to that in psoriasis. Key transcriptional programs activated in psoriasis, including IL1-related signalling and cholesterol biosynthesis, are replicated in the mouse model, suggesting that PPARβ/δ regulates these transcriptional changes in psoriasis. Finally, we identify phosphorylation of STAT3 as a novel pathway activated by PPARβ/δ and show that inhibition of STAT3 phosphorylation blocks disease development.

Conclusions: Activation of PPARβ/δ in the epidermis is sufficient to trigger inflammatory changes, immune activation, and signalling, and gene dysregulation characteristic of psoriasis.

Editor: Jacques Zimmer, Centre de Recherche Public de la Santé (CRP-Santé), Luxembourg

Funding: The work presented here was in part funded by Cancer Research United Kingdom (role: fellowship for JF), the Anonymous Trust (role: provision of funds for consumables), and Tenovus Scotland (role: provision of funds for consumables). The funders had no role in study design, data collection and analysis, decision to publish, or preparation of the manuscript.

Competing Interests: The authors have declared that no competing interests exist.

* E-mail: j.foerster@dundee.ac.uk

9 These authors contributed equally to this work.

Introduction

Psoriasis is one of the most frequent skin diseases world-wide, affecting appr. 2% in Caucasian, and 1% in African populations [1]. The disease represents a life-long affliction of affected patients. About 60% of psoriasis patients suffer from moderate to severe disease, i.e. more than 10% of the body surface area is covered by psoriatic plaques [2]. These patients are largely excluded from participation in activities involving public skin exposure due to stigmatization. Moreover, they exhibit increased rates of depression and alcohol consumption causing secondarily increased mortality [3,4]. Besides high direct treatment-related costs, absence from work-related indirect cost is enormous [5] and lack of employment is attributed to the disease in one-third of psoriasis patients [6]. Thus, psoriasis does not kill, but it impacts enormously on those affected and poses a huge financial burden on health care providers worldwide.

Among psoriasis patients, the prevalence of metabolic syndrome is increased [7] and an increased body mass index is a strong risk factor for psoriasis [8]. Although the molecular mechanisms underlying this association are unknown, it likely involves the existence of overlapping signalling pathways in psoriasis and other disorders of metabolism and chronic inflammation. The nuclear hormone receptor peroxisome proliferator activator (PPAR) β/δ has well established roles both in metabolism and in the skin. On the one hand, PPARβ/δ is a key regulator of adipogenesis and glucose metabolism [9]. On the other hand, it regulates keratinocyte differentiation [10]. The PPAR subfamily of nuclear hormone receptors also includes PPARα (target of fibrate class lipid lowering drugs) and PPARγ (target of the rosiglitazone-family of anti-diabetes drugs), all of which form heterodimers with the RXRα subunit of retinoid receptors and require binding of ligands in order to bind cognate promoters and transactivate distinct set of target genes. All three isoforms have been extensively reviewed elsewhere (e.g. [11]). Table S9 lists selected information on ligands. Several lines of evidence support a role for PPARβ/δ in psoriasis. It is upregulated in psoriatic skin [12,13], induced by TNFα [14,15], stimulates proliferation and blocks apoptosis in keratinocytes [16], and induces angiogenesis [17], all of which is consistent with a disease-promoting role in psoriasis. Thus, induction of PPARβ/δ in the context of metabolic dysregulation might underlie the observed clinical association of psoriasis with metabolic disease.

PPARβ/δ represents an isoform of the peroxisome – proliferator activator receptor subfamily of nuclear hormone receptors.

The inflammatory patches of psoriasis exhibit a number of characteristic properties which are important clues to the underlying pathogenesis. Macroscopically, they are inducible by wounding or other mechanical skin trauma, indicating that challenges to the skin barrier trigger specific response pathways. Histologically, they are marked by increased keratinocyte proliferation, as well as a block in terminal differentiation. Accordingly, markers of late differentiation, including fillagrin, are decreased [18]. Besides keratinocyte biology, psoriasis is marked by complex pattern of immune system activation, including expansion of CD11c[+] dendritic cells [19], upregulation of interferon signalling, and influx of T cells. Specifically, the Th17 subset of T cells has recently emerged as central for the disease [20]. In addition, endothelial cells are activated, bactericidal proteins accumulate, and a variety of soluble mediators are overexpressed (reviewed in [21]). Finally, the IL12/23p40 gene, the IL23 receptor, the β-defensin locus, as well as the HLA-C region harbour genetically predisposing variants [22], suggesting that quantitative differences in immune response pathways affect disease penetrance.

The combination of proliferative changes and a distinctive immune response pattern in psoriasis has long been recognized for its similarity to the wound response. Thus, like wound response pathways, the development of inflammatory psoriasis plaques are triggered by mechanical skin trauma, as well as infection. Therefore, in many respects psoriasis represents a proliferative wound response failing to terminate, suggesting the existence of molecular feed-forward circuits fuelling a vicious circle. In this regard, too, the upregulation of PPARβ/δ is notable since it is an important regulator of the wound response [10].

We report here that PPARβ/δ activation is sufficient to trigger a skin disease replicating many elements of psoriasis. Our findings identify PPARβ/δ as a molecular link between metabolism, keratinocyte differentiation, and the epidermal immune response.

Results

Overexpression of PPARβ/δ in psoriasis

We and others have previously shown that PPARβ/δ is overexpressed in psoriasis. In order to independently confirm those results, we re-analyzed two publicly available large gene expression datasets, totalling 58 paired lesional and non-lesional skin samples, for the expression of all PPAR isotypes. As shown in figure 1a, both data sets confirm highly significant upregulation of PPARβ/δ in psoriatic skin whereas both PPARα and PPARγ are downregulated, consistent with the notion that PPARβ/δ acts antagonistically to PPARγ in psoriasis, as previously proposed [12]. Furthermore, we localized the site of maximal PPARβ/δ accumulation in the skin by immunohistochemistry. As shown in figure 1b, PPARβ/δ is found in the cytosol of the lower epidermis both in normal skin and psoriasis. By contrast, strong nuclear

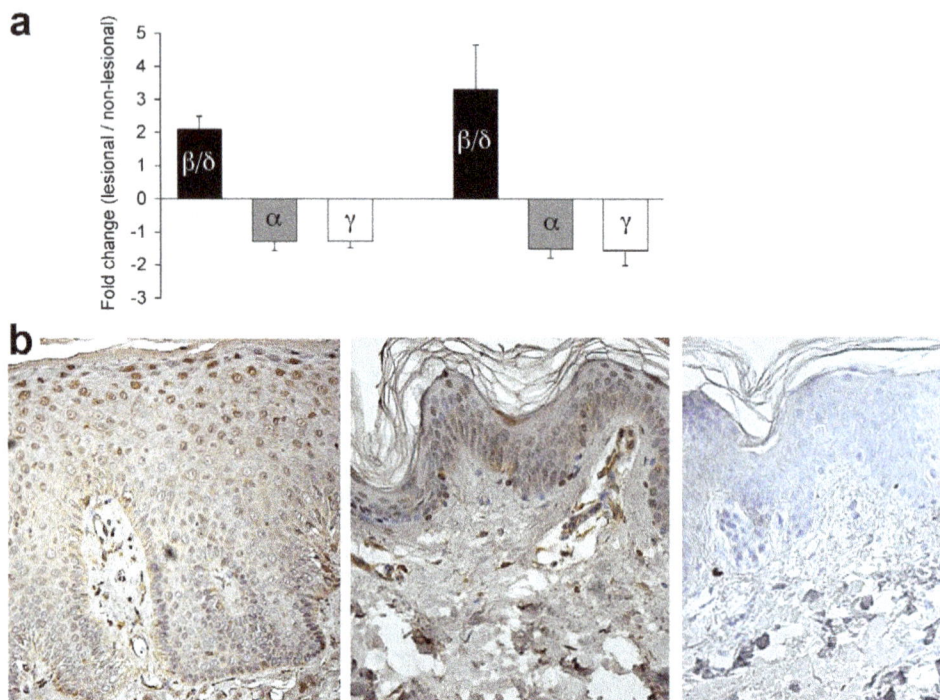

Figure 1. Overexpression of PPARβ/δ in psoriasis. A. Fold-change of mRNA expression of PPARβ/δ (black columns), PPARα (shaded), and PPARγ (white) between lesional and non-lesional skin. Data shown represent mean ± s.d. from the GAIN dataset (left, n = 30) and the GSE14905 dataset (right, n = 28). p<10[−3] for all data points shown. For each PPAR isoform, the probe yielding the highest hybridization signal was used to calculate the data shown (probesets 37152_at, 226978_at, 208510_at, respectively). **B.** Nuclear accumulation of PPARβ/δ in suprabasal epidermis in psoriasis skin lesions. Representative immunohistochemistry of paraffin-embedded lesional (left) and control (middle) skin samples stained with anti-PPARβ/δ, as well as staining control (right). Magnification 200×.

expression in the upper spinous layer was only seen in psoriasis. This pattern was highly reproducible (found in all eight lesional skin samples examined, figure S1a). These data confirm that upregulation of PPARβ/δ is a consistent feature of psoriasis and define the suprabasal epidermis as major site of its activation.

Targeting PPARβ/δ expression to suprabasal skin in mice in vivo

In mice, PPARβ/δ is not expressed in inter-follicular epidermis beyond the postnatal period [23]. To model the suprabasal expression of PPARβ/δ observed in psoriasis in humans, we initially intended to target transgenic PPARβ/δ expression using a "conventional" promoter active in suprabasal epidermis, e.g. the involucrin promoter. However, a transgenic line expressing PPARβ/δ under the control of the rat CYP1A1 promoter was already available, and turned out to afford skin-specific PPARβ/δ activation, as follows. The CYP1A1 promoter allows expression induced by the aryl hydrocarbon receptor (AhR) [24]. This promoter activity is mediated by a well-documented so-called "DXE/XRE" sequence cluster conferring responsivity to AhR [25]. In order to bind to the DXE/XRE cluster, the AhR must first be ligand-activated, which can be achieved by employing specific synthetic chemicals such as indole-3-carbinole (I3C). However, even in the absence of AhR activation and binding to the CYP1A1 promoter, a EGFP reporter gene placed under the control of the CYP1A1 promoter was found to be constitutively and strongly active in skin-associated sebaceous glands [26]. We were able to identify a G/C rich enhancer element most likely responsible for this sebaceous-specific expression, since this element had previously been shown to direct strong sebacous-gland specific expression in the keratin 5 promoter [27]. Indeed, a screen of the GEO database showed this G/C element to be highly conserved in the promoters of multiple genes belonging to the top 10% of all genes expressed in sebaceous glands (fig. 2a, bottom). Not surprisingly then, the CYP1A1 promoter also conferred high constitutive sebaceous-specific expression of PPARβ/δ in the absence of AhR activation (figure 2b). Human, rather than murine PPARβ/δ, was chosen as transgene to facilitate subsequent drug screening applications. We next observed that, unexpectedly, administration of the highly selective PPARβ/δ-agonist GW501516 to the chow of PPARβ/δ-transgenic mice induced subsequent additional expression of the PPARβ/δ-transgene in the epidermis (fig. 2c). Thus, functional activation of PPARβ/δ expressed at high level in the sebaceous glands causes secondary transgene expression in the epidermis. (RT-PCR analysis of PPARβ/δ -transgene expression revealed a borderline-detectable expression in whole-skin samples, consistent with the sebaceous glands forming a small minority of all skin associated cells, Figure S8). It is known that ligand-mediated activation of PPARβ/δ in the sebaceous gland triggers sebocyte differentiation [28,29] and delivery of sebum to the skin [30], containing lipoxygenase-derived bioactive lipids that can bind and activate the AhR, such as LXA4 or 5,6-DiHETE [31,32]. Once ligand-bound, the AhR is then able to transactivate the expression of the CYP1A1-controlled PPARβ/δ transgene in the epidermis via the AhR-responsive DXE/XRE element (shown in fig. 2d). In confirmation of this proposed mechanism, the transcriptional induction of the CYP1A1-controlled PPARβ/δ transgene in the epidermis could be replicated by direct topical cream application of the AhR ligand indole-3-carbinole (I3C) to the skin (I3C, fig. 2e). Furthermore, expression of transgenic PPARβ/δ was epidermis-specific and was not detectable in dermal fibroblasts, endothelia, skin – associated T cells, or any other organ screened, including intestine, muscle, liver, spleen (Fig. S1b), confirming that activation of AhR only occurred in the skin. Taken together, use of the rat

Cyp1A1-driven expression of PPARβ/δ and ligand-mediated activation by the specific PPARβ/δ agonist GW501516 promoter affords a tightly controlled epidermis-specific inducible expression of PPARβ/δ. Although we have not identified the endogenous AhR ligand(s) mediating secondary induction of the transgene in the epidermis, the net effect is a distribution and expression level of PPARβ/δ rather similar to that observed in human psoriasis (fig. 2f).

Psoriasis-like skin disease in PPARβ/δ transgenic mice

As early as seven days after initiation of PPARβ/δ - activation by GW501516 (GW), scaling, inflammation, and skin thickening was notable in all mice (figure 3a–c). Skin roughening ("hyper-keratosis") and concomitant hair loss was maximal in regions subjected to mechanical friction, such as abdomen (fig. 3b, S2), the paws (fig. 3a), or the chin (fig. S2). While psoriasis-like plaques also developed on the back in some mice (fig. 3c), changes on the dorsal skin were mostly limited to scaling (fig. S2). Thus, the overall distribution of skin changes suggest that mechanical friction contributes a trigger effect similar to that characteristic of psoriasis. Histology showed epidermal thickening (fig. 3e), dilation of dermal vessels (black arrowhead), and abundant lymphocytes (white arrowheads). Moreover, Ki67 staining demonstrated massive hyperproliferation in the basal layer of the epidermis (fig. 3g). All of these changes are highly similar to those found in psoriasis. In contrast to psoriasis, the granular layer was prominent (fig. 3f, white arrowhead), consistent with the known effect of PPARβ/δ on epidermal differentiation [33]. In order to exclude that AhR activation as such contributed to the development of skin disease, we also administered the AhR ligand I3C in the chow at a very high concentration (0.5% w/w) in the absence of GW501515 administration, which did not induce a skin phenotype. Likewise, skin disease could be effectively replicated by topical cream-based, instead of systemical, application of GW501516 + I3C to the skin, but not by I3C alone (fig. 3h), consistent with the observation that I3C induces transcription of the CYP1A1-driven PPARβ/δ transgene (fig. 2e), but does not activate it. Finally, C57Bl/6j wild type mice fed GW501516 did not exhibit skin changes. Thus, the psoriasis-like skin disease in PPARβ/δ transgenic mice is triggered solely by activation of PPARβ/δ overexpressed in the skin, but not by endogenous murine PPARβ/δ.

Immune system activation and involvement of Th17 cells in PPARβ/δ dependent skin disease

In order to further explore overlaps of the skin phenotype in PPARβ/δ transgenic mice with psoriasis, we next characterized immunological changes after disease induction. As shown in figure 4a, there was a massive influx of CD4$^+$ T cells into the dermis and, to a lesser extend, of CD8$^+$ T cells into the epidermis. CD11c+ dermal dendritic cells were abundant, while CD11c+ epidermal Langerhans cells were not found. Activation of endothelial cells was also evident by staining with CD31. All of these changes are highly consistent with those typical of psoriasis. Co-immunofluorescence studies revealed that the PPARβ/δ transgene was not found in either endothelial cells or dermal dendritic cells (fig. S3), further confirming that the skin disease in PPARβ/δ transgenic mice is driven by expression of the transgene in suprabasal epidermal keratinocytes, but not other cell types.

Th17 cells are required, but not sufficient, for phenotype development

Since the Th17-subset of T cells is of central importance in the immune activation of psoriasis, we next quantified these cells using intracellular FACS analysis. Indeed, Th17-cells, marked by

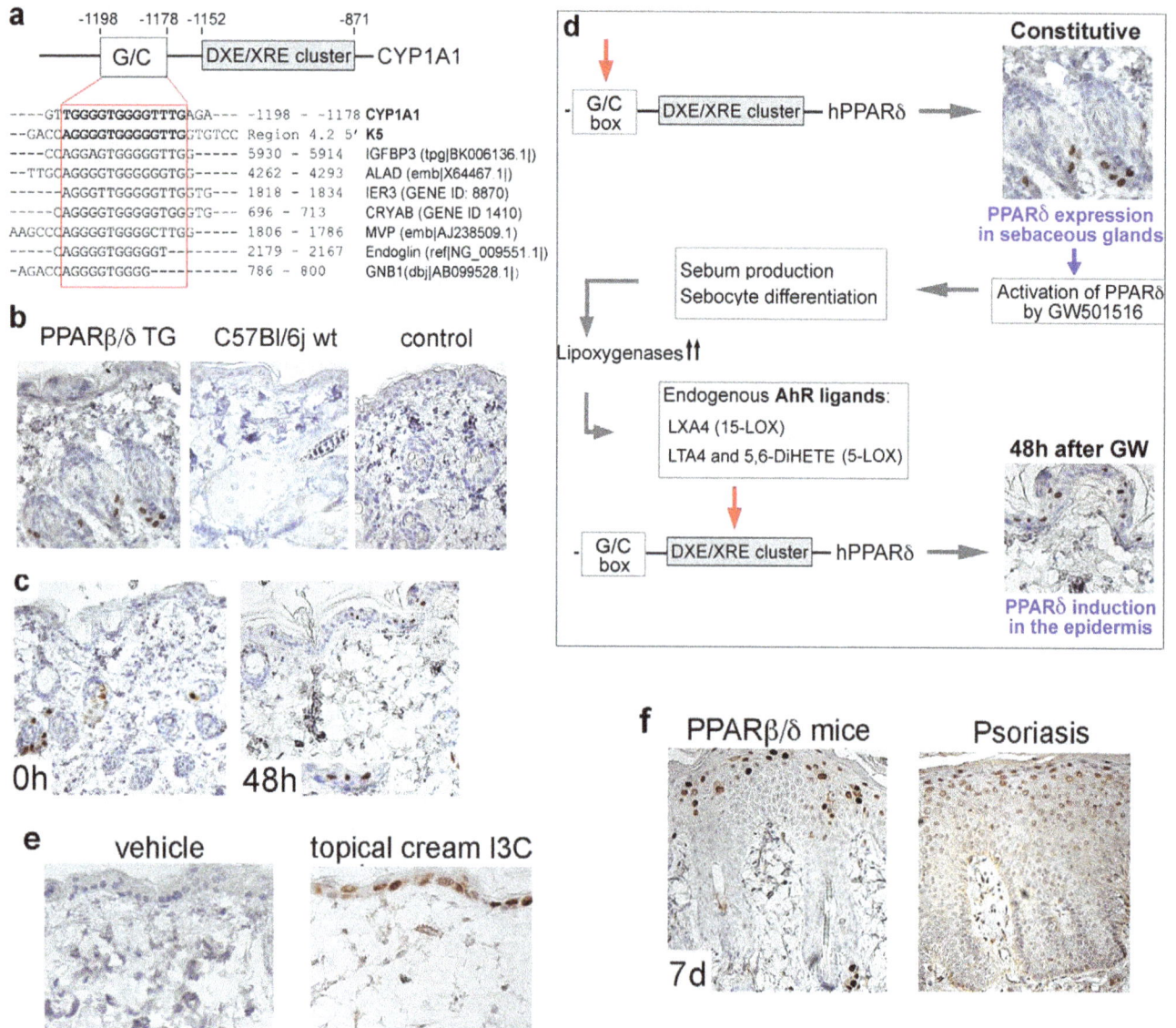

Figure 2. Inducible expression of PPARβ/δ in mouse epidermis. A. Cis-regulatory elements in the rat CYP1A1 promoter used to drive inducible expression of human PPARβ/δ. Upper panel: Map of the sebaceous – specific G/C-box element and the AHR – responsive DXE/XRE cluster in the cyp1A1 promoter as well as the human human K5 promoter. Bottom panel: ClustalW alignment of promoters identified by a BLAST search using the 20 bp G/C element of the Cyp1A1 promoter. All of the genes shown were found in the top 10% percentile of all transcripts expressed in human sebaceous glands (GDS3215 at the NCBI GEO website www.ncbi.nlm.nih.gov/geo/). **B.** Immunohistochemistry using anti-PPARβ/δ of mice transgenic for human PPARβ/δ driven by the rat CYP1A promoter (PPARβ/δ TG), as well as wild type mice. Magnification 200× **C.** Immunohistochemistry of skin samples from PPARβ/δ transgenic mice taken before, or 48 h after after initiation of PPARβ/δ activation by oral administration of the synthetic ligand GW501516 in the chow; (inset in "48 h": 400×); **d.** schematic illustrating the mechanism regulating constitutive expression of transgenic PPARβ/δ driven by the rat CYP1A1 promoter in sebaceous glands, as well as delayed PPARβ/δ expression in the epidermis after ligand-mediated activation of PPARβ/δ **e.** PPARβ/δ immunohistochemistry 48 h after topical cream application of indole-3-carbinole (I3C) to the skin of PPARβ/δ transgenic mice at 400× (right) magnification. **f.** Immunohistochemistry of PPARβ/δ in the skin of PPARβ/δ - transgenic mice after seven days of feeding of the PPARβ/δ ligand GW501516 in the chow (left) and in human psoriasis skin (right).

expression of IL17, were significantly expanded in the psoriasis-like plaques of PPARβ/δ mice, whereas the Th1 subset, marked by IFNγ[+] expression, was not (fig. 4b,c). A small, but statistically significant expansion of IL17[+] cells was also noted in peripheral lymphoid organs upon GW501516 stimulation (fig. S4). To assess the requirement of Th17 cells for PPARβ/δ - mediated skin disease, we depleted them *in vivo* by intraperitoneal injection of anti-IL12/23p40, analogous to the monoclonal antibody (ustekinumab) used to treat psoriasis. We extended this experiment to include the effect of injection using anti-TNFα. Blockade of TNFα

is an established treatment for psoriasis. Since TNFα itself induces PPARβ/δ expression [14], blocking of TNFα- should *not* be able to completely abrogate skin phenotype development in PPARβ/δ-transgenic mice since PPARβ/δ expression is enforced downstream of TNFα in this model. As shown in fig. 4d, treatment with anti-IL12/23p40, but not with anti-TNFα, effectively suppressed expansion of Th17 cells in GW501516-treated PPARβ/δ transgenic mice, verifying that the treatment had the expected effect. Strikingly, Th17-depletion caused a significant reduction of disease severity, as shown in fig. 4e and S5. By contrast, the effect

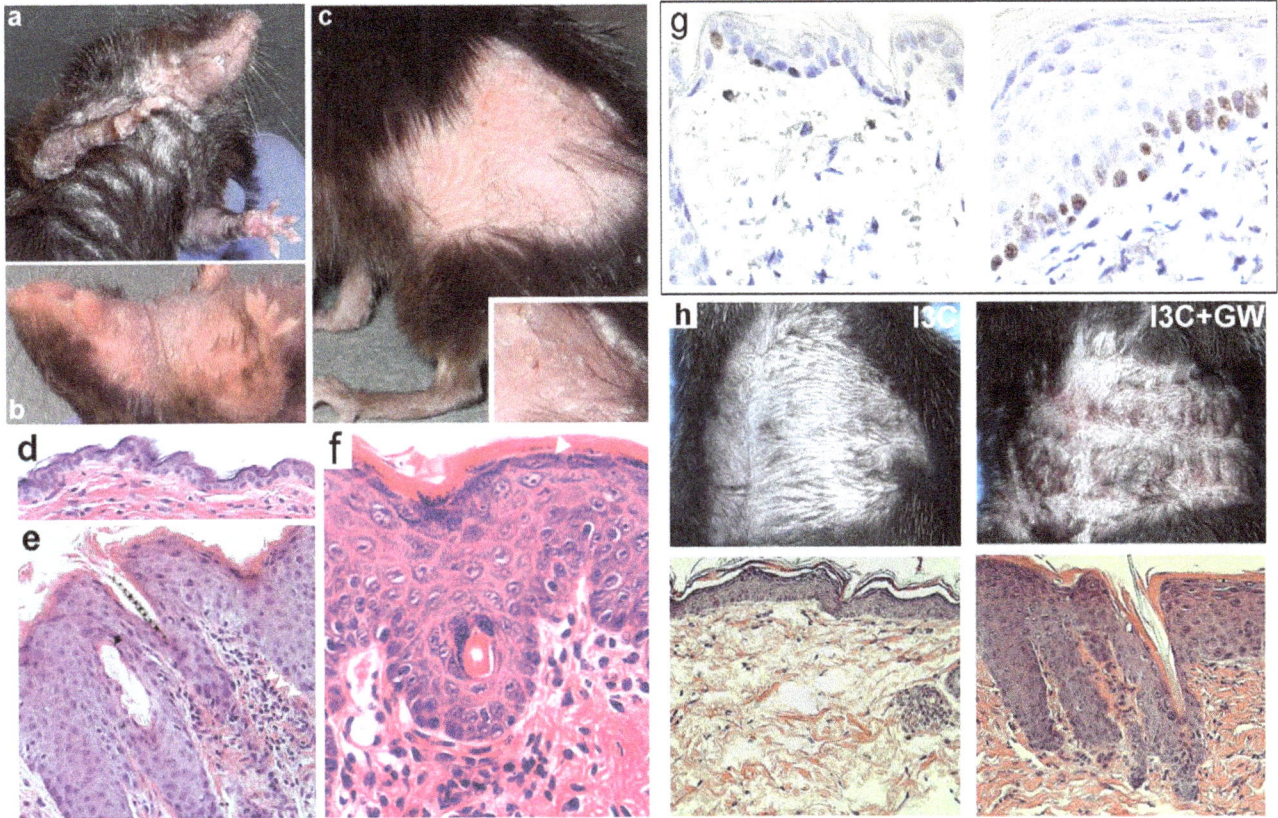

Figure 3. Skin phenotype in PPARβ/δ TG mice twenty days after GW501516 (GW) administration for twenty days. (a–c) Gross morphology, (d–e) H&E histology of control mice not treated with GW (d), or fourteen days after induction (e–g). Magnification 200× (d,e) or 400× (f). The white arrowhead in (f) denotes the granular layer. (g) Immunostaining for Ki67 of skin from PPARβ/δ TG mice maintained in the absence (left) or presence (right) of GW. Magnification 200×. (h) Induction of skin disease by topical application of either 0.3% of indole-3-carbinole (I3C, left) or I3C plus 0.3% GW501516 once daily to shaved abdominal skin. Gross macroscopic phenotype (top) and H&E histology of treated skin (bottom) was documented 10 days after beginning of treatment.

of anti-TNFα was much less pronounced, as expected. Thus, Th17 cells are required for full disease expression in PPARβ/δ transgenic mice. In order to clarify whether they are sufficient to trigger disease development, we performed adoptive transfer of splenocytes from PPARβ/δ transgenic mice with active disease to wild-type mice, which had previously been depleted of endogenous CD4+ cells. This treatment failed to induce any skin phenotype even after GW501516 administration to the recipient mice. Moreover, when GW501516 was administered to naïve wild type C57Bl/6j mice, they did exhibit a modest increase of Th17 cells in peripheral organs (fig. S4), indicating that endogenous murine PPARβ/δ also stimulates Th17 cell expansion. Wild type mice did not, however, develop skin disease. Thus, Th17 cells are required, but not sufficient for development of psoriasis-like disease in PPARβ/δ transgenic mice, although we cannot rule out that their presence in the skin in high numbers might allow disease development.

Psoriasis-like gene dysregulation in PPARβ/δ transgenic mice

Although psoriasis lesions are complex, involving various cell types and a multitude of dysregulated genes, the observed changes in gene expression are remarkably reproducible between different patients. This is demonstrated by the tight correlation between two large independent expression profiling datasets (Fig. S6), thus yielding a consistent psoriasis-specific pattern of global gene dysregulation. We studied to what extent this pattern is reflected in PPARβ/δ mice. As shown in figure 5a, most of the top 50 genes upregulated in lesional skin of PPARβ/δ mice were found congruently upregulated in human psoriasis. Quantitative real-time-PCR of selected genes confirmed that the changes observed by microarray-based expression profiling were reproducible (figure S7). Indeed, 56% of all upregulated and 33% of all downregulated genes in PPARβ/δ mice were found congruently regulated in psoriasis, respectively (figure 5b, clusters I and VI). Conversely, appr. 30% of all genes dysregulated in human psoriasis were found to be regulated congruently in PPARβ/δ mice (table S3). Geneset Enrichment analysis (GSEA) independently confirmed a highly significant enrichment of those genes upregulated in psoriasis (defined as gene-set) in lesional skin of PPARβ/δ mice (figure 5c). Only two small subsets of genes (8.3% of all, clusters III and IV) displayed inverse regulation between psoriasis and PPARβ/δ mice. When analysing the functional profile of these, we observed that cluster III, containing genes *up*regulated in PPARβ/δ mice but *down*regulated in psoriasis, was enriched for markers of late epidermal differentiation (e.g. FLG, PCDH21), indicative of cells in the so-called granular layer, which is prominent in PPARβ/δ mice (fig. 3f) but absent in psoriasis. Cluster IV, containing genes *up*regulated in psoriasis but *down*regulated in PPARβ/δ mice, was highly enriched for interferon-signalling (fig. 5b, table S3), where we were able to identify the mechanism underlying this discrepancy (see below). Taken together, expression profiling

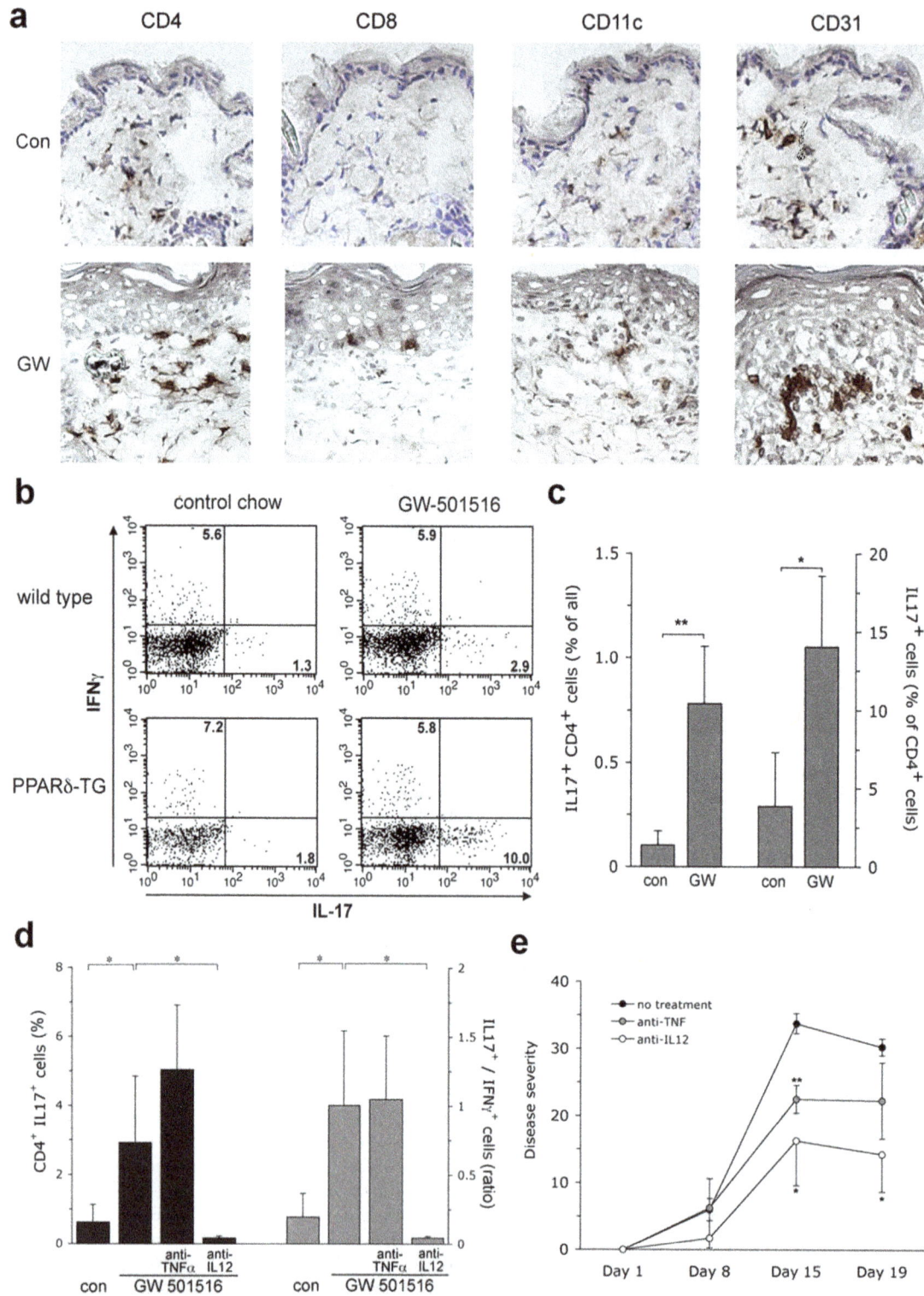

Figure 4. Immune activation in PPARβ/δ-mediated skin disease. (a) Immunohistochemistry for CD4, CD8, CD11c, and CD31 (Pecam 31) of skin from PPARβ/δ transgenic mice maintained in the absence (top) or presence of GW501516. Magnification 200×, (b) flow cytometry analysis showing intracellular FACS-staining for IFNγ and IL17 of skin cells (gated for CD4) from wild type and PPARβ/δ transgenic mice maintained in the presence or absence of GW501516, respectively. Numbers in quadrants indicate frequency of positive cells, (c) frequency of CD4$^+$IL17$^+$ of IL17$^+$ cells (expressed as percent of all CD4$^+$ gated cells) in PPARβ/δ transgenic and C57Bl/6 wild type mice maintained in the presence or absence of GW501516 (n = 4 per group), as determined by flow cytometry. * p<0.01; ** p<0.001, (d) frequency of CD4$^+$IL17$^+$ Th17 cells (left y-axis, black columns) and ratio of IL17$^+$ and IFNγ$^+$ cell frequencies (righ y-axis, grey columns) in the skin of PPARβ/δ mice maintained in the absence or presence of GW501516 with or without i.p. injection of anti-TNFα, or αIL12/23p40 (n = 4, see Methods), (e) disease severity, expressed as mean ± s.d., assessed by the degree of erythema, thickening, scaling, and hair loss (see Methods, representative photographs of mice on day 19 post induction are shown in figure S6) in PPARβ/δ transgenic mice GW501516 – containing chow with or without additional intraperitoneal injection of anti-TNFα or αIL12/23p40 (anti-IL12). * p<0.01, ** p<0.001 (treatment vs. control).

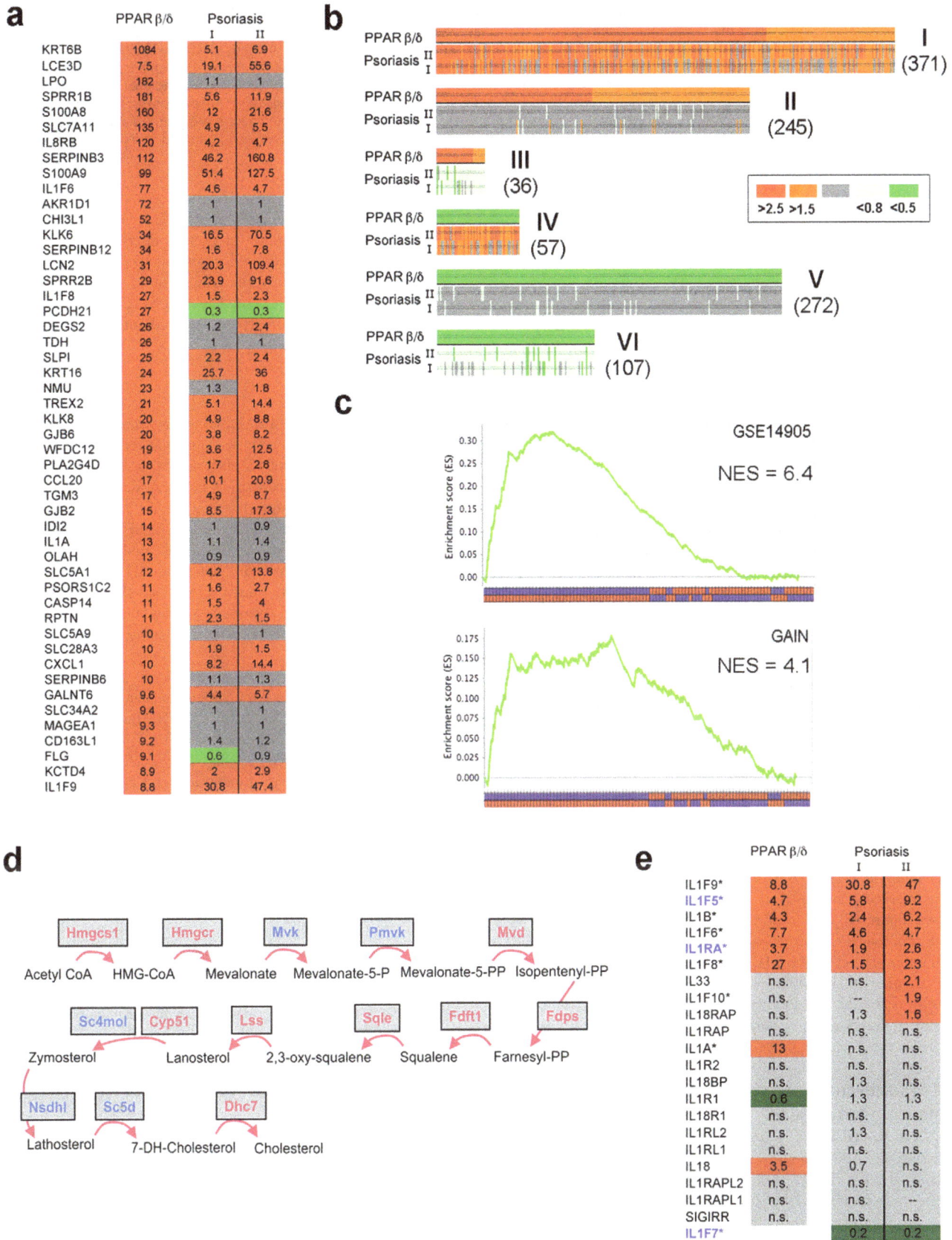

Figure 5. Congruent gene dysregulation in PPARβ/δ mice and psoriasis. (a) Fold-change between the lesional skin of PPARβ/δ mice after administration of GW501516 and control mice (n = 3 per group), and between lesional and non-lesional skin samples from psoriasis obtained through the GAIN (I) and the GSE14905 (II) datasets, respectively, as detailed in Methods. Red: FC >1.5, Green: FC <0.8. Shown are the top 50 upregulated genes. The complete dataset is given in table S1. (b) Heat map showing all genes dysregulated in GW501516-fed PPARβ/δ mice (n = 1077), clustered

by congruence with psoriasis. Color codes for –fold change are indicated. The genes in all clusters are detailed in table S2. (**c**) gene-set enrichment analysis (GSEA), performed using the top 500 genes upregulated in psoriasis lesions from the GSE14905 dataset (top), or the GAIN dataset (bottom), as genesets, respectively, and the complete mouse array collapsed to single genes as expression dataset. Analysis was run with 100 permutations and a classic statistic, NES = normalized enrichment score. The blue-red lines on the bottom represent heat-map of human genes found to be upregulated (blue on top) or downregulated in the mouse set. (**d**) Induction of cholesterol biosynthesis, conjugation, and channeling by PPARβ/δ. Red: upregulated in psoriasis and PPARβ/δ transgenic mice, blue: upregulated only in PPARβ/δ transgenic mice. Shaded boxes: repressed by Foxo1. (**e**) Induction of IL-1 signalling by PPARβ/δ. Datasets and color codes are as in (a). "n.s.": p>0.01; "--": fold change between 0.8–1.2., blue print: anti-inflammatory. * gene located within the IL1 cluster on chr. 2q between 113.2–113.7 Mb. (IL1F7 has only been identified in *homo sapiens* and *bos taurus*, the closest homologue in mice is IL1F5.).

confirms a large overlap in gene regulation between psoriasis and the skin disease in PPARβ/δ mice, strongly suggesting that the phenotype similarities described above are not a phenocopy but involve overlapping signalling pathways.

PPARβ/δ-dependent regulation of specific pathways

When extending analysis of gene expression to functional processes, we found that processes concordantly regulated in psoriasis and PPARβ/δ transgenic mice included lipid-metabolism, differentiation, and proliferation (table S4), which confirmed the expected, given the known activity profile of PPARβ/δ. Likewise, the complete set of genes involved in cholesterol biosynthesis was strongly co-upregulated (fig. 5d, table S6), as were a number of proliferation-associated kinases (table S8). Unexpectedly, however, both the human and the murine datasets exhibited a highly consistent upregulated IL1-signalling module, which, remarkably, not only includes pro-inflammatory transcripts but also the anti-inflammatory components IL1F5, and the IL1-receptor antagonist (fig. 5e, table S7). Importantly, wild type C57Bl/6 mice administered GW501516 did not exhibit these changes (table S1), but did show the expected upregulation of genes involved in lipid metabolism (table S5), thereby confirming that the observed induction of IL1-signalling was triggered by the transgene rather than endogenous murine PPARβ/δ. These results strongly suggest that a number of transcriptional programs known to be dysregulated in psoriasis are regulated by PPARβ/δ.

Critical role of STAT3 in PPARβ/δ dependent skin disease

STAT3 is phosphorylated in psoriasis [34], as well as in a wound-response type model of psoriasis induced by serum response factor-deficiency [35]. Accordingly, we analyzed STAT3 activation in PPARβ/δ mice. Tyr-705 phosphorylation of STAT3 was markedly increased in lesional skin of PPARβ/δ transgenic mice (figure 6a) and localized to the nuclei of suprabasal cells in the epidermis (figure 6b). Moreover, inhibition of STAT3 phosphorylation by the JAK2 inhibitor WP1066 led to a marked attenuation of skin disease, demonstrating the relevance of this pathway for the development of clinical disease, further demonstrating the overlap in pathogenesis between psoriasis and the current model (figure 6c).

STAT3 activation mediates suppression of interferon-target genes

As described above, the single group of genes upregulated in psoriasis but downregulated in PPARβ/δ mice were the interferon response genes (fig.5b, cluster IV). Strikingly, precisely this set of genes was previously shown to be repressed by STAT3 in vivo (fig. 6d, dark shaded columns). We therefore hypothesized that the notable repression of interferon-response genes in the skin of PPARβ/δ transgenic mice with skin disease was mediated by activation of STAT3. Indeed, repression of STAT3 activation by use of the JAK2 inhibitor significantly blocked the down-regulation of one of the most repressed transcripts, IFI27 (fig. 6e).

This STAT3-dependent effect was specific to interferon-response genes, since the dysregulation of another inflammatory pathway, exemplified by IL1β, remained unaltered by STAT3 inhibition (fig. 6e). These data show the inhibition of IFN signalling in PPARβ/δ transgenic mice is mediated by STAT3 as part of what has previously been termed the "anti-inflammatory response" [36].

Discussion

We here show that PPARβ/δ is activated in the upper epidermis of human psoriatic skin and that recapitulation of this event in mice is sufficient to elicit major elements of psoriasis. PPARβ/δ transgenic mice exhibit not only down-stream immunological changes but also psoriasis – specific gene dysregulation, thereby defining subsets of genes regulated by PPARβ/δ in psoriasis. Although the current transgenic model exhibits important differences to psoriasis (see below) and cannot recapitulate all features of a polygenetic disease, it does thus indicate that activation of PPARβ/δ in the upper spinous layer of the epidermis initiates a number of inflammatory and immunological changes seen in psoriasis.

One major implication of the present results is that they suggest a molecular explanation for the clinical overlap between psoriasis and metabolic, as well as cardiovascular disease [37]. Thus, PPARβ/δ expression is increased in chronic inflammation and regulated by caloric intake [38,39]. Specifically, factors such as TNFα which are known to directly induce PPARβ/δ expression are increased in the chronic inflammation accompanying metabolic syndrome [40]. Therefore, obesity, chronic inflammation, and dyslipidemia may increase the penetrance of psoriasis by inducing PPARβ/δ expression. Conversely, it is tempting to speculate that weight reduction or correction of other PPARβ/δ -inducing factors leads to suppression of PPARβ/δ expression in the skin, thus dampening disease severity. This may well be a contributory factor in the clinical observation that the response to low-dose cyclosporin, an established psoriasis treatment, is improved in psoriasis patients undergoing weight loss [41].

The role of PPARβ/δ in inflammation has been extensively and controversially studied, several papers suggesting anti-inflammatory properties (e.g. [42]), while others find that it stimulates pro-inflammatory cytokine synthesis including IL-8 and IL1β in macrophages [43]. Here, we show that, in the skin, PPARβ/δ induces a specific IL-1 signalling "module" both in human psoriasis and in PPARβ/δ transgenic mice. This module includes pro-inflammatory mediators such as IL1β, which is known to stimulate Th17 differentiation [44], and IL1F8, which stimulates pro-inflammatory mediators in fibroblasts [45], but also anti-inflammatory cytokines such as IL-1F5, which actually inhibits inflammatory skin disease [46], as well as the IL1 receptor antagonist (IL1RA). The latter has recently been shown to be a direct target of PPARβ/δ [47] and to be upregulated in psoriasis [48], thereby corroborating our findings. Thus, the PPARβ/δ -mediated induction of IL1-family cytokines in psoriasis defies a

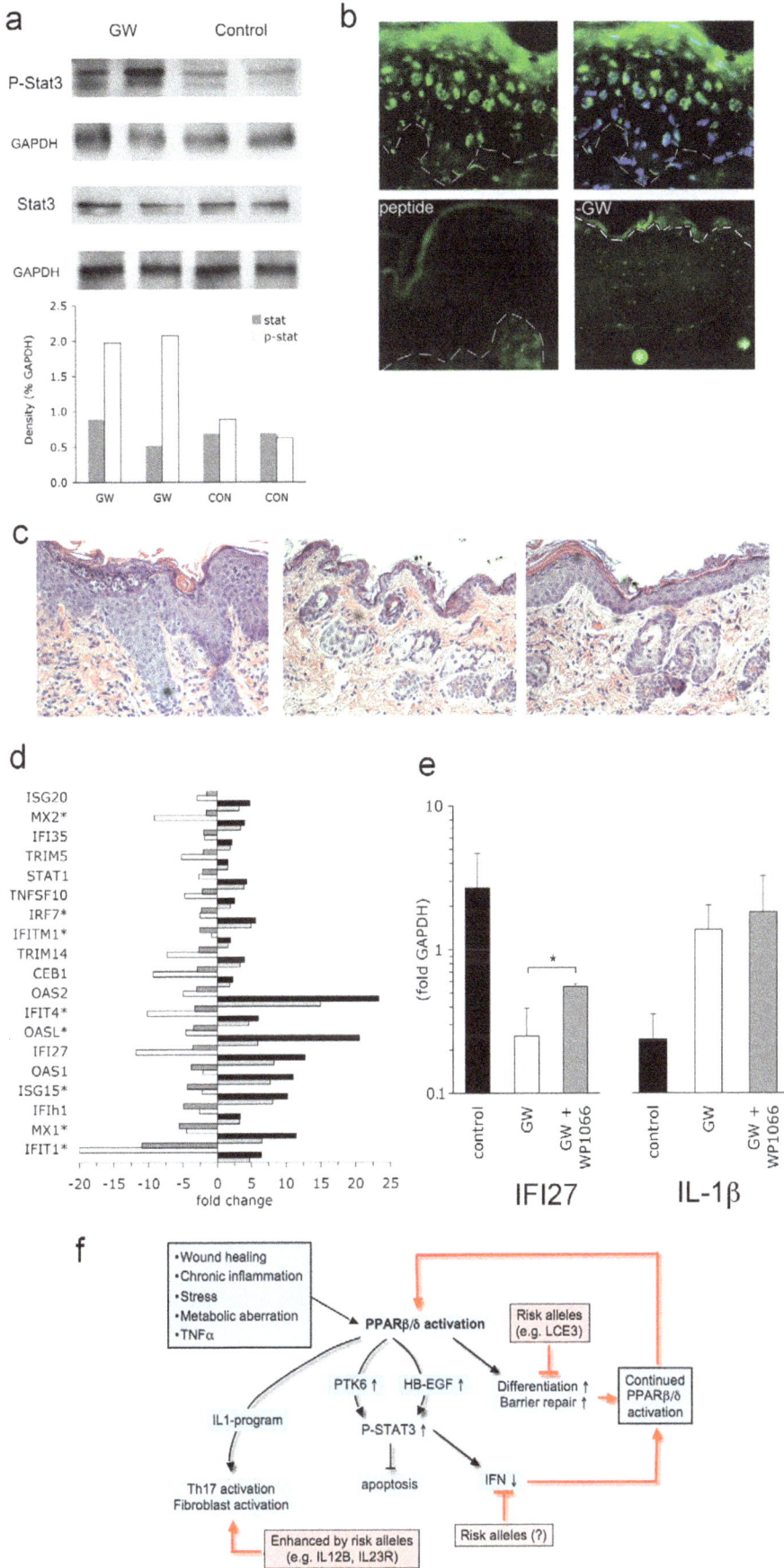

a

GW   Control

P-Stat3

GAPDH

Stat3

GAPDH

Density (% GAPDH)

2.5
2.0
1.5
1.0
0.5
0.0

GW   GW   CON   CON

stat
p-stat

b

peptide   -GW

c

d

ISG20
MX2*
IFI35
TRIM5
STAT1
TNFSF10
IRF7*
IFITM1*
TRIM14
CEB1
OAS2
IFIT4*
OASL*
IFI27
OAS1
ISG15*
IFIh1
MX1*
IFIT1*

-20 -15 -10 -5   0   5   10 15 20 25
fold change

e

10

(fold GAPDH)

1

0.1

control   GW   GW +
WP1066

IFI27

*

control   GW   GW +
WP1066

IL-1β

f

• Wound healing
• Chronic inflammation
• Stress
• Metabolic aberration
• TNFα

PPARβ/δ activation

PTK6 ↑   HB-EGF ↑

Risk alleles
(e.g. LCE3)

Differentiation ↑
Barrier repair ↑

Continued
PPARβ/δ
activation

IL1-program

P-STAT3 ↑

apoptosis

IFN ↓

Th17 activation
Fibroblast activation

Enhanced by risk alleles
(e.g. IL12B, IL23R)

Risk alleles (?)

Figure 6. Activation of STAT3 by PPARβ/δ. (a) Western blot of whole skin samples from two GW501516-treated (GW) and two control PPARβ/δ transgenic mice, respectively, probed with anti phospho-STAT3 (top) and anti-STAT3 (bottom) along with anti-GAPDH loading controls (top-band of the STAT3 doublet represents STAT3α, bottom-band STAT3β, respectively), semi-quantitative densitometry performed using ImageJ is included on the bottom, **(b)** immunofluorescence with anti phospho-STAT3 of GW-treated skin (upper left), upper right: same with DAPI counterstain to verify nuclear localisation, bottom left: control stain performed in the presence of blocking peptide, lower right: PPARβ/δ transgenic mouse not treated with GW. White dashed lines mark the dermo-epidermal boundary; all samples at 400× magnification. * = hair shaft **(c)** H&E histology of skin from GW-treated (left panel), untreated (middle), GW-treated mice concurrently receiving intraperitoneal injections of the STAT3 inhibitor WP1066 (right) at 200× magnification, **(d)** fold change of genes previously shown to be repressed by activated STAT3 (dark grey columns, data taken from [56]) and their regulation in GW501516-fed vs. control PPARβ/δ transgenic mice (white), lesional vs. non-lesional skin from psoriasis patients in the GSE14905 (black), as well as the GAIN (light grey) datasets, respectively. * denotes genes that are not contained in cluster IV (table S2) since they did not meet the p<0.01 cut-off. **(e)** Taqman-based qPCR of IFI27 and IL1β from whole skin of untreated (black columns), GW-fed (white), and GW-fed + WP1066-injected PPARβ/δ mice (grey), respectively (n = 3 mice per group), * p<0.05; **(f)** schematic illustrating the PPARβ/δ /STAT3 /IL-1 pathway identified here, the role of PPARβ/δ in maintaining chronically active psoriasis, as well as disease-enhancing role of predisposing genomic risk alleles. The box on the upper left lists factors known to trigger both PPARβ/δ induction as well as clinical psoriasis flares.

simplified concept of purely "pro-" or "anti-" inflammatory. Clearly, these results would signal some caution regarding the proposed use of PPARβ/δ agonists to treat a variety of conditions [49].

We here identify activation of STAT3 as a novel pathway targeted by PPARβ/δ. PPARβ/δ activation evidently causes psoriasis-like disease not solely through STAT3 activation since (i) the phenotype is not completely reversed by inhibition of STAT3 and (ii) overexpression of STAT3 alone causes a less widespread psoriasis-like phenotype with a much longer latency [34]. Regarding the mechanism of STAT3 activation, STAT3 can be phosphorylated by a number of kinases. Of these, at least two appear to be involved. First, the two EGF-family ligands TGFα and HB-EGF, previously identified as a direct transcriptional target of PPARβ/δ [12], are highly upregulated in PPARβ/δ as well as in psoriasis, suggesting that EGF-receptor activation contributes to STAT3 phosphorylation. Second, PTK6 kinase, which also phosphorylates STAT3 [50], is the most highly upregulated kinase in psoriasis and PPARβ/δ mice (table S8). Thus, at least two kinase pathways converge on STAT3 phosphorylation both in psoriasis and PPARβ/δ mice.

An obvious difference between the skin disease induced by activation of PPARβ/δ and psoriasis in humans is the regulation of IFN signalling. While IFN response genes are strongly induced in psoriasis they are repressed in PPARβ/δ transgenic mice. On the other hand, subsequent downstream events, including CD4+ and CD8+ T-cell influx, endothelial activation, dendritic cell accumulation, as well as Th17 activation are all recapitulated preserved in this model. Therefore, the present data suggest that upregulation of interferon response genes is not, as commonly assumed, required for sustained disease. Furthermore, while the upregulation of IFN response genes could be taken for granted in the milieu of a wound-response, our data show that they should actually be repressed by the so-called anti-inflammatory response mediated by STAT3 [36,51]. Their continuous upregulation despite STAT3 activation suggests the existence of as yet to be identified factors actively inhibiting STAT3 repression of IFN target genes (schematically shown in fig. 6f).

Psoriasis is a genetically determined disease and genomic variants at the PPARβ/δ genomic locus have not so far been associated with psoriasis. Although this might be regarded as evidence against a role for PPARβ/δ in psoriasis, our data clearly show that overexpression of PPARβ/δ in psoriasis skin lesions is a common phenomenon occuring in the vast majority of psoriasis patients (fig. 1). Thus, upregulation of PPARβ/δ appears to occur downstream of individually variable genomic risk, offering a potential target for treatment relevant for most patients.

Apart from interferon response genes, the other major difference in gene expression between psoriasis and the phenotype

in PPARβ/δ mice is terminal epidermal differentiation, which is blocked in psoriasis, but increased in the mouse model, which confirms the established pro-differentiation activity of PPARβ/δ [52] and the fact that it triggers differentiation in wound healing [28,53]. In psoriasis, on the other hand, late epidermal differentation is disturbed and the skin barrier disrupted. Based on the data presented here, one may speculate that the suppression of terminal differentiation and the block in skin barrier repair, aggravated by genomic risk alleles such as the recently described LCE3 variant [54], act as stimuli to maintain sustained upregulation of PPARβ/δ in the upper epidermal layers. The net effect would be the establishment of a vicious cycle, schematically shown in fig.6f, which is able to account for the chronic persistent course typical of psoriasis.

In conclusion, we here identify a central role for PPARβ/δ in the pathogenesis of psoriasis and identify IL1 and STAT3 signalling as novel pathways regulated by PPARβ/δ. Our data suggest novel approaches to psoriasis treatment. Finally, our results underscore that PPARβ/δ activation as a treatment strategy for metabolic diseases might harbour the risk of pro-inflammatory effects or autoimmune activation.

Methods

Ethics Statement

All work involving animals was approved by the Tayside Ethics Committee. Storage and use of all tissues included in the work presented here was approved by the Tayside Committee on Medical Research Ethics B (REC ref. Nr. 07/S1402/90).

PPARβ/δ immunohistochemistry

Paraffin-embedded samples were obtained from the Tayside Tissue bank. Prior to biopsy, patients gave written consent to storage and analysis of biopsy samples. Sections from paraffin embedded tissue (nominally 4 microns thick) were cut onto superfrost plus slides (VWR International Ltd) and dried for 1 hr at 60 °C before being de-paraffinised in Histoclear (National Diagnostics) and then rehydrated through a graded alcohol series. 10 mM Citric acid buffer, pH 6.0 was used as standard microwave-based antigen retrieval methods. Sections were microwaved in a pressure cooker for 15 min before being immunostained on a DAKO autostainer using Vectastain® ABC kits (Vector Labs) according to the manufacturer's protocol. Briefly, sections were blocked in either normal goat, rabbit or horse serum containing 10%(v/v) from stock avidin solution (Vector Labs) for 20 min followed by 1 hr incubation with anti-PPARβ/δ (R&D, PP-K9436) at 1:100 overnight at 4°C for human samples (incubation for 1 h at room temperature yielded comparable results.), and 1:1000 for murine samples. Sections were washed 3× for 15 min in TBS, pH 7.6, followed by anti-mouse-biotin, antibody for 30 min followed by Vectastain Elite ABC reagent for another 30 min. Liquid Diaminobenzidine (DAB) (DAKO) was applied for 5 min and sections were counterstained with Mayer's haematoxylin.

H&E histology

Paraffin-embedded samples were heated for 15 minutes. Samples were treated with 3 washes of Xylene, followed by a series of graded alcohol washes. Samples were washed with water followed with staining with Harris' Haematoxylin. Wash 2 with water. Samples incubated in 0.1% acid alcohol for 1 minute followed by a 3rd wash with water. Samples were then incubated in STWS for 1 minute followed by a 4th wash with water. Samples stained with Shandon Eosin for 30 seconds followed by a 5th wash. Samples were re-hydrated with a series of graded alcohol washes followed by 3 washes with Xylene. Sections were mounted with DPX.

Generation of PPARβ/δ transgenic mice

PPARβ/δ transgenic mice were generated by cloning full-length human PPARδ downstream of the human CYP1A1 promoter. Plasmids encoding human PPARδ were prepared as follows. The PPARδ coding sequence was amplified using primers PRMG15 (5′-CTAGTCTAGA**ATG**GAGCAGCCACAGGAGGAAGC-3′) and PRMG3 (5′-CTAGTCTAGATTAGTACATGTCCTTG-TAGATCTCCTG-3′), respectively (XbaI-sites underlined, ATG start codon in bold). PCR products were cleaved with XbaI and cloned in plasmid pUHD10-3 (M. Gossen, unpublished, Genbank accession number U89931) creating pMGD7 (PPARδ). The integrity of the inserts was confirmed by sequencing and cleaved out using BamHI and ligated into plasmid pAHIR1-β-gal (Campbell, 1996} cleaved with BglII, resulting in the plasmid pMGD72 (PPARδ). Proper insert orientation was confirmed by restriction endonuclease analysis and sequencing. Transgenic mice were generated by microinjection of the expression unit (NotI fragment) of the plasmid pMGD72 into pro-nuclei of C57BL/J6 x CBA F1 fertilized eggs. Mice were maintained under standard animal house conditions.

Disease induction

PPARβ/δ mediated skin disease was induced either by administration of powdered standard RMI-chow containing 0.003% GW501516 (w/w, custom – synthesized by AF-Pharmaceuticals, UK, to ≥98% purity), or topical application of 0.3% (w/w) GW501516 in 10% (w/w) DMSO in Hydromol ointment (Alliance, UK); for topical induction, control mice received 10% DMSO in Hydromol.

Flow cytometry and intracellular measurement of IL17

Skin samples were shaved, trimmed of associated fat, cut to appr. 10–15 mm^3 size using a scissor, incubated in 2 mg/ml collagenase IV (Roche, cat-nr. 110880855001), 1.1 U/ml dispase I (Roche, cat-nr. 04942086001) in HBSS for 30′ at 37°C. Subsequently, samples were incubated in RPMI incl. Pen/Strep and 10% FCS, 0.5 μg/ml PMA, 0.5 μg/ml ionomycin for 3 h. For the last hour, Brefeldin A was added at 2 μg/ml. Surface and intracellular staining for CD4-FITC (Pharmingen, clone RM4-4), CD8-PerCP/Cy5.5b (Pharmingen, 53–6.7), IFNγ-APC (Pharmingen, cat-nr. 554413), and IL17-PE (Pharmingen, cat-nr. 559502) and analysis on a FACS-Calibur was done according to standard procedures.

TNFα and IL-12 antibody treatment

70 μg of anti-TNFα (Millipore, cat-nr 05-168), anti-IL12/23p40 (BioLegend, Clone C17.8, cat-nr. 505304), or PBS, respectively, were injected on three times per week, beginning on day 1 of GW501516 administration. Mice were sacrificed on day 22 for tissue analysis. For disease severity, erythema, scaling, palpable hyperkeratosis, and hair loss were scored as absent (0), weak (1), moderate (2), or severe (3), respectively, and the sum calculated for index regions (chin, forepaws, abdomen) chosen in order to allow hand-held analysis of mice during on-going treatment.

Expression profiling was performed as detailed in the supporting information (Method S1).

Western blot STAT3, P-STAT3

Nuclear extracts were made using the NE-PER kit (Pierce). Protein concentration was determined by Bradford assay. 40 μg of protein loaded per well, subjected to SDS-PAGE gel and transferred to nitrocellulose membrane. Primary antibodies: 1:1000 dilution of Phospho-Stat3 (Tyr705) Antibody (New England BioLabs UK, 9131S) and 1:1000 dilution of anti-Stat3 (New England BioLabs UK, 9132) followed by HRP– conjugated anti-rabbit Ig, ECL Plus (GE Healthcare, Amersham), and detection using a CCD camera.

Immunofluorescence P-STAT3

5 μm thick sections of snap-frozen skin were fixed in methanol, followed by incubation with anti-Phospho-Stat3 (Tyr705) (D3A7) (New England Biolabs UK, 9145S) with or without blocking peptide (New England Biolabs UK, 1195) for 1 hour at RT. Secondary antibody was Alexa Fluro® 488 donkey anti-rabbit IgG (H+L) (Invitrogen). Coverslips were mounted using ProLong® Gold antifade reagent with DAPI (Invitrogen, Cat.no.: P-36931).

Treatment with WP1066

WP1066 (Calbiochem, order-nr 573097) was dissolved in DMSO/PEG 600 (20/80) according to [55] at 1.25 μg/μl. Mice were injected with WP1066 or vehicle at 75 μl intraperitoneally three times a week.

Supporting Information

Table S1 Synopsis of dysregulated genes in PPARβ/δ transgenic mice and psoriasis. Sheet "Changed in PPARd mice": all genes found dysregulated in PPARd mice, as detailed in the file Method S1. Sheet "PPARd mice vs psoriasis": all genes dysregulated in PPARβ/δ mice (orange shaded cells) that are also present on the two gene expression sets representing psoriasis (green shaded cells). FC = fold change lesional vs. non-lesional (psoriasis), or induced vs. non-induced (PPARβ/δ transgenic mice).
Found at: doi:10.1371/journal.pone.0009701.s001

Table S2 Clustering of genes dysregulated in PPARβ/δ transgenic mice. The table contains all 1077 genes listed in the synopsis between dysregulated genes in PPARβ/δ transgenic mice and psoriasis, color-coded as up- (red/orange) or down- regulated (light-green/dark green), as shown in Figure 5b.
Found at: doi:10.1371/journal.pone.0009701.s002

Table S3 Concordance of gene dysregulation between psoriasis and PPARβ/δ transgenic mice.

Found at: doi:10.1371/journal.pone.0009701.s003

Table S4 Genes concordantly regulated between PPARβ/δ transgenic mice and psoriasis, listed for the functional categories lipid-metabolism, differentiation, and cell-cycle.
Found at: doi:10.1371/journal.pone.0009701.s004

Table S5 Genes induced by the PPARβ/δ agonist GW501516 in the skin of C57Bl/6 wild type mice.
Found at: doi:10.1371/journal.pone.0009701.s005

Table S6 Expression of genes involved in cholesterol biosynthesis in PPARβ/δ transgenic mice and psoriasis.
Found at: doi:10.1371/journal.pone.0009701.s006

Table S7 Interleukin-1 related genes in PPARβ/δ transgenic mice and psoriasis.
Found at: doi:10.1371/journal.pone.0009701.s007

Table S8 Expression of kinase genes in PPARβ/δ transgenic mice and psoriasis.
Found at: doi:10.1371/journal.pone.0009701.s008

Table S9 PPAR isoforms and ligands.
Found at: doi:10.1371/journal.pone.0009701.s009

Method S1 Expression profiling.
Found at: doi:10.1371/journal.pone.0009701.s010

Figure S1 (a) Immunohistochemistry of PPARβ/δ in a panel of eight paraffin-embedded samples from psoriasis skin lesions, counterstained with hematoxilin. The inset in the right upper panel in addition demonstrates expression in dermal fibroblasts and endothelial cells. Magnification 200× in each case. (b) Immunohistochemistry of PPARβ/δ in PPARβ/δ- transgenic mice treated with GW501516 for seven days, counterstained with hematoxilin. Panels in lower row were taken fom slides stained with secondary antibody only. Magnification 200× for all panels.
Found at: doi:10.1371/journal.pone.0009701.s011

Figure S2 Macroscopic changes in PPARβ/δ transgenic mice upon ligand-mediated activation of PPARβ/δ by administration of the ligand GW501516 in the chow. Pictures shown were taken 14 (left) or 20 days (middle, right) after disease induction. Note the sharp demarcation of hyperkeratosis on the abdomen (middle). Panel on upper right represents illustrates the scalp, exhibiting heavy scaling, but no marked erythema.
Found at: doi:10.1371/journal.pone.0009701.s012

Figure S3 Confinement of PPARβ/δ transgene expression to suprabasal epidermal keratinocytes. Co-immunofluorescence with anti-PPARβ/δ visualized with Alexa288 and either CD11c, visualized with TexasRed, was performed as described in Methods. The white dashed line indicates the dermo-epidermal boundary. Magnification 400×.
Found at: doi:10.1371/journal.pone.0009701.s013

Figure S4 Expansion of Th17 cells upon activation of PPARβ/δ. PPARβ/δ transgenic mice were maintained in the presence (black columns) or absence (dark shaded) of GW501516, as were C57Bl6/j wild type (light shaded: GW; white: control) and Th17 cell frequencies determined by intracellular FACS, as described in

Methods. Data show mean ± s.d. of Th17 cells (top), as well as the ratio between IL17+ and IFNγ+ cells (bottom) in the lymphocyte gate for n = 3 mice per group. * p<0.05.
Found at: doi:10.1371/journal.pone.0009701.s014

Figure S5 Inhibition of PPARβ/δ-mediated skin disease by depletion of Th17 cells. PPARβ/δ transgenic mice were maintained in the absence (control) or presence (all other groups) of GW501516 and additionally treated by injection of either anti-IL12/23p40, or anti-TNFα, as described in Methods. Pictures shown were taken nineteen days after disease induction. Mice were manually restrained to allow for comparable positioning during photography, thereby causing artificial tightening of abdominal skin.
Found at: doi:10.1371/journal.pone.0009701.s015

Figure S6 Reproducibility of gene dysregulation in psoriasis. Fold-change of gene expression between lesional and non-lesional skin in two independent datasets. The left panel shows all genes, the right panel all genes significantly upregulated (p<0.001) in both datasets. R2 = 0.93 for both panels. The dashed line indicates theoretically equal up-regulation in the two datasets. Both datasets were obtained using the same platform (using the Affymetrix HU133 Plus 2.0 array). The dataset from the GAIN cohort was obtained from the dbGaP website (www.ncbi.nlm.nih.gov/sites/entrez?db = gap). The CEL files are also available at the GEO website of NCBI (GEO dataset GSE13355). In the initial release, whole-skin expression profiles from paired lesional/non-lesional samples of 31 psoriasis patients were available which was used for the present analysis. The CEL files containing the dataset GSE14905 (n = 28 patients) were also downloaded from the GEO website. The data show the extend of reproducibility of gene dysregulation across patients and also indicate that -fold changes obtained with the GSE14905 dataset are consistently slightly higher than those observed in the GAIN data.
Found at: doi:10.1371/journal.pone.0009701.s016

Figure S7 Upregulation of psoriasis-associated genes in lesional skin of PPARβ/δ transgenic mice. The expression level for the representative genes shown, previously found to be upregulated in the skin of PPARβ/δ mice treated with GW501516 by microarray-based expression profiling (see main text), was quantified using TaqMan-based real-time PCR using Assays-on-Demand kits obtained from ABI according to the manufacturer's instruction (LCE3f: Mm02605425, Il1β: Mm01336189, Hb-EGF: Mm004-39305, CRABPII: Mm00801693, ALOX12b: Mm00507782, m1: MM00436999, ATP12a: Mm00446786). The data shown represent mean ± s.d. of GAPDH-calibrated expression levels obtained from n = 3 mice for each group (GW-fed, red columns, vs. control, blue columns). For all genes, p<0.001 in a two-sided independent t-test.
Found at: doi:10.1371/journal.pone.0009701.s017

Figure S8 Expression of transgenically overexpressed PPARβ/δ in murine skin. Whole skin samples from C57Bl/6j wild type (WT) or PPARβ/δ transgenic mice fed control chow (Tg) or GW501516-containing chow (TG+GW) were taken, genomic DNA digested, and total RNA isolated, followed by cDNA synthesis. RT-PCR was performed for the indicated number of cycles using primers specific for the transgene. Two mice for each condition were used.
Found at: doi:10.1371/journal.pone.0009701.s018

Author Contributions

Conceived and designed the experiments: MR JF. Performed the experiments: MR LR JF. Analyzed the data: MR LR JF. Contributed reagents/materials/analysis tools: CNAP MCUG. Wrote the paper: JF.

References

1. Gelfand JM, Stern RS, Nijsten T, Feldman SR, Thomas J, et al. (2005) The prevalence of psoriasis in African Americans: results from a population-based study. J Am Acad Dermatol 52: 23–26.
2. Dubertret L, Mrowietz U, Ranki A, van de Kerkhof PC, Chimenti S, et al. (2006) European patient perspectives on the impact of psoriasis: the EUROPSO patient membership survey. Br J Dermatol 155: 729–736.
3. Wu Y, Mills D, Bala M (2008) Psoriasis: cardiovascular risk factors and other disease comorbidities. J Drugs Dermatol 7: 373–377.
4. Poikolainen K, Karvonen J, Pukkala E (1999) Excess mortality related to alcohol and smoking among hospital-treated patients with psoriasis. Arch Dermatol 135: 1490–1493.
5. Finlay AY, Coles EC (1995) The effect of severe psoriasis on the quality of life of 369 patients. Br J Dermatol 132: 236–244.
6. Schmitt JM, Ford DE (2006) Work limitations and productivity loss are associated with health-related quality of life but not with clinical severity in patients with psoriasis. Dermatology 213: 102–110.
7. Sommer DM, Jenisch S, Suchan M, Christophers E, Weichenthal M (2006) Increased prevalence of the metabolic syndrome in patients with moderate to severe psoriasis. Arch Dermatol Res 298: 321–328.
8. Naldi L, Chatenoud L, Linder D, Belloni Fortina A, Peserico A, et al. (2005) Cigarette smoking, body mass index, and stressful life events as risk factors for psoriasis: results from an Italian case-control study. J Invest Dermatol 125: 61–67.
9. Barish GD, Narkar VA, Evans RM (2006) PPAR delta: a dagger in the heart of the metabolic syndrome. J Clin Invest 116: 590–597.
10. Short B (2009) Time (and PPARbeta/delta) heals all wounds. J Cell Biol 184: 767.
11. Michalik L, Auwerx J, Berger JP, Chatterjee VK, Glass CK, et al. (2006) International Union of Pharmacology. LXI. Peroxisome proliferator-activated receptors. Pharmacol Rev 58: 726–741.
12. Romanowska M, al Yacoub N, Seidel H, Donandt S, Gerken H, et al. (2008) PPARdelta enhances keratinocyte proliferation in psoriasis and induces heparin-binding EGF-like growth factor. J Invest Dermatol 128: 110–124.
13. Westergaard M, Henningsen J, Johansen C, Rasmussen S, Svendsen ML, et al. (2003) Expression and localization of peroxisome proliferator-activated receptors and nuclear factor kappaB in normal and lesional psoriatic skin. J Invest Dermatol 121: 1104–1117.
14. Tan NS, Michalik L, Noy N, Yasmin R, Pacot C, et al. (2001) Critical roles of PPAR beta/delta in keratinocyte response to inflammation. Genes Dev 15: 3263–3277.
15. Di-Poi N, Michalik L, Tan NS, Desvergne B, Wahli W (2003) The anti-apoptotic role of PPARbeta contributes to efficient skin wound healing. J Steroid Biochem Mol Biol 85: 257–265.
16. Icre G, Wahli W, Michalik L (2006) Functions of the Peroxisome Proliferator-Activated Receptor (PPAR) alpha and beta in Skin Homeostasis, Epithelial Repair, and Morphogenesis. J Invest Dermatol 126 Suppl: 30–35.
17. Piqueras L, Reynolds AR, Hodivala-Dilke KM, Alfranca A, Redondo JM, et al. (2006) Activation of PPAR{beta}/{delta} Induces Endothelial Cell Proliferation and Angiogenesis. Arterioscler Thromb Vasc Biol.
18. van der Vleuten CJ, de Jong EM, van de Kerkhof PC (1996) Epidermal differentiation characteristics of the psoriatic plaque during treatment with calcipotriol. Arch Dermatol Res 288: 366–372.
19. Lowes MA, Chamian F, Abello MV, Fuentes-Duculan J, Lin SL, et al. (2005) Increase in TNF-alpha and inducible nitric oxide synthase-expressing dendritic cells in psoriasis and reduction with efalizumab (anti-CD11a). Proc Natl Acad Sci U S A 102: 19057–19062.
20. Di Cesare A, Di Meglio P, Nestle FO (2009) The IL-23/Th17 axis in the immunopathogenesis of psoriasis. J Invest Dermatol 129: 1339–1350.
21. Sabat R, Philipp S, Hoflich C, Kreutzer S, Wallace E, et al. (2007) Immunopathogenesis of psoriasis. Exp Dermatol 16: 779–798.
22. Nair RP, Duffin KC, Helms C, Ding J, Stuart PE, et al. (2009) Genome-wide scan reveals association of psoriasis with IL-23 and NF-kappaB pathways. Nat Genet 41: 199–204.
23. Di-Poi N, Ng CY, Tan NS, Yang Z, Hemmings BA, et al. (2005) Epithelium-mesenchyme interactions control the activity of peroxisome proliferator-activated receptor beta/delta during hair follicle development. Mol Cell Biol 25: 1696–1712.
24. Campbell SJ, Carlotti F, Hall PA, Clark AJ, Wolf CR (1996) Regulation of the CYP1A1 promoter in transgenic mice: an exquisitely sensitive on-off system for cell specific gene regulation. J Cell Sci 109 (Pt 11): 2619–2625.
25. Robertson RW, Zhang L, Pasco DS, Fagan JB (1994) Aryl hydrocarbon-induced interactions at multiple DNA elements of diverse sequence–a multicomponent mechanism for activation of cytochrome P4501A1 (CYP1A1) gene transcription. Nucleic Acids Res 22: 1741–1749.
26. Rowe JM, Welsh C, Pena RN, Wolf CR, Brown K, et al. (2008) Illuminating role of CYP1A1 in skin function. J Invest Dermatol 128: 1866–1868.
27. Kaufman CK, Sinha S, Bolotin D, Fan J, Fuchs E (2002) Dissection of a complex enhancer element: maintenance of keratinocyte specificity but loss of differentiation specificity. Mol Cell Biol 22: 4293–4308.
28. Michalik L, Wahli W (2007) Peroxisome proliferator-activated receptors (PPARs) in skin health, repair and disease. Biochim Biophys Acta 1771: 991–998.
29. Rosenfield RL, Kentsis A, Deplewski D, Ciletti N (1999) Rat preputial sebocyte differentiation involves peroxisome proliferator-activated receptors. J Invest Dermatol 112: 226–232.
30. Trivedi NR, Cong Z, Nelson AM, Albert AJ, Rosamilia LL, et al. (2006) Peroxisome proliferator-activated receptors increase human sebum production. J Invest Dermatol 126: 2002–2009.
31. Machado FS, Johndrow JE, Esper L, Dias A, Bafica A, et al. (2006) Anti-inflammatory actions of lipoxin A4 and aspirin-triggered lipoxin are SOCS-2 dependent. Nat Med 12: 330–334.
32. Chiaro CR, Morales JL, Prabhu KS, Perdew GH (2008) Leukotriene A4 metabolites are endogenous ligands for the Ah receptor. Biochemistry 47: 8445–8455.
33. Schmuth M, Jiang YJ, Dubrac S, Elias PM, Feingold KR (2008) Thematic review series: skin lipids. Peroxisome proliferator-activated receptors and liver X receptors in epidermal biology. J Lipid Res 49: 499–509.
34. Sano S, Chan KS, Carbajal S, Clifford J, Peavey M, et al. (2005) Stat3 links activated keratinocytes and immunocytes required for development of psoriasis in a novel transgenic mouse model. Nat Med 11: 43–49.
35. Koegel H, von Tobel L, Schafer M, Alberti S, Kremmer E, et al. (2009) Loss of serum response factor in keratinocytes results in hyperproliferative skin disease in mice. J Clin Invest 119: 899–910.
36. Murray PJ (2006) STAT3-mediated anti-inflammatory signalling. Biochem Soc Trans 34: 1028–1031.
37. Azfar RS, Gelfand JM (2008) Psoriasis and metabolic disease: epidemiology and pathophysiology. Curr Opin Rheumatol 20: 416–422.
38. Sun L, Ke Y, Zhu CY, Tang N, Tian DK, et al. (2008) Inflammatory reaction versus endogenous peroxisome proliferator-activated receptors expression, re-exploring secondary organ complications of spontaneously hypertensive rats. Chin Med J (Engl) 121: 2305–2311.
39. Masternak MM, Al-Regaiey KA, Del Rosario Lim MM, Bonkowski MS, Panici JA, et al. (2005) Caloric restriction results in decreased expression of peroxisome proliferator-activated receptor superfamily in muscle of normal and long-lived growth hormone receptor/binding protein knockout mice. J Gerontol A Biol Sci Med Sci 60: 1238–1245.
40. Sutherland JP, McKinley B, Eckel RH (2004) The metabolic syndrome and inflammation. Metab Syndr Relat Disord 2: 82–104.
41. Gisondi P, Del Giglio M, Di Francesco V, Zamboni M, Girolomoni G (2008) Weight loss improves the response of obese patients with moderate-to-severe chronic plaque psoriasis to low-dose cyclosporine therapy: a randomized, controlled, investigator-blinded clinical trial. Am J Clin Nutr 88: 1242–1247.
42. Barish GD, Atkins AR, Downes M, Olson P, Chong LW, et al. (2008) PPARdelta regulates multiple proinflammatory pathways to suppress athero-sclerosis. Proc Natl Acad Sci U S A 105: 4271–4276.
43. Hall JM, McDonnell DP (2007) The molecular mechanisms underlying the proinflammatory actions of thiazolidinediones in human macrophages. Mol Endocrinol 21: 1756–1768.
44. Kryczek I, Wei S, Vatan L, Escara-Wilke J, Szeliga W, et al. (2007) Cutting edge: opposite effects of IL-1 and IL-2 on the regulation of IL-17+ T cell pool IL-1 subverts IL-2-mediated suppression. J Immunol 179: 1423–1426.
45. Magne D, Palmer G, Barton JL, Mezin F, Talabot-Ayer D, et al. (2006) The new IL-1 family member IL-1F8 stimulates production of inflammatory mediators by synovial fibroblasts and articular chondrocytes. Arthritis Res Ther 8: R80.
46. Blumberg H, Dinh H, Trueblood ES, Pretorius J, Kugler D, et al. (2007) Opposing activities of two novel members of the IL-1 ligand family regulate skin inflammation. J Exp Med 204: 2603–2614.
47. Chong HC, Tan MJ, Philippe V, Tan SH, Tan CK, et al. (2009) Regulation of epithelial-mesenchymal IL-1 signaling by PPARbeta/delta is essential for skin homeostasis and wound healing. J Cell Biol 184: 817–831.
48. Debets R, Hegmans JP, Croughs P, Troost RJ, Prins JB, et al. (1997) The IL-1 system in psoriatic skin: IL-1 antagonist sphere of influence in lesional psoriatic epidermis. J Immunol 158: 2955–2963.
49. Kang K, Hatano B, Lee CH (2007) PPAR delta agonists and metabolic diseases. Curr Atheroscler Rep 9: 72–77.
50. Liu L, Gao Y, Qiu H, Miller WT, Poli V, et al. (2006) Identification of STAT3 as a specific substrate of breast tumor kinase. Oncogene 25: 4904–4912.
51. El Kasmi KC, Holst J, Coffre M, Mielke L, de Pauw A, et al. (2006) General nature of the STAT3-activated anti-inflammatory response. J Immunol 177: 7880–7888.
52. Schmuth M, Haqq CM, Cairns WJ, Holder JC, Dorsam S, et al. (2004) Peroxisome proliferator-activated receptor (PPAR)-beta/delta stimulates differ-entiation and lipid accumulation in keratinocytes. J Invest Dermatol 122: 971–983.
53. Michalik L, Desvergne B, Tan NS, Basu-Modak S, Escher P, et al. (2001) Impaired skin wound healing in peroxisome proliferator-activated receptor (PPAR)alpha and PPARbeta mutant mice. J Cell Biol 154: 799–814.
54. de Cid R, Riveira-Munoz E, Zeeuwen PL, Robarge J, Liao W, et al. (2009) Deletion of the late cornified envelope LCE3B and LCE3C genes as a susceptibility factor for psoriasis. Nat Genet 41: 211–215.

Permissions

All chapters in this book were first published in PLOS ONE, by The Public Library of Science; hereby published with permission under the Creative Commons Attribution License or equivalent. Every chapter published in this book has been scrutinized by our experts. Their significance has been extensively debated. The topics covered herein carry significant findings which will fuel the growth of the discipline. They may even be implemented as practical applications or may be referred to as a beginning point for another development.

The contributors of this book come from diverse backgrounds, making this book a truly international effort. This book will bring forth new frontiers with its revolutionizing research information and detailed analysis of the nascent developments around the world.

We would like to thank all the contributing authors for lending their expertise to make the book truly unique. They have played a crucial role in the development of this book. Without their invaluable contributions this book wouldn't have been possible. They have made vital efforts to compile up to date information on the varied aspects of this subject to make this book a valuable addition to the collection of many professionals and students.

This book was conceptualized with the vision of imparting up-to-date information and advanced data in this field. To ensure the same, a matchless editorial board was set up. Every individual on the board went through rigorous rounds of assessment to prove their worth. After which they invested a large part of their time researching and compiling the most relevant data for our readers.

The editorial board has been involved in producing this book since its inception. They have spent rigorous hours researching and exploring the diverse topics which have resulted in the successful publishing of this book. They have passed on their knowledge of decades through this book. To expedite this challenging task, the publisher supported the team at every step. A small team of assistant editors was also appointed to further simplify the editing procedure and attain best results for the readers.

Apart from the editorial board, the designing team has also invested a significant amount of their time in understanding the subject and creating the most relevant covers. They scrutinized every image to scout for the most suitable representation of the subject and create an appropriate cover for the book.

The publishing team has been an ardent support to the editorial, designing and production team. Their endless efforts to recruit the best for this project, has resulted in the accomplishment of this book. They are a veteran in the field of academics and their pool of knowledge is as vast as their experience in printing. Their expertise and guidance has proved useful at every step. Their uncompromising quality standards have made this book an exceptional effort. Their encouragement from time to time has been an inspiration for everyone.

The publisher and the editorial board hope that this book will prove to be a valuable piece of knowledge for researchers, students, practitioners and scholars across the globe.

List of Contributors

Suh-Young Lee and Seung-Eun Lee
Department of Internal Medicine, Division of Allergy and Clinical Immunology, Seoul National University Hospital, Seoul, Republic of Korea
Institute of Allergy and Clinical Immunology, Seoul National University Medical Research Center, Seoul, Republic of Korea

Sang-Heon Cho and Hye-Ryun Kang
Department of Internal Medicine, Division of Allergy and Clinical Immunology, Seoul National University Hospital, Seoul, Republic of Korea
Institute of Allergy and Clinical Immunology, Seoul National University Medical Research Center, Seoul, Republic of Korea
Seoul National University Hospital Regional Pharmacovigilance Center, Seoul, Republic of Korea

Min-Hye Kim
Department of Internal Medicine, Division of Allergy and Clinical Immunology, Seoul National University Hospital, Seoul, Republic of Korea
Institute of Allergy and Clinical Immunology, Seoul National University Medical Research Center, Seoul, Republic of Korea
Seoul National University Hospital Regional Pharmacovigilance Center, Seoul, Republic of Korea
Department of Internal Medicine, Ewha Womans University School of Medicine, Seoul, Republic of Korea

Min-Suk Yang
Department of Internal Medicine, Division of Allergy and Clinical Immunology, Seoul National University Hospital, Seoul, Republic of Korea
Institute of Allergy and Clinical Immunology, Seoul National University Medical Research Center, Seoul, Republic of Korea
Department of Internal Medicine, SMG-SNU Boramae Medical Center, Seoul, Republic of Korea

Jae-Woo Jung
Institute of Allergy and Clinical Immunology, Seoul National University Medical Research Center, Seoul, Republic of Korea
Department of Internal Medicine, Chung-Ang University College of Medicine, Seoul, Republic of Korea

Chang Min Park and Whal Lee
Department of Radiology and Institute of Radiation Medicine, Seoul National University College of Medicine, Seoul, Republic of Korea

Pablo Pinto, Ney Santos, Dayse O. Alencar, Sidney Santos and Ândrea Ribeiro-dos-Santos
Laboratório de Genética Humana e Médica, Instituto de Ciências Biológicas, Universidade Federal do Pará, Belém, Pará, Brasil

Claudio Guedes Salgado
Laboratório de Dermatoimunologia, Instituto de Ciências Biológicas, Universidade Federal do Pará, Bele´m, Pará, Brasil

Mara H. Hutz
Instituto de Biociências, Departamento de Genética, Universidade Federal do Rio Grande do Sul, Rio Grande do Sol, Brasil

Shervin Assassi, Maureen D. Mayes, Deepthi K. Nair, Ngan Nguyen and John D. Reveille
Department of Medicine, Division of Rheumatology, University of Texas Health Science Center at Houston, Houston, Texas, United States of America

Roozbeh Sharif
Department of Medicine, Division of Rheumatology, University of Texas Health Science Center at Houston, Houston, Texas, United States of America
Department of Medicine, University of Texas Medical Branch at Galveston, Galveston, Texas, United States of America

Astrud L. Leyva, Emilio B. Gonzalez and Terry A. McNearney
Department of Medicine, University of Texas Medical Branch at Galveston, Galveston, Texas, United States of America

Michael Fischbach
Department of Medicine, Division of Rheumatology, University of Texas Health Science Center at San Antonio, San Antonio, Texas, United States of America

Miriam Wittmann
Leeds Institute of Molecular Medicine, LMBRU LTHT, Division of Rheumatic and Musculoskeletal Disease, University of Leeds, Leeds, United Kingdom
Centre for Skin Sciences, School of Life Sciences, University of Bradford, Bradford, United Kingdom

Rosella Doble
Institute of Molecular and Cellular Biology, Faculty of Biological Sciences, University of Leeds, Leeds, United Kingdom

Malte Bachmann, Josef Pfeilschifter and Heiko Mühl
Pharmazentrum Frankfurt/ZAFES, University Hospital Goethe-University Frankfurt, Frankfurt am Main, Germany

Thomas Werfel
Division of Immunodermatology and Allergy Research, Department of Dermatology, Hannover Medical School, Hannover, Germany

Matthew B. Greenblatt and Kelly Tsang
Department of Immunology and Infectious Diseases, Harvard School of Public Health, Boston, Massachusetts, United States of America

Antonios O. Aliprantis
Department of Immunology and Infectious Diseases, Harvard School of Public Health, Boston, Massachusetts, United States of America
Department of Medicine, Division of Rheumatology, Allergy and Immunology, Brigham and Women's Hospital and Harvard Medical School, Boston, Massachusetts, United States of America

Vladimir Vbranac, Trevor Tivey and Andrew M. Tager
Center for Immunology and Inflammatory Diseases, Division of Rheumatology, Allergy and Immunology, Massachusetts General Hospital, Harvard Medical School, Charlestown, Massachusetts, United States of America
Ragon Institute of Massachusetts General Hospital, Massachusetts Institutes of Technology, and Harvard and Division of AIDS, Harvard Medical School, Charlestown, Massachusetts, United States of America

Kristen R. Taylor, Robyn E. Mills, Anne E. Costanzo and Julie M. Jameson
Department of Immunology and Microbial Science, The Scripps Research Institute, La Jolla, California, United States of America

Naoko Goto-Inoue, Takahiro Hayasaka and Mitsutoshi Setou
Department of Cell Biology and Anatomy, Hamamatsu University School of Medicine, 1-20-1 Handayama, Higashi-ku, Hamamatsu, Shizuoka, Japan

Nobuhiro Zaima
Department of Applied Biological Chemistry, Kinki University, Nara, Nara, Japan

Kimiko Nakajima and Shigetoshi Sano
Department of Dermatology, Kochi Medical School, Kochi University, Kohasu, Okocho, Nankoku, Nankoku, Japan

Walter M. Holleran and Yoshikazu Uchida
Department of Dermatology, School of Medicine, University of California San Francisco, Department of Veterans Affairs Medical Center, and Northern California Institute for Research and Education, San Francisco, California, United States of America

Kosuke Miyauchi, Yasutaka Motomura and Yoshie Suzuki
Laboratory for Signal Network, Research Center for Allergy and Immunology, RIKEN Yokohama Institute, Yokohama, Kanagawa, Japan

Ayako Uto-Konomi
Laboratory for Signal Network, Research Center for Allergy and Immunology, RIKEN Yokohama Institute, Yokohama, Kanagawa, Japan
Department of Molecular and Cellular Biology, Kobe Pharma Research Institute, Nippon Boehringer Ingelheim Co., Ltd., Kobe, Hyogo, Japan

Masato Kubo
Laboratory for Signal Network, Research Center for Allergy and Immunology, RIKEN Yokohama Institute, Yokohama, Kanagawa, Japan
Division of Molecular Pathology, Research Institute for Biological Science, Tokyo University of Science, Noda, Chiba, Japan

Naoko Ozaki and Shinobu Suzuki
Department of Molecular and Cellular Biology, Kobe Pharma Research Institute, Nippon Boehringer Ingelheim Co., Ltd., Kobe, Hyogo, Japan

Akihiko Yoshimura
Department of Microbiology and Immunology, Keio University School of Medicine, Tokyo, Japan

Daniel Cua
Schering-Plough Biopharma, Palo Alto, California, United States

Brett D.Thombs
Department of Psychiatry, McGill University, Montréal, Québec, Canada
Department of Epidemiology, Biostatistics, and Occupational Health, McGill University, Montre´ al, Québec, Canada
Department of Medicine (Division of Rheumatology), McGill University, Montréal, Québec, Canada
Department of Educational and Counselling Psychology, McGill University, Montréal, Québec, Canada
School of Nursing, McGill University, Montréal, Québec, Canada
Lady Davis Institute for Medical Research, Jewish General Hospital, Montréal, Québec, Canada

Erin Arthurs
Department of Psychiatry, McGill University, Montréal, Québec, Canada
Lady Davis Institute for Medical Research, Jewish General Hospital, Montréal, Québec, Canada

Russell J. Steele
Department of Mathematics and Statistics, McGill University, Montréal, Québec, Canada
Lady Davis Institute for Medical Research, Jewish General Hospital, Montréal, Québec, Canada

Marie Hudson and Murray Baron
Department of Medicine (Division of Rheumatology), McGill University, Montréal, Québec, Canada
Lady Davis Institute for Medical Research, Jewish General Hospital, Montréal, Québec, Canada

Mårten C.G. Winge and Maria Bradley
Dermatology Unit, Department of Medicine Solna and Center for Molecular Medicine, Karolinska Institutet, Karolinska University Hospital Solna, Stockholm, Sweden
Department of Molecular Medicine and Surgery and Center for Molecular Medicine, Karolinska Institutet, Karolinska University Hospital Solna, Stockholm, Sweden

Torborg Hoppe, Berit Berne, Anders Vahlquist and Hans Törmä
Department of Medical Sciences, Dermatology and Venereology, Uppsala University, Uppsala, Sweden

Magnus Nordenskjöld
Department of Molecular Medicine and Surgery and Center for Molecular Medicine, Karolinska Institutet, Karolinska University Hospital Solna, Stockholm, Sweden

Sonja Ständer, Dorothee Siepmann, Ilka Herrgott, Cord Sunderkötter and Thomas A. Luger
Department of Dermatology, Neurodermatology and Competence Center Pruritus, University of Mü nster, Münster, Germany

Bernardetta Maresca, Luisa Cigliano and Paolo Abrescia
Dipartimento delle Scienze Biologiche, Universita` di Napoli Federico II, Napoli, Italia

Maria Stefania Spagnuolo
Istituto per il Sistema Produzione Animale in Ambiente Mediterraneo, Consiglio Nazionale delle Ricerche, Napoli, Italia

Fabrizio Dal Piaz
Dipartimento di Scienze Farmaceutiche e Biomediche, Universitàdegli Studi di Salerno, Fisciano (Salerno), Italia

Maria M. Corsaro
Dipartimento di Chimica Organica e Biochimica, Universitàdi Napoli Federico II, Complesso Universitario M. S. Angelo, Napoli, Italia

Nicola Balato, Massimiliano Nino, Anna Balato and Fabio Ayala
Dipartimento di Patologia Sistematica - Sezione di Dermatologia, Università di Napoli Federico II, Napoli, Italia

Katrin Hack, Louise Reilly and Colin Palmer
Medical Research Institute, College of Medicine, Dentistry, and Nursing, University of Dundee, Dundee, Scotland

John Foerster
Department of Dermatology, College of Medicine, Dentistry, and Nursing, University of Dundee, Dundee, Scotland
Education Division, College of Medicine, Dentistry, and Nursing, University of Dundee, Dundee, Scotland

Kally Booth
Medical School Biological Resource Unit, College of Medicine, Dentistry, and Nursing

Kevin D. Read, Suzanne Norval and Robert Kime
Biological Chemistry and Drug Discovery Unit, College of Life Sciences, University of Dundee, Dundee, Scotland

Brian Argyle and Lindsi McCoard
Center for Therapeutic Biomaterials, University of Utah, Salt Lake City, Utah, United States of America

Jianxing Zhang, Xiaoyu Xu and Glenn D. Prestwich
Center for Therapeutic Biomaterials, University of Utah, Salt Lake City, Utah, United States of America
Department of Medicinal Chemistry, University of Utah, Salt Lake City, Utah, United States of America

Narayanam V. Rao and Thomas P. Kennedy
Department of Internal Medicine, University of Utah, Salt Lake City, Utah, United States of America

William J. Rusho
Department of Pharmaceutics and Pharmaceutical Chemistry, University of Utah, Salt Lake City, Utah, United States of America

Gerald Krueger
Department of Dermatology, University of Utah, Salt Lake City, Utah, United States of America

James V. Dunne
Department of Medicine, University of British Columbia, Vancouver, British Columbia, Canada

British Columbia Scleroderma Clinic, Vancouver, British Columbia, Canada

Stephan F. van Eeden
Department of Medicine, University of British Columbia, Vancouver, British Columbia, Canada, James Hogg Heart and Lung Institute, Vancouver, British Columbia, Canada

Kevin J. Keen
Department of Mathematics and Statistics, University of Northern British Columbia, Prince George, British Columbia, Canada

Nicolò Costantino Brembilla, Jean-Marie Ramirez, Rachel Chicheportiche and Carlo Chizzolini
Department of Immunology and Allergy, Swiss Centre for Applied Human Toxicology, University Hospital and School of Medicine, Geneva, Switzerland

Olivier Sorg and Jean-Hilaire Saurat
Department of Dermato-Toxicology, Swiss Centre for Applied Human Toxicology, University Hospital and School of Medicine, Geneva, Switzerland

Paul A. Cobine and Mary T. Mendonça
Department of Biological Sciences, Auburn University, Auburn, Alabama, United States of America

John D. Peterson
Department of Biological Sciences, Auburn University, Auburn, Alabama, United States of America
School of Biological Sciences, Washington State University, Pullman, Washington, United States of America

John E. Steffen
School of Science, Penn State Erie, Erie, Pennsylvania, United States of America

Laura K. Reinert
Department of Pathology, Microbiology and Immunology, Vanderbilt University Medical Center, Nashville, Tennessee, United States of America

Arthur Appel
Department of Entomology and Plant Pathology, Auburn University, Auburn, Alabama, United States of America

Louise Rollins-Smith
Departments of Pathology, Microbiology and Immunology and of Pediatrics, Vanderbilt University Medical Center and Department of Biological Sciences, Vanderbilt University, Nashville, Tennessee, United States of America

Wendy B. Bollag
Charlie Norwood VA Medical Center, Augusta, Georgia, United States of America
Department of Physiology, Medical College of Georgia at Georgia Regents University, Augusta, Georgia, United States of America

Ding Xie and Mutsa Seremwe
Department of Physiology, Medical College of Georgia at Georgia Regents University, Augusta, Georgia, United States of America

John G. Edwards
Apeliotus Technologies, Inc., Atlanta, Georgia, United States of America

Robert Podolsky
Center for Biotechnology and Genomic Medicine, Department of Medicine, Medical College of Georgia at Georgia Regents University, Augusta, Georgia, United States of America

Helga Sanner
Section of Rheumatology, Oslo University Hospital-Rikshospitalet, Oslo, Norway
Norwegian Competence Centre of Pediatric and Adolescent Rheumatology, Oslo University Hospital-Rikshospitalet, Oslo, Norway

Berit Flatø
Section of Rheumatology, Oslo University Hospital-Rikshospitalet, Oslo, Norway
Institute for Clinical Medicine, University of Oslo, Oslo, Norway

Maria Vistnes
Institute for Experimental Medical Research, Oslo University Hospital-Ullevål, Oslo, Norway
KG Jebsen Cardiac Research Center and Center for Heart Failure Research, University of Oslo, Oslo, Norway

Thomas Schwartz
Institute for Experimental Medical Research, Oslo University Hospital-Ullevål, Oslo, Norway
KG Jebsen Cardiac Research Center and Center for Heart Failure Research, University of Oslo, Oslo, Norway
Institute for Clinical Medicine, University of Oslo, Oslo, Norway

Ivar Sjaastad
Institute for Experimental Medical Research, Oslo University Hospital-Ullevål, Oslo, Norway
KG Jebsen Cardiac Research Center and Center for Heart Failure Research, University of Oslo, Oslo, Norway

Department ofCardiology, Oslo University Hospital-Ulleval, Oslo, Norway

Chien-Ya Hung and Fu-Shan Jaw
Institute of Biomedical Engineering, National Taiwan University, Taipei, Taiwan

Pei-Lun Sun
Department of Dermatology, Mackay Memorial Hospital, Taipei, Taiwan

Shu-Jen Chiang
Institute of Zoology, National Taiwan University, Taipei, Taiwan

Keiichi Yamanaka, Takehisa Nakanishi, Kenichi Isoda, Kenshiro Tsuda, Masato Kakeda and Hitoshi Mizutani
Department of Dermatology, Mie University, Graduate School of Medicine, Tsu, Mie, Japan

Hiromitsu Saito and Noboru Suzuki
Department of Animal Genomics, Functional Genomics Institute, Mie University Life Science Research Center, Tsu, Mie, Japan

Junko Maruyama
Department of Clinical Engineering, Suzuka University of Medical Science, Suzuka, Mie, Japan

Ayumu Yokochi and Kazuo Maruyama
Anesthesiology and Critical Care Medicine, Mie University, Graduate School of Medicine, Tsu, Mie, Japan

Kyoko Imanaka-Yoshida and Toshimichi Yoshida
Pathology and Matrix Biology, Mie University, Graduate School of Medicine, Tsu, Mie, Japan
Mie University Research Center for Matrix Biology, Tsu, Mie, Japan

Ryuji Okamoto, Satoshi Fujita and Masaaki Ito
Cardiology, Mie University, Graduate School of Medicine, Tsu, Mie, Japan

Yoichiro Iwakura
Division of Experimental Animal Immunology, Tokyo University of Science, Noda, Chiba, Japan

Esteban C. Gabazza
Immunology, Mie University, Graduate School of Medicine, Tsu, Mie, Japan

Motomu Shimaoka
Molecular Pathology and Cell Adhesion Biology, Mie University, Graduate School of Medicine, Tsu, Mie, Japan

Aline Rodrigues Hoffmann, Hoai Jaclyn Ly and Joanne Mansell
Dermatopathology Specialty Service, Department of Veterinary Pathobiology, College of Veterinary Medicine and Biomedical Sciences, Texas A and M University, College Station, Texas, United States of America

Malgorzata Romanowska, Louise Reilly and John Foerster
Division of Experimental Medicine, University of Dundee, Dundee, United Kingdom

Colin N. A. Palmer
Biomedical Research Institute, University of Dundee, Dundee, United Kingdom

Mattias C. U. Gustafsson
Department of Laboratory Medicine, Division of Medical Microbiology, Lund University, Lund, Sweden

Index

A

Ahr, 126-129, 131, 191-192

Anaphylactic Shock, 1-6

Anaphylaxis, 1-6

Aprepitant, 77-81

Atopic Dermatitis, 12, 49, 56, 69-70, 75-76, 80-81, 105, 127-128, 131, 156, 167, 176

C

Cathelicidins, 104, 106

Chronic Pruritus, 77-78, 80

Clavus, 149-152, 154

Cutaneous Inflammation, 104, 106, 108, 110, 114

Cutaneous Lupus Erythematosus, 22, 24, 29

Cytokine Signaling, 45, 57, 62-63, 68

D

Dermal Fibroblasts, 22-23, 25, 105, 191, 200

Differentially Expressed Genes, 71-73

Dioxin, 126-127, 131-132

Dorfman-chanarin Syndrome, 47, 49, 56

E

Eczema, 22, 24, 56, 69, 75-76, 81

Electrical Impedance, 149-151, 154-155

Eotaxin, 142-148

Epidermal Keratinocytes, 57, 94, 133, 135, 140, 156, 176-177, 191, 200

Epithelial Damage, 31, 35, 42

F

Fatigue Severity, 13-17, 19-20

Filaggrin, 69, 75-76

Flg Genotyping, 69-70

G

Glycosylation, 82, 84, 86, 88, 91-92

Graft-versus-host Disease, 24, 29, 123, 125

Gstm1 Gene, 9, 11

H

Haptoglobin, 82, 91-92

Homeostasis, 31, 35, 42-43, 45-46, 49, 56-57, 59-60, 62, 65, 68-69, 102, 133, 140, 175-177, 201

Hyperglycemia, 31-33, 35, 42-43, 45

Hypersensitivity, 1-6, 30, 68, 119, 123, 183

Hypotension, 1-5

I

Il-18 Binding Protein, 22, 29

Imaging Mass Spectrometry, 47, 54-56

Inflammatory Skin Disease, 23, 65, 93-94, 101, 189, 196

Inhospital Pharmacovigilance, 1-2

Insulin Resistance, 43, 45-46

Interleukin-20, 57, 59, 68

Intradermal Injection, 3, 104-106, 115

Iv, 69-75, 102, 193, 196, 198-199

J

Juvenile Dermatomyositis, 142, 144-148

K

Keratinocyte Proliferation, 75, 103, 133-140, 190, 201

L

L-selectin, 118-119, 121, 123-125

Leprosy, 7-12

Loss-of-function, 51, 53, 69-70, 76

M

Metabolic Abnormality, 47, 49

Metabolic Disease, 31-33, 35, 37, 42-43, 102, 190, 201

Metabolic Syndrome, 31, 33, 78, 93, 99, 102, 189, 196, 201

Monounsaturated Fatty Acids, 133, 136

N

Neurokinin Receptor, 77

Neutrophils, 58-59, 62, 65, 67, 118, 124, 180-183, 186-187

O

Obesity, 14, 31-33, 35, 37, 42-43, 45, 93, 156-157, 196

Organ Damage, 142-143, 145, 147-148

P

Phosphatidylglycerol, 133, 140-141

Polymorphism, 8, 12, 76, 91

Polyunsaturated Fatty Acids, 133, 135-140

Pruritus Intensity, 77-80

Psoriasis, 22-24, 27, 29-30, 49, 59-60, 63, 68, 82-84, 86, 88-91, 93-94, 96-97, 99-103, 105, 113, 117, 127-128, 131-133, 139-140, 156-157, 165, 167, 176, 189-193, 195-196, 198-201

R

Radiocontrast Media, 1, 3-4, 6

Rosacea, 104-106, 109-110, 112-116

S

Sclerodermatous, 123, 125

Skin Damage, 118-119, 124, 165

Skin Resident Cells, 22-23

Skin Test Positivity, 1, 4-6

Stat5 Signaling, 31, 33

Systemic Amyloidosis, 156, 163, 165

Systemic Sclerosis, 13, 20-21, 118, 123-125

T

T Cell Function, 31, 33, 35, 37, 40-42, 46

T Regulatory Cells, 126

V

Vascular Adhesion, 106, 115

Verruca, 149-152, 154

W

Wound Repair, 31, 33, 35, 45-46

www.ingramcontent.com/pod-product-compliance
Lightning Source LLC
Chambersburg PA
CBHW080650200326
41458CB00013B/4800